END MIGRAINES, BACKACHES,
ARTHRITIS PAIN, AND MORE ...

Relief at Last!

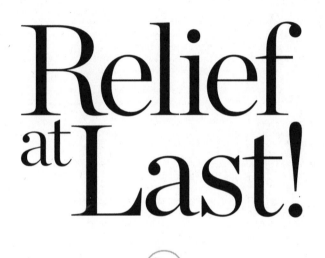

THE Prevention® GUIDE TO NATURAL PAIN RELIEF

Sarí Harrar
with the editors of Prevention®

RODALE.

Previously published for direct mail as *Your New Pain Prescription* in January 2011.
© 2011 by Rodale Inc.

Pain Scale illustrations adapted or reprinted with permission from "Challenges in Pain Management at the End of Life," October 1, 2001, *American Family Physician.* © 2011 by American Academy of Family Physicians. All rights reserved.

Photographs on pages 498–504 © 2011 by Mitch Mandel/Rodale Images; Water Workout photographs on pages 505–507 used with permission from The Arthritis Foundation, photographed by © 2011 Kevin Garrett.

Book design by Susan Eugster

Library of Congress Cataloging-in-Publication Data number: 2010049370

978-1-60961-047-0 paperback

2   4   6   8   10   9   7   5   3   1   paperback

Introduction

There's nothing small about chronic pain. On any given day, it's big news. Headlines in newspapers, on TV and on the Web trumpet new treatments to ease it, new discoveries about what causes it, and new tips for controlling it. It's big money: According to the National Institutes of Health, chronic pain costs a whopping $100 billion a year. That's money spent on everything from bottles of aspirin and heating pads to knee replacements, spine surgeries and IV drugs (as well as the cost of lost wages and lawsuits).

If you or someone you love lives with chronic pain, you know firsthand that it's a big deal—crowding out everyday pleasures, sending you to more and more doctors, getting in the way of work, relationships, running errands, taking care of your home and enjoying family and friends. It invades every corner of your life.

Too often, chronic pain is also a big mystery. The National Library of Medicine contains nearly a *half-million* studies of pain. Yet despite mountains of research, too many people live with long-lasting pain. Scientists are still unraveling the reasons it lingers (you'll read some of the latest findings in Chapter 1). But you don't have to wait for their final word in order to find big relief.

Throughout this book, you'll discover why combining old and new pain therapies into a new pain prescription has been the solution for so many people. Using conventional therapies (drugs and other treatments) along with alternative and complementary therapies (relaxation exercises, guided imagery, exercise, smart food choices and more) can work better than drugs alone. It can help when drugs fail and may even allow you to take less medication. It can brighten your mood, reduce stress, strengthen your body, let you get a good nights' sleep, help you return to work and give you better pain control. And best of all, let you step back into the life you love.

Contents

PART ONE

Therapies for Pain-Free Living

In Part One of *Relief at Last*, you'll find out why cutting-edge pain clinics are proving that you don't have to put up with chronic pain. The way out? Go beyond over-the-counter pain relievers and prescription pain-killers. New research shows that some old, even ancient, healing modalities have what it takes to ease pain—by attacking it on many levels.

In this section, you'll discover new thinking about what causes chronic pain—how it changes your nervous system and brain in ways that lower your pain threshold, changes the pain signals transmitted to your brain (so that small slights—like the rub of a sweater on your arm—suddenly feel agonizing), and increases pain intensity. You'll also find out about a vicious mind-body glitch that makes pain worse. Coping with everyday pain can increase your risk for depression and leave you feeling stressed and anxious. And these negative feelings, in turn, alter the way your brain interprets pain signals so that they're louder. The good news? Using a combination-care approach—smart pain relievers: medications targeted to your specific pain condition plus nondrug therapies—can break this cycle and bring relief.

You'll learn about four important nondrug healing modalities: food and supplements, exercise and movement therapies, touch therapies, and mind-body therapies proven to ease even the most tough-to-treat types of chronic pain. And you'll find smart advice on using pain relievers and other pain-condition medications safely and wisely.

Chapter 1

You Don't Have to Hurt

After the accident, I had burning pain that started in my foot and went up my leg and into my back. The pain should have eased off after a few weeks, but instead it got worse and worse.

I hate the pain inside me—it's an invader trying to take over. People can't see it, so they think I'm okay. But I'm not. I can't work. I can't play with my kids. I'm angry and depressed—and scared.

If you haven't lived with chronic pain, you can't imagine what it's like. Everything's taken away from you. The smallest things, like brushing your teeth, can be excruciating. I feel like I'm trapped in the body of a 90-year-old man.

Chronic pain. It gnaws and stabs, stings and aches, jabs and throbs—but it doesn't let up. We try to soothe it—with 30 billion over-the-counter pain pills and over 100 million prescriptions for narcotic painkillers every year.[1, 2] We spend over $100 billion on relief,[3] and make over 70 million doctor visits a year[4]—often seeing three, four, five, or even dozens of doctors in search of real help.

Yet 76 million of us continue to live with chronic pain.[5]

Defined as any pain that lasts more than 3 to 6 months, chronic pain includes headaches, backaches, joint pain, nerve damage, digestive problems, cancer-related pain, and more. It's the bad back that keeps flaring up. The nerve damage from diabetes that sends stinging, shooting pains into your toes and fingertips. The cramping and bloating of irritable bowel syndrome. The deep aches of fibromyalgia and cancer. The migraine headaches that leave you flat on your back in a dark room pressing a bag of ice to your temples. The arthritis in your knees that makes sitting down, standing up, or running after your toddler-age grandchildren excruciating instead of fun. Or the mystery pain that started after an accident or injury and hasn't stopped.

There's plenty about chronic pain that doesn't make sense. Why does pain keep ringing alarm bells long after an injury has healed? Why do depression and fear make pain so much worse? Why do so many doctors ignore, misunderstand, or undertreat pain in the twenty-first century?

But one thing about chronic pain is crystal clear: It doesn't have to rule your life.

Beyond Pills and Needles

I feel like a new person!

I not only have less back pain, I am more aware of my life and am learning to live it to the fullest.

My pain isn't completely gone, but I'm amazed by how I'm able to deal with it. Pain relievers help take the edge off. And I also know how to relax my whole body; thanks to biofeedback and muscle relaxation, I'm controlling my pain with my mind. I'm exercising, too, even though at first I really didn't want to. I feel less stressed. I'm stronger and more confident. I'm in control now.

Pain researchers and pain specialists say there's better evidence now than ever before that if you're coping with chronic pain, you can get the relief you need and reclaim your life. The secret? Using the right pain medications and medical treatments along with a smart mix of complementary therapies. We're talking about dietary therapies (including supplements), movement therapies (such as exercise, physical therapy, yoga, and more), mind-body therapies (from guided imagery and meditation to hypnotherapy and beyond), and touch therapies (acupuncture, massage, and others).

These aren't just nice add-ons. Plenty of well-designed studies show that these healing modalities work on many levels to reduce pain and give you back a sense of control. As pain researchers understand more about how chronic pain wreaks havoc in your nervous system and even in the circuitry of your brain, the importance of these nondrug therapies for getting real relief is growing stronger. Many address pain in ways that pain relievers, surgery, and other treatments cannot.

We're not suggesting you ditch your medications or cancel your next doctor's appointment. The combination approach—what the nation's cutting-edge pain clinics call multidisciplinary pain management—almost always includes drugs as well as other medical treatments as needed. Research shows that combining these conventional pain therapies with unconventional approaches brings more relief than drugs alone.

In studies, adding one, two, or three of these new pain relief modalities fills the comfort gap when medicine falls short. Some people even reduce their drug doses or eliminate medications entirely. But these therapies do more than mute pain.

The therapies you'll find in *Relief at Last* are proven to help your medication work better, relieve the depression that so often comes with chronic pain, ease stress, restore your memory and ability to focus, and to help you sleep better, stop feeling afraid or hopeless, and get back to working, enjoying your relationships, and getting what you want out of your life.

Best of all, they're proven to work.

The New Science of Pain Relief

In the past, the way we feel pain was seen as a simple, three-step process:

1. You hit your thumb with a hammer.

2. Pain-sensing nerves, called *nociceptors*, telegraphed loud "ouch" signals to your spinal cord, which relayed them to your brain.

3. Your brain told your hand to stop swinging the hammer and suggested it was high time you got some ice and a Band-Aid.

But thanks to a tidal wave of new research—including thousands of brain scan studies—scientists now know that chronic pain doesn't follow that neat script. It's bigger, crazier, and therefore tougher to control. In fact, there are at least three basic types of pain:

Nociceptive pain: The most common, caused by an injury to your body's tissues—skin, connective tissue, muscles, joints, and organs. Back pain, joint pain, cancer pain, digestive pain, and others are examples of nociceptive pain.

Neuropathic pain: Caused by damage to nerves, the spinal cord, and/or the brain that alters pain signals. As a result, your pain threshold drops, so that small twinges legitimately feel huge, even nonpain sensations become painful, and pain spreads to other parts of your body. Diabetic neuropathy, nerve pain after a bout of the shingles virus, complex regional pain syndrome, and others are examples. Sometimes, pain that begins with an injury becomes neuropathic pain, as damaged nerves change the way they transmit pain signals.

Psychogenic pain: A very real type of pain with roots in regions of your brain that receive and interpret pain signals from your body. Truth is, many chronic pain conditions contain a mind-body element—as fear, stress, and depression work together to make pain truly feel worse. Don't misunderstand. We're not dismissing this kind of pain as "all in your head." More and more research shows that brain changes associated with pain and with emotional reactions to pain work to make pain feel worse, and that by managing your thoughts and emotions you can really ease pain.

Your New Pain Mix

When pain lingers, there's a good chance all three types of pain become part of the picture. New research shows that changes in your brain and in your nervous system alter the way you experience pain when it becomes chronic. It's fascinating, and it also explains why simply easing nociceptive pain (the old approach to pain relief) isn't enough. Among the new insights that are changing the way pain is seen and treated are:

Chronic pain rewires your brain. Five to ten different regions of the brain play important roles in how you perceive pain, and many of these brain regions also process feelings. These include the amygdala, a region involved in your emotional responses to pain and in turning pain intensity up or down; the anterior cingulate cortex, which processes both physical pain and emotional pain; and the periaqueductal gray, which normally turns down pain intensity in the presence of strong emotions.

Links between feelings and pain may seem odd but they make a lot of sense. If a saber-toothed tiger was gnawing on your leg 700,000 years ago, feeling scared and getting motivated to sprint in the opposite direction had real survival advantages.

But when pain becomes chronic—thanks to an ongoing medical condition, nerve damage, joint problems, or as a result of an injury, for example—this circuitry somehow rewires itself. Emotional responses triggered by ongoing pain—such as depression, stress, helplessness, loneliness, and loss of hope—alter your

Better Together

Which therapy is right for you? When it comes to relieving chronic pain, new research says it's smart to think in multiples. Don't stop with one approach. Try two . . . or three . . . or more. Combination care gets the best results because it addresses pain on many levels at once.

The proof? In one study of 70 people with back pain, those who followed an exercise program and got counseling to help meet the emotional and practical, everyday demands of living with pain were 56 percent less likely to need prescription pain relievers and 55 percent more likely to return to work a year later than those who got treatment as usual—pain relievers and advice to take it easy.[6] In another study, people with fibromyalgia who combined mild exercise, relaxation training, stress management skills, biofeedback, and cognitive behavior therapy got significant pain relief even though they stopped their prescription and over-the-counter pain drugs before starting the combination-care program.[7]

In one study that looked at the results of the combination-care pain programs, researchers found that compared to standard treatments this smart approach reduced pain by 20 to 60 percent and helped two-thirds of people with chronic pain cut their use of prescription pain drugs. These innovative programs also tripled the odds that people in pain could return to work, doubled the chances they would be physically active, and helped with better sleep and brighter moods.[8]

The best combination-care program—what we call Relief at Last—depends on your specific chronic pain. If you have irritable bowel syndrome, the best combination care might include keeping peppermint oil capsules on hand for flare-ups; and when you're feeling better slowly adding more fiber to your diet, taking a probiotic supplement to boost levels of beneficial bacteria in your digestive tract, and finding a medical hypnotherapist for a few sessions of "gut-directed" hypnotherapy aimed at using your mind to encourage better digestion. If you're coping with cancer pain, medication for pain control and for stopping breakthrough pain is a cornerstone of combination care, to which you might add acupuncture, guided imagery, mindfulness meditation, and/or yoga.

brain's responses to signals from your body. Pain becomes more intense and your brain begins interpreting mild pain signals and sensations that otherwise wouldn't feel excruciating.

Negative feelings can crank up pain. Chronic pain triples your odds for depression. Deep in your brain, that's going to make things hurt worse. In one study from England's University of Oxford, people who listened to depressing

Portraits of Pain

76.5 million: Number of Americans whose chronic pain flares up for more than 24 hours at a time[10]

1 in 2: Odds that a person with chronic pain doesn't feel they've got any control over it

42: Percent of people with chronic pain who can't work because of it

1 year (or longer): Time it takes most people who get pain relief to find it

3 or more doctors: Number seen by one in four people seeking relief from chronic pain

2 out of 3: Older people who say pain makes cooking, housework, and hobbies impossible

86: Percent whose pain keeps them from sleeping well

3 out of 4: People with chronic pain who feel depressed and have low energy

25 million: Number of people with headaches, migraines, and facial pain

26 million: Number of people with low back pain

46 million: Number of Americans with arthritis, gout, and/or fibromyalgia

music and recordings of negative thoughts had greater sensitivity to pain than those who weren't subjected to all that gloom.[9] In another study of people with fibromyalgia—a chronic pain condition marked by deep muscle aches and tender, sore spots—those who also felt the most depressed showed the most activity in the amygdala and another brain region called the insula. Both regions process how pain feels.[11]

Worry, fear, and the anticipation of pain turn up the volume, too. At the University of California, San Diego, brain scans revealed that people expecting intense pain felt it—even when the experimental pain they received (a hot jolt from a probe attached to the skin) was actually mild.[12]

"I think when people say pain is 'all in my head,' it suggests it's not real," one researcher noted. "These studies don't say it's not real, they show that brain activity can create a situation that produces real pain." These findings help explain why standard pain treatments so often fail—why, for example, half of the people who take strong painkillers like morphine get surprisingly little relief, with pain dropping by just 30 to 40 percent. The problem isn't just the pain signals. It's the way the brain interprets them. And pain pills may do little to adjust that aspect of pain.

Pain changes nerve endings in the rest of your body, too. Damaged nerves don't know when to call it quits. Harmed by high blood sugar, by the shingles virus, by an accident, or even by some medications, injured nerves send distress signals to the brain. But instead of quieting down as they heal, they start sending pain signals in response to the slightest pressure; the brush of a T-shirt across your arm or the whisper of a breeze on your neck can feel excruciating. Nearby areas that weren't damaged start also sending the same over-the-top messages to your brain.

Ouch.

What's going on? The process is called *sensitization*. New research shows that after an injury nerves may begin growing tiny new supersensitive fibers. Not only do they signal the brain when something touches you, they may create their own pain signals out of nothing at all, ratcheting up the aches even more.

Therapies That Soothe

What does all this research mean for you? The good news is that researchers have also been busy discovering that many nondrug therapies tackle chronic pain in new ways. Some can literally change your brain, reducing stress, lifting depression, and easing worry so that pain is less intense. Others alter your brain's response to pain-reducing drugs and pain-easing brain chemicals so they become more effective. Still others (including some new drug and drug-free strategies) have the power to soothe frazzled nerve endings so your pain threshold is higher.

This good news about pain relief is the flip side of new pain research. There's plenty of solid proof that by going beyond painkilling pills, you can tackle pain in meaningful ways and on many fronts. The result? Not only do you feel fewer aches, but you also feel more in control, more relaxed, more positive, and more able to jump back into family life, personal interests, work, and the other joys and necessities of everyday life.

One of the most fascinating aspects of this new research involves mind-body therapies and the placebo response. The power of positive thinking—believing something works—creates brain changes that can turn down the intensity of pain signals. Researchers first noticed the placebo response decades ago when people in medical studies who got the fake treatments—like sugar pills instead of the real drug—also improved. Of course, a placebo response is no substitute for real treatment for the physical side of many chronic pain conditions. We'd never recommend using sugar pills instead of migraine prevention drugs or inflammation-soothing medications for inflammatory bowel disease, for example. But science is showing that when positive, upbeat belief replaces the dark tunnel of worry, fear, and depression experienced by many people with unrelenting pain, aches become less intense and less frequent.

Some examples of strategies you'll find in *Relief at Last* (tailored to your specific pain condition, of course):

- **Acupuncture** made the brains of women with fibromyalgia more receptive to painkilling medication and to the body's natural pain relievers, called endorphins, report researchers from the University of Michigan's Chronic Pain and Fatigue Research Center. This traditional Chinese healing art increased the number of receptors for pain-stopping compounds—called mu-opioid receptors (MOR)—in an area of the brain that receives pain signals from the spinal cord.

- **Meditation** soothes many types of chronic pain and may help by changing the way your brain thinks about pain. Brain scans show that people who meditate have more activity in brain regions associated with optimism; less activity in areas involved with anticipating and fearing pain; and have a thicker anterior cingulate, an area of the brain that regulates pain and emotions.

- **Yoga** could help you reduce your pain medication dose. In one study of 101 people with chronic low back pain, 6 weeks of yoga allowed 75 percent of those who had been using painkillers to stop taking them. How does it help? Experts suspect yoga works because it strengthens and relaxes muscles, reduces stress, and improves mental focus.[13]

- **Guided imagery plus stress-busting progressive muscle relaxation** helped ease joint pain and improve flexibility in one study when practiced twice a day for 12 weeks by 28 women with osteoarthritis.[14]

- **Biofeedback** teaches you to control stress levels in your body. Studies have shown that it eases the persistent throbbing of tension headaches, the tough-to-soothe agony of complex regional pain syndromes,[15] and the deep aches of fibromyalgia,[16] too.

- **Acupressure** was better than physical therapy for relieving low back pain—and keeping it away—in one recent Taiwanese study.[17] Practitioners say it improves the flow of energy in the body.

- **Cognitive behavior therapy** teaches you effective new ways to think about and cope with chronic pain. It eased chronic face and mouth pain in six studies, say researchers from England's University of Manchester.[18] In another study, it improved joint pain and helped people with arthritis get better sleep, too.[19] People with chronic pain who've gone through CBT feel less hopeless and afraid, and stop thinking of their pain as never ending and uncontrollable.

- **Massage** lessened pain by 20 percent in one University of Colorado study of 380 people with advanced cancers by relaxing tight muscles and delivering the profound stress-relieving power of human touch. Study volunteers had cancers of the lung, breast, pancreas, colon, and prostate—all of which had spread to other organs or to their bones.[20] Just a couple of half-hour massages over two weeks helped. In another study of over 1,200 cancer patients, any type of massage—deep Swedish muscle work, light-touch massage, or even just foot rubs—eased pain a whopping 40 percent.[21]

- **Exercise** can diminish pain by unkinking tight, spasm-wracked muscles and by building muscle strength to help take pressure off joints. It is emerging as an important pain relief therapy for nearly all chronic pain sufferers. The reason? The drop in stress and the feeling of control you get from seeing the results of a regular routine contribute to its pain-erasing powers.

- **Capsaicin cream and other new topical pain-stopping products** work by stopping pain signals before they can whiz to your brain. Options include over-the-counter creams and prescription-only patches containing capsaicin (the same compound that gives red peppers their fiery zing) as well as prescription creams containing strong pain drugs such as the potent nonsteroidal anti-inflammatory drug diclofenac or the numbing lidocaine. The advantage of these topical (meaning they're applied to the skin) remedies is that active ingredients reach your nerve endings but you don't have to take pills, which reduces the risk of many side effects. That's relief you can cheer about!

Is Your Pain Plan Working?

It's hard to remember exactly how intense your pain was last week, last month, or last year. Our memories of pain are notoriously faulty. In one study of people with chronic jaw pain, those whose pain was low before their treatment later remembered it as more intense than it really was. But those whose pain was really intense remembered it as "not so bad." Even odder: All the study participants later remembered their treatment as a success, even though pain checks by their doctors revealed that it didn't work at all for some.

This isn't just an odd fact—it's big trouble. If you don't know whether you're truly feeling better, you won't know whether the drugs you're taking or the other therapies you're trying are helping, hurting, or doing nothing at all. You can get stuck with pain instead of finding real relief. If you're the kind of person who tries her best to soldier on or work through her pain, or who denies he's in pain at all, you may even lose touch with how much pain you're feeling—another obstacle to getting real relief.

The solution? An easy (we mean really easy!) way to keep track of your real pain level. Tracking your pain is crucial as it's the only way to know whether the medications and other therapies you're using really work. Tracking regularly will also help you communicate more effectively with your doctor so that she or he can assess whether medications and other medical interventions are working. That's important, because studies show that doctors tend to underestimate their patients' pain and only get it right when you can set the record straight. In one study from Johns Hopkins University, 120 doctors watched silent videotapes of people undergoing painful procedures and were asked to evaluate their pain level. The doctors almost always got it wrong, but were closest to getting it right when they could also review the patients' own pain ratings.

Tracking your pain with a pain rating scale gives you and your doctor a common language and set of measurements for discussing your pain and your progress. You'd use it in different ways for different pain conditions. If you tend to get migraine headaches, for example, you might track how frequently you have them, how long they last, how intense they are, and whether any medications you took relieved your pain. If you have irritable bowel syndrome, you might track how often you feel gassy or bloated, whether you're having constipation or diarrhea, and how long it lasts. For all these conditions, adding information about activities and stress levels as well as food, supplements, and medications you've ingested in the hours before a flare-up can help you find triggers, too.

Rating your pain is an important part of tracking, a measurement you can compare to other days and share with your doctor to assess your treatments. Fortunately, you don't have to make up your own rating system. The pain scale here is widely used and relies on numbers (**0**, a smiley face, is no pain, to 10, a distressed and crying face, the worst possible pain). You can photocopy it or simply add the number or face that best describes your pain each day to a journal or calendar to keep track. It's that easy, and could be the tool that makes all the difference for pain relief.

Tracking your pain is even more important if your pain is unexplained. Without a good diagnosis, treating the root cause is impossible. Unexplained pain can affect any part of your body, from your feet and legs to your abdomen, back, shoulders, and face. It may be burning and tingling, a constant ache or knifelike jabs. But if you've got it, you know how tough it is to live with it. In one recent study from the Netherlands, up to one in eight people with pain couldn't get a good diagnosis, which in turn meant they couldn't get targeted, effective treatment either.[22]

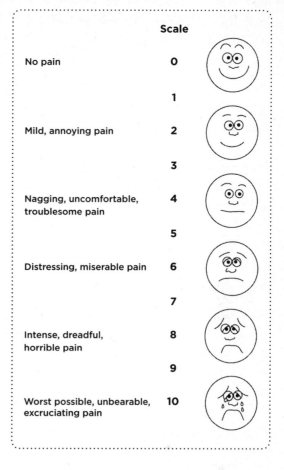

Scale

No pain	0
	1
Mild, annoying pain	2
	3
Nagging, uncomfortable, troublesome pain	4
	5
Distressing, miserable pain	6
	7
Intense, dreadful, horrible pain	8
	9
Worst possible, unbearable, excruciating pain	10

The journey to a good diagnosis and a good treatment plan can be long and frustrating. In one national survey, nearly 30 percent of people with a type of inflammatory bowel disease called Crohn's disease said they saw five or more doctors over more than 3 years in their quest for a diagnosis. Nearly half were misdiagnosed first with another condition, and understandably, half were frustrated by the experience.[23]

If you're coping with mystery pain, don't give up. Keep a pain diary (you'll find a sample page in Part Three of this book.) Rate your pain level daily. The information will help your doctor figure out what's going on. Ask for a referral to a specialist if your family doctor hasn't been able to pinpoint the cause. By listening to your own pain, you can help solve a mystery and start feeling better.

RATE YOUR PAIN:
Relief at Last Quiz

Do you know the cause of your chronic pain? Have a great treatment plan? Are your pain pills letting you down? Or are you avoiding medications altogether? How much does chronic pain intrude on your everyday activities, your relationships, your sleep? Find out with a revealing quiz that will show you how pain is affecting your life and how this book can help.

1. I've got a clear diagnosis of the cause of my chronic pain.

a. True

b. False

What your answer means: A clear understanding of the cause of chronic pain is essential for finding the right treatments. Yet many people spend months or years, and see three, five, ten or more doctors searching for a good diagnosis. If your chronic pain has not been diagnosed yet, don't give up hope. Use the pain diary and pain scales described in this chapter to help you track symptoms and pain levels. The more information you have, the better your chances for success. Consider asking your primary care doctor for a referral to a pain specialist, too. These specially trained doctors can look for clues and order tests that pinpoint pain's source and help you get relief at last.

2. I work closely with my doctor to be sure my chronic pain treatment plan is working.

a. I call or visit several times a year so my doctor can assess my pain, adjust my medications, or add other therapies.

b. I have some prescriptions but not a real plan. I rarely (less than once a year) discuss my pain with my doctor.

c. I've never mentioned my pain to my doctor. I take care of it myself.

What your answer means: A treatment plan that includes strategies for immediate relief, ways to prevent flare-ups in the future, and drug and nondrug therapies aimed at treating your underlying condition and controlling pain on many levels is essential for gaining control of chronic pain. So is reviewing the plan with your doctor regularly so that she can make adjustments. If you don't have a pain management plan, ask your doctor about one, and read about the latest combination-care strategies for your condition in Part Two. If you do have a plan, the information you'll find there can help you find new strategies that may ease pain more fully, treat your condition more thoroughly, and perhaps even allow you to reduce the amount of pain medication you take.

3. I use these medications for pain relief:

a. Over-the-counter pain relievers only

b. Prescription pain relievers and muscle relaxants

c. Prescription drugs for my specific type of pain (such as migraine-stopping triptan drugs or antidepressants and antiseizure drugs for nerve pain) and pain relievers as needed

d. No drugs for me. I only use natural remedies.

What your answer means: Although mild or infrequent pain may respond to over-the-counter pain relievers alone—and occasionally to natural therapies alone—many people with chronic pain do better with prescription pain relievers and medications targeted to their specific pain condition and nondrug therapies such as exercise, mind-body therapies, touch therapies, healthy eating, and wisely chosen supplements. In *Your New Pain Prescription,* you'll find plenty of proven nondrug therapies, but you'll never be encouraged to stop taking drugs that treat your condition or ease pain.

If you're still experiencing pain despite drugstore or health food store remedies, you owe it to yourself to investigate this smart, proven mix.

Don't fool yourself. Pain medication isn't for wimps, but used wisely and safely it usually doesn't trigger serious side effects or lead to addiction, and it can allow you to get back to the life you want to lead.

4. On average, the medications I take ease my pain this much:

a. Not at all. I'd give them a zero

b. A little—about 10 to 20 percent

c. Somewhat—about 30 to 40 percent

d. Pretty well—about 50 to 70 percent

e. Significantly—about 80 to 100 percent

What your answer means: If your pain drugs are failing you, it's time for something new, but the answer may not be a bigger dose or a stronger drug. The latest pain research is finding that adding other therapies—such as exercise, relaxation, guided imagery, and others—addresses pain in ways that medications cannot. The result? The aches are eased. Of course, everyone's situation is unique. We encourage you to try the well-rounded strategies in this book and to work with your doctor to be sure you're taking the right medications at the right doses for your condition.

5. The nondrug pain therapies I use include (circle as many as apply):

a. Movement therapies such as exercise, physical therapy, water routines, yoga

b. Touch therapies such as massage, acupuncture, chiropractic

c. Mind-body therapies such as muscle relaxation, guided imagery, meditation or deep breathing, hypnotherapy, counseling (such as cognitive behavior therapy)

d. Diet changes and supplements

e. None

What your answer means: The more the merrier. Adding these therapies to your pain reduction tool kit can help you stop pain faster and keep it away more effectively. From guided imagery for irritable bowel syndrome to stress reduction for tension headaches, from water exercise for fibromyalgia to hypnotherapy for cancer pain, these techniques have been shown, in well-designed studies published in serious, peer-reviewed medical journals, to bring real, measurable relief. The bonus? You not only have less pain, you feel more in control. Less stressed. Happier. And healthier. You deserve nothing less.

6. Chronic pain has changed my life in these ways (circle all that apply):

a. My relationship with my spouse or partner, my kids, and other family members isn't what it used to be.

b. I rarely do the things I love anymore. It's just too difficult.

c. I don't get a good night's sleep very often.

d. I have trouble walking and exercising.

e. I'm struggling at work, have had to change jobs, cut back my hours, or stop working altogether because of my pain.

f. It's made life more challenging, but I've found ways to cope, adjust, and continue.

What your answer means: Chronic pain is truly life altering. If you circled one of the first five answers, you need a better relief strategy, and you deserve to judge how well your relief plan works by how much it allows you to return to the life you love. That's the real measure of success. It may mean going way beyond pain pills to include exercise or physical therapy, stress reduction, counseling to learn new coping strategies, and relaxation and guided imagery to help you deal with the physical and emotional fallout of pain flare-ups.

7. Since my pain started, my moods have been (circle all that apply):

a. Lower. I often feel depressed.

b. Anxious. I'm filled with worry and fear.

c. Stressed out. Pain and worries about what it's doing to my life keep me really upset.

d. Up and down. I'm working hard to keep my spirits up and use emotional support from family or a counselor, good times with good friends, and relaxation techniques to help me.

What your answer means: Pain can make anyone feel depressed, worried, and stressed. But did you know that these feelings can, in turn, make your pain feel even worse? It's hardly fair, but new research shows that the areas of your brain that process pain and emotions are often linked (or are the same). Tension, depression, and fear—such as anticipating the next wave of pain—change the way your brain processes pain signals so that they're more intense. It's not "all in your head." This pain feels real. Understanding the mood-pain connection helps explain why pain medications alone can't always erase pain, and why adding mind-body approaches like relaxation, meditation, deep breathing, hypnotherapy, and guided imagery really helps. (Yes, new research also shows that these techniques help reverse the effects negative mood states have on your pain.)

Relief at Last

Throughout *Relief at Last*, you'll discover the latest about the most effective medications and medical interventions for your type of pain, including important treatments your doctor may be overlooking. You'll also learn how to combine them with other therapies proven to help stop flare-ups and prevent future pain for your specific condition. In this book you'll find:

- **Research-proven strategies for more than 60 top pain conditions:** These include ways to ease flare-ups quickly as well as approaches that prevent future pain.

- **Tips for taking common pain relievers safely and effectively:** These days there are plenty of drug side effects to worry about. Among them are concerns about heart attacks, strokes, and gastrointestinal bleeding with nonsteroidal anti-inflammatory drugs (ibuprofen, naproxen, Celebrex), the risk of liver damage or even failure if you take too much acetaminophen, as well as fears of dependence and even addiction with strong opioid-based prescription pain drugs. You'll find advice on taking common painkillers and pain blockers safely and effectively, along with the latest research-proven information on nonpain medications for specific conditions that may work better than relying on pain drugs alone.

- **Gentle exercise routines:** We want you to get moving, at your own pace. To get you started, we've got a simple walking program, a yoga stretching routine, an easy-does-it strength-building program, and even a basic water exercise plan, all designed to be safe and effective for people with chronic pain. Give one a try and find out why pain experts recommend movement to almost everyone who comes to the nation's top pain clinics. (Of course, it's always wise to check in with your doctor before beginning a new exercise program.)

- **The latest, study-based advice on how to use foods and supplements to support your journey to relief:** Separating the hype from the truth about diets and dietary supplements for pain relief isn't easy, especially with supplement shelves loaded with products that promise to cut pain and with bookstores brimming with pain relief diets. The science behind these is ever-changing. Ahead, you'll learn what works best for your specific condition and what popular supplements aren't living up to their early promise.

- **Help assessing your pain and talking to your doctor about it:** The only way to know whether a new therapy is working for you is to track your pain and look for signs of improvement. Researchers say the only way to be sure you're communicating about your pain so that your doctor understands is to find a common language—a pain rating scale to use for tracking your pain, then describing it to your doctor. You'll get better care and become more aware of what's working and what's not if you use a scale. You'll find several to choose from in the resource section at the end of this book.

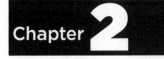
Food and Supplements

Could a special diet or a brand new supplement spell the end of your chronic pain forever? Although health food stores and Internet Web sites are loaded with pills, potions, and diet books that promise to erase your aches, well-designed research tells a different story.

Truth is, some dietary strategies can relieve flare-ups or prevent future pain problems in a few pain conditions. And some well-studied supplements have good track records, too. But too often, the advertised promises are wishful thinking at best. At worst, they're lures designed to make you reach for your credit card or open up your wallet.

Throughout *Relief at Last*, we've made a commitment to sticking with well-researched food and supplement strategies for chronic pain relief. You'll also find the latest about popular supplements that haven't lived up to their potential. Here's what you need to know about how far dietary therapies can go to ease your pain.

Food

From the "back pain diet" to the "fibromyalgia diet" to the "pain-free arthritis food plan" and beyond, bookstores and the Internet are crowded with meal plans touting food as the answer to chronic pain. It's an interesting theory. But while some types of chronic pain—such as migraines, tension headaches, and digestion-related conditions like irritable bowel syndrome and inflammatory bowel disease—do respond to dietary changes, the real connections between your plate and your pain are more complex and more subtle than proponents of pain diets might suggest.

There's no proof that highly restrictive eating plans offer real pain relief, and experts warn they could leave you with dangerous nutrition gaps. For example, "arthritis-relief" diets with no real science behind them include plans that eliminate nightshade vegetables (like tomatoes and eggplant), exclude vitamin C–rich foods (the "alkaline" diet), or even advocate snacking on gin-soaked raisins (a popular folk remedy).

It's true that eliminating specific ingredients and trigger foods can relieve or prevent pain for some people and some conditions. It's also true that adding foods to your diet—such as fiber and probiotics—may help, too, especially for some digestive conditions. But food really shines as a support system rather than as a direct pain reliever. Eating a healthy diet can help you achieve or maintain a healthy weight, for example, which is important because being overweight or obese can make many chronic pain conditions worse. Good food choices also maintain your energy throughout the day and keep your immune system strong, key for avoiding fatigue and illnesses that make coping with pain even more difficult.

Dietary changes can help with chronic pain in three ways.

Eliminating trigger foods could ease symptoms. Cutting out red wine and cheese might help you avoid another migraine. A low-fiber diet can help you ease pain during a flare-up of diverticulitis. Avoiding sulfite-rich foods like red meats and many types of wine could cut your odds for a flare-up of inflammatory bowel disease. If you have a food sensitivity or intolerance—such as to dairy products or to grains containing the protein gluten—avoiding offenders can keep you more comfortable. The catch: Steer clear of diets that ask you to eliminate large groups of foods, which can lead to nutritional deficiencies. If you suspect a food is causing flare-ups, test it by cutting it out for 2 weeks. If you feel better, skip it. Some experts recommend confirming the reaction before you eliminate a food permanently by eating a tiny bit and seeing how you react.

Eliminating trouble foods works if you customize your strategy instead of cutting out huge categories of healthy foods that may not really be bothering your body at all. In one study of 150 people with irritable bowel syndrome (IBS) published in the journal *Gut*, those who stopped eating their personal trigger foods experienced a 26 percent reduction in pain and other symptoms.[1] But the list of potential trouble foods is huge—alcohol, chocolate, caffeinated beverages such as coffee and sodas, sugar-free sweeteners such as sorbitol or mannitol, and high-fat foods may set off diarrhea and pain. IBS gas and bloating may even get worse after eating otherwise healthy foods like beans, broccoli, cabbage, and cauliflower. It makes sense to spend time tracking down your personal pain culprits rather than cutting so much out of your diet.

Adding healthy stuff could soothe symptoms. Fiber for irritable bowel syndrome. Yogurt packed with beneficial bacteria for inflammatory bowel disease. Blood sugar–steadying foods of all sorts for type 2 diabetes, as lower blood sugar can improve nerve pain slightly. Sometimes add-ons spell relief. Throughout this book, you'll read about research-proven, beneficial foods that can help specific conditions.

Some examples: Drinking plenty of water can cut your risk for kidney stones by 32 percent,[2] important news if you've already experienced these painful little rocks and want to avoid a second round. Getting more good bacteria—such as the probiotics found in yogurt and some supplements—helped 77 percent of people with inflammatory bowel disease feel better, according to one study. People who kept their blood sugar under tight control slowed the progression of painful diabetic nerve damage by an impressive 57 percent in another study.[3]

The catch: Steer clear of miracle foods that promise to ease all sorts of pain. There's no evidence they work. After careful research, we can't promise that any single food is a pain cure. Even omega-3 fatty acids, long recommended to ease the inflammation of everything from rheumatoid arthritis to inflammatory bowel disease, don't have a research-proven track record for pain relief (though it makes sense for plenty of health reasons to get these good fats into your diet).

Controlling your weight may be the best pain-relieving benefit of all. Extra pounds put pressure on your joints and make muscle-strengthening, joint-easing exercise more difficult. In addition, researchers now suspect that carrying extra fat around your midsection may ratchet up bodywide inflammation enough to make many pain conditions feel worse.

Does weight loss matter? You bet. In one recent, eye-opening University of California, San Diego, study of 3,471 people, being overweight increased risk for a surprising array of pain types including low back pain, tension or migraine headache, fibromyalgia, abdominal pain, and chronic widespread pain.[4] Other research shows that being overweight triples or even quadruples your risk for knee pain; every additional 10 pounds you carry puts an extra 30 to 60 pounds of pounding pressure on your knees with every step.[5] The good news? Losing weight takes the pressure off.

What about inflammation? As we said earlier, we can't promise that any food or diet will cool off this danger enough, on its own, to soothe pain. But we do think the healthiest eating plan for anyone with (or without) chronic pain is one that keeps a lid on this health problem. Following a Mediterranean-style diet may be your best bet. This eating plan is packed with fruits and vegetables and full of whole grains, lean protein, low-fat or fat-free dairy, and good fats from fish, nuts, and olive and canola oils. Good fats can reduce inflammation— and they're helped in that endeavor by the produce and grains—as well as the lack of inflammation-raising saturated fats and refined grain products. We think it's a winner for overall health.

Several small studies are beginning to find that a Mediterranean diet may improve some pain conditions somewhat. In one small Swedish study, 51 people with rheumatoid arthritis followed that eating plan or their regular diet for three months. Researchers report a 56 percent improvement in disease activity; participants felt less pain and had less joint swelling.[6]

»More Research Needed

Homeopathy

You'll find plenty of personal testimonials on the Internet claiming that homeopathic remedies from creams and gels to premade formulas and customized treatments can ease everything from back pain to arthritis to fibromyalgia. This alternative medicine system, developed 200 years ago in Germany, is based on the notion that cure comes when you ingest tiny doses of substances that produce symptoms similar to your medical problem. It's an interesting theory, but when researchers from 14 major US medical centers evaluated the evidence they found no proof that homeopathy eases chronic pain. Yes, some small studies have been done, but the scientists say they've found little benefit and, for the most part, were not well designed.[7] Our advice: If you're curious about this form of alternative medicine, try it as an add-on to therapies with a proven track record. Don't use it in place of treatments that really work!

Fitting dietary changes into your relief at last plan: Smart, healthy food choices that promote good health and that target your specific health needs are always a good idea. A new eating plan is a great addition to a multifaceted pain control plan, but remember that food can rarely tackle pain on its own. In Part Two of this book, you'll find plenty of specific, research-proven strategies that use food to help ease the pain of specific conditions and to prevent flare-ups. And if you suspect that something in your diet is triggering pain, we've got advice on how to use a food diary to track food choices and pain to look for real patterns.

What you should know: Often, the best way to use food as a pain-relief tool is by enjoying healthy calorie-controlled meals and snacks that will help you lose weight and/or maintain a healthy weight.

Supplements

Americans spend billions of dollars a year on supplements that promise to erase chronic pain, but do the hundreds of pills, powders, and liquids crowding drugstore and health food store shelves really work? When researchers looked at the evidence for an exhaustive Department of Veterans Affairs review of alternative pain remedies in 2007, most supplements got low marks. An analysis of 91 supplement studies found that although many supplements claim to work, most of the supporting studies were too brief and/or involved such a small number of people that the results weren't reliable proof of effectiveness or safety.[8]

From vitamins and minerals to herbs, amino acids, enzymes, and beyond, supplements are big business. While some have a proven track record, new research has recently overturned long-held beliefs about widely used pain remedies such as the herb feverfew for migraines and fish oil for inflammatory bowel disease. That's a good thing. Through well-designed studies, we can discover what really works and what really doesn't. At the same time, they can confirm that other supplements show real promise.

More disturbing are the dozens of supplements that make big claims based on little or no solid evidence. These waste your money and your time by keeping you away from treatments proven to help. At worst, they may raise your risk for side effects and interactions.

Supplements that really work to ease pain do so in many different ways. Some ease inflammation; others short-circuit pain signals. Others directly address condition-specific sources of pain, such as calming spasm-prone muscles, protecting joints from damage, and supporting healthy digestion.

The evidence: New research is proving that some popular supplements do little to ease pain and uncovering others with real promise. At this point, for example, there's no good evidence that magnesium helps with fibromyalgia, that feverfew or coenzyme Q10 prevents migraines, that vitamin D actually eases back and joint pain, or that fish oil is beneficial for inflammatory bowel disease. We'd like to see more good research on some other widely used yet understudied supplements. Among the remedies we think still belong in the wait-and-see category are ASU (avocado soybean unsaponifiables), bovine cartilage, bromelain, CSO, devil's claw, ginger, MSM (methylsulfonylmethane), shark cartilage, and wild yam.

That said, there's good evidence for many supplements, and you'll read more about them in Part Two. They include:

Peppermint oil: In nine small studies, enteric-coated peppermint oil capsules eased symptoms of irritable bowel syndrome by as much as 75 percent.

Choosing a High-Quality Dietary Supplement

Throughout *Relief at Last* you'll find up-to-date, science-based information about dietary supplements worth trying—and those you should avoid—for your particular chronic pain condition. If you're ready to buy one—online, or at a drugstore, health food store, or supplement store—be prepared. You may find dozens of products to choose from at a wide variety of prices. Use these guidelines for finding top-quality supplements.

Mention it to your doctor or ask the pharmacist before you buy. Even if a supplement has proven benefits for your condition, it's worth checking in with your physician or pharmacist first. You may have other health conditions that would make it a less than terrific choice or you may be pregnant or nursing, scheduled for surgery, or on medications that could interact with it.

Double-check drug/supplement interactions. If you take medication regularly for a chronic condition, or even for a short-term medical problem, it's smart to educate yourself about potential interactions with supplements. For example, melatonin may interact with steroids, and tetracycline-based antibiotics and the thyroid drug Synthroid may interact with calcium supplements. For more information, check the National Institutes of Health Dietary Supplement Fact Sheets.

Peppermint may work by relaxing smooth muscle cells in the walls of your intestines so you don't have painful spasms.[9] These special capsules survive stomach acids to release their oils in your intestines. It's not clear that this remedy is safe during pregnancy.

Fiber supplements: A diet rich in whole grains, fruits, and vegetables can supply all the fiber you need in a day, but a supplement will bridge the gap if you can't quite hit your daily fiber quota of 25 to 30 grams (twice what most of us get). Soluble fiber such as psyllium (Metamucil and other brands) is proven to ease digestive pain for many, but not all, people with IBS and diverticulitis. It forms a soothing gel in your gastrointestinal tract that can help you stay regular, reducing diarrhea and easing constipation. Two teaspoons a day cut pain and other IBS symptoms 59 percent in one Dutch study.[10] Getting plenty of fiber kept people with diverticulitis symptom free for years in a British study.[11]

The more scientists research fiber, the more benefits they discover. It turns

Check for the "USP Verified" logo. Products with this designation have been reviewed by the nonprofit US Pharmacopeia, which sets standards for the purity, potency, and quality of supplements or their ingredients. This ensures that a product contains the ingredients listed on the label in the listed quantities, is free of tested contaminants, and will be absorbed by the body. The USP also monitors the manufacturing processes of supplement makers who request it and performs random, off-the-shelf tests of verified products to ensure their continued quality. The program is voluntary and not all supplement makers use it. Other seals to look for: GMP (Good Manufacturing Practices) or TruLabel, both awarded by the Natural Products Association.

Skip megadoses. Don't assume that if a little is good, a higher dose is even better. More and more research shows, for example, that high-dose antioxidants don't work and can even be harmful; the same is true of many other dietary supplements. Stick with recommended supplement doses.

Store the smart way. Cool and dark is best. Research shows that bouts of high humidity—like a steamy bathroom after you shower or take a bath—can reduce the potency and quality of supplements quickly. A kitchen cabinet or shelf in a bedroom or hall closet (out of reach of children) is smarter. Be sure the expiration date is far enough in the future that the product won't expire before you finish taking it.

out that soluble fiber also creates a good home for "good bacteria" in your intestines, which soothe inflammation and calm down pain signals zinging from nerves in your intestinal walls to your brain. If you're new to fiber, go slowly and drink plenty of water.

Probiotics: Powders and capsules containing good bacteria are becoming major players in easing several types of chronic digestive pain including IBS and inflammatory bowel disease (IBD), and for good reason. These friendly critters cool inflammation and turn down pain signals beamed from your intestines to your brain. They even seem to calm overactive immune responses in your intestines that can make IBS worse.[12] There are many types of probiotic supplements on the market, each containing a different mix of bacteria with a bewildering variety of high-tech names, so follow the advice in Part Two of this book to find the types that work best for your condition.

Capsaicin cream: Packed with the substance that gives chile peppers their fiery, tongue-searing bite, capsaicin cream is an improbable pain soother. Rub it on stiff, painful joints or sensitive, painful skin after a bout of shingles and it desensitizes nerve fibers that send pain signals. Capsaicin cuts arthritis pain in half for 40 percent of people who try it and reduces neuropathic pain by the same amount for 60 percent of people with postshingles pain called postherpetic neuralgia, say pain experts from the University of Oxford.[13]

Glucosamine and chondroitin: Are these popular joint pain pills worthless duds, as some experts now say, or can they deliver? A landmark National Institutes of Health study in 2006 of 1,583 people with mild to severe osteoarthritis revealed that the combination of these two substances—which are found naturally in the cartilage cushion between joints—eased pain by a respectable 25 percent for people with moderate to severe arthritis. There was no benefit for people with mild pain.[14] Other research suggests it may help with arthritis-related pain of the hands, spine, and jaw, too.[15] These two compounds may also protect joints against progressive wear-and-tear damage related to osteoarthritis.

SAMe (S-adenosylmethionine): According to the government's Agency for Healthcare Research and Quality, this supplement's osteoarthritis-soothing power is on par with drugstore and prescription pain relievers like ibuprofen and celecoxib (Celebrex). SAMe works by increasing cartilage thickness, but it takes a while to feel the benefits. In one study, celecoxib provided better pain relief for the first two months of treatment, but after that SAMe was just as effective.[16] It is safe and may even have a better safety profile than NSAID pain relievers, which can raise your risk for gastrointestinal bleeding and ulcers. But because it may increase available levels of feel-good brain chemicals like serotonin and dopamine (which may also help ease pain), it shouldn't be used along with mood-raising antidepressants without first consulting your doctor.

Turmeric: A compound called curcumin in this traditional curry powder ingredient has anti-inflammatory properties that might ease the aches of osteoarthritis. We'll be honest—the research isn't quite solid yet, but well-credentialed pain experts say turmeric is the best of the anti-inflammatory herbs touted for pain relief. (Others, which need more study, include devil's claw, willow bark, cat's claw, rosemary, and green tea.)

Alpha-lipoic acid: This strong antioxidant helped lessen back pain significantly for people who were also in an exercise program, in one recent Italian study.[19] It has also been shown to ease pain and other symptoms of diabetes-related neuropathy, say Dutch researchers who reviewed six studies investigating this supplement.[20] Used for decades in Europe to treat nerve pain, it also shows promise for carpal tunnel syndrome[21] and burning mouth syndrome.[22]

Alpha-lipoic acid is found naturally in every cell in your body, where it protects against damage by free radicals—destructive molecules produced naturally in the body when you digest food. Side effects are uncommon but you should skip this drug if you're pregnant or breast-feeding. Talk to your doctor before taking alpha-lipoic acid if you have diabetes; it can lower blood sugar and could lead to dangerous blood sugar lows when combined with your medications.

L-carnitine: The amino acid L-carnitine shows promise for easing the pain of diabetes-related nerve damage; in one study, people with this type of peripheral neuropathy saw nerve function improve after taking it for a year.[23] In another, it also eased pain and improved nerve sensitivity in people with diabetes.[24]

Carnitine, found naturally in the human body, helps cells convert fat into energy, but it also reduces damage to tissues by free radicals, which can harm cells. L-carnitine is generally safe, but don't take it without talking first with your doctor if you have peripheral vascular disease, diabetes, high blood pressure, or kidney disease. Avoid "D-carnitine." It can interfere with L-carnitine's benefits in your body.

Fish oil capsules: In one University of Pittsburgh study of 250 people with back and neck pain, daily fish oil capsules reduced pain for 60 percent and let 59 percent stop taking other pain relievers.[25] Rich in inflammation-cooling omega-3 fatty acids, fish oil capsules may also take the edge off the pain of rheumatoid arthritis and improve nerve functioning in people with nerve damage resulting from diabetes. In one study, researchers found it eased coldness and numbness and improved perception.[26]

But fish oil isn't always a winner. Although many people with inflammatory bowel disease take fish oil in the hope that it will ease inflammation and prevent flare-ups, one large, yearlong study found that it did not help keep people in remission after all.[27]

How to fit supplements into your Relief at Last plan: Be skeptical and demanding about any supplement you're going to ingest for the short-term or the long term. The supplements you choose should have proven pain-relieving benefits and little to no risk for side effects. That's the standard we've used in *Relief at Last.*

Avoid remedies that make promises based on laboratory studies, on a single study, or on little evidence, and steer clear of any that sound too good to be true or claim to be quick fixes. Just as there's no single medical treatment that's a magic cure for chronic pain, no supplement can fix pain on its own either.

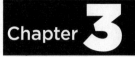

Chapter 3

Exercise and Movement Therapies

Move? Getting up to take a walk, do an exercise routine, work out with an exercise band, or slip into a swimming pool may be the last thing you want to do when you're in pain. But, yes, we want you to move. Exercise is emerging as an important therapy for nearly all types of chronic pain, as researchers, pain specialists, and people living with chronic pain see the benefits of physical activity. Among them? Keeping muscles strong and flexible, helping stiff joints become more mobile, reducing stress, and even lifting depression.

We're not suggesting you train for the Boston Marathon or do anything that's beyond your physical abilities at this point. Simple moves performed while sitting in a chair or even lying in bed may be all you can do and all you need to do. What counts is finding activity that fits your needs and fitness level, then fitting a little in most days of the week. Depending on your pain condition, your doctor may also recommend that you see a physical therapist, which is a great opportunity to get an exercise plan tailored to your needs. Your sessions will likely incorporate many of the types of movement described here, so read on for some ideas.

Exercise

It's free, strengthens your muscles, helps you feel happier and more energetic, and is proven to help control many types of chronic pain, from migraines and fibromyalgia to cancer pain and aches associated with digestive disorders. Small wonder, then, that exercise tailored to your personal needs is a cornerstone treatment at the nation's top-notch pain-relief programs.

The catch? Outside of those cutting-edge programs, exercise may be the best-kept secret in chronic pain management. When researchers from the University of North Carolina at Chapel Hill recently surveyed 684 people with chronic back or neck pain (a type of pain for which exercise has a very long track record), they found that slightly less than half had a "prescription" for

"Slow-Motion" Movement Therapies for Chronic Pain

Exercise that makes you slow down and become more aware of your body are popping up at more and more pain management centers. The reason? There's growing evidence that this type of physical activity soothes pain and gives you unique tools for controlling it on your own.

Alexander Technique: A gentle method of retraining your physical and emotional responses, the Alexander Technique improves balance, posture, and alignment in everyday activities. But it goes beyond that, focusing on how emotional responses affect the way we hold our bodies. You learn new, healthier ways to stand, sit, and move, and as a result feel lighter and freer. There's plenty of anecdotal evidence that taking a series of Alexander Technique classes or lessons can help with back pain, neck pain, shoulder pain, even carpal tunnel syndrome. In one large British study of 579 people with back pain, this therapy was even better than exercise (which you already know is highly effective) for reducing pain.[1] Of course, that doesn't mean you should skip physical activity. Doing both could double your relief!

Feldenkrais: This method helps you become more aware of your body and your posture through movement. In studies, it shows promise for easing fibromyalgia and is also widely used for back pain and other chronic pain conditions affecting the muscles and joints.[2]

Hatha yoga: Slow, simple, and flowing, this progression of easy yoga postures exercise.[3] It was recommended most often to those who were already seeing a physical therapist. In contrast, physicians recommended exercise to just 15 percent of people in the survey.

That's a troubling gap. Exercise belongs in the pain prescription of virtually every person with chronic pain. It could be as simple as a gentle routine you perform in a chair, in bed, or in a pool; it might be a program adapted to your limitations if you've got foot pain or shoulder pain, or, if you're in great shape, a challenging routine of strength training, cardiovascular exercise, and stretching. The important thing is to get moving. The benefits are just too essential to miss out on.

The moves best for you may involve one or more of the following types of physical activity.

helped people with chronic low back pain ease aches and lift depression in a study of one 12-week program.[4]

Pilates: Pronounced "puh-LAH-teez," this low-impact fitness method can help with back pain, fibromyalgia, weight loss, and more, and as a result Pilates classes are becoming a feature at pain clinics around the country. Done on mats or with special equipment, it usually involves a series of flowing exercises and stretches coordinated with your breathing. Instead of lots of repetitions, this technique focuses on doing a stretch or exercise a few times very well. In a recent study of 50 Turkish women with fibromyalgia, those who took an hour-long Pilates class three times a week saw pain diminish.[5]

Qigong: A component of traditional Chinese medicine practiced daily by millions of people around the world, qigong is a series of flowing movements that combine breathing, meditation, and specific postures to strengthen your life force, or *qi* (pronounced "chee"). They also increase strength, balance, and flexibility and can reduce stress. Qigong is showing promise as a gentle, pain-relieving movement therapy for fibromyalgia and is used in some chronic pain management programs for other types of pain as well.

Tai chi: The flowing movements of tai chi look like a slow-motion dance routine, but the grace of this ancient, joint-friendly exercise hides a multitasking marvel. Tai chi can help you improve strength, balance, and posture as well as bring more relaxation and mental focus into your life. In one recent study, it was as effective as water exercise for relieving the pain and stiffness of arthritis.[6]

Cardiovascular exercise: Walking, riding an exercise bike, swimming, taking an exercise class, or even running are all cardiovascular exercises that burn calories and boost endurance and fitness by helping your heart and lungs work more efficiently, reduce stress, and lift your mood. If you're trying to lose weight (often an issue for people with chronic pain conditions), cardiovascular activity will help.

Strength training: Muscle-building moves that use hand weights, weight machines, resistance bands, or your own body weight build strength (especially important if you've got muscle or joint pain), help with balance, and help you lose weight. Stronger, denser muscles burn more calories around the clock.

Stretching: It feels good, helps you stay flexible (important if you have joint pain, muscle pain, or bodywide aches and pains), and helps balance the tug of connective tissue on your joints so they stay in better alignment.

How it helps: Exercise can reverse many of chronic pain's most damaging effects on your body, as well as on your mind and mood. Sitting still is a natural reaction to pain. But over time it weakens muscles, making everyday activities more difficult and raising your risk for other health problems like overweight, heart disease, diabetes, and brittle, fracture-prone bones. Sedentary living— some doctors call it "sitting disease"—can also make some pain conditions, such as back pain, neck pain, and osteoarthritis of the knees and other joints, worse because out-of-shape muscles can't keep your spine and joints in proper alignment and can't act as shock absorbers when you walk across a room, head down a flight of stairs, or twist your torso to get out of the car.

Pain also takes a toll on your emotions, raising your odds for anxiety and depression. Exercise can help here, too. Studies show that just a half-hour of exercise can help lift depression for many people.

The evidence: Exercise is so essential for reversing knee pain that experts even say it can stop the progression of osteoarthritis in its tracks. An easy routine helped 62 percent of people with knee pain make a full recovery in one Dutch study; in contrast, just 51 percent of those who got the usual care—rest and advice to avoid activity that causes pain—felt better.[7] And when 439 people with arthritis followed one of three programs for 18 months—strength training, aerobic conditioning, or healthy living advice with no exercise component— researchers found big gains for both exercise groups. Pain fell 8 to 12 percent; the distance that volunteers could walk in 6 minutes improved dramatically; and the time it took to get out of a car and to lift and carry a 10-pound weight also dropped significantly. These gains may sound small, but all are proof positive that a little exercise can make everyday life much easier, say the researchers from Bowman Gray School of Medicine.[8]

Your Optimal Exercise Routine

There's no one best exercise for easing chronic pain. Tailoring a routine to fit your own needs means taking into account the type of pain you have, your fitness level, muscle strength, other medical conditions, and your personal likes and dislikes. (If you just can't stand swimming or being in the water, a pool routine isn't right for you even if it's touted as the top routine for your condition!)

Your doctor may be able to help point the way, or even better, refer you to a physical therapist who can help design a program to meet your needs. Another option is to use routines endorsed by organizations for people with your specific condition. A good routine may include one or more of these types of exercise:

Stretching or range-of-motion moves: These keep joints and muscles flexible, which is important as you age or if you've been sedentary as a result of your pain.

Options: Gentle stretches, yoga, tai chi, and Pilates.

Note: It's smart to work with a physical therapist at first to avoid overstretching. Gentle is best!

Aerobic or cardiovascular exercise: These activities boost the power of your lungs and the strength of your heart. You become more fit and better able to do all the things you want and need to do every day. You build endurance and coordination, tone your muscles, and you can even lose weight.

Options: Walking, riding an exercise bike, swimming or water exercise, an exercise DVD, or aerobics class.

Note: Everyday activities like gardening, cleaning, shoveling snow, raking leaves, washing windows, and waxing the car can also help you build fitness and burn calories. It's important to include these nonexercise moves with some formal exercise for maximum fitness and weight control.

Strength-training or resistance exercise: These moves build up strength in your muscles. Everyone's muscle mass begins to decline after about age 30; if you're sedentary, declines can be even greater, which can intensify many chronic pain conditions.

Options: Moves that use your own body weight (such as crunches) for resistance, or that use resistance bands, light hand weights, or weight equipment (usually found at a gym).

Note: Start slowly; you'll build strength by doing strength-training moves for a few minutes several times a week. Use light weights or light resistance bands; increase slowly as you build up strength.

Exercise has also proven to be better than shockwave therapy for improving shoulder pain.[9] It also eases fibromyalgia's debilitating symptoms[10] and reduces the intensity and frequency of migraine[11] and tension headaches.[12] It can even treat symptoms of Crohn's disease and ulcerative colitis. When people with these inflammatory bowel disorders walked three times a week for 12 weeks, their symptoms improved significantly, and people with Crohn's disease had no flare-ups at all. In contrast, those who didn't walk said symptoms grew worse.[13, 14]

The benefits of exercise reach beyond physical comfort. In one University of Georgia review of chronic pain studies involving 3,000 people, researchers found that those who exercised regularly had 20 percent fewer symptoms of anxiety than those who didn't,[15] and anxiety eased up in as little as 3 weeks. That's important, because when you're feeling calm it's easier to take all the other

Physical and Occupational Therapy

There's plenty of evidence that physical therapy helps with everything from back and neck pain to knee pain and beyond. Traditionally, people who need a physical therapist have seen one on the advice of their physician, but in most states you can now make your own appointment with a physical therapist. Physical therapy is usually covered by insurance. That's good news, because a physical therapist can create a custom exercise program that takes into consideration your current pain condition.

Occupational therapists, on the other hand, can help you adapt everyday activities (such as cooking, getting dressed, and sitting at a keyboard) so that they're easier and don't cause pain. Even if you're seeing a physical therapist, adding an OT to your pain care team can give you extra insights and practical know-how that make daily living less painful and more satisfying.

Once you've learned some basic movements that ease your pain, you can safely exercise on your own or join classes at your local gym. You may also want to work with a personal trainer to give you more exercise ideas. Just be sure to let any instructors or trainers know about your pain condition before you begin, and if any particular moves cause pain, don't be shy about speaking up.

Part Three provides more information about finding physical and occupational therapists, as well as certified personal trainers and fitness instructors.

steps that help you cope with and vanquish pain, like getting good sleep, following a healthy diet, and keeping up with medication and nondrug therapies.

Fitting exercise into your relief at last plan: Start slowly. Keep your moves gentle. And be sure to talk with your doctor about exercises customized to your pain condition, fitness level, and any other limitations (and likes and dislikes) you may have. Plenty of organizations for people with specific chronic conditions offer easy routines online. A few, such as the Arthritis Foundation, have even sponsored community exercise programs. Of course, you can also find exercise classes offered at any gym or health club, you can work with a personal trainer who knows how to modify a routine to meet your needs, or you can exercise along to many DVDs (look for types designed for people with your pain condition; you'll find suggestions throughout this book). Just be careful not to aggravate your condition. Let the instructor know your needs, learn from your doctor or a physical therapist what types of moves you definitely should not try, and listen to your body. Gentle yoga, easy stretches, slow walking, water walking and water exercise programs, and beginning strength-training moves are all great options. You'll find four easy exercise programs—a walking routine, a strength-building program, a simple yoga sequence, and a water workout—in Part Three.

Hydrotherapy

Take the soothing, buoyant, easy-on-your-joints pleasure of a warm pool and add gentle stretches, easy strength-training exercises, and simple calorie-burning moves. Now you've got hydrotherapy, a fancy way to describe water-based exercise routines for people with chronic pain conditions such as osteoarthritis.

How it helps: Water, according to the Arthritis Foundation, "is a safe, ideal environment for relieving pain and stiffness." Great for joint problems and low back pain, hydrotherapy increases strength and flexibility while it decreases pain and stiffness. You'll feel better fast, especially in the muscle-loosening, joint-pampering warm water used in the aquatic programs aimed specifically at people with arthritis.

Exercising in water supports your body weight, taking pressure off joints, muscles, and connective tissue; if you're in water up to your neck, it supports 90 percent of your weight. That makes it easier to do exercises that might otherwise hurt. It also provides resistance so that even simple movements—like easy leg raises—work your muscles more than they would on dry land. That boosts muscle strength.

The evidence: In one review of six well-designed studies of hydrotherapy for knee pain, researchers found that it improved pain by 22 percent and also made daily living easier.[16] Women with fibromyalgia who signed up for an easy "deep water running" class saw the intensity of their pain subside by 36 percent.[17]

How hydrotherapy fits into your relief at last plan: If chronic pain has tightened your muscles and/or made your joints stiff so that regular exercise seems too difficult, hydrotherapy might be a great alternative.

What you should know: You don't have to be able to swim to do hydrotherapy. Many classes are held in shoulder-deep water. Others, in deeper water, use buoyancy belts and other flotation devices to keep you upright. Classes developed jointly by the Arthritis Foundation and the YMCA are offered at pools across the United States.

Yoga

Ease stress. Become more flexible. Get in touch with your body. And just feel terrific. Those are just some of the benefits of even the gentlest, simplest yoga routines, making this ancient, meditative exercise perfect for easing chronic pain.

How it helps: Yoga is a profound stress reducer and can interrupt the pain/stress/more pain/more stress cycle that makes everything feel worse when you're living with a chronic pain condition.

Yoga poses, called *asanas*, can also relax your muscles, which brings welcome relief from tightness and spasms. As you practice yoga, your awareness of your own body grows so that you notice muscle tension—such as in your neck or lower back—sooner and can take steps to reverse it. But that's not all. Yoga can also improve sleep; although insomnia and interrupted sleep make pain feel worse, a refreshing night of deep sleep leaves you ready to cope in healthy ways. And yoga can also improve your posture, taking the stress off muscles, ligaments, and joints that contributes to back, neck, and shoulder pain, and even to headaches.

Yoga also simply helps you to slow down so that you can notice how you're feeling physically and emotionally. Its focus on breath can help you break a common chronic pain habit: holding your breath. Many people in pain do this, setting off a chain reaction of stress hormones. Calm, mindful breathing can melt this stress and, over time, help you avoid stressed-out reactions to pain.

The evidence: In one study conducted at West Virginia University of 90 people with low back pain, those who attended yoga classes several times a week for 6 months had significantly less pain and reported that they could go about their daily lives more easily; a control group that didn't do yoga saw no improvement.[18]

Fitting yoga into your relief at last plan: If you're a newcomer to yoga, look for a class or DVD featuring gentle, easy poses and stretches. It can be helpful to work with a yoga instructor, at least at first, to help you learn how to adapt the poses to your own body (such as by using pillows and other supports if you have stiff, achy knees) and to avoid mistakes that could put extra stress on your body or even cause an injury.

What you should know: Yoga classes are available in communities across America. There are many styles of yoga out there, from slow-moving Iyengar yoga that focuses on holding each pose and using props to flowing types like Hatha yoga and athletic "power yoga," called *Ashtanga*. There are even hybrids that combine yoga with Pilates or weight training. If you're just starting out, a beginner Iyengar class or DVD may be best for you. It will focus on learning the fundamentals of one pose at a time. Many DVDs of yoga routines designed specifically for people with chronic pain are also available online. If you take a class, talk with the instructor ahead of time to see if she or he has experience working with people with chronic pain and can help you can adapt poses for your particular condition.

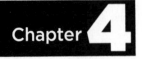

Touch Therapies

The soothing touch of a massage therapist, or even of a family member gently rubbing your shoulders. The ancient healing art of acupuncture, updated with 21st-century technology and techniques. Acupuncture's decidedly low-tech yet powerful cousin acupressure, which uses fingertip pressure to keep your natural energy flowing.

These touch therapies can ease many types of chronic pain, from headaches and fibromyalgia to intractable cancer pain and back pain. In fact, acupuncture worked better than pain relievers in one large, recent study of people with ongoing low back pain. New research shows that these therapies work on many levels to ease pain. Massage, for example, lowers levels of substance P, a brain chemical linked with higher pain intensity in people with low back pain, fibromyalgia, and arthritis. Acupressure seems to trigger the release of your body's own natural pain relievers. Here's what you need to know.

Massage

A good rubdown is always a luxurious treat, whether you're in the hands of a family member who's massaging your neck while you sit in the living room recliner or a masseuse who's kneading your sore muscles with scented aromatherapy oils in the hush of a beautiful spa. But when it comes to pain relief, massage is more than a soothing retreat; it has unique and lasting effects.

Massage brings welcome relief from headaches if neck muscles are tight, eases backaches, and even soothes cancer pain. It can help you sleep better so that coping with pain and getting on with your life are easier. The unique, prolonged human contact also brings a sense of well-being and calm that's hard to find when you spend your days (and nights) fending off pain, restoring a sense of peace so that pain is no longer the center of your life.

How it helps: In addition to relaxing stiff muscles, boosting circulation, reducing swelling, and bringing you the comfort of compassionate human touch, researchers suspect massage erases pain on deeper levels, too. It can relieve pressure on nerves, turn off trigger points—the highly sensitive areas that may refer pain to other parts of the body—and reduce stress. There's evidence it raises levels of feel-good brain chemicals serotonin and dopamine. It promotes deeper sleep, which reduces levels of pain-sensitizing substance P. Massage can also send signals along pressure-sensitive nerves, which may block competing pain signals before they can reach your brain.[1] No wonder people with cancer pain who had massage said afterward, "It's like a vacation from cancer," and "I'm overcome by the most amazing feelings of acceptance and peace."

The evidence: Research suggests that massage can help with back and shoulder pain, cancer pain, and tension headaches and may also ease fibromyalgia and neck pain.[2] And by helping you relax, it eases the stress that can make any type of chronic pain feel even worse.

Rubbing your temples with mint oil can melt the immediate pain of a tension headache, and regular massage can do far more, cutting in half the number of headaches suffered by chronic head pain sufferers in one study published in the *American Journal of Public Health*. After receiving two half-hour massages that focused on tension-prone areas of the head, face, and neck, participants' headaches were several hours shorter and significantly less intense, too.[3] In one study of women with fibromyalgia, massage lifted pain and even reduced the number of tender points (a hallmark of fibromyalgia) on the body.[4]

Perhaps the most dramatic benefits are for people living with deep, tough-to-treat cancer pain, the type that can flare up at any time despite regular pain medication. In one University of Colorado study of 380 people with advanced cancers, those who received several half-hour massages felt pain ebb significantly, dropping nearly 2 points on a 10-point scale. Study volunteers had cancers of the lung, breast, pancreas, colon, and prostate, all of which had spread to other organs or to their bones.[5] In another study of over 1,200 cancer patients, any type of massage—deep Swedish muscle work, light-touch massage, or even just foot rubs—eased pain a whopping 40 percent.[6]

Fitting massage into your relief at last plan: Massage works best in combination with other chronic pain treatments including medications, acupuncture, exercise, and mind-body therapies. You probably won't be able to trade in your pain-relieving drugs for an hour on a comfy massage table, but combining this hands-on therapy with your current treatment regimen may help ease pain more than drugs alone can. And it might even allow you to reduce your dose.

What you should know: There are many types of massage out there (150, according to some experts!). What's best for pain? In one study of people with cancer pain, four types of rubdowns—classic deep-tissue massage, the long gliding strokes of Swedish massage, light-touch massage, and simple foot rubs—all helped people feel better.[7] Another type, myofascial release, targets tight spots in the fascia—a stringy, spongy tissue that connects muscles, skin, and organs throughout your body—to ease muscle-, joint-, and nerve-related pain conditions such as back pain, carpal tunnel syndrome, fibromyalgia, shoulder problems, headaches, jaw pain, foot pain, facial pain from trigeminal neuralgia, and more.

It's important to work with a licensed and/or certified massage therapist with experience and training in chronic pain. Talk with your doctor about types of massage that are right (or not) for you and any areas of your body the therapist should skip. For example, if you have cancer pain, your therapist should avoid tumor sites, areas that have received radiation, and incisions.

Acupuncture

Acupuncture is one of the world's oldest healing arts; archeologists have uncovered 5,000-year-old stone acupuncture needles in Inner Mongolia. Today, practitioners of this Chinese healing technique insert sterile, hair-thin needles (it's nearly painless, we promise!) at precise points on the body to unblock "energy"—called *qi* (pronounced "chee"). Traditionally, the needles are twirled or heated. But modern practitioners may also use laser beams, sound waves, and mild electric currents to stimulate qi. Some even practice a special type of ear, or auricular, acupuncture in which thumbtack-shaped needles are left in place for days or weeks.

More Touch Therapies to Try

Chiropractic: Visit a chiropractor for back, shoulder, or neck pain and your spine will be pushed, pulled, and twisted—adjustments intended to fix "subluxations" (misalignments) of the vertebrae in your spinal column. There's something to it: In one study of 2,780 people with lower back pain, researchers found that those who got chiropractic treatments had better pain reduction and less disability than those who received standard medical care (medication, exercise, and physical therapy), and at a slightly lower cost.[8]

Hot/cold therapy: Heat and cold can both help ease the pain, stiffness, and inflammation of arthritis, joint pain, and muscle pains. Which is better? That's up to you. Experts say it's smart to try both and see. Heat therapy—with adhesive heat patches, a warm bath or shower, or a warm, moist towel—expands blood vessels, boosts circulation, and relaxes tense muscles. In contrast, cold therapy—with a cold pack, a sealed bag of ice cubes, or a bag of frozen vegetables wrapped in a towel—can numb deep muscle pain and prevent or soothe inflammation. Some people find alternating is best; others prefer one over the other. It's a personal choice.

The MELT method: Short for Myofascial Energetic Lengthening Technique, this cross between self-massage and exercise uses rubber balls and foam rollers to relieve tight, restricted areas in your fascia—the whole-body connective tissue that joins skin, muscles, and organs. Tight spots in your fascia can contribute to muscle and joint pain.

Reiki: This ancient Japanese healing art—the name means "universal life energy"—is said to release "stuck" energy, allowing pain to ebb and tense muscles to relax. You lie down, fully clothed, and the Reiki practitioner works to free up the energy flowing through and around your body by lightly touching, tapping, or moving his arms above your body and focusing on seven key areas called "chakras."

TENS: Transcutaneous electrical nerve stimulation (TENS for short) is a system that sends low-level electric currents into your skin to ease pain. Although a 2009 review concluded that TENS units don't help lower back pain in large studies,[9] the researchers note that these portable systems may relieve back pain for some people by interfering with pain signals from nerves in the back to the brain. They also say this drug-free option may help with pain caused by diabetes-related nerve damage.

Acupuncture has been proven to play an important role in relieving many types of chronic pain, including back pain, cancer pain, carpal tunnel syndrome, knee pain, fibromyalgia, headache,[11] myofascial pain, neck pain, osteoarthritis, and shoulder pain.

How it helps: Traditional acupuncturists say that this ancient healing technique restores the healthy flow of life energy in the body. Removing blockages relieves symptoms such as pain and helps correct underlying health problems.

Scientific research shows that stimulating acupuncture points can trigger the release of pain-relieving compounds called *opioid peptides* in the brain and spinal cord.[12] It also seems to increase the number of receptors on brain cells in areas that process and mute pain signals—a good thing, because more receptors means more places for your body's natural pain relievers and for pain-relieving drugs to dock and get to work. Magnetic resonance imaging (MRI) scans show that brain activity related to pain calms down by 60 to 70 percent during an acupuncture treatment.[13]

The evidence: Acupuncture can help with nerve, bone, and muscle pain caused by tumors and cancer treatments, providing relief when drugs alone cannot.[14] In one French study of people with advanced cancer whose nerve pain wasn't fully controlled with medication, ear acupuncture decreased aches by 36 percent.[15] In another study of people who'd had surgery for colon cancer, those who received acupuncture and massage therapy along with pain medication got more relief than those who received only drugs.[16]

In 2009, a groundbreaking study of 683 people with ongoing lower back pain concluded that acupuncture worked better than pain pills or physical therapy, report researchers from the Group Health Center for Health Studies in Seattle. Sixty percent of those who received acupuncture got meaningful relief, compared to 39 percent of those who had usual back pain treatments. A year later, 65 percent who had been helped by acupuncture were still feeling better compared to just half of those who got a break from pain with conventional care.[17]

Tension headaches and migraines also respond to this drug-free therapy with lasting results. One review of 22 acupuncture studies found that headache sufferers were still enjoying a break from pain 9 months after their acupuncture treatments ended. In one study of 24 Norwegian women with neck and shoulder pain, those who got 10 acupuncture treatments over 3 to 4 weeks had 50 percent less pain, slept better, and felt less anxious and depressed. And things kept improving over the next three years.[18]

How acupuncture fits in your relief at last plan: Acupuncture is used along with medication and drug-free therapies such as massage, cognitive therapy, meditation, and relaxation to create a multifaceted plan of attack against severe pain, such as cancer pain. It may be used along with migraine-preventing drugs to help stave off big headaches, or stand alone as a back pain treatment if you'd like to avoid long-term use of medication or if other strategies fail.

Yes, needles are involved. But they're so thin, and are inserted only to a depth of about 1 inch, that acupuncture is usually painless. You may feel relaxed or you may get a tingling, energetic feeling during and after a treatment. Will it work for you? Researchers and practitioners say that about 15 to 30 percent of people with ongoing pain do not respond to acupuncture. No one's quite sure why, but some experts suspect that it may be a result of higher levels of compounds called cholecystokinin octapeptides, which seem to block acupuncture's pain-relieving powers.[19]

Acupuncturists tailor the treatment to match each person's unique set of symptoms, as there's no single, one-size-fits-all prescription. You may have one or two sessions (each lasting up to 30 minutes or so) a week for several weeks or months. Relief may be immediate or it may take a while.

Acupressure

Think of acupressure as a hands-on, needle-free version of acupuncture. Both forms of traditional Chinese medicine stimulate special points on the head, arms, legs, and torso so that energy flows freely in the body. Instead of needles, acupressure relies on firm finger or thumb pressure. In the hands of a trained practitioner, acupressure is a sophisticated and complex healing art. But it is also one you can use at home just by pressing a few well-chosen points to relieve the pain of sinus headaches.

Research suggests it may help you reduce the amount of medicine you need for headache pain[20] and that it may help ease many of the same types of pain that respond to acupuncture, such as low back pain and carpal tunnel syndrome. The advantage? Unlike acupuncture, which must be performed by a qualified practitioner, acupressure can be practiced anywhere, at no charge, whenever you need it.

How it works: Acupressure relieves pain for the same reasons that acupuncture does, experts suspect. It encourages circulation and may encourage the release of the body's natural pain-relieving substances, peptide opioids, in the brain and spinal cord. It can also relieve specific types of pain in other ways—clearing sinus congestion to stop a sinus headache, easing muscle tension to soothe a sore back, boosting energy to help make the aches and pains of chronic fatigue syndrome easier to live with, easing insomnia so that you can sleep and wake up feeling less achy in the morning.

The evidence: In one case study from the University of California, Los Angeles, David Geffen School of Medicine, an elderly woman whose knee arthritis wasn't helped by a long list of pain medications finally got relief using a combination of acupuncture and at-home acupressure.[21] The pain had been so severe she couldn't walk. Five months after starting her combination treatment, she

Press Here for Relief

Wondering whether you'll be able to hit the right spot if you give acupressure a try at home? The good news is that acupressure points are fairly large—about 1½ inches in diameter—so you don't have to worry about finding a tiny, precise spot. (Some practitioners say you'll know you're at the right spot because it will feel more tender than surrounding skin.) No need to press hard; just use enough force so that you can feel the muscle you're pressing on relax. You can also use the knuckle of your first finger, or even a pencil eraser, to press a point. Some acupressure experts recommend increasing the pressure while you hold on to a point. Hold each one for about a minute. You can repeat the process as often as you like.

was off her pain drugs and walking again. The researchers suspect acupressure helped by relieving muscle spasms.

Acupressure has also been proven in many studies to help ease severe menstrual cramps and labor pain, lessen pain after surgery, and mute dental pain. In one Taiwanese study of 129 people with low back pain, six sessions of acupressure did more to relieve back pain immediately after the treatments, and 6 months later,[22] than physical therapy.

How acupressure fits into your relief at last plan: If your pain will respond to acupuncture, it's worth finding out about at-home, do-it-yourself care with acupressure. Your acupuncturist can suggest specific acupressure points to press on. For some conditions, such as sinus headaches and neck pain, we've included suggestions later in this book.

Don't use acupressure points that are located where you've got a mole, wart, varicose vein, or a bruise or break in the skin. And skip acupressure if you're pregnant, as practitioners say stimulating some points could trigger early labor or other pregnancy problems.

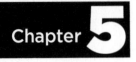

Chapter 5

Mind-Body Therapies

S oothing stress, easing muscle tension, restoring a sense of peace and control to your life: These benefits were once seen as nice extras in the battle to ease chronic pain. Now, they've taken their place at center stage. And the results are impressive.

Mind-body therapies feel good on their own. In combination with other pain-relief therapies—such as exercise, medication, and well-chosen supplements and dietary strategies—they can improve pain more than drugs alone. Counseling, meditation, guided imagery, and other techniques can help you cope better and lift the fear, stress, and hopelessness that make everyday life with chronic pain so difficult.

The bonus? Easing negative emotions, it turns out, flips switches in your brain that tone pain down and make it easier to bear. (Read Chapter 1 for more on pain and emotions.)

Here's what you need to know about five mind-body therapies that belong in your relief at last plan.

Cognitive-Behavioral Therapy

Ever feel overwhelmed by pain? You're not alone. It's a natural response when the simplest movements—getting out of bed, loading the dishwasher, petting the dog, or driving the car—hurt a lot. When feelings of hopelessness and helplessness about pain move into your mind, it's time to push back. That's why the newest chronic pain prescriptions go beyond soothing aches to helping you hold on to optimism and develop powerful new strategies for living your best life despite the pain.

One of the best ways to keep pain from defining you and your life is a short course of cognitive-behavioral therapy (CBT, for short). This practical approach to therapy won't leave you rehashing your past for months on a therapist's couch. Instead, in a few sessions you'll learn to manage stress, find solutions to personal challenges related to pain (such as feeling too achy to exercise or keep up with your interests), set tangible goals, and assert yourself when necessary to reach your goals. You'll feel hopeful, capable, and ready to take action.

CBT can help with any type of chronic pain. Researchers have documented its unique ability to ease pain by reducing stress and changing your thinking about pain, and to improve the quality of life of people with everything from cancer, fibromyalgia, and osteoarthritis, to back pain, headaches, pelvic pain, carpal tunnel syndrome, and mouth and face pain.

How it helps: CBT challenges your old assumptions about pain and teaches you practical, powerful new ways to cope. You'll learn new ways to think about, respond to, and even perceive pain so that it's no longer overpowering. Over time, CBT can help you master your pain so that it interferes as little as possible with your life. You'll go from automatic responses to pain ("pain is endless," "I can't cope," "here we go again") to having a personalized set of problem-solving skills that let you rise to any challenge pain throws your way. You'll learn to plan, be persistent, and be positive, and to identify and sidestep thoughts and feelings that would otherwise allow pain to defeat you. In short, CBT puts you back in control.

For example, if you have low back pain, one of your goals might be to stop the cycle of doing too much, then being physically inactive for days or weeks due to muscle spasms and pain flare-ups. Instead, CBT can teach you to plan out your activities so that they won't aggravate your back and to recognize when you are reaching your limits so that you stop before you trigger a flare-up.

Because CBT reduces stress, it can also have a direct and beneficial effect on painful conditions like irritable bowel disease, as well as help turn down the volume on pain perception in your brain.

The evidence: One review of 40 CBT studies concluded that this mind-body approach has the best track record of all psychological therapies for chronic pain.[1]

When researchers from the University of Manchester School of Dentistry in England reviewed six well-designed studies of CBT for chronic face and mouth pain, they found that it eased pain significantly, both when used on its own and when used in combination with conventional medical care and with complementary therapies such as biofeedback. They conclude that it's effective on its own and also when combined with conventional care, such as medication.[2]

In a Dutch study, people with fibromyalgia who got 16 weeks of CBT and

Counseling for Chronic Pain: It's Not "All in Your Head"!

If your doctor—or friends or family— suggest a counselor to help you cope with chronic pain, it doesn't mean they think you're crazy or that your pain is all in your imagination. Truth is, pain affects your thoughts and feelings as much as it affects your body. The toll it takes on your emotions can get in the way of your efforts to take good care of yourself. It can even raise stress levels so much that pain feels worse.

Counseling—including cognitive-behavioral therapy, one-on-one work with a psychologist or psychiatrist, or even group support, telephone counseling, or therapy over the Internet—can help you understand and reverse thoughts and assumptions about your pain that can keep you isolated and sap your motivation to take good care of your health. A few sessions can help you feel supported, understood, and in control again.

If you find yourself thinking thoughts like these, consider asking your doctor for a referral to a therapist who works with people with chronic pain:

- I'm a failure. My pain means I can't do anything right.

- I can't provide for my family because of my pain. I have no value.

- No one understands what's happening to me. I'm all alone.

- I'm a wimp if I complain about my pain.

began gentle exercise programs saw big improvements in pain, fatigue, anxiety, and mood.[3] Eight weeks of CBT helped people with joint pain and insomnia caused by osteoarthritis sleep 27 minutes longer each night in one University of Washington study—a good thing, because lack of sleep can make pain feel worse. CBT helped them challenge unrealistic beliefs and fears about their insomnia and motivated them to make better use of other sleep-promoting habits such as regular exercise, getting sun exposure (morning sun helps reset your body clock), and limiting caffeine.[4] In addition to getting more shut-eye, they also felt less pain, leading researchers to speculate that improving sleep has a direct and beneficial effect on pain.

CBT works for many types of pain, including the bloating and cramps of irritable bowel syndrome. In a University of Buffalo study, people with IBS who learned CBT at home or from a counselor got an amazing 90 percent reduction in pain and an 80 percent reduction in bowel symptoms such as constipation and diarrhea.[5]

Fitting CBT into your relief at last plan: CBT is flexible. It works when you see a counselor one-on-one, in group therapy, and in self-study programs. It may not replace medication (though it may help you cut back your dose); in some studies, CBT worked best along with IBS medications. CBT is often used in conjunction with many other therapies in a holistic pain control plan. This might include progressive muscle relaxation, physical therapy, pain relievers, guided imagery, and perhaps even biofeedback for even deeper stress relief.

What you should know: CBT is a brief, results-oriented therapy; most people go for 16 sessions. You'll be asked to work hard trying out new solutions at home between sessions, identifying challenges so that you and your therapist can find solutions, and challenging your own feelings and beliefs about pain.

Guided Imagery

Imagine a single chocolate chip melting slowly on your tongue. The splash of waves breaking on a quiet beach. The sharp scent of pine trees in the summer sun. We bet you're feeling more relaxed already! That's the power of guided imagery, which calls on all of your senses to imagine an experience so completely that you might just think it's real!

How it helps: The ability to transport yourself to a soothing, beautiful place whenever you'd like to or need to is a valuable tool for coping with chronic pain. First, it can distract you during a flare-up. Second, it can be used with stress-reduction exercises to send you into a deep and delicious state of relaxation that

Rethinking the Meaning of Pain

It's easy to think of pain as never-ending when you have a chronic pain condition— even if it waxes and wanes or disappears entirely sometimes. This disheartening viewpoint can color your whole life. The fix? Guided imagery to help you rethink your relationship with pain. In one study published in the journal *Pain Management Nursing*, people who did guided imagery exercises for 4 days shifted their view of pain from unending to changeable. This switch may seem small, but it brings hope and the expectation that you'll get breaks from the hurt, and that can lift you up when pain tries to get you down.[6]

could cut your risk for new episodes of hurt. By reducing tension, fear, and worry, guided imagery can help dial down the intensity of pain.

Useful for any type of chronic pain, it may be especially helpful for inflammatory bowel disease and irritable bowel syndrome, cancer pain, chronic fatigue syndrome, arthritis, fibromyalgia, and nerve and burn pain.

The evidence: Guided imagery made everyday life easier for women with painful osteoarthritis in one Purdue University School of Nursing study.[7] In a related study, listening to a 10- to 15-minute tape with a guided imagery and progressive muscle relaxation exercise twice a day for 12 weeks helped women with arthritis reduce pain significantly.[8] And in a study from the University of Wisconsin, severe cancer pain improved for 62 percent of study volunteers who listened to a guided imagery exercise. Pain levels stayed lower for an hour.[9]

Guided imagery is often incorporated into hypnotherapy so that suggestions for reducing stress, for paying less attention to pain, even for a healthier body are delivered in imaginative ways. For example, gut-focused hypnotherapy used to control inflammatory bowel disease and irritable bowel syndrome might ask you to imagine your digestive tract as an orderly garden with wide paths.

How to fit guided imagery into your relief at last plan: Guided imagery works best along with other stress-reduction techniques such as progressive muscle relaxation or breathing exercises. Using imagery to put yourself into a state of bliss gives you a break from day-to-day concerns (like paying the bills and cooking dinner); that will cut stress all by itself. But pulling yourself away from daily distractions also frees you up to focus more fully on relaxing, which is a real bonus if you tend to have trouble letting go of tension. As we noted earlier, guided imagery is also a great tool for healthy distraction when pain strikes or when you face a painful or worrisome medical procedure.

What you should know: You can take guided imagery classes, listen to recorded exercises, or get one-on-one attention in sessions with a trained guided imagery leader to learn and practice this technique. Using it once or twice a day for a few weeks is more helpful than practicing once in a while. Best times? Some experts say first thing in the morning and last thing at night before bed.

Hypnotherapy

Inside Las Vegas's glitzy nightclubs, hypnotism is a crazy spectacle. Hypnotists seem to send volunteers into deep trances, make them melt to the floor in sudden deep sleep, then command them to do crazy stuff they'd never do in real life. But in medical hypnotherapy—the type of hypnosis proven to ease chronic pain dramatically—you'll never be asked to quack like a duck or pretend a chair is your favorite pet.

Instead, you'll tap into your mind's amazing ability to change the way you experience pain—so that you hurt less and can do more with your life every day. It feels effortless, but the results can be huge. Pain becomes less intense, less frequent, and more short-lived. Some people lower their doses of pain relievers.[10] Stress and depression ebb. Days become more productive and satisfying. Nights are, at last, a time for deep, uninterrupted sleep, which we know makes pain easier to deal with! No wonder the National Institutes of Health recommends hypnotherapy for chronic pain.[11]

Proven to help with a wide range of conditions—including arthritis, cancer, digestive pain like irritable bowel syndrome, fibromyalgia, jaw pain, and low back pain—it helps 70 percent of people ease pain immediately and helps 20 to 30 percent get long-lasting reductions.[12] In studies, it has also helped make painful procedures such as bone marrow aspiration and chemotherapy easier to get through.[13] An impressive track record for a healing modality sometimes seen as a party trick!

How it helps: In a hypnotherapy session, you'll be put into a deeply relaxed yet alert state. Your unconscious mind will be receptive to suggestions from your hypnotherapist for easing pain and improving the medical condition causing it. She may also make suggestions for continuing the benefits once the session is over.

Hypnotherapy seems to retrain your brain so that it pays less attention to pain, by temporarily rewiring it so that it's open to suggestion. In the past decade, researchers have begun using brain scans to unravel just how it works. Areas of the brain involved with daydreaming and letting your mind wander become less active because you're extremely focused. An area called the precuneus that processes mental images revs up, presumably because you're receiving hypnotic suggestions. And regions involved with perceiving pain, such as the somatosensory cortex and anterior cingulate cortex, become less active.[14]

The evidence: A single, 20-minute hypnotherapy session eased pain in a study of 45 people with fibromyalgia. The best results came for those whose sessions included a suggestion that they imagine a blue stream of pain relief flowing into painful areas of their bodies.[15] Powerful imagery really helps: In a study of women undergoing breast biopsies or lumpectomies, those who had a 15-minute hypnosis session before surgery needed less pain medication. They also spent less time in the operating room than women who didn't receive hypnosis. Sessions included peaceful visual imagery, relaxation, and suggestions to decrease pain.[16]

Hypnotherapy also seems to have the power to help our bodies function better. In one study of 81 people with irritable bowel syndrome, those who got five half-hour sessions of gut-directed hypnotherapy tailored to each person's symptoms saw pain decrease more than those who got usual medical care.[17] Pain not only lessened after people with the jaw pain of temporomandibular disorder listened daily to taped self-hypnosis exercises, but the benefits lasted for at least 6 months afterwards.[18]

Fitting hypnotherapy into your relief at last plan: Hypnosis can't cure medical conditions. But it's worth adding to your tool kit of strategies if drugs alone aren't keeping your pain in check, if you'd like to explore ways to reduce your dose, or if you're looking for ways to ease stress and anxiety. It can help you follow an exercise or physical therapy program without letting pain get in the way and simply make everyday life more productive and satisfying despite chronic pain. In other words, it can give you back your life.

In fact, if you're using other mind-body therapies (like guided imagery, relaxation techniques, or cognitive therapy) to help you relax and cope with pain, you may be getting the advantages of hypnotherapy without even knowing it. All these techniques may draw on the power of suggestion to help your mind ease your pain. In one study, cognitive-behavioral therapy was more effective when combined with hypnotherapy for 70 percent of volunteers.[19]

What you should know: Treatment may take several sessions; many insurance companies will cover 50 to 80 percent of the cost if you see a qualified practitioner.

Plan on practicing at home, too. Self-hypnosis CDs or materials from your hypnotherapist can help. University of Washington researchers say doing a little every day will help you get the most pain-relief benefits.

Meditation

You don't have to join a mountaintop monastery, twist your body into pretzel shapes, or sit on a rock-hard cushion for hours on end to get a pain-relief boost from meditation. While researchers and pain specialists have known for years that settling into a refreshing, still place within yourself can ease aches, in mid-2010 a new study made it clear that the benefits are for everybody, not just longtime meditators.

The proof? In a study from the University of North Carolina at Charlotte published in the journal *Consciousness and Cognition*, people who meditated for just 20 minutes a day saw their pain tolerance rise in 4 days.[21] Volunteers learned a technique called *mindfulness meditation* that taught them to focus on their breath and stay in the present moment. Researchers tested their pain thresholds with mild electric shocks and found that the shocks that the volunteers considered "high pain" before learning to meditate were ranked as mild pain afterward.

That's great news. Meditation is proven to help a wide range of chronic pain types including back pain,[22] cancer pain,[23] and pain from arthritis,[24] tension headaches,[25] and inflammatory bowel disease.[26] In one survey of people with chronic pain, 85 percent who had tried meditation said it was helpful.[27]

How it helps: Meditation seems to help by reining in the stress hormones that fool your brain into interpreting small pain signals as big ones. In a study from England's University of Manchester, meditation also eased pain by helping volunteers' brains stop anticipating it.[28] Relaxing and letting yourself be in the moment also helps you feel more in control; pain no longer controls you. Less stress can also mean better sleep,[29] more motivation to exercise, and even less depression—all of which also take the edge off pain.

This quiet healing art also boosts alpha and gamma brain waves, which

Best Meditation for Chronic Pain

There are many types of meditation, but two of the most widely practiced are mindfulness meditation and transcendental meditation. Which is right for you? Some pain experts vote for mindfulness for two important reasons: It's proven to help ease pain and may be easier for people with chronic pain to practice.

Transcendental meditation is all about focusing your attention and senses on one thing—a word, image, or object—in order to rise above everyday thought. It's like using the zoom lens on your camera to concentrate on one small point. In contrast, mindfulness meditation is like a wide-angle lens, meditation researchers say. Your goal is to remain aware of your thoughts, feelings, and physical sensations without judging them. By simply observing your thoughts and feelings you can begin to separate the physical sensation of pain from your emotional and intellectual reactions to it. Instead of magnifying it, you diminish it. This gentle, accepting form of meditation requires patience rather than lots of intense concentration.[30]

Staying in the present moment may be the last thing you'd like to do when pain flares up. But having the courage to try it can actually ease pain, melt stress, and boost your mood—a pretty good payback for sitting quietly for a few minutes a day!

5 Minutes of Mindfulness

Ready to try mindfulness meditation? Follow these instructions to get started.

Close your eyes; it will help you stay focused. Breathe in and out, slowly and naturally (no need to hyperventilate!), paying attention to how each inhalation and exhalation feels. Observe the thoughts, feelings, and physical sensations in your body, but don't judge them or get wrapped up in them. Keep gently returning your focus to your breath. After a few minutes, begin to notice your surroundings as you breathe calmly, then plan to go about your day with this feeling of calm awareness.[31]

increase feelings of well-being and help regulate the nervous system. And it lifts anxiety and depression,[32] states of mind that create brain changes that make pain feel worse.

The evidence: In one Drexel University College of Medicine study of 133 people with a variety of pain conditions, those who meditated at home saw pain improve. People with arthritis got the biggest benefits, followed by those with fibromyalgia and migraines.[33] Meanwhile, three studies of meditation specifically for fibromyalgia showed that it relieved pain significantly.[34] In other research, meditation has been shown to thicken the anterior cingulate, an area of the brain that regulates pain and emotion. As a result, 17 regular meditators were less sensitive to pain than 18 nonmeditators, report researchers from the University of Montreal in Canada.[35]

In another study, 37 people with lower back pain who practiced a guided meditation for 90 minutes a week for 8 weeks felt better, and most kept practicing meditation on their own. The benefits are lasting. When University of Massachusetts researchers got back in touch with 225 people with chronic pain who had practiced mindfulness meditation for 8 weeks, 60 percent said meditation was still responsible for a "moderate to great improvement" in their pain 4 years later.[36] Eight out of ten were still meditating. Brain scans showed another benefit: more activity in areas of the brain associated with optimism.[37]

Fitting meditation into your relief at last plan: Anyone who has stress in their lives, and that certainly includes everyone coping with stubborn pain, could benefit from learning how to meditate. It may not replace medicine or medical therapies, but it is an add-on therapy that, like other mind-body techniques, can help you continue to live the full life you want to have and not find yourself defined and limited by chronic pain.

What you should know: The deep relaxation that comes with meditation can start relieving pain quickly. The more you meditate, the better the benefits. Once you begin practicing this soothing technique, you may also discover something that people in one study realized: They could perform "minimeditations" anytime, in any place, which is great for staying stress free when you're caught in a traffic jam, stuck in a long line at the supermarket, feel the start of a pain flare-up, or need to take the edge off the day's accumulation of little annoyances. All it takes is stopping to follow your breath, in and out, for a moment or two.

Even when mindfulness meditation doesn't ease pain, it can lift the emotional distress brought on by a painful condition. That's exactly what happened for 63 people with rheumatoid arthritis in a 4-month study. Those who practiced mindfulness meditation regularly saw distress fall 35 percent, a sign they felt more peaceful and in control of their lives.[38]

Progressive Muscle Relaxation

Tensing your muscles is a natural response to chronic pain. Sometimes, such as when muscles spasm in your back, the tightness is your body's attempt to immobilize and protect an area that seems injured. Other times, tightening up

»More Research Needed

Aromatherapy

A lavender-scented bath can help you relax. Sniffing mint or orange might boost your energy. But can aromatherapy ease chronic pain? Early evidence suggests the right scent might help. In one New York University Medical Center study, weight-loss surgery patients who sniffed lavender needed smaller doses of painkillers during recovery;[39] in another study, some people with migraines who sniffed a green apple fragrance had shorter, less painful headaches. (But most of the study volunteers didn't like the scent!)[40] We think of aromatherapy as a pleasant "extra," but not as a first-choice therapy for chronic pain. If you like a scent, use it to help you wind down or recharge, but don't use scents in place of proven pain-relieving therapies.

High-Tech Relaxation: Biofeedback

Plenty of mind-body therapies can help you relax, but only one takes the guesswork out of the process: biofeedback. By training to take control of muscle tension, blood pressure, heart rate, or skin temperature—factors that are normally regulated automatically by your body—you can figure out which relaxation techniques really work for you and exactly how to do them to get the best results.

In a biofeedback session, electrodes attached to your skin send information about one or more of these body processes to a computer. The results appear on a computer monitor as an image, a line, or a sound. A therapist trained in biofeedback will lead you through exercises designed to help you relax while you track how well you're doing.

Experts aren't sure how it works, but it does. Studies show that biofeedback may help reduce tender points and muscle aches of fibromyalgia[41] and chronic tension headaches,[42] and may help with complex regional pain syndrome,[43] too. It can also relieve jaw pain and rheumatoid arthritis.

is an emotional reaction related to anger, frustration, fear, or stress. It hurts, so you draw inward, pulling taut muscles around you like a protective cocoon. Trouble is, all of that tension can make pain feel worse.

That's where progressive muscle relaxation comes in. Proven to help ease everything from arthritis and headaches to ulcerative colitis and cancer pain, the practice of slowly and methodically relaxing every muscle group in your body eases muscle tension and reduces mental stress. It's even recommended for pain relief by the National Institutes of Health.

How it helps: Relaxation techniques can work at a deep level to de-stress your mind and body. They soothe activity in the sympathetic nervous system, the part of your nervous system that makes you feel stressed when your "fight-or-flight" response kicks in in response to perceived danger. Your heart rate, blood pressure, and breathing slow down.[44] Reducing stress is proven to reduce the perception of pain.

Relaxing your muscles may also change the way nerves transmit pain signals. In one Ohio State University study, researchers tested the pain thresholds of 55 people before and after they did a progressive muscle relaxation exercise. The result? After relaxing, their pain thresholds were higher.[45]

The evidence: Cutting stress so that you feel calm and peaceful is a benefit that belongs in every pain prescription. When 28 women with osteoarthritis joint pain listened to guided imagery tapes that included progressive muscle

De-Stress Today: Progressive Muscle Relaxation Exercise

If you've got 10 minutes, you can teach your body and your mind to relax deeply. Doing this exercise once or twice a day relieves tension. It also increases your awareness, so that you'll be able to spot and reduce stress quicker. Learning how to relax your body on command is a wonderful skill you'll be able to use anytime, anywhere, even if you're in pain.

Practice in a quiet room as you sit in a comfortable chair with both feet flat on the floor. Relax your arms and put your hands in your lap. Or lie down on the floor or on your bed. Choose a time and place where you can be alone and undisturbed for 10 minutes.

You'll tense each group of muscles for about 5 seconds, relax for 10 seconds, then repeat. You may do one side of the body, then the other, or tense both sides (such as your left and right arms) at the same time. As you tense up your muscles, don't strain. If your muscles are already tight as a result of pain, stress, or disuse, it's okay to skip the tensing part of the exercise and focus instead on relaxing each muscle group. When you relax, let go of all the tension at once, so that you feel it flowing from your body. Stay relaxed for a full 10 seconds before tensing again. Enjoy this feeling! When you've finished, you can repeat the whole routine or focus in on areas of your body that are still holding stress.

Let's begin:

● **Feet:** Point or curl toes as you tighten foot muscles.
  Tense for 5 seconds, then release and relax for 10 seconds. Repeat.

● **Lower legs and feet:** Clench big muscles in your calves.
  Tense for 5 seconds, then release and relax for 10 seconds. Repeat.

● **Thighs:** Tighten muscles in your upper legs from knee to hips.
  Tense for 5 seconds, then release and relax for 10 seconds. Repeat.

relaxation twice a day for 12 weeks, they saw significant improvements in pain and mobility.[46] After surgery for colorectal cancer, people who learned how to do progressive muscle relaxation at home reported that they felt less stressed and that daily life was easier.[47] Other research shows that inflammatory bowel disease,[48] rheumatoid arthritis,[49] and lower back pain[50] respond, too.

● **Buttocks:** Squeeze together.
Tense for 5 seconds, then release and relax for 10 seconds. Repeat.

● **Back:** Squeeze shoulder blades together.
Tense for 5 seconds, then release and relax for 10 seconds. Repeat.

● **Abdomen:** Clench those tummy muscles.
Tense for 5 seconds, then release and relax for 10 seconds. Repeat.

● **Chest:** Tense muscles of upper chest.
Tense for 5 seconds, then release and relax for 10 seconds. Repeat.

● **Hands:** Clench fists.
Tense for 5 seconds, then release and relax for 10 seconds. Repeat.

● **Forearms:** Extend your arms with your elbows locked.
Tense for 5 seconds, then release and relax for 10 seconds. Repeat.

● **Upper arms:** Bend your arms at the elbows and flex your biceps.
Tense for 5 seconds, then release and relax for 10 seconds. Repeat.

● **Neck and shoulders:** Clench muscles tightly.
Tense for 5 seconds, then release and relax for 10 seconds. Repeat.

● **Jaw:** Open your mouth wide and stick out your tongue.
Tense for 5 seconds, then release and relax for 10 seconds. Repeat.

● **Mouth:** Press your lips together firmly.
Tense for 5 seconds, then release and relax for 10 seconds. Repeat.

● **Eyes:** Close tightly.
Tense for 5 seconds, then release and relax for 10 seconds. Repeat.

● **Forehead:** Wrinkle forehead and eyebrows.
Tense for 5 seconds, then release and relax for 10 seconds. Repeat.

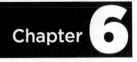

Chapter **6**

Using Pain Medications and Medical Treatments Wisely

N ot too long ago, choosing a pain reliever for chronic pain was fairly simple—even if it wasn't always as effective as you may have hoped. Maybe you started with aspirin, acetaminophen, or ibuprofen at home, then made an appointment to see your doctor if these over-the-counter pills didn't bring relief. Your doctor considered the cause and severity of your pain, perhaps asked about your budget or prescription drug plan, and soon you were leaving the pharmacy with a prescription painkiller as well as a potent muscle relaxer, a steroid, or other medications aimed at a specific type of chronic pain.

That was before a spate of serious health warnings about pain relievers turned trips to the pharmacy into a frustrating and confusing game of Risk.

The new dangers? In recent years, researchers have discovered that most OTC and prescription nonsteroidal anti-inflammatory drugs increase your odds of heart attacks and stroke. For many people, they also boost odds for silent yet deadly gastrointestinal bleeding and ulcers. Some NSAIDs even make arthritis worse! But that's not all. New research shows that acetaminophen, long considered one of the safest pain relievers in the drugstore, could damage or even shut down your liver if taken too often or in too large doses—leading the US Food and Drug Administration to issue new warnings and consider limiting pill strengths and recommended doses.

Widely used prescription narcotics—strong opioid painkillers like hydrocodone, Oxycontin, Vicodin, codeine, and morphine—are getting a bad rap, too. New warnings about addiction and new worries about prescription painkiller abuse and theft have scared many chronic pain patients and their doctors away from these potent and highly effective pain stoppers. And if you're taking opioids for headaches, migraines, back pain, or other types of noncancer pain, you should know that they could eventually erode your pain threshold to the point where the pain itself is worse. And for some conditions, like nerve pain and fibromyalgia, opioids don't even work well, it turns out.

Meanwhile, surveys show that many people with chronic pain aren't getting the targeted, nonpain drugs that relieve specific pain condition symptoms and even address the medical condition underlying their aches so there's simply less pain! These range from antidepressants (which have pain-relieving effects) and antiseizure drugs to migraine prevention drugs, special antibiotics, and high-tech "biologics."

If your pain plan includes older, well-established pain condition medications such as muscle relaxants or steroids (alone or in addition to pain relievers), you still may not be getting the relief you deserve if you and your doctor aren't reviewing your pain plan on a regular basis. For example, newer medications could help you reduce or eliminate the use of steroids if you have inflammatory bowel disease, but many people with IBD aren't getting these effective, low-side-effect replacements for steroids. If you rely on muscle relaxants for back, neck, or shoulder pain, you may not be taking advantage of nondrug therapies that could reduce your need for these often potent pills.

What if your condition is so severe that you're considering surgery or another invasive medical treatment? Should you hold back or rush ahead? Sometimes deciding in favor of a surgical procedure early on is wise; other times, it makes sense to consider the procedure's track record and to be sure you've exhausted all other options. We'll help you with a series of questions you can ask yourself and your doctor to help decide what's right for you.

Basic Steps to Smarter, Wiser Medication Use

Recently experts from the American Pain Society (APS) and the American Academy of Pain Medicine (AAPM) joined forces to work out guidelines that pain specialists and family doctors could use to help their chronic pain patients get the most from their medications with the fewest risks. Their advice? Before using strong, prescription painkillers, try other drugs and nondrug therapies (the type you'll find throughout *Relief at Last*) first.

Pain specialists recommend this process when it comes to using medications for chronic, noncancer pain.

- **If your pain flares up fewer than four times per week:** Start with OTC pain relievers or prescription nonsteroidal anti-inflammatory drugs, or NSAIDs (such as ibuprofen, Motrin, or Advil). Experts now recommend making acetaminophen (such as Tylenol) your very first choice; it doesn't raise risk for gastrointestinal bleeding, heart attacks, and strokes the way prescription and OTC NSAIDs can. If that isn't effective, use NSAIDs with care (read on for the smartest strategies) and don't rely on them alone. At the same time, go for physical therapy, exercise, and training in pain control techniques like distraction, guided imagery, meditation, and muscle relaxation. If the pain medications don't work and pain is severe, a short-acting opioid could help.

- **If pain is persistent and severe:** Use nonpain drugs that work best for your condition, such as antidepressants and antiseizure drugs for nerve pain, migraine-preventing and -stopping drugs, and aminosalicylates (ASAs), immunomodulators, and biologics for inflammatory bowel disease. Add pain-relieving creams such as capsaicin and other prescription pain-stopping creams. At the same time, start physical therapy or an exercise routine and add a wide range of mind-body, nondrug pain relief strategies like relaxation, meditation, and guided imagery. These may allow you to skip stronger pain drugs and get relief with an OTC medication. Consider a long-acting opioid drug if these steps don't bring enough relief for you to get back to your normal life.

- **If you have cancer pain:** Talk with your doctor about taking a long-acting opioid to control pain and adding shorter-acting drugs for break-through pain.

You'll find details about nondrug strategies in the rest of this book. Here's what you need to know about the safe and wise use of the four levels of pain medications recommended by experts: acetaminophen, NSAIDs (OTC and prescription types), nonpain medications used to treat specific chronic pain conditions, and opioids.

Basic Pain Relief Begins with Acetaminophen

At recommended doses, acetaminophen (Anacin Aspirin Free Extra Strength Tablets, Genapap, Genebs, Goody's tablets and powders, Tylenol, and other brands) has the best safety profile for people who need ongoing pain relief. Why? It won't increase your risk for gastrointestinal bleeding, ulcers, heart disease, or strokes the way aspirin and other NSAIDs like ibuprofen and the prescription drug Celebrex (celecoxib) can. According to the Arthritis Foundation, most people can safely take 325 to 1,000 milligrams every 4 to 6 hours—up to 4,000 milligrams per day—without raising the risk for liver problems. (The FDA recommends limiting yourself to 650-milligram doses every 4 to 6 hours up to four times per day.)

You've probably heard that acetaminophen, long considered the safest and gentlest pain-easer, can cause big trouble. Overdoing this popular OTC pain reliever can overwhelm your liver, leading to damage and even fatal liver failure. The risk is highest for people who take large doses or who also overindulge in alcohol, but experts say that liver problems can begin if you take just a little extra or mistime doses so they're too close together. Acetaminophen poisoning sends 56,000 people to American emergency rooms each year and leads to more than 100 unintentional deaths annually. As a result, the US Food and Drug Administration was, at press time for this book, considering a reduction in the recommended maximum single and daily doses of acetaminophen.

You should know that acetaminophen won't help with inflammation or swelling, an issue if you've got arthritis or joint or muscle pain. It's crucial to limit or stop drinking alcohol while using acetaminophen; having more than three drinks a day increases odds for liver damage even at safe drug doses.

A Safer Strategy for NSAIDs

Americans take 30 billion NSAID tablets and capsules a year for everything from minor aches to long-term relief of back, knee, and hip pain. This group of drugs includes the OTC NSAIDs aspirin, ibuprofen (Advil, Motrin, Nuprin), and naproxen (Aleve, Anaprox, Naprosyn), as well as the prescription COX-2 inhibitor celecoxib (Celebrex) and the prescription NSAIDs diclofenac (Cataflam, Voltaren), ketoprofen (Actron, Orudis KT), oxaprozin (Daypro), and piroxicam (Feldene).

Once considered safer and more effective than plain aspirin, OTC and prescription NSAIDs got a careful second look in 2004 when research revealed that the prescription NSAIDs Vioxx and Bextra raised risk for fatal heart attacks. These drugs—COX-2 inhibitors once called "super aspirins"—were quickly pulled from the market. But new research shows that NSAIDs still available may also boost risk for heart attacks and strokes in people with heart disease and in people with healthy cardiovascular systems. In the summer of 2010, a landmark Danish study of over one million people revealed that taking ibuprofen or prescription NSAIDs increased odds for a stroke by 29 percent and for a heart attack by as much as 91 percent.[1]

Warnings about NSAIDs don't stop there. These pain relievers switch off enzymes that protect the lining of your stomach, raising the risk for ulcers and life-threatening bleeding in some people. Experts estimate that NSAID-related bleeding sends up to 100,000 people to hospitals each year, killing 16,500.[2] It's important to understand that not everyone is at risk for this side effect. You may be if you take higher than recommended doses or if you're over age 65, have a history of stomach ulcers, or if you also take steroids, low-dose aspirin (for heart attack prevention), or blood thinners. The scary part? Eight out of ten people who've developed serious gastrointestinal bleeding have no warning signals, which means using NSAIDs as safely as possible is important.[3]

Follow these smart steps to get the best pain-stopping results with the fewest risks.

If you have (or have had) a stomach ulcer or gastrointestinal bleeding or are at high risk, skip NSAIDs or ask about stomach protection. Try acetaminophen, or talk with your doctor about other options such as nonpain drugs for your specific chronic pain type, as well as nondrug strategies. If you're at risk for GI problems but need the kind of pain relief you can get from an NSAID, your doctor may recommend that you protect your stomach by also taking an acid-blocking proton pump inhibitor (Prilosec, Prevacid, Aciphex, Protonix, and Nexium)[4] or a stomach-guarding prescription drug called misoprostol.

If you have heart disease or are at high risk for it, talk with your doctor before taking NSAIDs long term. You may be better off with acetaminophen.

If you only use NSAIDs once in a while, stick with the lowest dose of naproxen for the shortest period of time. Follow the label directions carefully. Studies show that for people with and without heart disease, OTC naproxen (Aleve, Naprosyn) doesn't raise heart disease, heart attack, and stroke risk the way aspirin, ibuprofen, diclofenac, and celecoxib do.[5, 6]

According to the American College of Gastroenterology, it's safe to take one to three naproxen pills a day—up to 660 milligrams a day if you're under 65. Limit yourself to two a day—up to 440 milligrams—if you're 65 or older.[7] Take it for the shortest amount of time possible and skip alcohol while using it. Beer, wine, and spirits raise the risk for GI bleeding if you're using it or any other NSAID.

Diclofenac: Skip the Pill, Get the Gel for Joint Pain

In pill form, the prescription NSAID diclofenac (Cataflam, Voltaren-XR) raised heart and stroke risk the highest in studies, and it may make arthritis worse. In a Dutch study of 1,695 people with arthritis of the knees and hips, those who used this drug for more than 6 months saw arthritis-related damage to their joints increase significantly. Those who took naproxen saw no damage and those who took ibuprofen saw minimal changes.[8]

A pain-relieving prescription gel containing diclofenac (Voltaren Gel) may be a good alternative to pain pills if you have pain in just a few joints that are close to the surface of the skin, such as knees, hands, elbows, and ankles. It cut knee and hand pain by at least 40 percent in two studies of people with arthritis.[9] Researchers say very little of the active ingredient is absorbed into the bloodstream, a plus if you can't use an NSAID. However, it's not a good option if you plan to continue using NSAIDs because it could increase your risk for NSAID side effects. The gel may not be a good choice if you have widespread pain because spreading it over large areas may be impractical and messy.

If you need something stronger, ask your doctor about a prescription for Celebrex, which was also safer than other NSAIDs in recent studies.

Talk with your doctor if you use NSAIDs several times a month or more often. You may need the kind of pain relief an NSAID can provide if you have osteoarthritis or joint pain that's not eased by exercise and acetaminophen, if you need pain relief for rheumatoid arthritis, or if you have nonsevere chronic pain—like regular backaches—and you don't want to use an opioid or a strong muscle relaxer.

Invest in a healthy lifestyle: Gentle exercise and weight loss may reduce or even eliminate your need for pain relievers if you have joint or back pain. For example, dropping 15 pounds can cut knee pain in half. Exercise builds muscles that act as shock absorbers for knee joints and can protect knees from further damage, pain, and disability.

Condition-Specific Drugs for Chronic Pain

One of the biggest strides in chronic pain management in the past 15 years has been the rise of more medications that effectively treat the symptoms and root causes of specific pain conditions. Often, these drugs are more effective than acetaminophen, NSAIDs, or opioids at preventing pain and stopping flare-ups. Other times, your doctor may prescribe these drugs along with a pain reliever for better pain coverage.

Pain specialists say that if you experience pain more than a few times a week and/or if pain is moderate to severe, these medications should be your first-line treatment. Over-the-counter pain relievers and even prescription nonsteroidal anti-inflammatories may not be enough to control it and these drugs, in many cases, help relieve underlying conditions so they can stop a pain flare-up before it starts. If you have noncancer chronic pain, consider medications like these, tailored to your pain condition, before relying on stronger opioid-based pain-killers alone. (Although you may also use some of these for cancer pain, this severe type of pain is often treated with opioids at the same time.)

If you're not taking one of these medications or another condition-specific drug for your pain condition, it's worth asking your doctor why. You'll find more details about disease-specific drugs throughout this book. For now, here's an overview of some of the most widely used pain condition medications that may be options for you.

Antidepressants: Often prescribed for cancer pain, nerve pain, and fibromyalgia as well as for tension headaches, migraines, and low back pain, these drugs help even if you're not depressed. Antidepressants increase levels of available neurotransmitters in your brain such as serotonin and norepinephrine, which in turn reduces pain intensity. The catch? It may take several weeks for the pain-relieving effects to kick in.

Duloxetine (Cymbalta) is often prescribed for nerve pain resulting from diabetes. The tricyclic antidepressant amitriptyline (Elavil, Tryptizol, Laroxyl, Sarotex) is often the first choice for nerve pain after a bout of shingles, but drugs such as imipramine (Tofranil), desipramine (Norpramin, Pertofrane), venlafaxine (Effexor), bupropion (Wellbutrin), paroxetine (Paxil), and citalopram (Celexa) are also prescribed for nerve pain.

Antiseizure drugs: Prescribed for nerve and cancer pain, antiseizure drugs used to have a bad reputation for serious side effects like liver damage, double vision, and headaches. The good news? Newer types are just as effective with a lower risk for problems. Two out of three people who try antiseizure drugs for nerve pain can expect to get relief, researchers say.[10]

These drugs block nerve pain, possibly by muting signals from oversensitive nerve fibers so they can't transmit "ouch!" messages to your brain. Newer types now widely used include gabapentin (Neurontin) and pregabalin (Lyrica) (approved by the FDA for diabetic neuropathy). Doctors also sometimes recommend oxcarbazepine (Trileptal), tiagabine (Gabitril), and topiramate (Topamax). An older type called carbamazepine (Tegretol, Carbatrol) can trigger side effects including fatigue, nausea, vision problems, and dizziness, especially in people of Asian and South Asian ancestry.

Aminosalicylates (5-ASAs): These medications help about 80 percent of people with ulcerative colitis[11] and 55 percent of people with Crohn's disease stay symptom free.[12] Mesalamine (Asacol, Rowasa, and others), olsalazine sodium (Dipentum), sulfasalazine (Azulfidine), and others contain the active ingredient 5-aminosalicylic acid (5-ASA), which helps control inflammation in your gastrointestinal tract. Available as pills and as enemas, foams, and suppositories, 5-ASAs are considered first-line treatments for inflammatory bowel disease and may be used alone or with a steroid or antibiotic to better control inflammation, stop bacterial overgrowth, and prevent flare-ups.

Antibiotics: Bacteria-killing medications are being deployed more often these days for two gastrointestinal pain conditions, Crohn's disease and irritable bowel syndrome, but not to wipe out conventional infections. It turns out that the antibiotics metronidazole (Flagyl, Protostat) and ciprofloxacin (Cipro) can help reduce levels of inflammation-promoting bacteria that harm the lining of the intestines and cause pain and other symptoms in Crohn's disease. Research shows that these antibiotics can help about half the people who use them go into remission.[13]

Meanwhile, a special, nonabsorbable antibiotic called rifaximin (Xifaxan) is being used to knock back bacterial overgrowth that may be responsible for the pain and bloating of IBS. Benefits lasted long after treatment ended in one study.[14]

Biologics: A cutting-edge treatment for rheumatoid arthritis, other types of arthritis, and inflammatory bowel disease, biologics work by targeting specific immune system compounds, and so are considered safer than steroids, which suppress the entire immune system. Given by injection or intravenous infusion, these genetically-engineered drugs include adalimumab (Humira), certolizumab pegol (Cimzia), golimumab (Simponi), infliximab (Remicade), and natalizumab (Tysabri). They're developing a strong track record for helping with severe IBD that doesn't respond to other treatments.[15]

Corticosteroids: Steroids—including prednisone (Deltasone and Orasone), prednisolone (Prelone), and dexamethasone (Decadron)—ease inflammation faster and more effectively than any other drug, and so are used for everything from back pain to osteoarthritis, rheumatoid arthritis, joint pain, cancer pain, and inflammatory bowel disease. Available as pills, creams, sprays, inhalers, and injections, they work by mimicking cortisol, a hormone produced naturally by your adrenal glands. The downside? Because corticosteroids suppress your entire immune system, they can leave you more vulnerable to infection. Long-term use can lead to serious side effects including raised blood pressure, weight gain, mood swings, weakened bones, sleep problems, and even cataracts.

Disease-modifying antirheumatic drugs (DMARDs): These medications, including leflunomide (Arava), methotrexate (Rheumatrex), sulfasalazine (Azulfidine), and the biologics mentioned above, stop the underlying causes of inflammation in rheumatoid arthritis and other types of inflammatory arthritis such as ankylosing spondylitis. They are sometimes even prescribed for cancer pain and inflammatory bowel disease. Older DMARDs are sometimes combined with low-dose steroids for better results.

Immunomodulators: Potent immunosuppressants like azathioprine (Imuran), mercaptopurine (Purinethol), and methotrexate (Rheumatrex) can put severe Crohn's disease and ulcerative colitis into remission when aminosalicylates fail.

These medications work by reducing inflammation. They can also help people who've become dependent on steroids to control inflammatory bowel disease stop taking them or reduce doses without flare-ups. Like steroids, they can make you more vulnerable to infection but are still considered safer for long-term use.

Migraine-prevention drugs: If you get two or more moderate to severe migraines a month despite your best efforts to cut migraine triggers (like some foods, not enough sleep, stress) out of your life, it's worth asking your doctor about drugs that can prevent these headaches. These aren't a special type of drug; instead, seven medications normally used for other health issues—including the high blood pressure drugs verapamil (Calan, Verelan) and propranolol (Inderal), the antiseizure drugs divalproex sodium (Depakote) and topiramate (Topamax), and the tricyclic antidepressant amitriptyline (Elavil)—have been proven to reduce the odds for future migraines by 50 to 90 percent.[16, 17] The catch? Different drugs work for different people; you'll have to use trial and error to find the best one for you.

Muscle relaxants: Sedatives like cyclobenzaprine hydrochloride (Flexeril), diazepam (Valium), metaxalone (Skelaxin), and methocarbamol (Robaxin) can unkink tight muscle spasms fast, but can leave you drowsy, with a dry mouth, and even with trouble urinating. They can also cause dependence. In a recent review of 30 well-designed studies, researchers affiliated with the evidence-based medicine organization The Cochrane Collaboration found that muscle relaxants relieve low back pain 80 percent of the time within 2 to 4 days (often sooner), but risk for side effects is high. They're best for short-term use and should be taken only at night, never when you need to drive a car or operate machinery.

Pain patches: Infused with the numbing drug lidocaine (Lidoderm), pain-relief patches can reduce nerve pain from shingles or diabetes significantly in as little as 30 minutes. The catch? Pain relief extends only as far as the patch itself. Each one is slightly bigger than an index card and you can wear up to three at a time. Lidocaine seems to help by preventing the transmission of nerve signals from your skin to your spinal cord and brain. Another new pain patch, made with high-dose capsaicin—the red pepper ingredient found in OTC capsaicin creams—is showing promise for nerve pain.

Pain-relief creams: Prescription and OTC pain creams can help with joint pain, arthritis, back pain, sore muscles, and even nerve pain. Off-the-shelf creams include types that heat or cool your skin (like Biofreeze and IcyHot), those that use the aspirin-like ingredient salicylate to ease pain (like Bengay and Aspercreme), and those containing capsaicin (such as Capzasin-HP, Ther-all Capsaicin-HP, and drugstore brands). They diminish pain over several weeks by depleting a pain-transmitting chemical found in nerve endings in the skin. The prescription NSAID pain cream diclofenac (Voltaren), described above, may also help, but it shouldn't be used if you're taking NSAIDs by mouth; the combination could increase your risk for side effects.

Triptans: These medications can stop, or abort, a migraine quickly, especially if you take one as soon as you feel the telltale signs that a big headache is coming on. Triptans such as sumatriptan (Imitrex)[18], zolmitriptan (Zomig),[19] and sumatriptan plus naproxen (Treximet)[20] work better than OTC pain relievers to stop pain if you get severe, frequent, or disabling migraines. They're also available as nasal sprays and tablets that melt under your tongue, which are good for people whose migraine-related nausea makes swallowing pills impossible.[21, 22]

Opioids: Strong Pain Relief Minus the Fears

Wild and beautiful, red poppy flowers are the source of one of the strongest and most effective pain relievers in the world: opium and its refined, prescription drug form, morphine. These drugs latch onto pain-sensing receptors on nerve cells in your gastrointestinal tract and your spinal cord and on neurons in your brain, blocking pain signals. They're extremely effective. Today, people coping with severe chronic pain are more likely to use drugs such as fentanyl (Duragesic patch and other brands), oxycodone (Oxycontin), hydrocodone (Vicodin), and tramadol (Ultram and Ultracet), all of which contain active ingredients based on the chemistry of this highly addictive pain-erasing elixir.

Pain specialists say that these medications can ease the burden of stubborn and agonizing pain such as cancer pain, and as a result, eight million American adults now use opioids to control chronic pain. But these miracle drugs have downsides. Severe constipation is a nearly universal side effect. They can also cause physical dependence or even addiction, though perhaps less frequently than you've heard. Prized as street drugs and sometimes overused by people who don't really need them, opioids are now at the center of a huge controversy involving people living with legitimate chronic pain, their doctors, law enforcement officials, drug abusers, and politicians.

The problem? Politicians and police say opioids may be overprescribed, allowing more to fall into the wrong hands. Attempts to tighten rules for prescribing and dispensing these drugs have led some doctors to stop prescribing them. Unfounded fears about addiction have also frightened away people whose chronic pain isn't controlled with anything else. The result? Pain specialists say opioids are actually underprescribed and underused by those who need them, and that tens of thousands of people live unnecessarily with pain that could be eased if they and/or their doctors would take a chance with an opioid.

Choosing long-acting types (rather than those that wear off in just a few hours) and adding other drugs and other pain therapies can help you avoid developing a higher tolerance to your drug—meaning you'd need more to get the same pain relief. We'll be honest. Even if you develop a physical dependence on an opioid, your doctor will be able to help wean you off your drug when you need to. That's very different from an addiction, which involves drug cravings, compulsive use whether you need it or not, using a drug even if it's causing you physical or mental harm, and becoming so impaired by the drug itself that you can't control your use.

But the opioid story isn't simple or clear cut. With more people using them than ever before, overdoses are on the rise, and tripled between 1999 and 2006.[23] An estimated 14,000 people die annually in the United States as a result of unintentional opioid overdoses; another 100,000 suffer nonfatal overdoses. Despite these scary statistics, experts in the pro-opioid camp say that just 3 percent of people who take these drugs for pain abuse their prescriptions or develop dependence. The risk for addiction is very low if you take them as your doctor recommends and if you don't have a history of substance abuse. Keeping these drugs out of the hands of people who need them, they say, isn't the way to solve other troubles, such as illegal sale and use of stolen opioids.

There's plenty of evidence that opioids bring much–needed relief from stubborn back pain, burns, wounds, and cancer pain. But these drugs aren't perfect. They can become less effective when used long term. In addition to causing severe constipation, they can slash your body's production of sex hormones (making libido plummet), weaken immunity, and even increase pain sensitivity.

If your doctor suggests an opioid or if you're considering asking about these medications, these steps can help you make an informed choice about whether these painkillers are right for you.

Try other strategies first. Be sure to follow the steps outlined earlier in this chapter before adding an opioid. Acetaminophen and short-term naproxen may be all you need, especially if you follow a multifaceted pain control strategy that also includes exercise, physical therapy, stress reduction, and counseling, as well as strategies and medications tailored to your specific condition. Nonpain drugs such as antidepressants, muscle relaxers, steroids, and others could help you avoid opioids or keep your dose low. Be sure to ask about medications that target your specific pain type. Migraine-stopping drugs called triptans, for example, are more effective at stopping severe head pain. Researchers say nerve pain and fibromyalgia may also respond better to other medication strategies as outlined above. The result? Less pain without the risks posed by opioids.

If pain persists, have a frank talk with your doctor or consider seeing a new one. Many people who need strong pain relief can't get it, surveys show, because doctors are reluctant to prescribe opioids. The truth is, risk for addiction and abuse are extremely low. You may develop some physical dependence, which can be overcome simply by tapering off when you're ready to stop taking the drug.

Agree on pain relief goals and a maintenance strategy. Opioids won't completely erase your pain and on their own won't lift the emotional fallout of chronic pain, such as depression, worry, and frustration. But by lessening your pain, they can help you reach some practical and important goals, including starting a gentle exercise program, getting a better night's sleep, and being able to enjoy your family life and other relationships.

In one study of 100 people taking opioids, 51 percent got significant pain relief, another 28 percent got partial pain relief, and everyone reported that they could function better in their daily lives.[24]

Talk with your doctor about some reachable goals that matter to you and judge how well your opioid is working based on whether it helps you get there in a reasonable amount of time—several weeks or months. If not, you may need a different pain-relief strategy.

Talk to your doctor about how often you should check in about your dose, tolerance, and side effects.

Deal with side effects. Constipation, daytime sleepiness, itchy skin, and nausea are common complaints among people taking narcotic drugs. For constipation, drink plenty of water, eat a high-fiber diet, and follow your doctor's recommended action plan. It may involve taking an over-the-counter or prescription laxative. Sleepiness usually goes away in a few days. If it persists, call your doctor. It may be caused by another medication you're taking or a change in your medical condition. If nausea continues, medications may help.

Less is more. Taking opioids on a regular schedule helps prevent flare-ups; waiting until you're in pain often means taking bigger doses for longer periods of time and losing precious minutes or hours while you wait for relief. If your doctor recommends that you take your medications on an around-the-clock schedule to prevent breakthrough pain, understand that this strategy probably means you'll use less than if you waited for the pain. One example: Stalling on taking a dose of an opioid that takes 2 hours to work leaves you vulnerable to breakthrough pain you could have avoided. Or it could mean you'll have to use a fast-acting opioid (often used by people with severe breakthrough pain) that you could have avoided with continuous long-acting drugs.

If one type isn't effective, work with your doctor to find one that is. Often, different opioids work better for different people. Your doctor may also prescribe two at lower doses, or ask you to take an over-the-counter pain reliever, too, to increase effectiveness. Be sure to talk with your doctor, however, before adding an OTC pain drug on your own. Some opioids already include acetaminophen in the formula. Adding an extra dose increases your risk for liver damage.

Skip that cocktail. Alcohol can increase the effects of opioids and may even put you at risk for breathing problems.

Be responsible. Keep your medication in a safe place, don't share it with anyone else and stop using it when you and your doctor decide it's time to taper off. Also know that your pharmacy may ask you for identification or even require a waiting period before filling your prescription, a standard safety precaution that's no reflection on you.

Know the signs you've crossed the line. If you're using someone else's prescription drugs, buying them on the street, getting prescriptions from multiple doctors in order to have enough, lying or hiding your pills, or find yourself always thinking about when you can take your next dose or get your next refill, you may be developing a prescription drug abuse problem. Talk with your doctor about the best way to taper off and find alternatives to address your pain.

Medical Interventions for Pain

From back surgery to knee and hip replacement, from gallbladder stone removal to procedures that sever or mute overactive nerves, hundreds of medical procedures hold out the promise to quiet severe pain that doesn't respond to medications, exercise, and drug-free therapies. Throughout *Relief at Last*, you'll find the latest on procedures that work, and those that you should think twice about, for specific pain conditions.

We've done the homework so you get the most current information in this ever-changing and often controversial area of pain management. There are no hard-and-fast rules about whether to say yes, no, or something in between about surgeries and other medical interventions for pain. Sometimes it makes sense to opt early for surgery in order to stop a progressive pain condition. A good example is diverticulitis. It can eventually trigger infection and inflammation throughout your abdomen, leading some experts to recommend surgery for anyone under age 50 who's had just one or two attacks.

Other times it pays to wait. In the nation with the world's highest rates of surgery for low back pain, new research suggests that skipping the scalpel is sometimes the best route. In one study from Dartmouth Medical School, researchers compared the results of surgery and nonsurgical treatments for herniated disks with sciatica, nerve pain in the buttocks and leg. The result? Waiting was as good as surgery for herniated disks. Although the surgery group felt better in the first few months, the group that opted against surgery felt just as good within two years.

Either way, make sure you consider all your options for surgery. Case in point: surgery for spinal stenosis, a narrowing of parts of the spine, usually at the neck or lower back, that puts extra pressure on the spinal cord or the nerves that lead away from it. This painful problem is the most common reason for spine surgery in people over age 60. But another recent Dartmouth study found that the usual procedure—fusing the bones of the spine together to minimize motion and wear and tear on nerves—doesn't work as well for many people as a less invasive procedure called decompression surgery, which relieves pressure on nerves. Decompression surgery was better than nonsurgical treatment with pain pills, anti-inflammatory drugs, and exercise, too.

The bottom line? Think about what matters to you most: You want pain relief, but what is your risk tolerance? Is recovery time an issue for you? What are the odds that surgery will ease pain significantly? Then gather as much information as you can, talk the matter over with a relative or trusted friend (or two), and work with your doctor to make an informed decision you can feel good about.

Along the way, it may make sense for you to seek a second opinion, too. You need one if your doctor suggests surgery or wants to prescribe a long-term drug with serious side effects or if you have a medical condition that's simply not improving. Getting one can ease doubts and build your reassurance that you're doing the right thing. It can also reveal treatment options you hadn't heard about from your first doctor.

Want one? Turn to an experienced doctor affiliated with a different hospital or practice for a fresh point of view. Look to a major medical center or university hospital for more information on new procedures or if you have a rare or complex medical condition. Don't overlook online services like MyConsult (my.clevelandclinic.org) or similar programs offered by Johns Hopkins and the hospitals affiliated with Harvard Medical School. For a fee, you get access to the institution's top doctors, who review your medical records and provide detailed reports. You can also find online resources to help you gather and organize the information you need to make this important decision. You'll find details about these resources in Part Three.

Pain-Relief Prescriptions

In Part Two of *Relief at Last*, you'll discover proven ways to stop pain fast, prevent flare-ups, and treat medical conditions underlying pain.

This section includes detailed information on more than 60 conditions including arthritis and knee pain, lower back pain, digestive system pain, nerve pain, cancer pain, fibromyalgia, and chronic fatigue syndrome. Arranged by body system, the information here can help you better understand the type of pain you have, which is the first step to freedom from pain. Too often, people with chronic pain spend months or years trying to get a diagnosis that will open the door to effective treatment. In the pages that follow, you'll discover telltale symptoms and important tests that can help you and your doctor reach this starting point.

That's just the beginning. You'll also find the latest combinations of alternative and complementary therapies, prescription and over-the-counter drugs, and other treatments proven to stop your specific pain type quickly and effectively. You'll discover a world of proven strategies that address flare-ups and breakthrough pain, tackle the root causes of pain to help prevent its return, and help you get better relief without relying on bigger and bigger doses of pain pills. You'll find out how pain specialists use a wide variety of nonpain drugs to treat chronic pain effectively, learn which combinations of conventional and complementary therapies best ease your pain type, and discover the latest research-backed news about long-trusted therapies that don't work.

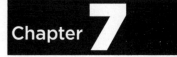
Head Pain

Migraines, tension headaches, sinus headaches

Stroll the pain-reliever aisle at the drugstore, watch TV for more than 15 minutes, or flip through a magazine, and you'll quickly see that fixing head pain is big business in America. Today, pain relievers come in a wider variety than ever before and make big promises to fix everything from garden-variety tension headaches to sinus headaches to the throbbing agony of a migraine. We spend billions of dollars on headache remedies every year, yet all too often, headaches still happen.

Now that could change. A rising tide of research shows that by targeting the real causes of head pain, most migraines and tension headaches can be avoided and the rest can hurt less and end sooner. Researchers have learned some surprising things about head pain in the past decade that have revolutionized relief.

- Migraine pain is much more than throbbing blood vessels in your temples. That's old thinking. Now headache specialists know it all begins deep in your brain when something—from food to stress to last night's second glass of wine—sets off a cascade of events involving nerves, brain chemicals, and even waves of electrical activity. The good news is that a sensible, nondrug strategy of finding and eliminating triggers can cut brain pain significantly.

- Sinus headaches, the subject of countless TV commercials and dozens of special pain pills, are actually quite rare. Most are really misdiagnosed migraine headaches. Knowing the difference can get you relief at last.

- Tension headaches and migraines are often caused by the pain relievers you're popping to stop them. Experts say medication overuse headaches are extremely common—meaning your first step toward relief may be to quit your painkillers.

- Relief isn't all about drugs anymore. Acupuncture, yoga, progressive muscle relaxation, and even a regular sleep schedule have proven themselves to be effective, drug-free ways to sidestep head pain.

Read on for research-proven strategies that can halt head pain at last.

When to Call the Doctor

Get medical help immediately if you or a loved one has any of these headache symptoms, no matter what type of headache you're prone to.

- Sudden, severe head pain unlike anything you've felt before
- Head pain with loss of consciousness, dizziness, weakness, balance problems, numbness, vision changes, trouble speaking, or mental confusion
- A headache with a fever, shortness of breath, stiff neck, or rash
- Head pain that wakes you up at night
- A headache after a head injury or accident
- A headache that's worse when you're lying down
- A headache that's not helped by treatments that have worked in the past
- Headaches when you're pregnant or think you might be pregnant (some head pain drugs shouldn't be used by pregnant women, and your doctor can suggest alternatives)

Migraines

If you're among the 29.5 million women and men who've experienced the knife-sharp agony of a migraine, you probably know deep down and firsthand that there's something different about the migraine-prone brain.

Science is now catching up with your hunch. The old view of migraine pain focused on swollen, throbbing blood vessels in your temples, head, and face. These do cause pain, but fixing a migraine means going deeper, into the brain itself.

The new thinking: Big headaches happen because, for some people, a brain region called the somatosensory cortex is exquisitely sensitive, 24/7. This area processes nerve signals for pain, temperature, touch, and other stimuli. If yours is on a hair trigger, even a tiny irritant like too much coffee or a change in the weather could kick off a migraine by setting off cascades of electrical activity, altering levels of brain chemicals like serotonin, and creating feedback loops in nerves that carry pain signals. From this storm inside your cranium come all the classic symptoms of a migraine: strange flashing lights and other visual disturbances; sensitivity to light, sounds, and the slightest touch (even combing your hair can be too painful); nausea and vomiting; deep fatigue; a wrung-out, hungover feeling when it's all done; and, of course, all that pain.

This new view isn't just gee-whiz science trivia. Understanding the roots of severe head pain can mean fewer and less painful migraines and faster relief when you do get one. You cannot "cure" the cause of migraines, but there's plenty you can do—often without drugs—to raise your tolerance level for your pain triggers. Strategies range from getting off pain pills that make your brain more vulnerable to boosting your pain threshold with regular sleep, meals, and exercise. But there's more, so read on!

Is It a Migraine?

Half of all people who get migraines think their head pain is something else—such as a sinus headache or a regular tension headache—or simply try to cope when pain arrives rather than getting a diagnosis and taking steps to turn down migraine-related brain sensitivity.

You most likely have migraines if you have had any of these symptoms along with your headaches in the last 3 months.

- Nausea or feeling sick to your stomach

- Extra sensitivity to light

Talk Therapy

Feel like migraines are making your life spin out of control? Someday your doctor may write you a prescription for counseling along with pain prevention or pain-stopping medications for migraine relief. No, we're not suggesting this pain is "all in your head." It's real. But in a recent study, people who got help developing migraine-coping strategies—everything from steps that prevent pain to the best strategies for relieving it—felt more confident about controlling their head pain than those who only received prescription drugs.[2]

● Pain that kept you from working, studying, or going about your activities for a day or longer

If you've had two of these, there's a 93 percent chance you're having migraines. If you have all three, the odds are 98 percent![1] Other symptoms that may signal a migraine include sensitivity to sound or odors and moderate to severe throbbing on one side of the head that gets worse when you move or bend over. In addition, if you've had at least five attacks that last from 4 hours to 3 days (if untreated), see your doctor as soon as you can.

To get a diagnosis, be ready to tell your doctor all about your symptoms—how often and how severe the pain is, how long it lasts, and whether you have other classic migraine symptoms such as visual disturbances (such as seeing wavy lines) before an attack or being ultrasensitive to lights, smells, and touch during one. Describe the steps you take to treat or prevent pain, including how often you use pain relievers. Your doctor may offer you migraine-aborting medications or suggest you try healthy lifestyle changes first to reduce triggers. Or he may refer you to a headache specialist. Either way, expect a migraine relief and prevention plan, including advice on when to check back in so you both can evaluate whether it's working.

Fast Pain Relief

Feel a migraine coming on? Take these steps as soon as you notice warning signs of an impending migraine, such as flashes of light, tunnel vision, or other visual disturbances called auras; sensitivity to noise, odors, or lights; a prickling or burning sensation on your skin; food cravings; thirst; unusual fatigue; or mood changes.

1. **If your migraines tend to be mild to moderate, take an over-the-counter pain reliever or migraine formula.** Acetaminophen, ibuprofen, naproxen, and aspirin have all been shown to stop migraine pain, as have OTC

migraine formulas that combine acetaminophen, caffeine, and aspirin, such as Excedrin Migraine formula.

Caution: Taking pain relievers more than once or twice a week or more than 10 times per month can trigger medication overuse headaches, a major cause of chronic migraines. See page 88 for details.

2. **For moderate to severe migraines, ask your doctor about a higher dose of aspirin plus the prescription antinausea drug metoclo-pramide (Reglan).** In a 2010 review of 13 studies involving 4,222 people who get migraines, researchers found that 1 in 4 got complete relief within 2 hours if they took 900 to 1,000 milligrams of aspirin (three regular strength 325-milligram tablets) and 10 milligrams of metoclopramide.[3] Another 28 percent got significant relief but still had some pain.

3. **If you know that your migraines don't respond to OTC pain relievers, take a migraine-stopping prescription drug called triptan pronto.** These drugs, such as sumatriptan (Imitrex),[4] zolmatriptan (Zomig),[5] and sumatriptan and naproxen (Treximet)[6], are usually a better choice than an OTC pain reliever if you have severe, frequent, or disabling migraines. If you're too nauseous to swallow a pill, use a triptan nasal spray or tablets that melt in your mouth.[7, 8] *Caution:* Taking a triptan more than 15 days per month can trigger medication overuse headaches. Skip these drugs if you have had or are at risk for heart attack or stroke. Be careful with them if you're taking antidepressants called selective serotonin reuptake inhibitors (SSRIs) such as citalopram (Celexa), escitalopram (Lexapro), fluoxetine (Prozac), paroxetine (Paxil, Paxil CR, Pexeva), or sertraline (Zoloft), or if you take a serotonin and norepinephrine reuptake inhibitor (SNRI) like venlafaxine (Effexor) or the antidepressant and smoking cessation medication bupropion (Wellbutrin, Zyban). The combination can cause serotonin syndrome—an overload of serotonin that can make you feel restless, confused, uncoordinated, and headachy, or even cause a high fever, seizures, and heart palpitations.

4. **Retreat to a dark, quiet room and cool off your head.** Lie down in a dark room with a cool, damp washcloth over your eyes. Or use a "cool cap"—a hoodlike hat containing a gel that can be chilled ahead of time in your freezer. These help by cooling all sides of your head, including your forehead and your upper neck, at the same time.[9] No more

balancing several ice packs at once! Some even have eye covers. In one small study published in the journal *Evidence-Based Complementary and Alternative Medicine*, migraine pain was reduced by about a third within 25 minutes for people who used a gel cap.

There's a reason plenty of people retreat to a dark place when a migraine begins. New research from Beth Israel Deaconess Medical Center in Boston has found that even dim light quickly activates migraine-related neurons deep in the brain and can fuel migraine pain.[10]

Relief at Last

Cutting-edge migraine treatment is aimed at preventing headaches, not waiting to treat the pain when it shows up. There's plenty you can do protect the migraine center in your brain so that it's less likely to respond to everyday headache triggers. Below are a number of migraine control approaches.

Follow them in this order for best results.

Step 1: Stop medication overuse headaches. Half of all chronic migraines may be triggered by overuse of pain drugs.[11] If you're taking too many pain relievers (read on for details), this absolutely must be your first step toward freedom from head pain. Other strategies won't be very effective if you're caught in a cycle of pain/pills/more pain.

Step 2: Identify your personal migraine triggers. Figuring out what sets off your migraines customizes your pain prevention plan for best results.

Step 3: Raise your pain threshold with exercise, relaxation, and healthy eating habits. These steps keep your brain's migraine center from becoming more vulnerable to the headache triggers you encounter in

Botox for Frequent Migraines

Long recommended to prevent headache pain, injections of the wrinkle-smoother Botox (onabotulinumtoxinA) won US Food and Drug Administration approval for the prevention of frequent migraines in late 2010. The regimen could help people who get migraines more than 14 days out of the month, but isn't approved for less-frequent migraines or for other types of headaches. The shots are given about every 3 months, in several spots around the head and neck, to dull future pain. Most common side effects? Neck pain and . . . headaches.

everyday life. (Turn to the Mind/Body Therapies section of "Tension Headaches" further on in this chapter for relaxation techniques that can help your head, too.)

Step 4: Still getting headaches? Look to supplements, acupuncture, and pain-preventing prescription medications. For many people, the first three steps in this strategy work to stop or control head pain. If yours persists, these additional approaches can make your days pain free.

Pain Prevention Strategies

Food and Supplements

BUTTERBUR SUPPLEMENTS: Also known by its Latin name, *Petasites hybridus,* butterbur is a shrub that grows along riverbanks in Germany. Specially formulated supplements made from the roots of this plant have been used in Europe to prevent migraines since the early 1990s.

The evidence: Several studies have found benefits.[12] In one, of 245 people with migraines, 68 percent who took 75 milligrams of a butterbur product twice a day saw the number of migraines they experienced drop by at least 50 percent, report researchers from Albert Einstein College of Medicine in New York.[13]

How it works: Compounds from butterbur root seem to reduce inflammation; this botanical may cut migraine risk by discouraging blood vessel swelling.

What you need to know: Butterbur roots also contain liver-damaging compounds called pyrrolizidine alkaloids (PAs for short). If you try this herb, it's important to use only PA-free products, such as Petadolex.[14] Follow label directions.

Exercise and Movement Therapies

GENTLE EXERCISE: For many people, migraines make exercise difficult, thanks to fears that bursts of activity will switch on head pain. The good news? Gentle activity can help you stay in shape even if you're migraine prone and help keep pain in check.

The evidence: In one large Swedish study, nonexercisers were 14 percent more likely to have head pain than those who got regular physical activity.[15] In another by the same team of researchers, 26 migraine sufferers who rode exercise bikes three times a week for 12 weeks reported that their headaches became less frequent and less intense.[16] In an Austrian study of 30 women with migraines, pain was milder after a 6-week program of twice-weekly aerobics and muscle relaxation.[17]

How it works: Exercise helps buffer you against migraines in several ways: reducing stress, improving sleep, and boosting levels of endorphins, your feel-good brain chemicals.

What you need to know: Your goal? Eat meals on time, set a regular time for going to sleep and getting up in the morning, and aim for a half-hour of activity most days of the week. If you're worried that exercise will set off a migraine, follow these steps: Drink water before, during, and after your workout; warm up gradually; exercise in a cool environment; and avoid exercises that make your head bob up and down, such as running on a treadmill or doing step aerobics. If you're prone to exercise-induced head pain, try taking ibuprofen or naproxen 30 to 60 minutes before you work out.

YOGA: Relaxing mind and body with a slow, easy yoga routine can also help raise your threshold for migraine pain. While few studies have looked at whether and how well it works, there's some evidence that it does.

The evidence: In one study from India's University of Rajasthan, migraine sufferers who performed easy yoga postures along with breathing exercises had significantly fewer and less painful migraines.[18]

How it works: Gentle yoga poses and breathing exercises that focus on relaxation may help ease stress and muscle tension that can trigger a migraine or ratchet up the pain.

What you need to know: For some people, physical activity itself can trigger a migraine. If you try yoga, stick with gentle poses. Look for books, CDs, and classes described as "gentle," "mild," or "restorative." See Part Three for suggestions and for a simple yoga routine you can start with.

Touch Therapies

ACUPUNCTURE: A growing stack of research shows that this ancient healing art is good medicine for people with migraines. It prevents some migraines completely, reduces the pain and length of headaches you do get, and even short-circuits new headaches if you can get to a practitioner as soon as a migraine begins. If healthy lifestyle changes and relaxation aren't enough to bring your pain under control, this type of touch therapy may be a good next step for you.

The evidence: In a study of 401 headache sufferers (most of whom had migraines) from Memorial Sloan-Kettering Cancer Center in New York City, researchers report that 12 acupuncture treatments over 3 months let people reduce their use of pain relievers by 15 percent and make 25 percent fewer visits

Migraine Treatments That May Not Work

Touted on the Internet and in health food stores as natural migraine remedies, claims about these five famous head pain treatments haven't withstood scientific scrutiny.

Feverfew: A popular herbal headache remedy, feverfew didn't stand up to the test when British scientists reviewed the evidence. Their conclusion: Its benefits were "mild and transient."[19] But this is a case that may work for some people but be a dud for others. Taking 50 to 82 milligrams per day of feverfew was somewhat effective in another review.[20] If it works for you, don't stop taking it, but if it's not helping, be sure to try the better-established strategies in this chapter.

Melatonin: Melatonin really doesn't have much of a track record against migraine pain. One oft-quoted Brazilian study found some benefits, but it was small—just 34 people—and they knew they were taking it, so some of the pain reduction may have been wishful thinking.[21]

Homeopathy: Skip it. In one study, migraine sufferers who used customized homeopathic remedies for 3 months were no better off than those who got fake remedies.[22]

Magnesium: Researchers have found that the brains of people who get migraines are low on magnesium, but in two out of three studies, this mineral didn't prevent head pain.[23]

Coenzyme Q10: In a review of 24 studies of alternative medicine for migraines, researchers from Park Nicollet Health Services in Minneapolis were on the fence about CoQ10.[24] Maybe it helps, maybe it doesn't. That's not a good enough reason to take a supplement!

to the doctor.[25] The researchers concluded that "acupuncture leads to persisting, clinically relevant benefits for primary care patients with chronic headache, particularly migraine." Results seem long lasting, too. German scientists who reviewed 22 well-designed acupuncture studies found that people still had less pain 9 months after acupuncture treatments ended.

How it works: Hair-thin needles inserted at points along your arms, legs, head, or torso restore the free flow of the life energy called *qi* (pronounced "chee").

What you need to know: Acupuncturists tailor the treatment to match each person's unique set of symptoms. There's no single, one-size-fits-all prescription for treating migraines.

You may have one to two sessions (each lasting up to 30 minutes or so) a week for several weeks or months; relief may be immediate or it may take a while. Turn to Part Three for information on finding a trained, certified acupuncturist near you.

Pain Medications and Medical Treatments

MIGRAINE PREVENTION MEDICATIONS: If you're still enduring two or more moderate to severe migraines per month, you may be a candidate for a drug that prevents the pain. And you're not alone. In one 2007 study of over 162,000 Americans, researchers from the Albert Einstein College of Medicine determined that 39 percent of migraine sufferers might get relief with one of these medications, yet just 12 percent were getting them.[26]

The evidence: Ranging from the high blood pressure drugs such as propranolol (Inderal) to the antiseizure drugs divalproex sodium (Depakote) and topiramate (Topamax) to the tricyclic antidepressant amitriptyline (Elavil), these medicines can cut your odds for future migraines by 50 to 90 percent.[27, 28]

How they work: Each works differently. Antidepressants keep more feel-good neurotransmitters in play in your brain, seizure drugs seem to calm nerve cells, and beta-blocker drugs for high blood pressure relax blood vessel spasms, for example.

What you need to know: These drugs must be taken daily in order to be effective. You'll have to work closely with your family doctor or a headache specialist to find the right one. It's a matter of trial and error. All are effective, but not every one works for every person.

Other Strategies

STOP OVERUSING PAIN RELIEVERS: If you get 15 or more migraines per month and take prescription pain relievers (triptans, ergotamines, or opioids) or OTC headache remedies such as migraine or sinus headache formulas on at least 10 days each month, your medicine may be causing your headaches.[29] Even using plain aspirin, ibuprofen, or acetaminophen more than 15 days a month could trigger head pain.[30] Signs that your drugs are causing problems include frequently waking up in the morning with a migraine, or discovering that your usual pain relievers aren't working as well as they used to. If any of those situations describes you, its time to stop taking your pain medications.

The evidence: We know. It's not easy. But studies show that for 7 in 10 people,

Pain Free This Month: Menstrual Migraine Relief

Plummeting estrogen levels just before menstruation set the stage for migraine by making you more sensitive to pain. The result can be a migraine that keeps coming back month after month. These steps can help you stay pain free.

● **Keep other triggers under control.** Hormone shifts set the stage for a migraine, but steering clear of triggers like stress and poor sleep might help you avoid developing one. Get enough sleep, eat regular meals, drink plenty of fluids, exercise, reduce stress, and avoid notorious trigger foods like red wine, Cheddar, and blue cheese, Harvard Medical School headache experts recommend.

● **Skip birth control pills or switch to a low-dose formula.** Most oral contraceptives can trigger migraines; the old theory that regulating hormones with them would stop menstrual migraines hasn't held up. Many versions of the Pill trigger migraines because they actually deliver different hormone doses at different points in a pill cycle. If you want to use this method of birth control, try a low-dose monophasic formula that has a consistent dose and is taken continuously, such as Lybrel (90 mcg levonorgestrel/20 mcg ethinyl estradiol).

● **Take an NSAID.** Start taking a nonsteroidal anti-inflammatory pain reliever such as ibuprofen 2 to 3 days before your period begins and continue until it ends.

● **Need something stronger? Use a migraine-stopping triptan.** Triptan has been shown to help with menstrual migraines. Try frovatriptan, naratriptan, or sumatriptan instead, but follow the directions for an NSAID. If you're still in pain, ask your doctor about stronger pain medicines called ergot derivatives, available as tablets or a nasal spray.

quitting pain pills reduces migraine intensity and frequency significantly.[31, 32] Quitting also allows other steps you're taking to work effectively to prevent future migraines.

How it works: Overusing pain drugs makes your brain more vulnerable than ever to migraine triggers. Quitting allows your brain to recover, so that it's less bothered by small, everyday insults (like a whiff of perfume, an extra cup of coffee, or a short night of sleep).

Pain-easing drugs wind up provoking pain in several ways. Migraine-stopping triptans, for example, normally help brain cells use more of the pain-blocking, feel-good brain chemical serotonin.[33] But serotonin levels drop when the drug wears off, leaving you more vulnerable than before to whatever triggers your migraines.[34] Caffeine in OTC migraine formulas and decongestants in OTC sinus headache drugs tighten swollen blood vessels, but afterward they swell up bigger than before. Strong opioid pain drugs like codeine mute pain receptors on brain cells but leave them more sensitive to pain signals when they wear off.

What to do: Stop taking pain relievers. It can take 10 days to 2 weeks for the pain to subside. The good news? You may be able to safely use a few types of medication to make the transition more comfortable, so it's worth talking with your doctor before you stop using your pain medications and staying in touch with her during the process. Medications that can help (without prolonging problems) include a short course of steroid pills or shots, a few doses of a longer-acting triptan such as frovatriptan (Frova), or a little bit of aspirin or ibuprofen. Experts say they all may tide you over without fueling new headaches.

IDENTIFY AND CONTROL YOUR PERSONAL MIGRAINE TRIGGERS: Does a slice of Cheddar cheese or a glass of red wine set off your head pain? What about stress, a change in your sleep schedule, strong odors, or a

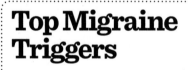

Top Migraine Triggers

Foods, situations, and medications can all set off migraines. In one survey of 916 women and men conducted by the Headache Center of Atlanta, triggers included:

- Stress: 80 percent
- Hormonal fluctuations for women: 65 percent
- Sleep disturbances: 50 percent
- Perfumes or odors: 44 percent
- Neck pain: 39 percent
- Lights: 38 percent
- Smoke: 36 percent
- Sleeping late: 32 percent
- Heat: 30 percent
- Exercise: 22 percent
- Sex: 5 percent[35]

medication you're taking for another health condition? Figuring out your personal pain triggers can help you avoid them or cope better when you simply can't avoid them, reducing your odds for future head pain. This therapy is really all about *not* doing something, by skipping offenders.

The evidence: For one in four people who get migraines, experts say food is a potent trigger. Which edibles or drinks? Culprits can include caffeine, the additive monosodium glutamate, chocolate, processed meat and fish, cheese (particularly aged cheeses like Cheddar and blue cheese), nuts, and alcohol (especially red wine, champagne, and dark-colored drinks like rum).

But that's not all. Weather changes—temperature shifts and changes in barometric pressure—may trigger your headaches. For some people, medications provoke migraines. These include bronchodilator drugs for asthma such as albuterol (Proventil) and salmeterol (Serevent), birth control pills, diet pills, the acne drug isotretinoin (Accutane), and SSRI antidepressants like fluoxetine (Prozac).

How it works: Nobody knows why a single slice of aged Vermont Cheddar sets off a thundering migraine for you, yet leaves your migraine-prone aunt blissfully unaffected. Triggers are personal, but all cause trouble by somehow creating changes in brain chemicals that irritate the nerves responsible for migraine pain. Obviously, avoiding them reduces the odds of your next headache.

What you need to know: To figure it all out, keep a headache diary. You can copy the blank diary pages in Part Three or make your own. For a week or two (or longer), note your headache symptoms, intensity and duration of pain, nausea or light sensitivity, and any potential triggers like foods and beverages, stressful situations, sleep changes, other medications you've taken, or where you are in your menstrual cycle, for example. Include whether or not you exercised and weather changes, too.

Then look for patterns. Sometimes the links are clear. You drank orange juice this morning and the throbbing started by noon. Other times it takes a combination of triggers (a stressful work deadline plus lack of sleep plus the bright lights of oncoming traffic during your commute home) to get things started.

Once you notice triggers, avoid those that you can. If a medication seems responsible, ask your doctor about alternatives. Stop eating any foods that you can pinpoint as probable triggers. Although some headache specialists recommend special migraine diets that eliminate a host of potential trigger foods, others say starting out by eliminating personal triggers is simpler. Don't know which foods are behind your pain? Start by cutting out the trigger foods listed above.

What about triggers you can't sidestep, like a stressful day at the office, a bad night's sleep, or the inevitable hormonal ups and downs of your menstrual cycle? The good news is that when you take charge of controllable triggers, the ones you can't control may have less of an effect. Be very careful to avoid other triggers at these times. Resist the urge to drink an extra cup of coffee, be sure to drink plenty of water and eat meals on time, choose a route home that won't leave you facing an endless line of headlights, and get plenty of sleep. Following a regular schedule for meals helps prevent pain-provoking swings in blood sugar, and getting into a steady sleep schedule insures your brain can produce plenty of pain-preventing brain chemicals like serotonin and dopamine.

Tension Headaches

Whether your head hurts every once in a while or all too frequently, the skull-busting pain of a tension headache can hijack every aspect of your life. In national surveys from the National Headache Society, 74 percent of participants said head pain made them miss work, 84 percent said it led them to skip family functions or social events,[36] and over 40 percent said head pain got worse while traveling—something you definitely don't need on a special, long-anticipated vacation or important business trip.[37] That's why fast relief and preventing future brain pain are so important.

These headaches are very common, affecting more than 80 percent of adults. Yet they're often misunderstood, misdiagnosed, and mistreated, which ratchets up the pain instead of helping you get out from under it.

For example, you may not know that the pain relievers you take for frequent headaches may actually be setting you up for new brain aches tomorrow and the next day, keeping you stuck in a cycle of pain, pills, then more pain. Stress can trigger pain, perhaps by tightening muscles in your shoulders, neck, and face; but it's just as likely that what you do under stress—like getting less sleep, drinking more coffee, and reaching for foods that make blood sugar swing wildly—plays an even bigger role in how much pain you get. The good news? A whole host of proven yet often overlooked strategies and treatments (from relaxation and exercise to medications) can help.

The latest on garden-variety tension headaches? Specialists now suspect that "tension headaches," "episodic headaches," and "chronic headaches" are, at their core, fueled by the same forces that drive migraines. Although your head pain may not fit the classic description of a migraine—it may not throb on one side of your head, make you sensitive to lights and sounds, leave you nauseated, or compel you to retreat to a dark room—there's evidence that similar triggers cause both types of pain by activating the same brain areas. The same strategies that prevent big migraine pain could help you steer clear of future headaches and make those you do get more manageable.

Is It a Tension Headache?

Tension headaches usually bring pain on both sides of your head and may come with a feeling of pressure on your forehead, temples, or the back of your head or neck. They're usually not set off or made worse by exercise or other physical activity and usually don't make you feel sick to your stomach or sensitive to lights, noises, or odors. (If you are, you may actually have migraine headaches.) There are three types of tension headaches, and knowing which type you tend to get can help guide your pain-relief choices.

- **Episodic tension headaches:** You get this type if your headaches come less than once a month and are usually a result of stress, tiredness, or even strong emotions.

- **Frequent tension headaches:** These happen 1 to 15 times per month. Although drugstore pain relievers can melt the pain, be careful. Using them too often could turn your headaches into a chronic problem. It's important to deploy other strategies to control them.

- **Chronic tension headaches:** Occur 15 or more days per month. If you're taking pain relievers 10 to 15 days per month, waking up with a headache, or getting less and less relief from each dose, it's very likely that the drugs you're taking are causing these headaches. Chronic tension headaches boost your risk of sleep problems and depression. Medications like the tricyclic antidepressant amitriptyline can help prevent chronic tension headaches, not because you're depressed, but because they help stabilize levels of important brain chemicals called neurotransmitters. But there's plenty of evidence that weaning yourself from pain medications, avoiding pain triggers, and adopting drug-free pain prevention strategies can reduce headache frequency significantly.

Fast Pain Relief

It pays to have pain-stopping tools on hand so that you can block a tension headache as soon as possible. (Who wants to go to the drugstore with a

Stopping Cluster Headaches

Cluster headaches are so excruciating that the people who live with them often call them "suicide headaches" or "red migraines." They're so frequent that they're also called "clockwork headaches" because they return regularly—at the same time of day for weeks, months, or even years on end.

No one's sure what causes this agonizing pain, but researchers know that brain activity that excites the trigeminal nerve, which carries pain signals to and from the brain to the face and head, is involved. They suspect the hypothalamus, a brain region involved with daily rhythms in the human body, also plays a role, perhaps explaining the cruel regularity of this uncommon brain pain. About a million people in the United States get cluster headaches; 9 out of 10 are male. And for 1 in 5, the pain is chronic, happening all year long without a break.

As the name suggests, this head pain comes in groups. Each headache lasts just 30 minutes to a few hours, but you may have several a day for several weeks or months. They're more common in spring and fall. Yet although an attack may include symptoms that seem like an allergic reaction—like a runny nose and watery eyes—these headaches don't seem to be triggered by pollen or other allergens. In fact, little is known about what sets them off.

Controlling these "red migraines" involves using medication to prevent attacks and to abort new headaches when they begin. The most widely used drug for preventing cluster headaches, verapamil, is effective but carries risks. In one study of 30 people, 12 out of 15 who got the drug had fewer attacks in just 2 weeks. But other research shows that it raises the risk for irregular heartbeats significantly, so you'll need regular heart checks if you choose it.[38] But other options may be better for fast relief.

Sumatriptan: This migraine medicine, used as a nasal spray or injection, works fast. Injections stopped pain within 15 minutes for 96 percent of volunteers in one study. In another, 47 percent of headache sufferers who used a sumatriptan nasal spray were pain free in 30 minutes.[39, 40, 41]

Oxygen therapy: In a recent British study of 109 cluster headache sufferers, 78 percent who tried inhaling oxygen were pain free within 15 minutes.[42] Study participants used the oxygen at home. If you get this type of headache, ask your doctor about oxygen for home use.

head-banger?) Stock up on ibuprofen or acetaminophen, a cold pack you can keep in the freezer, some peppermint essential oil, then follow these steps.

1. **Take ibuprofen liquid gel capsules or acetaminophen with a glass of water.** Follow the dosage directions on the label. Choose acetaminophen if you can't take ibuprofen because of the risk of gastrointestinal upset or bleeding. If you have medication overuse headaches, follow the advice under "Relief at Last" on page 96. Have a full glass of water; mild dehydration can cause or exaggerate head pain.

   Important note: If you have frequent or chronic tension headaches, pain relievers can trigger new headaches. It's important to stop using them—read on for advice.

   OTC pain relievers mute head pain by short-circuiting the release of inflammation-causing compounds responsible for swollen blood vessels in your head and face. Although all of them—acetaminophen, aspirin, ibuprofen, and naproxen—cut the ache by at least 50 percent, Dutch researchers who analyzed 41 headache remedy studies recommend that most people start with ibuprofen because it is less likely to cause gastro-intestinal upset when taken occasionally. The liquid in gel capsules is absorbed more quickly than solid pills and tablets, research suggests.[43] In one study, gel capsules eased pain 14 minutes faster than acetaminophen in a study of 154 headache sufferers published in the journal *Headache*.[44]

   If you can't take ibuprofen or other NSAIDs (because you're using the anti-clotting drug warfarin or are at high risk for gastrointestinal bleeding), start with acetaminophen.[45]

2. **Add caffeine for faster relief.** Caffeine helps by shrinking swollen blood vessels in the face and head.[46] Get yours by having a mug of coffee or strong tea with your ibuprofen, or by taking an OTC migraine formula such as Excedrin Migraine that combines acetaminophen, aspirin, and caffeine. Studies show that this mix works better than acetaminophen or ibuprofen alone.[47] In one study of 345 people conducted at the Diamond Headache Clinic in Chicago, a 200-milligram dose of caffeine plus ibuprofen eased headache pain for 71 percent. In contrast, just 60 percent of those who took either caffeine or ibuprofen got relief. Skip the caffeine, however, if you get medication overuse headaches.

3. **Massage this acupressure point.** Using your right hand, squeeze and rub the webbing on your left hand between thumb and index finger for one minute. Then switch sides.

   Practitioners say the "LI-4" point—located where your finger bones meet under your skin in the webbing between thumb and index finger—relieves inflammation. For best results, press toward your index finger. (Skip if you're pregnant or think you might be; some acupressure practitioners consider this a "forbidden point" during pregnancy.)

4. **Ice your head.** Hold a cold pack, wrapped in a towel, on your forehead or on the back of your head (depending on where the pain is strongest).

   Ice packs helped ease pain in just 15 minutes in a University of Illinois study of 45 people prone to tension headaches and migraines. Cold shrinks swollen blood vessels but probably won't cut discomfort on its own. Researchers say it was mildly to moderately effective for about half the volunteers in one study and completely stopped pain for just 9 percent.[48] So be sure to use other pain-relieving techniques listed here, too.

5. **Massage your temples and forehead with a peppermint oil blend.** Use a 10 percent mixture of peppermint (*Mentha x piperita*) essential oil and massage oil, made by blending 1 drop of peppermint essential oil with 9 drops of jojoba or another massage oil. Keep away from your eyes and out of the reach of children. Peppermint essential oil is not intended for internal use.

In one study, a minty massage worked nearly as well as acetaminophen to lift headache pain.[49, 50] Researchers say more study is needed, so consider this an add-on therapy.

Relief at Last

If your headaches are few and far between—less than once a month—a pain reliever may be all that you need. But if you get more frequent aches, use these steps as a guide to which headache-stopping strategies to try first.

Step 1. Stop medication overuse headaches. About one in four people with chronic tension headaches pops too many pain relievers, triggering a new headache each time a dose wears off. Stopping this cycle is your top priority for pain relief.

Step 2. Use food therapy to soothe your brain's headache center. Cutting out your personal pain-provoking trigger foods and keeping yourself hydrated and fueled for steady blood sugar all help prevent headaches.

Step 3. Cut stress and boost feel-good brain chemicals with regular sleep, exercise, and relaxation. You can also prevent headaches by easing stress associated with eye strain and with posture problems at your desk and on the sofa.

Step 4. Still experiencing head pain? Try treatments like acupuncture or medication. For some people, chronic tension headaches respond to this ancient healing art as well as to antidepressant drugs.

> ## Quick Tip
> No pain pills handy? Grab an 8-ounce cup of strong coffee or tea. In one study, 200 milligrams of caffeine eased head pain 30 minutes faster than ibuprofen. You'll also get that amount from two cups of well-steeped black tea (leave bag in the cup for about 3 minutes).[51] Skip soda. With 30 to 60 milligrams in 12 ounces, it is probably not strong enough.

Pain Prevention Strategies

Food and Supplements

PAIN-PREVENTING EATING HABITS: If you don't have medication overuse headaches or still have head pain after getting off the pain reliever merry-go-round, lower your odds for aches with a gentle diet makeover. This form of food therapy is aimed at avoiding pain triggers like dehydration and blood sugar swings, as well as removing any food triggers that may fire up a headache for you.

The evidence: Headache specialists say getting plenty of water, eating regular meals, and avoiding personal food triggers can all reduce the number of headaches you get and make the ones that do strike shorter and less intense.

How it works: Low blood sugar and even mild dehydration can irritate the brain centers where headaches originate, setting off the cascade of inflammatory chemicals that leads to headache pain. Food triggers work the same way. Avoiding these pitfalls can help prevent pain.

What you should know: Following these healthy eating strategies can help.

- Sip six to eight 8-ounce glasses of water through the day.

- Aim to eat meals on a regular schedule. Don't wait more than 4 to 5 hours in between, and less if you find that hunger pangs set off pain. Include a healthy mix of blood sugar–steadying foods. Fill your plate with whole grains, fiber-rich fruits and vegetables, lean protein, and good fats (found in olive and canola oil, fish, nuts, and avocado). These can all help keep blood sugar levels stable for hours after a meal. Cut back or skip refined carbohydrates like white bread as well as sugary drinks and sweets; these can make blood sugar spike, then drop.

- Keep an eye out for food triggers. Chronic headaches can be triggered by the same edibles that ignite migraines. Big offenders can include caffeine, chocolate, alcohol, monosodium glutamate, and even aged cheeses, nuts, and processed meats and fish. If you suspect that a food triggers your headaches, track the effects with the Pain Diary in Part Three. Once you've figured out your triggers, eliminate them for 2 weeks and see if headaches stay away.

LESS CAFFEINE: Yes, the same wake-you-up ingredient that helps fight headaches can, when consumed regularly in extra-large doses (like that *venti latte* from the coffee shop), increase headache risk.

The evidence: In a Swedish study of 50,483 people, those who got a whopping 500 milligrams of caffeine a day—the amount in about 2½ to 5 small cups of coffee—were 18 percent more likely to have headaches a few times per month than those who had about 1 cup a day.[52]

Why it works: Caffeine shrinks blood vessels slightly, which is the reason it can make a headache feel better. But vessels can swell up bigger as it wears off. Frequent doses put you on a shrink/swell/shrink/swell cycle that causes pain.

What you need to know: Like quitting pain relievers, cutting out (or even cutting back on) caffeine could cause some pain before it helps you feel better. Try a gradual switch to decaf—mix caffeinated and caffeine-free coffee half and half, then gradually adjust the balance until you're sipping an all-decaf drink. The good news? Complete abstinence may not be necessary; a cup in the morning may be okay.

Exercise and Movement Therapies

REGULAR EXERCISE: Aiming for at least 30 minutes of exercise, like walking or riding an exercise bike, most days of the week is a proven headache stopper. Keep it at a moderate pace, though; intense exercise can set off migraines and might trigger a tension headache, too.

The evidence: Getting a half-hour of exercise most days of the week can cut headache pain and frequency by an impressive 50 percent, say headache experts from the University of Maryland. In a Swedish study of 22,397 people, those who were the least active were 14 percent more likely to get headaches than those who were the most active.[53]

Why it works: Physical activity fights headaches two ways: It boosts feel-good endorphins and eases stress.

What you need to know: Exercising with a buddy can help you stick with physical activity. If you find that working out later in the day makes getting to sleep more difficult, fit your walk in before work or at lunchtime. You can try splitting it into several 10-minute sessions scattered throughout the day.

Touch Therapies

ACUPUNCTURE: In the hands of a trained and licensed practitioner, acupuncture could cut the number of headaches you get by half, one German study found, and the benefits of this ancient and advanced form of touch therapy could last for months after treatment ends.

The evidence: In a recent review of 11 well-designed studies, German researchers concluded that acupuncture "could be a valuable non-pharmacological tool in patients with frequent episodic or chronic tension-type headaches."

Why it works: This ancient healing art is believed to restore the healthy flow of life energy, called qi, in the body.

What you need to know: Acupuncturists tailor treatment to an individual's unique symptoms, then insert fine-gauge needles into the skin of the arms, legs, torso, and head to stimulate the flow of energy. Expect one to two sessions per week for at least 8 weeks. Turn to Part Three for information on finding a qualified practitioner.

Mind/Body Therapies

RELAXATION TECHNIQUES: Simple, do-it-yourself relaxation techniques like deep breathing and progressive muscle relaxation can deliver big pain prevention benefits. These mind-body therapies truly live up to their name—easing your mind and lessening your odds for brain pain.

The evidence: A recent Harvard Medical School study found that simple stress reducers worked as well as or better than pricey biofeedback sessions in a study of 64 tension headache sufferers.[54] Italian office workers who took brief relaxation breaks every 2 to 3 hours got 41 percent fewer headaches in one University of Turin study. And when Ohio University researchers tracked 203 adults with chronic daily tension headaches, 35 percent of those who got five sessions of stress management advice saw headache frequency fall by more than 50 percent.

Why it works: Tight muscles can send pain signals to your brain, starting a headache. Relaxation may help simply by easing tension in your face, neck, shoulders, and back. Headache experts say it also reduces levels of stress hormones, which can trigger headaches and make your brain more sensitive to other pain triggers.

What you should know: A few minutes of slow breathing, a progressive relaxation session (follow our routine in Chapter 5), or some gentle relaxing or restorative yoga (try the routine on page 502) can all move you from tense to tension free.

Pain Medications and Medical Treatments

ELIMINATE MEDICATION OVERUSE HEADACHES: Pain relievers may be causing head pain if you get headaches 15 or more days each month and use regular pain relievers 15 times per month or an OTC migraine or sinus headache formula (or prescription pain stopper such as a triptan) 10 or more times per month. Medication overuse headaches are surprisingly common. Experts say that at least 27 percent of people with chronic headaches unwittingly fuel their pain with pain relievers. Quitting allows your brain to bolster its pain protection defenses, and will allow other pain prevention strategies to work effectively.

The evidence: In one Danish study of 175 people with medication overuse headaches, the number of headaches they suffered dropped 46 percent when they quit taking pain relievers. They also found that other measures they took to prevent future headaches became more effective.[55]

How it works: Overuse hurts your head two ways: When the decongestants in sinus headache remedies and the caffeine in migraine formulas wear off, blood vessels swell up with a vengeance. As other pain relievers are metabolized, pain receptors in your brain become very sensitive, and the smallest trigger can set off your next headache.[56]

What you need to know: Quitting pain meds isn't easy. It could take 10 days to 2 weeks, or longer, for rebound pain to wear off when you do. But it's proven to reduce the number of headaches for many people. And getting rid of the rebound effect of pain meds allows other pain prevention strategies to work. It's important to work with your doctor while going off pain remedies; she may be able to prescribe a short course of steroids, a long-acting triptan, or advise you about whether it's okay to take a few doses of plain aspirin, acetaminophen, or ibuprofen to blunt the pain.

AMITRIPTYLINE (ELAVIL): If nondrug approaches aren't enough to stop frequent headaches, ask your doctor about the depression-lifting drug amitriptyline (Elavil). Taken daily, this tricyclic antidepressant cuts the number and intensity of headaches for about 65 percent of the people who take it.

> *Quick Tip*
>
> St. Louis University researchers found that pent-up anger was a more potent headache trigger than anxiety or depression in one study of 171 people. They recommend brisk walking to melt the tension stirred up by angry feelings. Also worthwhile: Ask yourself what's ticking you off, then try to find ways to resolve it.[57]

The evidence: In a recent review of 10 well-designed studies, Spanish headache researchers concluded that this antidepressant is effective.[58]

Why it works: It seems to help the brain make better use of serotonin, and low levels of this feel-good brain chemical are associated with headaches.[59]

What you need to know: Doctors usually recommend taking amitriptyline at bedtime because it can make you feel groggy. Other side effects include weight gain and blurry vision.[60] This drug seems to work best if you also use relaxation techniques on a regular basis.

Other Strategies

KEEP A REGULAR SLEEP SCHEDULE: A steady routine that allows for 7 to 8 hours of shut-eye per night, ideally with the same bedtimes and wake-up times every day, keeps you and your brain well rested.

The evidence: Risk for tension headaches was 2.3 times higher in women who had trouble falling asleep or staying asleep in one recent study of 310 women from Hong Kong.[61]

Why it works: Your brain needs a full night's sleep for optimal functioning. Without it, neurons can't release as much of the feel-good chemicals serotonin and dopamine, and low levels could make your head hurt. A regular doze dose also regulates the hormone melatonin, which may trigger headaches when levels are out of balance.[62] Setting a sleep schedule will, most likely, also lead to a more regular breakfast routine, eliminating the dips in blood sugar and morning caffeine withdrawal that increase headache risk.

Rescue Plan for Six Surprising Head Pains

The exercise headache: Vigorous activity can activate nerves in the brain that lead to a migraine after a sweaty workout. If you're susceptible, don't give up on physical activity; it has too many important benefits for weight control, health, and stress reduction.

The fix: Protect your head by warming up slowly and taking ibuprofen or acetaminophen a half-hour before you begin.

The ponytail headache: A tightly pulled ponytail tugs on muscles in your scalp, irritating nerve endings in connective tissue. In a study of these hairdo headaches in the journal *Headache*, a researcher from the City of London Migraine Clinic noted that the pain can spread across the forehead, temples, and neck.[63]

The fix: As the researcher noted, "the remedy is obvious." Loosen your hair!

The roller-coaster headache: Brain-rattling amusement park rides can set off a "posttraumatic migraine."

The fix: Most go away with a dose of an OTC pain reliever. But if your headache persists for hours, days, or weeks after you leave the amusement park, see your doctor. Researchers have found that in rare cases, the sudden speed changes on a roller coaster can tear tiny veins and cause bleeding in the brain.[64]

The sex headache: In one survey, 5 percent of migraines were triggered by making love. Coital headaches may be caused by a buildup of pressure in head and neck muscles.

The fix: Taking ibuprofen beforehand should help.

The weather headache: Changes in temperature, humidity, barometric pressure,[65] and even wind speed[66] can alter brain chemicals in ways that irritate nerves, causing pain. In one study of 7,000 people who came to a Boston emergency room with head pain, every 9-degree increase in the outdoor air temperature boosted headache rates by 8 percent.[67]

The fix: If you get weather-related migraines, take a pain reliever at the earliest sign a headache is on the way.

The weekend headache: Your head hurts every Saturday morning? The culprit could be oversleeping, a hangover from Friday's happy hour, a letdown from the week's stress, or a delay in getting that first cup of morning coffee.

The fix: Try to keep the same routines for meals and sleep on weekdays and weekends, and go easy on the alcohol next time.

What you should know: If you wake up with a headache, ask your bed partner if you grind your teeth, snore loudly, or seem to stop breathing during sleep. A morning headache may be a sign of tooth-damaging bruxism or sleep apnea, conditions that deserve a check with your dentist (for bruxism) and your doctor (for apnea).[68]

PRACTICE GOOD POSTURE: Computer jockeys and sofa slumpers: Give your muscles a break. Lounging on the couch or slouching and hunching over a computer keyboard tenses back, shoulder, and neck muscles, leading to head pain. Fight back by adopting picture-perfect posture that relieves muscle tension.

The evidence: In one study of 200 people with chronic headaches caused by tense neck and shoulder muscles, 76 percent of those who did muscle-loosening exercises and learned about good posture cut the number and intensity of their headaches by half or better; 42 percent got complete relief.[69]

Why it works: Good posture eliminates muscle tension.

What you should know: For better posture while sitting at a computer, first be sure your monitor is at the right height—your eyes should be in line with a point 2 to 3 inches from the top. When you sit down, plant your feet on the floor (instead of crossing your legs). Your thighs should be parallel to the floor and your knees should be bent at a 90-degree angle. Roll your pelvis forward slightly so that the backs of your thighs and your buttocks support your weight. Your lower back should press against the back of your chair. You can use a small pillow behind your lower back for support. Your core muscles should help support your torso, and your head and neck should be in line with your spine.

Take a break every hour or so and walk around your office to relieve muscle tension.

Spend a lot of time on the couch? Try sitting up straight, feet planted on the floor, spine aligned as described above.

Or try these exercises, designed to relax tight muscle groups that can contribute to tension headaches.

Chin tuck: Sitting tall in your chair, tuck your chin until you feel a slight stretch (but no pain) in your neck muscles. Hold for a second or two, then relax. Repeat 10 times.

Neck turn: While sitting in your chair, tuck your chin slightly and turn to look over your right shoulder. You should feel a little stretch in the right side of your neck (but no pain). Hold for a second or two, then relax. Repeat 10 times on each side.

Shoulder squeeze: Sit or stand with your arms bent at a 90-degree angle as if resting on the armrests of a chair. Squeeze your shoulder blades together and push your elbows back until you feel tension (but no pain) between your shoulder blades. Hold for 4 to 5 seconds, then relax. Repeat 10 times.

ELIMINATE SCREEN GLARE: Eye strain is a growing cause of headaches, thanks to the hours we spend using computers and smart phones, playing video games, and catching up with old movies and new reality shows on TV. Taking steps to eliminate glare and strain make screen time more pleasant and erase head pain, too.

The evidence: In one 2009 survey sponsored by the National Headache Foundation, top headache triggers included eye strain, glare from computer monitors, and bright, flickering, or fluorescent lighting at work.[70] (Flickering lights could even trigger a migraine if you're prone to those big headaches.[71])

Why it works: Eye strain may cause muscle tension that can bring on a headache. For some people, it may even trigger brain chemical shifts that kick-start a headache.

What you need to know: Eyeglasses with antiglare coatings can help. When working at a computer or watching TV, be sure there are no bright lights or other sources of glare (like a sunny window or light from another room) behind or above the screen. Going to the movies? If eye strain causes headaches, consider opting for 2-D rather than 3-D versions of blockbuster hits. Vision researchers say 3-D effects require our eyes and brains to focus on near and distant objects at the same time, a task that makes vision blurry and could cause headaches.

Sinus Headaches

An aching head, pressure in your cheeks, and a runny, stuffy nose: the text-book-perfect definition of a sinus headache? Maybe not. In fact, "sinus headache" is not an accepted diagnostic term. There's a good chance it's a migraine in disguise. In an eye-opening study from the Headache Care Center in Springfield, Missouri, of 2,991 women and men who thought they had chronic sinus headaches, researchers found that nearly 90 percent really had migraines.[72]

There's a good reason for the confusion. It turns out that the trigeminal nerve, which conducts pain signals from the brain to the face during a migraine, can also cause congestion and facial pressure when activated. If you're taking sinus headache remedies and not getting any relief, a better diagnosis may be the ticket to showing pain the door. Read on for ways to tell the difference and get real relief.

Is It a Sinus Headache?

Your head pain may be a sinus headache if you have one or more of these signs and symptoms: fever, pressure, and/or pain in your cheeks or behind your eyes (on one or on both sides); green, yellow, or brownish nasal discharge; fatigue; reduced sense of taste and/or smell; a cough; dental pain; and/or bad breath. Timing is also a clue. Real sinus headaches usually come on a few days to a week after you catch a cold, when mucus trapped in swollen nasal passages becomes infected.

In contrast, your headache is more likely to be a migraine if you haven't had a cold in the past week or so and if your pain throbs, is located on just one side of the head, gets worse if you move or bend over, and if you also feel nauseous and/or sensitive to lights, sounds, or odors.[74] Remember, not all migraines are severe enough to send you into a dark room for hours or days on end. If you think you're getting migraines, see your doctor and follow the advice in the Migraines section of this chapter.

Fast Pain Relief

Doctors usually don't prescribe antibiotics for sinus infections (and sinus headaches) because most of the time the cause is a viral infection, not a bacterial infection that would be wiped out by an antibiotic. The new strategy: Do all you can to encourage your sinuses to drain. This will relieve the pressure and help clear up the infection. If you've got a sinus headache right now, take these steps.

1. **Use an over-the-counter decongestant nasal spray.** Decongestant nose sprays containing the active ingredients phenylephrine hydrochloride or oxymetazoline (such as Afrin or Dristan) shrink swollen blood vessels in the lining of your nose almost instantaneously, allowing trapped mucus to drain. Limit yourself to 3 days of spray use;

any longer can cause "rebound congestion"—worse swelling and more head pain as a dose wears off.

2. **Ask for a decongestant pill.** If you don't like sprays, ask the pharmacist for a decongestant containing pseudephedrine, but only use it during the day. Pseudoephedrine is nonprescription, but it is kept behind the pharmacy counter to avoid misuse. It's more effective than the phenylephrine in decongestants and sinus headache combination remedies out on the shelves. Be careful: Pseudoephedrine can make you jittery or even keep you awake, so don't take it at night. Limit your use to about 3 days to avoid rebound head pain when blood vessels swell up again. (For more on the best decongestants, see the Pain Prevention Strategies on the opposite page.)

3. **Take a plain pain reliever, not a combination sinus remedy.** Ordinary aspirin, ibuprofen, and acetaminophen can all take the edge off sinus pain without putting you at risk for a rebound headache the way combination sinus remedies containing decongestants can. And there's another advantage: By using a separate decongestant product you can get the most effective ingredients at the most effective dose, and only use it when you need it. Combination remedies often contain less than 60 milligrams of pseudoephedrine, the recommended adult dose, and many use a less effective decongestant called phenylephrine.[75, 76]

4. **Warm your sinuses.** Placing a warm, moist washcloth across your eyes and cheeks is soothing and encourages the microscopic hairs in your sinuses, called cilia, to move faster. Cilia slow down during a cold, leaving mucus in your sinuses and nasal passages longer. Giving them a boost helps sweep away congestion and infection.[77]

5. **Use steam to thin trapped mucus.** Stand in a hot shower, get out your vaporizer, or drape a towel over your head and lean over a bowl or sink of hot water for 10 minutes. Inhale deeply, and repeat three to four times a day. Inhaling steam can improve sinus drainage by thinning thick mucus.

6. **Try a mucolytic.** These contain the active ingredient guaifenesin (Mucinex) and may help thin mucus. They don't work for everyone, but experts say they're worth a try. If you don't notice better drainage or less pressure in 2 to 3 days, they may not be for you.

Relief at Last

Preventing sinus headaches is all about keeping mucus from becoming trapped in your sinuses where it becomes a breeding ground for viruses or bacteria and causes pressure and pain. If you're prone to sinus infections and sinus headaches after a cold or even after a bout with a respiratory allergy like hay fever, here are your best strategies.

Step 1: Use a daily saline rinse. This may feel odd at first, but a mild saltwater rinse is a proven way to flush out viruses and bacteria that cause sinus infections, to dislodge dried mucus that can block sinus passages, and to thin out mucus for better drainage.

Step 2: Keep a drainage-promoting decongestant on hand to use at the first sign of a cold. Used wisely, a decongestant spray or pill can keep your sinus passages open, preventing a backlog of trapped mucus that becomes a breeding ground for infection.

Step 3: Ask your doctor about a steroid nasal spray if you get chronic sinus infections or your colds and allergies almost always turn into sinus infections. You can't use over-the-counter decongestants for more than 2 to 3 days at a time, so if you're prone to sinus infections it makes sense to ask your doctor about prescription types that can be used long term.

Step 4: Practice gentle nose-blowing. This can actually protect against sinus problems. Yup, your mom was right. High-velocity honking can make things worse by propelling germs deeper into your sinuses instead of getting rid of them.

Step 5: Take the herb *Andrographis paniculata* at the first sign of a cold. This herbal remedy is putting together a better track record than echinacea for relieving cold symptoms fast, and could help you short-circuit a sinus infection before it starts.

Pain Prevention Strategies

Food and Supplements

ANDROGRAPHIS PANICULATA: This herbal remedy isn't as well known as other herbs used to fight colds, but it may be one of the most effective.

    The evidence: In one well-designed Chilean study of 158 adult cold sufferers, nasal secretions dried up significantly for those who took 1,200 milligrams of andrographis extract daily for 5 days.[78] Other studies are also finding benefits.[79]

How it works: Andrographis contains anti-inflammatory compounds that might help shrink swollen nasal passages.[80]

What you should know: Look for this botanical in health food stores. Follow label directions. The usual dose is 400 milligrams three times a day.

Pain Medications and Medical Treatments

DECONGESTANT SPRAYS OR PILLS: Keep one ready in your medicine cabinet and use it at the first sign of a cold. It won't shorten your cold but will help keep nasal passages from swelling up and trapping mucus inside.

The evidence: Congestion eased 30 percent after just one dose in a British study of 283 women and men with stuffy noses who used a decongestant.[81]

How it works: Decongestants shrink swollen nasal passages so trapped, infected mucus can drain.

What you should know: If you use a spray, stop after 3 days—longer use can

---

Sinus Pain? Press Here

Could simply pressing special points along your eyebrows and cheekbones relieve sinus pressure and aches? Practitioners of acupressure—a traditional healing therapy that uses finger pressure to stimulate the flow of energy in the body—say yes. And there's plenty of anecdotal evidence that it might help. Here are two ways to give it a try.

Press the hollows at the bridge of your nose. These little indentations are located near the inner corner of your eyebrows, where the upper ridge of your eye sockets ends. Use your thumbs to press here for 1 minute. Close your eyes and relax your head so it's supported by your thumbs. These points, called B2 in modern acupressure and Drilling Bamboo by traditional practitioners, are believed to relieve sinus congestion and headaches.

Press the lower edge of your cheekbones. Put your middle fingers in the space beside the lower edge of your nostrils. Place your index fingers beside them, on the lower edge of your cheekbones. Close your eyes, relax, and slowly press up and in for a minute. This activates two points: ST 3 (also called Facial Beauty) and LI 20 (Welcoming Perfume). Both also ease congestion and sinus pain.

cause rebound congestion, worse swelling and more head pain as each dose wears off. If you opt for a decongestant in pill form, go to the pharmacy counter in your drugstore and ask for one containing pseudoephedrine. It's more effective than the phenylephrine found in the types out on the drugstore shelves. Pseudoephedrine is kept behind the counter to discourage its use in the production of illegal drugs, and you may need a photo ID to buy it. The only drawback? It can keep you awake at night or make you feel jittery, so don't use it in the late afternoon or the evening.

STEROID NASAL SPRAY: If you have chronic sinus infections or if your colds or allergy attacks tend to turn into sinus infections, a prescription nasal steroid spray could help prevent the next one.

The evidence: In one large study from the Allergy and Asthma Medical Group and Research Center, San Diego, 981 people with sinus infections got an antibiotic or used a steroid nasal spray. Researchers found that using the spray twice a day improved symptoms faster and more effectively than the antibiotic. Volunteers began feeling better, with less sinus pressure and head pain, by the second day.[82]

How it works: These drugs soothe inflammation, shrinking swollen nasal and sinus passages so that they can drain, without the side effects of OTC decongestant sprays.

What you should know: Sprays include beclomethasone (Beconase and Vancenase), fluticasone (Flonase), triamcinolone (Nasacort), and flunisolide (Nasalide).

Other Strategies

USE A SALINE NOSE RINSE: If you're prone to sinus infections, a daily rinse with mild saltwater could lower your odds for the next one.

The evidence: British researchers who analyzed eight studies found that a daily saline rinse reduced odds for sinus infections significantly.[83]

How it works: A mild saltwater rinse helps wash away viruses and bacteria, removes dried mucus that can block sinus passages, and also thins mucus so it can drain.

What you should know: You can buy premade saline or make your own by mixing $1/2$ teaspoon un-iodized salt such as pickling or canning salt (it's less irritating than iodized salt) and 1 pinch of baking soda in 8 ounces of warm water.[84]

To rinse, pour the saline into a neti pot (available at health food stores and online) or use a clean bulb syringe. Lean over the sink with your head down and tilted slightly to the right. Insert the neti pot spout into your right nostril and inhale the saline (or insert the syringe tip and squeeze gently). The saline will run down into your mouth; spit out the fluid that drains into your mouth. Gently blow your nose. Repeat until you've used up half the saline, then repeat on the other side.

One caution: Rinsing your nose too frequently might increase sinus infection risk, new research suggests. The reason might be that it could strip away beneficial bacteria. Experts recommend using a rinse a few times a month, not daily.

BLOW YOUR NOSE GENTLY: Blowing your nose too hard might cause a sinus infection! A gentler approach is still effective.

The evidence: Researchers from the University of Virginia found that vigorous honking sends mucus flying backward, deeper into your sinuses.[85] Experts say it can also trigger "reflex nasal congestion," actually making your nasal passage swell.

How it works: Blowing hard creates a vacuum deep in your sinuses that sucks some mucus deeper inside.

What you should know: To clear your nose with finesse instead of force, place a tissue over both nostrils. Close one nostril and blow the other gently. Switch sides. Repeat if necessary.

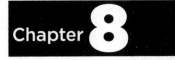

Chapter 8

Face, Mouth, and Respiratory System Pain

Sinusitis and sinus infection, temporomandibular disorders, dental pain and tooth sensitivity, burning mouth syndrome

F acial pain affects millions of people every year. From burning mouth syndrome to sinusitis to sensitive teeth and temporomandibular joint (TMJ) disorders, it can be a real pain . . . in the mouth.

Your face may only be a small part of your body, but even when you exclude the many different types of headaches (see Chapter 7), chronic facial pain comes in a number of different forms. Some of the most common include:

- **Sinusitis:** Inflammation of the sinus cavities of the skull that causes pain to spread from your forehead to your ears, your nose, and even your upper jaw

- **Temporomandibular disorders:** A group of disorders of the jaw hinge that can lead to symptoms from a mild clicking when you open your mouth to tension headaches and ear pain

- **Dentin hypersensitivity:** Tooth and gum damage that leaves your teeth sensitive to cold, certain foods, and touch

- **Burning mouth syndrome:** A strange tingling or burning sensation that can cover all or part of your lips, palate, and tongue

Fortunately, no matter what's causing your facial pain, you'll have plenty of options for tackling it. Treatment options for burning mouth syndrome, dental pain, TMJ pain, and sinusitis have exploded over the past few years, and these days your pain-relief choices span everything from the ancient art of acupuncture to the futuristic technology of lasers.

Read on to learn more about some of the many strategies that can give your facial pain an about-face.

Sinusitis and Sinus Infection

Sinusitis affects more than 31 million people each year, making that horrible feeling of an aching head, pressure in your face, and a runny nose one of the most common health complaints in the United States. Billions of dollars are spent annually on treatment and almost half a million sinus surgeries are performed every year. In addition, there are estimates that one out of every five antibiotic prescriptions is given to someone with a sinus infection.[1]

This may all amount to a whole lot of overtreatment. There is a growing consensus that antibiotics are only useful for an extremely limited number of sinus infections,[2] and many doctors believe that surgery is almost never

When to Call the Doctor

Although sinusitis is often something that you can handle on your own, you should call your doctor if:

1. You have mild sinusitis symptoms that haven't improved by 10 days or that continue to get worse over time

2. You have serious pain in your facial sinuses that lasts for more than 2 to 4 days

3. Your face becomes swollen, particularly around the eyes

4. You have a fever or colored discharge from your nose

5. You experience sinusitis more than four times a year

necessary for sinusitis unless it results from a physical obstruction such as nasal polyps or a deviated septum.[3]

That's why the new thinking for sinusitis treatment is that patients and doctors need to get back to the basics. When it comes to treating sinus pain, most of the time doctors should ditch the surgery and the antibiotics and go back to simpler times. Nasal irrigation with a commercial treatment or a neti pot can actually help people as much as or more than many drug treatments. Even better, it doesn't create antibiotic resistance in bacteria or any side effects other than a bit of a mess.

For people with chronic sinus pain, doctors have also become increasingly aware of the importance of environmental effects on individuals' health. Allergies are a major cause of chronic sinusitis; reducing their effects on the body can greatly improve a patient's quality of life, including sinus pain.

Is It Sinusitis?

When your nose is stuffed up, the hollows under your cheekbones ache, and your ears feel like they're full of fluid, there's a good chance you may have sinusitis. Symptoms of sinusitis include:

- Nasal congestion and discharge

- Postnasal drip

- Facial pain, pressure, or fullness

- Headache

Sinusitis comes in two forms: acute and chronic. Acute sinusitis is short lived, lasting less than 4 weeks, and is usually the result of a sinus infection. Although most cases of sinusitis will resolve on their own with self-care, there are times when you should bring your symptoms to the attention of your doctor.

Most of the treatments your doctor will recommend for a sinus infection you can take care of yourself. Based on new scientific evidence, very few doctors these days will even consider prescribing antibiotics until your symptoms have lasted at least a week, so there's little point in going to the doctor before at least that much time has passed unless your symptoms are unusually severe.

If you do visit your doctor, make certain to let her know if you were sick with an upper respiratory infection before you began to experience sinus pain. Knowing the time course of your infection will help her determine whether your sinusitis is more likely to be bacterial or viral so that she can recommend appropriate treatment.

Unlike acute sinusitis, chronic sinusitis, which lasts for more than 8 weeks without improvement or recurs more than four times a year, does require medical attention. Chronic sinusitis can be the result of an underlying health problem—such as allergies, gastric reflux, immunodeficiency, or even dental disease—that it could be important to treat.

Fast Pain Relief

If your face is aching, your nose is running, and you want relief right now, here are some quick sinus pain-relief steps.

1. **Use a saline wash to clean out your sinuses.** Whether you use a neti pot or a commercial saline wash like Ocean, saline irrigation of your sinuses can provide fast relief. It not only clears trapped mucus out of your nose and your sinuses, it can also relieve local inflammation. This should reduce the feeling of facial pressure that can be the most unpleasant part of sinusitis pain.

2. **If you have allergies, make certain you've taken your drugs.** Sinusitis can be a complication of allergic rhinitis. Prescription allergy medications, particularly nasal sprays, can reduce the swelling in your head, relieve the pain, and prevent it from coming back.

3. **Consider an over-the-counter decongestant for short-term relief.** Decongestants help relieve swelling in the nasal passages and may improve the feeling of pressure in your head. However, although doctors frequently recommend these drugs for short-term symptom relief, there is very little research evidence that they are effective treatments for sinusitis.[4]

Relief at Last

The cutting edge of sinusitis treatment is aimed at preventing pain before it occurs. That means keeping your sinuses from getting irritated by allergens or infections so that they don't swell up and start to cause you pain. Here are some steps you can take to try to keep your sinuses under control.

Step 1: **When you're sick, give yourself time to heal.** Acute sinusitis often occurs after you've experienced an upper respiratory infection, and such infections can also set off a flare of chronic pain. If you give

If It's Not Sinusitis

There are several conditions that can be easily mistaken for a sinus infection or chronic sinusitis. They include:

1. **Migraine:** If your headache includes nausea or light or sound sensitivity, then a migraine is the more likely culprit for your pain.

2. **TMD:** The pain from temporomandibular disorders can spread out from your jaw to your ears and under your eyes. If your pain increases when you chew or if you hear a clicking in your jaw, TMD may be more likely than sinusitis.

3. **Cold or flu:** If your nose is running like crazy, you're coughing up a storm, and you are going through tissues so fast you think you should buy stock in Kleenex, but your face doesn't hurt, you probably don't have sinusitis. Not every runny nose is attached to a sinus infection, although, left untreated, a stuffed-up nose can sometimes lead to a stuffed-up head.

yourself time to heal when you have a cold or the flu, you may be able to stop sinusitis before it starts.

Step 2: If you have chronic sinusitis, figure out what triggers your pain. Is your sinusitis worse during allergy season? Does it go away when you're on vacation and not at your house and job? Try to identify any environmental factors that are contributing to your sinus pain so that you can reduce your exposure.

Step 3: Keep your head clean. Whether your sinusitis is acute or chronic, nasal irrigation is a great way not only to treat symptoms but to prevent new sinus infections from taking hold.

Pain Prevention Strategies

Food and Supplements

STAY HYDRATED: It doesn't need to be chicken soup, but you should take in a lot of fluids when you're sick with a sinus infection. Even if your sinusitis is caused by allergies, drinking plenty of water is still a good idea.

The evidence: There's no research on staying hydrated to help improve your sinus symptoms, but that's because doctors recommend it as a matter of course.[5] Besides, drinking enough water is such an important part of overall good health that it's hard to imagine how anyone could ethically study it.

How it works: When you are well hydrated, the mucus in your body becomes thinner and it's easier for your body to remove it from your sinus cavities.

What you need to know: Eight glasses of water a day may not be necessary, but your body will thank you if you keep it replenished. Instead of waiting until you're thirsty to start drinking, try to drink water regularly throughout the day.

Movement Therapies

EXERCISE: Mild to moderate aerobic exercise may be able to help some people with sinusitis clear their heads, at least for a little while. The effects don't usually last that long, but sometimes it can make you feel better to simply get up and go.

The evidence: There is very little scientific evidence for the use of exercise in treating sinusitis. Although historically it has been a standard recommendation,[6] most support is anecdotal. For example, in one study of complementary therapy use, 81 percent of sinusitis patients used exercise to relieve their symptoms.[7]

How it works: Exercise improves blood flow to the sinus regions, which can thin mucus, dilate nasal pathways, and promote drainage. It also increases the activity of cilia in the upper airways, which can help remove trapped mucus from the sinus cavities[8]—a major component of chronic sinusitis.

What you need to know: Exercise is a double-edged sword. If working out makes you feel worse, then stop, but if it makes you feel better, then you shouldn't let your sinusitis stop you. Just be careful. For some patients with sinusitis, particularly those with asthma, an overly vigorous workout can actually make symptoms worse. Overstressing your body when you have sinusitis could lead to serious complications.[9] If your sinusitis comes with a fever or body aches, skip the exercise altogether and go to bed!

Pain Medications and Medical Treatments

ORAL AND NASAL STEROIDS: Much of the pain from sinusitis arises from inflammation of the lining of the sinus cavities, which can also trap mucus and increase pressure. Steroids, both oral and nasal, can help with inflammation and provide symptom relief.

The evidence: A large randomized controlled trial comparing 200 micrograms of mometasone furoate nasal spray twice daily to amoxicillin pills or a nasal spray placebo found that people using the nasal spray had significantly fewer sinus headaches and less facial pain than those in the other two groups. Symptom relief was fast, starting within 2 days of using the spray, and although the placebo spray also improved symptoms, the steroid was more effective.[10]

How it works: Steroids interact with cells to reduce production of the proteins that cause inflammation. Nasal steroids work both locally and systemically (since much of the drug ends up swallowed), and oral steroids affect the whole body at once.

What you need to know: Nasal steroids are generally doctors' first choice of prescription treatment for sinusitis. Steroid sprays direct the medication where it's most needed and reduce the risk of full-body side effects associated with oral steroid medications.

Why You Shouldn't Ask for Antibiotics

The first thing many people do when they think they have a sinus infection is go to the doctor and ask for antibiotics. However, many cases of sinusitis are caused by viruses or allergies and, in these cases, antibiotics will do absolutely no good. Even when sinusitis is caused by bacteria most people will be able to kick the infection on their own. A recent meta-analysis found that 64 percent of sinus infection patients would be cured within 2 weeks with no treatment at all.[11] Furthermore, even when bacterial infections are present, symptom relief is probably faster with treatments such as nasal steroid use or nasal irrigation than antibiotics.

There are certainly some instances in which antibiotic treatment may be appropriate for a sinus infection, but in general most patients will do just as well with rest, relaxation, and other therapies. Current evidence-based guidelines[12] suggest that doctors should not even consider prescribing antibiotics until symptoms have lasted at least 7 to 10 days, and even then the benefit is small.

If you think you have a sinus infection and your doctor tells you that antibiotics aren't right for your treatment, don't push for a prescription. When antibiotic use is restricted to only when it is really necessary, it becomes substantially more effective. Overuse of these drugs can lead to antibiotic-resistant bacteria and serious treatment problems for you as well as other patients down the line.

ANTIHISTAMINES: Somewhere between 10 and 30 percent of the population is affected by nasal allergies[13] that, when left untreated, can progress to sinusitis. Nasal allergies occur because we take in uncountable numbers of small particles every time we breathe, and if we happen to be allergic to some of them, our bodies fight back. These particles can move from the nose into the other sinus cavities and spark inflammation there directly, or the inflammation caused by allergic rhinitis can simply spread.

The evidence: Most of the evidence for antihistamine treatment focuses on treating allergic rhinitis before sinusitis even becomes an issue. A recent randomized trial comparing 5 milligrams of levocetirizine to placebo for the treatment of allergic rhinitis found that the antihistamine significantly reduced symptoms and improved quality of life, although it did cause sleepiness in a small percentage of users.[14]

How it works: Antihistamines interrupt the body's reaction to an allergen. When you are allergic to a substance, your body produces a compound known as histamine, which stimulates inflammation. When left untreated, swelling from nasal allergies can proceed into the sinus cavities and lead to sinusitis.

What you need to know: Antihistamines are only a useful treatment for sinusitis if your sinus pain is caused by an allergic response. The inflammation of the sinus cavities that occurs after infection is a response to different biological signals that will not be interrupted by antihistamines. These drugs should always be taken with a lot of water, since they can cause a thickening of the mucus that may worsen symptoms and also lead to fatigue.[15]

Other Strategies

USE A SALINE NASAL RINSE: Washing out the inside of your sinuses by pouring, or squirting, saltwater up your nose sounds like a really unpleasant idea, until you try it and discover that it works. Although the sensation of water moving through your head can feel somewhat odd, it can provide almost immediate relief for sinusitis symptoms. Most people find enough of a benefit to get past any dislike of the method. Having a glass of regular water handy to wash the taste out of the back of your throat can really reduce the "ick" factor.

The evidence: Numerous randomized controlled trials have shown that nasal irrigation is an effective way to reduce sinusitis symptoms. A recent meta-analysis looking at eight such studies found that, when compared to placebo, nasal irrigation substantially reduced symptoms and improved patients' quality of life. Nasal irrigation also improved patients' quality of life when they combined it with their use of oral antihistamines.[16]

How it works: In addition to the fact that using a nasal rinse can wash mucus out of the sinus cavities, there is some evidence that saline may also have direct effects on inflammation in the sinuses.

What you need to know: Nasal irrigation is so effective at relieving sinus symptoms that in many clinical trials patients don't want to stop using the products they were testing after the study is over!

Nasal irrigation can be used as a treatment on its own or in combination with other sinusitis therapies, and there are commercial products and homemade options available. The main advantages of commercial saline sprays and rinses over neti pots are that they're sterile and already mixed to contain the right amount of salt. Still, many people who have been taught to use neti pots swear by them. They may be a little more work up front, but you can't beat the convenience and cost. It is worth noting that some experts think that rinsing your nose too frequently might increase the risk of sinus infection by stripping away beneficial bacteria, so it is probably a good idea to irrigate your nose only as often as you need to for symptom relief.

CHANGE YOUR ENVIRONMENT: Allergies and irritations are a major cause of sinusitis suffering. Children who live with smokers are particularly prone to sinusitis[17] and other upper respiratory diseases, and other allergens in the house or workplace can also contribute to chronic sinusitis.

The evidence: One case control study found that people with chronic sinusitis were 2.3 times more likely to be exposed to secondhand smoke than people without sinusitis. Furthermore, those cases who had been exposed to smoke had more severe nasal obstructions and discharge and more headaches.[18]

How it works: Irritants and allergens such as cigarette smoke, mold, and pollen cause a reaction in the lining of the sinus cavities that leads to swelling and pain. Limiting your exposure to triggering substances decreases the assault on your body and gives it time to heal.

What you need to know: If your home is the source of allergens, a thorough, deep cleaning may help, particularly if you choose mild, nonirritating cleansers. Limiting the number of soft surfaces that can hold on to dust, pollen, and other irritants is also a good idea. If you're being exposed at work, simply moving your desk to a place with increased airflow might improve your symptoms. In addition, some workplace exposures can be reduced through the use of masks that decrease your inhalation of allergens through the air.[19]

Temporomandibular Disorders (TMD)

Millions of Americans are afflicted with pain in the temporomandibular joint (TMJ)—the hinge of the jaw—and for some of them it is disabling. Scientists estimate that jaw pain causes almost 18 million workdays to be lost each year for each 100 million working adults.[20] Like many other joint diseases, TMJ pain disproportionately affects women, but it tends to hit much earlier in life, between the ages of 18 and 45. Fortunately for most people with TMJ pain, the condition is only a minor concern; only 5 to 10 percent require medical treatment.

TMJ pain can be caused by several underlying conditions, and disorders of the temporomandibular joint are extremely common. In some studies, one-third of adults in the United States report that they've experienced the symptoms of temporomandibular disorders (TMD), and the proportion with asymptomatic damage to the joint is even higher. On physical examination, doctors have found at least one sign of TMD in 40 to 75 percent of the population![21]

Historically, treatment for TMJ pain simply focused on bringing the jaw into proper alignment, but more recent therapies recognize the wide variety of factors that can contribute to jaw pain. TMD is now treated with everything from the newest anti-inflammatory drugs for rheumatoid arthritis to laser therapy and massage. There have also been many surgical advances in the treatment of TMJ pain, but the good news is that the vast majority of sufferers can treat their symptoms without ever needing to go under the knife.

Is It TMD?

Although there are many conditions that can lead to jaw pain, the classic signs of TMD are pretty easy to recognize. Symptoms include:

- **Pain on one side of your face:** Although this pain is usually localized in the jaw, it can spread to the temples, and even the base of the neck.

- **A dull, aching pain that may become more severe when you move your jaw:** The pain may be constant or intermittent, and TMJ pain often varies with the time of day.

- **Limited motion of your jaw:** Sometimes it is difficult to open your mouth as wide as you once could, and activities such as yawning, chewing, and even talking may increase your pain.

- **Locking of your jaw, either in the open or closed position:** TMD is sometimes known as lockjaw because of this disconcerting symptom.

Causes of TMJ Pain

Numerous types of damage to the temporomandibular joint can lead to TMJ pain. Some of the most common include:

1. **Disk derangements:** The intra-articular disk is the cartilage structure that separates the bones of the jaw. If it moves out of proper alignment, the jaw won't function properly, which can cause significant amounts of pain.

2. **Myofascial pain disorders:** This type of TMJ is caused by tension in the muscles of the jaw and may be related to grinding of the teeth. It is most commonly seen in women, and there is a strong association between myofascial pain disorders and affective disorders such as depression, anxiety, and post-traumatic stress.[22]

3. **Osteoarthritis:** This is a type of TMJ that usually only occurs in patients over 50 years of age. It results from wear and tear on the bones and other structures of the jaw and is more likely to cause pain on both sides of the face than other forms of TMJ.

4. **Rheumatoid arthritis:** The temporomandibular joint is not the most common joint affected in individuals with rheumatoid arthritis, but about 17 percent of RA patients do have swelling and pain there.[23]

- **Clenching or grinding of your teeth:** These types of involuntary movements can occur while you are awake or asleep.

- **Clicking or popping sounds when you move the joint:** These sounds are often felt more than heard. Grinding and crackling sounds can be a problem as well. However, noise alone is not a sign of TMD and is actually quite common in the general population.

- **Soreness in the muscles of the jaw and the neck:** When TMD leads to problems with chewing, it can then lead to muscle tension in the jaw, neck, and even shoulders.

It's a good idea to check with your dentist or primary care physician if you think you have TMD because some of the causes of jaw pain can be serious. When diagnosing your jaw pain your doctor will rule out cavities and gum disease and check to make certain that you don't have any other systemic diseases, localized infections, or cancer that could be causing the pain. Your doctor may

When to Call the Dentist

TMD is one of the most common chronic health conditions that prompt you to make an appointment with your dentist. Although TMJ pain usually isn't an emergency, it is a good idea to consult your doctor or dentist if:

- You cannot open or close your jaw all the way, or your jaw does not open equally on both sides
- Your jaw locks in position, even for short periods of time
- Jaw pain is severe enough to affect your quality of life
- You find yourself unable to chew the foods you are used to
- TMJ pain is accompanied by loose teeth or pain in your teeth or jawbones

In addition, if your TMJ pain is constant, lasts for more than a few days, or gets progressively worse, it's a good idea to make an appointment with your doctor or dentist. You don't have to rush, but you don't want to wait any longer than necessary to fix your pain.

also use various imaging techniques to look inside your jaw to see if it contains any structural abnormalities or damage that could be contributing to your TMJ pain. Surgical diagnosis is not generally recommended unless you have been treated for at least 3 months without success.

When you go for a diagnosis, make certain to tell your doctor if you hear noises when you move your jaw as well as whether the pain affects how wide you can open your mouth or causes your jaw to lock in place. It's also a good idea to keep a record of what time of day the pain is at its worst. If it's first thing in the morning, you may be grinding your teeth in your sleep!

Fast Pain Relief

If your jaw aches after every meal or if you have trouble opening your mouth when you get up in the morning, there are some tricks that may be able to help you stop your pain in its tracks.

1. **Take a mild painkiller, preferably an NSAID, according to the directions on the bottle.** Not only are over-the-counter painkillers one of the easiest and most effective ways of dealing with pain of TMJ, but depending on the cause of your pain, NSAIDs may be able to help with any swelling that is contributing to the severity of your symptoms. NSAIDs such as aspirin and ibuprofen block the release of

pro-inflammatory proteins known as prostaglandins, which play an important role in the painful effects of rheumatoid arthritis.

2. **Apply heat.** Heat can be a very effective way to soothe jaw pain and is often recommended by doctors as a first-line treatment for TMD.[24] Both dry heat and moist heat have been shown to be effective at treating jaw pain, so use whatever method is most convenient for you—whether it's a heating pad or a wet washcloth popped in the microwave for a few seconds to steam it up. By applying heat to your jaw, you're causing local blood flow to the area to increase, which promotes healing.

3. **Massage your jaw.** Start off by gently stroking your jaw and then slowly increase the pressure. Like heat, massage stimulates blood flow to the muscles of the jaw, which both relieves pain and helps you to relax and prevent the pain from getting worse.[25] Massage also releases endorphins, hormones that can keep the feeling of pain at bay.

Relief at Last

Cutting-edge TMD treatment is aimed at preventing pain before it starts, particularly for individuals with myofascial pain disorders. There are several easy steps you can take to reduce the effects of TMJ pain on your life, or even stop pain in its tracks.

Step 1: Watch your mouth. Paying attention to your mouth can help you catch bad habits before they cause real problems. Tooth grinding, cheek biting, chewing on pens, and other activities that stress the muscles of the jaw can increase your risk of TMJ pain.

Step 2: Relax and limit your stress. When people are stressed and anxious, they tense up. Excess muscle tension in the face, as well as the tooth grinding that may accompany stress, can encourage TMJ symptoms. Depression and anxiety are also associated with TMD in other ways that remain poorly understood.

Step 3: Use gentle exercise to retrain the muscles of your jaw. If your jaw is tense and tight, gentle stretching exercises can help it relax and open more fully. You should also make certain to chew on both sides of your mouth so that the muscles are evenly worked.

Step 4: Eat smart. If you have TMD, it can be painful to put too much pressure on the muscles of your jaw. Therefore, when chewing hurts, consider restricting your diet to soft foods to give tired muscles a rest. Limiting caffeine is also a good idea since it can increase muscle tension.

Step 5: Practice good posture, awake and asleep.[26] Good posture reduces stress on the muscles of the neck and jaw. Paying attention to your posture while you're awake and sleeping on your back or on your side—with your jaw in proper alignment—can help stop TMJ pain before it starts.

Pain Prevention Strategies

Movement Therapies

JAW EXERCISES: One of the many complications of TMJ pain is difficulty opening and moving the jaw. Fortunately, exercises designed to stretch the muscles of the jaw and improve posture can reduce TMJ pain and improve jaw mobility.

The evidence: One randomized controlled trial of 60 people with TMJ pain originating in their chewing muscles found that the patients in the posture training group had large and statistically significant reductions in their pain. They also increased the mean opening width of their jaw by more than 5 millimeters compared to a 1.2-millimeter improvement in the control group.[27] Several randomized controlled trials of jaw stretching have also shown significant improvements in both pain and jaw opening.[28]

How it works: Jaw-stretching exercises focus on relaxing the muscles of the jaw in order to decrease pain and increase range of motion. In contrast, postural exercises use repetitive movements to improve the alignment of the structures of the jaw. Both reduce pain by making sure everything is working the way it should and also improve the strength and flexibility of the muscles of the jaw.

What you need to know: Talk to your doctor before starting postural or jaw exercises so that you can learn how to do them safely. You should never push these exercises to the point of pain since doing so can make your symptoms worse instead of better.

Touch Therapies

MASSAGE: Both self- and professional massage of the muscles of the neck and jaw can reduce the pain associated with TMD, particularly pain of the myofascial variety. Gently stroking the skin of your jaw and then slowly increasing pressure will increase blood flow to tense and painful muscles and also identify trigger points, which are small knots or painful spasms in the muscle.[29]

The evidence: Much of the evidence for the use of massage in the relief of TMJ pain comes from studies of self-care, in which people report using self-massage for pain relief and prevention,[30] as well as small observational studies.[31] One randomized controlled trial of physical therapy for TMJ pain found that a massage-containing protocol had positive effects, but the study was too small to draw definitive conclusions.[32]

How it works: Massage increases blood flow to the muscles and releases endorphins, which together produce a feeling of warmth and relieve pain. Massage may also help to release spasms in the jaw and relieve the pain associated with them.

What you need to know: Learning to massage yourself means that you have pain relief quite literally at your fingertips. While professional massage can also be a useful therapy, once you know how to massage your own jaw you can ease your TMJ pain at any time.

ACUPUNCTURE: Acupuncture is often recommended for TMJ pain, particularly pain of muscular origin. It is used so frequently, in fact, that several new types of acupuncture for TMD have been developed, including a laser-based technique.

The evidence: Evidence for acupuncture's effectiveness in treating TMJ pain is somewhat mixed. Of four recent randomized controlled trials comparing acupuncture to sham acupuncture, one showed significant decreases in facial pain, neck pain, and headache;[33] one showed improvements in both pain and various indices of joint function, including mouth-opening width;[34] one showed improvements in pain but not mouth opening;[35] and one showed equal improvement in both the treatment and control groups—raising the concern of a placebo effect.[36] Still, recent reviews have concluded that there is moderate evidence to support acupuncture for TMD pain relief.[37]

How it works: The theory behind acupuncture is that precise needle placement improves the flow of energy in the body. However, because of the study that showed an improvement in both the treatment and control groups, placement may not be as important as skin penetration. In that study, the sham acupuncture involved inserting needles shallowly into "nonactive" sites. In the other studies, sham acupuncture did not involve needle penetration.

What you need to know: Although the studies examining its effects have been small, it seems that acupuncture can be a good option for short-term pain relief from TMJ. In particular, local acupuncture of the LI-4 point between the thumb and first finger seems promising, although more research is clearly needed to explain the nature of the effect.[38]

Mind-Body Therapies

COGNITIVE-BEHAVIORAL THERAPY: Cognitive-behavioral therapy (CBT) helps patients develop habits they can use to improve their health and gives them the skills they need to deal with their pain in a positive way. For example, therapies might contain instructions to check and correct jaw posture regularly, practice relaxation techniques, and engage in breathing exercises.

The evidence: A randomized controlled trial comparing a CBT protocol with more general health care information sessions found that at 1 year after treatment 35 percent of TMJ patients could go about their life without interference from pain compared to only 12 percent of the control group. Patients who received CBT training also had less pain, less depression, and significantly improved jaw function.[39]

How it works: Cognitive behavioral therapy teaches pain management skills, such as massage and postural exercises, as well as techniques for emotionally and practically coping with pain. With the help of a trained professional, individuals with TMD develop self-care plans that they can use to improve their quality of life. CBT sessions may also incorporate practice with relaxation techniques that it may be difficult for people to manage on their own.

What you need to know: Cognitive behavioral therapy won't improve your TMJ pain overnight. It takes hard, consistent work to develop the skills you need to live your life to the fullest. In addition, you have to practice the relaxation, exercise, and attention techniques outside of the therapist's office for this type of therapy to do the most good.

BIOFEEDBACK AND RELAXATION THERAPIES: Jaw tension is a significant contributor to TMJ pain. Biofeedback and other relaxation techniques can help people release tension and exercise some control over their pain.[40]

The evidence: An early study comparing biofeedback and relaxation found that both techniques were effective at long-term symptom relief. Two years after patients completed treatment, 60 percent of the relaxation group and 54 percent of the biofeedback group were still experiencing either significant improvement in their symptoms or were symptom free.[41] It is difficult to evaluate the precise nature of the effect since the study did not contain a control group; however, several additional studies have also found benefits in different biofeedback techniques for the reduction of pain.[42]

How it works: Biofeedback uses measurements of physiological signals either to encourage overall relaxation or to help patients retrain the muscles involved in chewing. Audio or visual signals give objective feedback about whether a person is achieving the desired physical state.

What you need to know: Looking at the effects of relaxation on TMJ pain, biofeedback does not necessarily improve outcomes over relaxation training alone. However, biofeedback may make relaxation training more fun. There are several commercial biofeedback devices and games available that enable individuals to work on relaxation techniques outside of the clinic setting while still getting the advantage of real-time feedback.

Pain Medications and Medical Treatments

JOINT INJECTIONS: Injections of painkillers and anti-inflammatory drugs directly into the temporomandibular joint allow the medications to act quickly because they're immediately available at the site of pain.

The evidence: In one randomized controlled trial comparing injections of morphine, saline solution (placebo), or a topical anesthetic (Carbostesin), scientists found that all patients experienced pain relief within an hour after injection. However, the patients in the placebo and anesthetic groups found that their pain levels quickly returned to normal, while pain relief in the morphine patients lasted for at least a week.[43]

How it works: Injections may include painkillers such as morphine, anti-inflammatory drugs such as corticosteroids, or drugs designed to lubricate the joint. Multiple types of drugs may also be combined to broaden an injection's effects. In addition, beyond the effects of individual drugs, simply injecting fluid of any kind into the joint increases the space between the bones, which can reduce pressure and relieve pain.

What you need to know: Some patients experience serious side effects after this type of injection, including further damage to the joint. Furthermore, how long the effects of intrajoint injections last varies based on the drug used. Although you will likely experience immediate pain relief, the effects may wear off over the course of hours, days, or weeks, necessitating additional injections. Scientists are currently working on alternate methods for delivering drugs into the temporomandibular joint, including investigations into time-release gels.[44]

ORAL PAINKILLERS: The painkillers most often prescribed for TMD are chosen for their ability to relieve pain and to reduce inflammation. NSAIDs— nonsteroidal anti-inflammatory drugs, which include painkillers such as aspirin, ibuprofen, and naproxen sodium—are widely recommended for TMJ pain, although there are few clinical trials that demonstrate their effectiveness.

Botox for TMJ Pain

Botulism toxin is a neurotoxin made by the bacterium *Clostridium botulinum*. It is best known by the trade name Botox, for its use in cosmetic surgery to eliminate forehead lines. However, it has also been used as a treatment for muscle pain and spasm for many years. Botulism toxin works by interrupting the signals that cause muscles to contract, preventing or reducing both the conscious ability to move the muscle and involuntary spasm.

Although Botox is not a front-line therapy for TMJ pain, some doctors do use it for patients who have not responded to more conservative therapies.[45] There have been several studies demonstrating its effectiveness in reducing pain. One randomized controlled trial found reduced pain in 91 percent of individuals and increased pain-free mouth opening. But the treatment can have unpleasant side effects including difficulty chewing hard food, temporary paralysis, and facial asymmetry. While some studies reported no such adverse events, others saw them in more than half of all treated patients.[46]

The evidence: In one noncontrolled study, the maximum suggested dose of diclofenac—50 milligrams, three times a day—reduced pain in patients with arthritic TMJ by more than 50 percent over 3 months;[47] however, a shorter placebo-controlled study showed no effect.[48] A high-quality randomized controlled trial of 500 milligrams of naproxen sodium twice daily also reduced TMJ pain by more than 50 percent compared to placebo, but only after 3 weeks of treatment.[49]

How it works: NSAIDs interrupt the manufacture of pro-inflammatory cytokines. They are also painkillers, but since randomized controlled trials of several NSAIDs have shown them to be effective only after extended use, it seems likely that it is their anti-inflammatory properties that cause the reduction in TMJ pain.[50]

What you need to know: Long-term use of NSAIDs can cause side effects that range from mild stomach upset to kidney damage. See Chapter 6 for more information on how to use NSAIDs safely.

MUSCLE RELAXANTS: Muscle tension is associated with certain types of TMJ pain, as is stress. Some doctors will prescribe muscle relaxants to reduce physical tension and jaw pain.

The evidence: A small randomized controlled trial compared the effects of an antianxiety medicine (clonazepam/Klonopin, 0.5 milligrams at night) and a muscle relaxant (cyclobenzaprine/Flexeril, 10 milligrams at night) to placebo for the reduction of morning jaw pain. Although all three treatments resulted in a significant reduction in pain, in part a result of the placebo effect, the muscle relaxant did significantly improve pain reduction over the placebo.[51]

How it works: Muscle relaxants decrease the pressure on the temporomandibular joint as well as relieving pain in the chewing muscles.

What you need to know: Although doctors often prescribe muscle relaxants for TMJ pain,[52] there are very few studies demonstrating their effectiveness or establishing appropriate dosing. If the medication your doctor recommends is too strong or too weak, don't be shy about asking him to adjust the prescription.

TRICYCLIC ANTIDEPRESSANTS: These drugs affect the processing of three neurotransmitters in the brain: serotonin, norepinephrine, and dopamine. They are used to treat depression, anxiety, and other affective disorders such as post-traumatic stress, all of which are strongly linked to certain types of TMJ pain. These types of conditions can affect the way that pain is processed in the brain, and treating them can have both direct and indirect effects on a person's experience with TMD.

The evidence: In a small randomized trial, 12 female patients with chronic TMJ pain were treated for 2 weeks with either 25 milligrams a day of the antidepressant amitriptyline or a placebo. Seventy-five percent of the patients in the treatment group experienced a significant reduction in pain compared to only 28 percent in the placebo group.[53]

How it works: For some patients, chronic pain appears to be mediated by changes in the brain that can be treated effectively with antidepressant drugs, which increase serotonin production and affect pain perception. Reducing psychological stress may also lower jaw tension and relieve pressure on the joint.

What you need to know: Many people with anxiety and other affective disorders are also troubled by chronic pain. Although there is not sufficient evidence to recommend widespread use of antidepressants for TMD patients,[54] they may be a useful treatment resource for those whose pain seems to be related to depression and similar conditions.

Other Strategies

REMOVABLE ORTHODONTIC APPLIANCES: Mouth guards, bite blocks, and splints are all types of orthodontic appliances used to keep people's jaws in alignment and stop them from grinding their teeth. Although these devices are usually custom made by dentists, in recent years less expensive over-the-counter options have been made available for home treatment.

The evidence: Both soft and hard removable orthodontic appliances are widely used in clinical practice, although the evidence for their benefit is mixed.

How it works: These devices stabilize the temporomandibular joint, discourage tooth grinding, and redistribute the forces on the jaw.

What you need to know: At this point, scientists believe that these appliances are mostly useful for patients with myofascial TMJ pain rather than for those individuals whose TMD is caused by problems with jaw alignment.[55] Their main benefit may be in reducing nighttime tooth grinding.

Types of TMJ Surgery

Most people with TMJ pain can be treated successfully without surgery, and surgery is usually not considered until all other options for medical care and self-care have been exhausted. However, for some people, surgery can sometimes be an effective choice for relieving TMJ pain.[56] There are several types of TMJ surgery.

1. **Arthrocentesis:** This is the simplest form of TMJ surgery and involves injecting fluids into the joint to wash or lubricate it. It may also involve dislodging a stuck disk with a blunt instrument. Arthrocentesis is most often tried when someone's mouth has suddenly locked closed despite her having no previous history of TMJ pain.

2. **Arthroscopy:** This type of surgery is used to visualize problems in the temporomandibular joint and move a dislocated articular disk back into place. Depending on what the doctor finds and on the patient's TMD history, inflamed tissue might also be removed or an artificial anchor might be inserted to hold the disk in place and prevent further movement.

3. **Diskectomy:** This procedure removes a damaged articular disk from a person with severe TMD to improve pain; however, failure to insert a replacement disk can cause long-term wear and tear on the joint.

4. **Joint replacement:** Seen as a last resort option for TMJ pain that cannot be resolved by any other method, joint replacement surgery replaces all or part of the temporomandibular joint with artificial constructs.[57]

Dental Pain and Tooth Sensitivity

The good news about most dental pain is that it's treatable. The bad news is that it's extremely common. There are estimates that between 25 and 38 percent of people have sensitive teeth, and the prevalence of toothaches may also be as high as 30 percent.[58]

After cavities, broken teeth, and other acute problems that require an immediate dental visit have been eliminated—along with TMJ (see page 120) and referred pain from other health conditions—most of the tooth pain that remains is attributable to dentin hypersensitivity. Tooth sensitivity most often comes from damage to the gums, either from surgery or gum disease, that leaves the nerves at the base of the teeth more exposed. However, it can also be caused by damage to the visible surfaces of the teeth.

The good news is that technology has been a great boon for people suffering from sensitive teeth. There is an ever-expanding number of options for prevention and symptom relief, both in the drugstore and at the dentist's office. Still, the best way to prevent this type of chronic tooth pain is to practice good dental hygiene from an early age. If you can avoid damage to your teeth and problems with your gums, you're unlikely to develop hypersensitivity in the first place.

Is It Dental Pain or Tooth Sensitivity?

If you wince in pain every time you drink a glass of really cold water or find that eating ice cream makes your teeth ache, then there's a good chance you're suffering from dentin hypersensitivity. Sensitivity to heat, cold, touch, and sweet or spicy foods usually comes in the form of a sharp pain that may be followed by a dull ache.

Although dentin hypersensitivity doesn't necessarily require a dentist's intervention, you should always see a dentist if you start experiencing pain in your teeth. Tooth pain other than hypersensitivity can and should be treated professionally because leaving dental infections untreated can lead to serious health problems. Tooth pain can also be caused by serious problems; in a small number of people it's the first sign of coronary heart disease.[59]

Fast Pain Relief

The single best thing you can do for a toothache is make an appointment with your dentist. However, if your teeth are in pain because of sensitivity to cold or other substances, there are also several things that you can do to relieve your pain right now.

Understanding Tooth Sensitivity

Teeth are made up of several different layers of materials. The visible outer later, the enamel, covers a secondary layer of a material known as dentin. This dentin layer is full of tiny holes, called tubules, through which sensations can be transmitted to the dental nerves contained in the pulp below.

Normally the dentin tubules are protected by enamel, but tooth enamel only extends to the gum line. In individuals whose gums have receded because of age, gum disease, or dental surgery, the dentin tubules are still covered by a material known as cementum, but this layer is easily worn away by simple toothbrushing and exposure to acidic foods.

When a tooth is sensitive, it's because its dentin tubules have become exposed to all the substances you put in your mouth. Drinking cold or hot liquids, eating sugar, or putting pressure on your teeth can cause the fluid inside those tubules to move. This leads to pressure changes around the dental nerves, which respond by signaling pain.

In order to short-circuit the pain of sensitive teeth, treatment involves either coating teeth with a substance that blocks the entrances to the dentin tubules or deadening the sensitivity of the nerves.[60]

1. **Brush your teeth with a desensitizing toothpaste containing potassium nitrate.** Potassium nitrate can depolarize the dental nerves[62] and stop them from sending pain signals to your brain. These products don't generally provide long-term pain relief or help prevent pain in the future, but they can be a great way to short-circuit an intense sensitivity episode when it occurs.

2. **Take a painkiller.** Although painkillers don't solve the underlying problem of tooth sensitivity, they can be a good option if your teeth are in severe pain. Painkillers recommended for the treatment of acute dental pain[63] include:

   Ibuprofen: 200–400 milligrams every 4 to 6 hours, with the possibility of going up to 600 milligrams every 4 to 6 hours

Tylenol: 325–1000 milligrams every 4 to 6 hours, not more than four times a day

Oruvall: 200 milligrams every 6 to 8 hours

Actron: 12.5 milligrams every 4 to 6 hours

Vioxx: 50 milligrams 4 times a day

3. **Avoid the triggers of your pain.** If your teeth are primarily sensitive to extremes of temperature, then avoid very hot or very cold foods. Brush your teeth gently with lukewarm water. Always have water around to drink if you're going to eat a food that you know can trigger a pain signal. In addition, since tooth sensitivity affects individual teeth rather than your whole mouth, you can try to direct problematic substances away from the most sensitive teeth. In general, however, it's important to chew with both sides of your mouth since uneven chewing is associated with TMJ pain and other dental problems.[64]

When to Call the Dentist

Although sensitivity to hot or cold probably isn't a dental emergency, there are types of dental pain that merit an immediate call to the dentist. Dental pain may not only signal a health emergency, such as cardiac disease, but some information suggests that dental disease may contribute to such serious problems as well.[61] It's a good idea to call your dentist right away if you have:

● Dental pain associated with swelling or heat in the jaw

● Sudden, severe dental pain

● A toothache that is not associated with temperature changes or food

● Ulcers or pus in your mouth

● Unexpected pain following dental surgery

More mild forms of dental pain, such as dental sensitivity, should also be checked out by your dentist, although they do not usually require urgent care.

Relief at Last

The best way to avoid the pain of sensitive teeth is to prevent the damage that causes it. That means doing everything you can to optimize the health of your teeth and gums.

Step 1: Brush your teeth twice a day with fluoride toothpaste. The fluoride protects the enamel from damage, which helps keep your dentin tubules safely under cover.

Step 2: Floss once a day. Flossing removes food and bacteria that can get stuck between teeth and irritate your gums. Healthy gums make an enormous difference in preventing the development of dentin hypersensitivity.

Step 3: Visit your dentist regularly. Not only can your dentist do a more thorough job of cleaning your teeth than you can, but by visiting regularly you can try to arrest any dental damage before it becomes severe. In addition, if you already have sensitive teeth, your dentist has access to a whole array of long-acting coating products and desensitizing treatments that can help you deal with your pain.

Pain Prevention Strategies

Food and Supplements

AVOID ACIDIC FOODS AND BEVERAGES: If your mother told you that drinking soda was bad for your teeth, she was right. Soda and other acidic foods can break down the protective coatings that cover your teeth and help block pain.

The evidence: Numerous in vitro studies[65] have directly demonstrated that exposure to acidic food products, such as citrus juices[66] and vinegar,[67] can wear down the coating on the dentin surface. Dietary studies in humans also seem to support that conclusion. For example, drinking juice seemed to be tightly linked to dental erosion in one study of Canadian athletes.[68]

How it works: Acidic drinks and other liquids can dissolve the outer layers of the tooth, exposing the dentin tubules and causing an increase in tooth sensitivity.

What you need to know: Popular beverages and foods containing acids include orange juice (ascorbic and citric acid), cola (phosphoric acid), white wine (tartaric acid), sports/energy drinks (various), and vinegar (acetic acid). Limiting the amount of these foods may help preserve the health of your remaining dentin and slow the progress of your tooth sensitivity. Rinsing your mouth with water after eating may help reduce pain, but you should try to avoid brushing your teeth right after eating acidic foods, since doing so can increase their damaging effects.[69]

Pain Medications and Medical Treatments

TOOTH COATINGS: Resins, varnishes, and sealants sound more like products you'd find in a hardware store than in your dentist's office, but these coatings can be a good way of protecting your sensitive teeth.

The evidence: One 2009 study looking at the effect of a single application of a 5 percent fluoride varnish found that patients' pain scores from exposure to compressed air and ice dropped from 35 (air) and 68 (ice) to 26 and 55 at 2 weeks after treatment and 21 and 35 at 6 months.[70] Other studies have shown similar effects for other types of coatings.[71]

How it works: Although the different types of tooth sealants work in different ways, they all are based on the same principle: coating the outside of the tooth so that the dentin tubules are no longer exposed.

What you need to know: Long-acting sealants can only be applied in your dentist's office, but once applied, they last for years. Right now there is no significant evidence to suggest that one particular sealant is better than any other.

Tooth Whitening and Sensitivity

Tooth whitening is a cosmetic procedure performed to reduce the appearance of stains on the teeth. It can be done either in a dentist's office or with commercially available products in the home. Most whitening techniques use a hydrogen peroxide solution, sometimes in combination with light treatments or other adjunct therapies.

Depending on the strength of the product used, whitening procedures often lead not just to color changes in the teeth but increased sensitivity. This sensitivity is usually minor and short lived, but it can occasionally be severe and last for a month or more.

If you are already suffering from tooth sensitivity, you may want to avoid tooth-whitening procedures unless you have extreme amounts of staining that are significantly impacting your quality of life.[72]

Afraid of the Dentist?

One of the biggest new directions in dental research is looking for ways to encourage people to get into that chair. The first step? Reducing fear. Anxiety about dental care not only makes people experiencing dental symptoms suffer for longer than they need to because they avoid a visit, it can also make any pain they experience in the dentist's chair worse.[73]

That's why you should never be afraid to ask for anesthesia if you need it. If pain during a dental visit is going to make you unwilling to return for further care, then talk to your dentist about what can be done to prevent it before the visit starts. Some dentists will be willing to do their work using sedation or general anesthesia, which can be a great resource for particularly nervous children and adults.[74]

TOPICAL DESENSITIZERS: Toothpastes and other topical desensitizing agents applied in a dental office are often stronger or longer-lasting versions of the products you can find in the drugstore.

The evidence: In one study looking at a single in-office application of a desensitizing paste containing 8 percent arginine and calcium carbonate, researchers found that, compared to those who received a control paste, people who received the active paste immediately became less sensitive to pain from air pressure and cold. The effect wore off sometime between 1 and 3 months after application.[75]

How it works: Some desensitizers partially block the openings of the dentin tubules. Others, particularly those containing potassium salts, interfere with nerve cell signaling. Most in-office products use the first mechanism, since the action of potassium salts tends to be short lived.

What you need to know: There are a lot of desensitizing products out there, but studies suggest that in general they have similar effects.[76] Research is complicated by the fact that teeth may also become naturally less sensitive over time, even without treatment. This can make accurate estimates of a product's strength somewhat difficult to make.

Other Strategies

CHOOSE THE RIGHT TOOTHBRUSH: Brushing your teeth twice a day is an important part of your dental care routine. Always use an ADA–approved toothpaste containing fluoride to reduce your risk of cavities and choose a soft-bristled toothbrush that is comfortable to use in your mouth.

The evidence: One study examining the effects of providing a specially designed "sensitive" toothbrush to patients with dentin hypersensitivity found that using the gentle toothbrush significantly reduced sensitivity to both pressure and cold. However, since the study had no control group and no information about what previous types of toothbrush were used, it is difficult to say how much of the change was a result of the particular brush that was studied.[79]

How it works: Hard toothbrushes and bad brushing technique can cause unnecessary wear and tear on the surfaces of your teeth. Using gentle strokes and a soft toothbrush allows you to clean your teeth without damaging them.

What you need to know: Any ultra-soft or soft-headed toothbrush should do a good job of safely cleaning your teeth. Just stay away from the brushes labeled medium or hard.

USE A DESENSITIZING TOOTHPASTE:

Picking a good toothbrush is only the first step to optimizing your brushing habits when you have dentin hypersensitivity. It may also help to use one of the many toothpastes designed to reduce the sensitivity of your teeth.

The evidence: Using scanning electron microscopy, scientists recently measured the effects of several sensitivity toothpastes in vitro—two containing potassium (Sensodyne Freshmint and Colgate Sensitive) and one containing a bioactive glass (Novamin). All three products greatly reduced tooth permeability, although the Novamin was slightly more

On the Horizon

Laser Therapy for Tooth Sensitivity

In recent years there has been a growing interest in the potential medical uses of lasers. Early studies suggest that they may be a viable option for the treatment of dentin hypersensitivity. One study of 40 patients treated with either a fluoride varnish, a high-intensity laser, or a combination of both found that, compared to controls, sensitivity to a cold air blast was reduced by 43, 50, and 83 percent, respectively.[77] Combining the laser and the varnish was even more effective.

Both high-intensity and low-intensity lasers can be used for dentin hypersensitivity treatment. Although high-intensity lasers work by melting the surface of the tooth to block off dentin tubules, the mechanism by which low-intensity lasers reduce pain is not well understood. Some scientists think low-intensity laser radiation increases production of hard surface products, while others think that it alters conduction.[78]

effective than the other two. It was also better at protecting teeth from a 24-hour immersion in artificial saliva. Sensodyne, however, was the most effective at preventing tooth damage by a 1-minute treatment with citric acid.[83]

How it works: Like other desensitizing products, desensitizing toothpastes work either by reducing the amount of fluid that flows through the dentin tubules or by interrupting the way that nerves signal pain. Desensitizing toothpastes also usually contain fluoride to help build strong teeth.

What you need to know: There are several over-the-counter desensitizing toothpastes currently available in the United States. Just follow the directions on the package. Your dentist may also be able to prescribe a stronger option if the commercially available toothpastes don't work for you, but try several different brands before giving up. One specific combination of active and inactive ingredients may work better for you than another.

Burning Mouth Syndrome

If you are suffering from a burning or tingling sensation in your mouth that has no obvious cause, your doctor may diagnose you as having burning mouth syndrome. This is a relatively common problem. It affects more than one million people in the United States,[84] mostly women of middle age and older. In fact, in postmenopausal women, the prevalence may be as high as 33 percent.[85]

Current treatments for burning mouth syndrome focus on finding the reason that a person's mouth is burning so the source of the pain can be eliminated. For many people, mouth pain seems to be linked with affective disorders such as anxiety and depression, and treating those problems can be the fastest route to improving their symptoms. In other patients, burning mouth syndrome seems to be linked to medication side effects or food allergies, and looking at when symptoms started can give doctors a clue about how to make them go away. What if you're one of the many people whose burning mouth syndrome remains unexplained? Some scientists think nerve or circulatory problems may be causing your pain. But even without an explanation, there are still treatments available, such as clonazepam, that may help.

Is It Burning Mouth Syndrome?

The one symptom all patients with burning mouth syndrome have in common is, as the name of the disorder implies, a burning sensation in their mouths. While most burning mouth syndrome symptoms occur on the tongue, they can also affect the lips and the palate. People's experience of the timing of burning mouth pain also varies; sometimes it's constant, sometimes it's intermittent, and sometimes it increases in severity throughout the day.[86]

Burning mouth syndrome usually isn't diagnosed until you have experienced pain for several months. In part, this is because doctors primarily diagnose burning mouth syndrome by looking for underlying causes of your pain. If there's no good reason for your mouth to be burning, you may end up being diagnosed with the condition by default.

That's why it's a good idea to keep a diary of your pain symptoms to discuss with your doctor or dentist. Be sure to record where the pain appears in your mouth, what times during the day you experience it, if anything improves your symptoms, and when the pain first appeared. The more information your doctor has about your burning mouth symptoms, the better chance she has of finding an effective way to treat them. In fact, if your pain is intermittent, you might even want to keep track of the food you eat and the medications you take to see if there is a correlation between the timing of your symptoms and something you're putting in your mouth. The Pain Diary in Part Three may help you zero in on the cause of your pain.

Fast Pain Relief

If you've been suffering from burning mouth syndrome for long enough to get a diagnosis, you know that there's no quick fix for your pain. Still, there are a few tricks you can try that may reduce the toll that burning mouth syndrome takes on your mind and body.

1. **Keep your mouth moist.** When your mouth is dry, the sensations of burning and pain can increase. Drinking water or sucking on a hard

candy can help; but if dry mouth is a frequent problem for you, it's worth asking your doctor to prescribe a lubricating solution.

2. **Work on your oral habits.** If you tend to clench your teeth, chew on your lips, bite your tongue, or otherwise play with your mouth, make a real effort to stop. These activities can dry out your mouth and irritate or damage your skin, increasing your pain rather than making you feel better.

3. **Find new ways to deal with depression and stress.** Anxiety, stress, and depression are closely linked to many people's experiences with burning mouth pain, both because these conditions affect the way that sensations are processed in the brain and because people have reduced saliva production when they're stressed.[91] If you can improve your mental health through therapy, medication, or a combination of both, it may also have the pleasant side effect of relieving your physical pain.

Relief at Last

The best thing you can do to relieve your burning mouth pain is to identify its underlying cause. Although your doctor is an excellent resource, there is also some research and experimentation you can do on your own.

Step 1: Try to figure out what's causing your pain. Check your prescriptions in a *Physicians' Desk Reference* to see if any of them has the side effect of mouth pain. See if your mouth is sensitive to the food you're putting into it by selectively eliminating foods from your diet for 2 weeks. Eliminate mouthwash from your regimen since it can dry you out. Switch to a new toothpaste to make certain that it isn't the source of irritation.

Step 2: Reduce your stress. Stress can make burning mouth pain worse, so finding ways to reduce your stress can also help you treat your pain. Whether this means taking time to go for a walk each day, adjusting your workload, or seeing a doctor for professional help, anxiety reduction can both reduce your pain and make it easier to cope with.

Step 3: Try supplementation. Experimenting with zinc supplementation is a relatively low-cost and low-risk technique for treating burning mouth at home. Zinc supplements are available over-the-counter and as a component of multivitamins. Just don't take more than the recommended dose.

Pain Prevention Strategies

Food and Supplements

ZINC: Zinc is the second most abundant mineral in the body after iron. Several studies have suggested that zinc deficiency[92] may play a role in burning mouth syndrome for a subset of patients.

The evidence: A study of 276 patients with burning mouth syndrome found that approximately 25 percent of them had low blood zinc levels. When they were treated with 14.1 milligrams a day of zinc and a steroid gargle, 72 percent of the patients experienced partial or complete pain relief compared to 52 percent of the controls, who received only the gargle.[93]

How it works: Zinc plays a role in the function of the nervous, immune, and reproductive systems. It is also associated with good mental health. In people with zinc deficiency, dietary supplementation can help raise levels to normal and improve overall health. Zinc may also improve taste perception,[94] which is a problem common in individuals with burning mouth syndrome.

What you need to know: Follow-up studies are definitely indicated to see how well zinc replacement works in larger populations of individuals with burning mouth syndrome, including those who are not noticeably zinc deficient. However, adding a zinc-containing multivitamin to your diet if you are not already

Acupuncture for Burning Mouth Syndrome

A small study investigating the use of acupuncture for burning mouth syndrome may also have uncovered some of the reasons why individuals experience burning mouth pain. The study, which was designed as a controlled trial to examine the relationship between the circulation of the tongue and burning mouth symptoms, found that acupuncture seemed to improve certain circulatory problems seen in the mouths of people experiencing discomfort that were not present in the mouths of people without pain. The average pain that patients experienced dropped from an 8 before acupuncture treatment to a 2 afterward. Six months after the end of the therapy their pain had increased slightly, to a 3, but it remained stable at that level for another 18 months of follow-up. Control patients without burning mouth syndrome experienced an average pain level of zero for the whole study period.[98]

taking one poses minimal risk to your health as long as you stay below the tolerable upper limit, which for adults is 40 milligrams a day.[95]

CAPSAICIN: Capsaicin is the substance that makes hot peppers burn your mouth. That's why it's slightly ironic that it may also be an effective treatment for burning mouth syndrome.

The evidence: A small, placebo-controlled trial involving 50 patients with burning mouth syndrome found that swallowing capsaicin caplets significantly reduced mouth pain.[96] Another small study of 14 patients found that a thrice daily mouth rinse with 250 milligrams of red pepper emulsion in 50 milliliters of water could also be effective.[97]

How it works: Capsaicin causes a burning sensation in the mouth, but that sensation can desensitize the nerves of the mouth to pain by overloading their response cycle.

What you need to know: Capsaicin pills can cause serious stomach upset when used too often. Although topical capsaicin treatments such as "hot" candies and Tabasco sauce have been shown to be useful for the treatment of other oral pain syndromes, there have been few studies of their efficacy in treating burning mouth.

Mind-Body Therapies

PSYCHOTHERAPY: There is some evidence that certain types of oral habits—including pressing the tongue against the teeth, clenching or grinding the teeth, and biting the tongue or lips—may predispose individuals to burning mouth syndrome.[99] In addition,

»More Research Needed

Alpha-Lipoic Acid

Alpha-lipoic acid is an antioxidant that, unlike the essential fatty acids found in fish oil, can be made by the body. However, it is also found in certain foods such as spinach, broccoli, brewer's yeast, and organ meats, and it can be purchased as a supplement.

Although it was initially considered to be an extremely promising treatment for burning mouth syndrome,[100] the evidence for alpha-lipoic acid has recently come under fire. Three early randomized controlled studies of alpha-lipoic acid that seemed to demonstrate its efficacy at reducing symptoms were all published by the same research group. The two most promising of these were both open-label, meaning that subjects knew whether they were receiving a drug or a placebo. When patients were blinded to what drug they were taking, the supplement's effects were diminished as the placebo effect became more pronounced. Three later studies published in 2009 found that alpha-lipoic acid had no greater effect on pain than a placebo.[101, 102, 103]

burning mouth syndrome has been linked to anxiety, depression, and other affective disorders.[104, 105, 106]

The evidence: A study comparing group psychotherapy to the use of a placebo pill found that pain scores improved in 70 percent of the patients in the psychotherapy group but only 40 percent of patients in the placebo group.[107]

How it works: Different types of psychotherapy can be a useful way not only of adjusting problematic habits but also of improving people's ability to deal with their pain. In addition, since burning mouth syndrome is linked to affective disorders such as anxiety and depression, for many patients treating those disorders may also improve symptoms by eliminating their underlying cause.

What you need to know: Both individualized cognitive-behavioral therapy[108] and group psychotherapy have been shown to improve the pain that people experience from burning mouth syndrome. It may, however, take several months for therapy to have an effect.

Pain Medications and Medical Treatments

CLONAZEPAM: Clonazepam (Klonopin) is an antiseizure drug that is also used for the treatment of panic attacks. It is one of a class of medications known as benzodiazepines.

Could My Medicine Be Causing My Burning Mouth Syndrome?

Burning mouth symptoms have been reported as a side effect of several types of prescription medications. If you are on one of these drugs and burning mouth syndrome is affecting your quality of life, ask your prescribing doctor if there may be an alternative treatment that will work just as well.

Medications That Have Been Associated with Burning Mouth Syndrome:[109, 110, 111]

- Antiretrovirals: nevirapine (Viramune), efavirenz (Sustiva)

- Anticonvulsants: topiramate (Topamax), clonazepam (Klonopin)

- Antidepressants: fluoxetine (Prozac, Sarafem), sertraline (Zoloft), venlafaxine (Effexor)

- Antihypertensives: captopril (Capoten), enalapril (Vasotec), lisinopril (Prinivil, Zestril), eprosartan (Teveten), candesartan (Atacand)

- Hormone replacement therapy

If your burning mouth syndrome started shortly after starting a new medication that is not on this list, it is worth talking to your prescribing doctor about the possibility that your symptoms might be a side effect. An alternative medication might be able to treat your original illness without making your mouth ache.

The evidence: A randomized controlled trial of 48 patients with burning mouth syndrome found that sucking on a 1-milligram tablet of clonazepam reduced pain scores by four times as much as sucking on a placebo tablet.[112]

How it works: It is thought that clonazepam might reduce burning mouth syndrome pain by altering the reactivity of GABA nerve receptors in the mouth; however, its mechanism of action is still poorly understood.

What you need to know: Clonazepam is probably the most widely accepted medical treatment for burning mouth syndrome; however, it can also cause burning mouth syndrome when used in some patients. In addition, there is a risk that clonazepam can be habit forming with prolonged use, which means that it should not necessarily be your first choice for treatment.[113]

Other Strategies

WATCH WHAT YOU PUT IN YOUR MOUTH: Sometimes burning mouth syndrome is caused by underlying health problems, but other times it seems that the pain is caused by the things that go into your mouth.

The evidence: Although allergy does not seem to be responsible for most cases of burning mouth syndrome, it may play a role in some people's pain.[114] In addition, some foods and products may cause irritation without an allergic reaction. Therefore, changing your diet and the oral care products you use may be an effective way to deal with your pain.

How it works: Low-level allergies and contact hypersensitivity[115] can make your mouth feel like it's starting to burn. Figuring out what products irritate your mouth and keeping them far away is a good way to stop your pain and keep it from coming back.

What you need to know: The American Dental Association recommends[116] that people with burning mouth syndrome try eliminating gum, tobacco, and acidic foods (soft drinks, coffee, some fruit juices) from their diets for at least 2 weeks to see if their symptoms improve. It also suggests removing mouthwash entirely from your oral care routine, since it can dry out your mouth, and switching toothpaste brands in case additives are responsible for your symptoms.

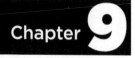
Back, Neck, and Shoulder Pain

Strains and sprains, disk-related pain, arthritis, slipped vertebrae, spinal stenosis, scoliosis and kyphosis

P ain in your back or neck and shoulder is about as common as sun in San Diego (odds are around 90 percent, to be exact). When you consider everything these complex structures do for your body, it's no wonder that they sometimes lead to problems.

Your back is a symphony of bones, spongy disks, muscles, ligaments, and nerves that are responsible for a dizzying array of functions. Your upper back provides stability and connects to your ribs to make up the cage that protects your heart and lungs, and your lower back helps control the movement of your lower body. The spinal column houses and carries the nerves to all parts of your body, and is responsible for getting pain messages to and from your brain. Let's not leave out the neck and shoulders, which help to support, twist, and turn your 10-pound head.

Unfortunately, in our sedentary society this work of art is treated more like a workhorse. Sitting too much makes muscles weak and puts triple the load on your lower back than when you are standing. Sixty-five percent of Americans are overweight; excess weight heavily burdens their backs, making them more susceptible to injury, strains, sprains, and herniated disks, just to name a few possible results. To make matters worse, less than a quarter of American men and women get their daily quota of moderate exercise (at least 30 minutes of walking, jogging, swimming, or other activity most days of the week).

Add all this to the fact that the average person sits and stares at one type of screen or another (from laptops to flat-screen televisions) for about $8\frac{1}{2}$ hours a day, and you can clearly see why back, neck, and shoulder problems are on the rise.[1]

Shutting Off the Pain

The good news is that there's a solid and ever-expanding silver lining when it comes to treating the back and neck pain that plagues more than 26 million men and women in the United States.[2] In the old days, your doctor would tell you to pop a couple of painkillers and stay in bed until the pain eases up. If things didn't get better quickly, you'd probably be referred for surgery. Today, doctors know that a combination of nondrug therapies and lifestyle changes is the way to go when managing chronic neck or back pain—not lying in bed, taking drugs, or going under the knife.

Of course, there are instances when surgery is appropriate. Sometimes, a compressed nerve will cause extreme pain or a disk can get ruptured. Spinal deformities caused by conditions like scoliosis also require surgery. But according to many of the experts we spoke with for this chapter, surgery is often overused and many patients who have surgery don't get relief from their pain. "Many back pain specialists are surgeons," says Thom Lobe, MD, founder and medical director of the Beneveda Medical Group in Beverly Hills. "When you get referred to an orthopedist or neurosurgeon, their bias may be toward surgery. Pain specialists often opt for procedures and injections. Physical therapists lean toward exercise and strength training."

Treating your pain successfully means focusing on the following:

- **Use a combination of therapies.** People who use multiple treatments, including acupuncture, chiropractic care, massage, stretching techniques, yoga, cognitive-behavioral therapy, and meditation have less pain and fewer flare-ups than those who use the conventional therapies above. The beauty of taking a bountiful dose of these therapies? No muddled thinking, risk of addiction or abuse, liver damage, or other unsavory side effects. When Swedish researchers had adults with neck or back pain attend either traditional care (doctor visit, advice about staying active, and exercise samples), or traditional care plus a combination of chiropractic care and massage, they found that the combo group's pain improved 21 percent more than the traditional care group.[3] Other studies have shown similar findings when chiropractic care and physical therapy, yoga and traditional care, or acupuncture and meditation are combined. All these—as duos, trios, or more—seem to be more powerful than traditional care alone.[4]

- **Get into your head.** Living with chronic back or neck pain is frustrating, depressing, and worrying, so it isn't really surprising that therapy would help. What is surprising, though, is that people with neck pain seem to do the best by combining several therapies, such as joining a support group, banishing negative thinking, and having coping skills and strategies in place.

- **Start moving.** The old view of back pain called for lots of bed rest and no exercise, but today's experts know that it's essential (barring complications) for your body to move as soon as possible after an injury to have the best chance of a successful recovery. We realize that moving when you are experiencing sharp or aching pain can be a hard sell. But if you understand what you need to do first to get pain under control, you can get back on your feet much faster.

What Is Causing My Back, Neck, or Shoulder Pain?

Pain can come from damage to soft tissues such as muscles, ligaments, or tendons; bones in the back and neck; and the disks that support and protect the vertebrae in the spine.[5] The first step in treating your pain correctly and effectively is to figure out what's causing the aching, throbbing, or stabbing sensations.

The easy part is pointing to where it hurts. It's a bit trickier terrain from there, but thinking about how your pain feels, when it hurts worst, and what activities trigger painful flare-ups can help you zero in on the cause of your pain. Keeping a pain diary can help; try the one in Part Three of this book or create your own.

Whether your pain is in your neck, shoulders, or lower back, often the treatments can overlap. That's because you can have a disk problem way up high in your cervical spine (the neck), or down in the lumbar region (lower back). The same goes for strains, sprains, pinched nerves, and other back and neck problems.

When you consider the entire area of the body, low back pain is most common, with neck pain coming in second, and pain in the upper back taking third place. When Australian researchers monitored more than 1,000 adults with low back pain for a year, they found that less than 1 percent had more severe issues such as vertebrae fractures or cancer-related pain.[6]

Below you'll find an overview of the causes of back, neck, and shoulder pain, from the more common causes to the more obscure.

- **Low back pain:** Low back pain costs about $100 billion a year in related health care costs and the costs have doubled since the 1990s, according to University of North Carolina researchers.[7] The researchers aren't sure of the cause, but they suspect that obesity and overweight are the main suspects. Many people have trouble figuring out why they hurt; they could have slipped and fallen, lifted something improperly, or twisted too fast. Poor muscle tone, chronic strain from poor posture, and excess weight, not to mention degenerating bones and disks in your back, can all contribute to low back injury and pain. Low back pain is often caused by strain, sprain, other types of injury, and also by age. The disks in the low back break down over time and can cause nerve-related pain, and the bones of the spine itself can break or grow painful spurs that can irritate nerves. The spinal cord itself can become infected or the victim of disease. In very rare cases, your low back pain may be caused by cancer. Ruling out one in favor of another can be tricky because expensive scans aren't always helpful. The American College of Physicians and the American Pain Society both recommend scans only if they feel a serious nerve pain or cancer is suspected. (For more on cancer-related back pain, see Chapter 16.)

- **Neck pain:** As with low back pain, neck pain is an extremely common complaint and most of us can expect a bout of it at one time or another in our lives. If you have one bout of neck pain, you have a 50 to 85 percent chance of it occurring again anywhere from 1 to 5 years later.[8] When it comes to your neck, pain is often a result of your occupation (athlete, writer, or computer technician) or your poor habits (slumping and slouching). Most people with neck pain don't completely recover. It can also be tricky to distinguish between upper back pain and neck pain since they often occur together.

- **Upper back pain:** The most telling clue that your pain originates in your upper back is a consistent feeling of tension and pain in the middle of your back that often encompasses most of the area around your upper back. Sometimes the pain can radiate to the chest area because the thoracic spine (a fancy term for the upper back) connects to your ribs. People with upper back pain may also feel an intense shooting pain if they try to twist toward the side of the pain. Often the cause is a strain or a sprain from day-to-day poor posture, a quick twist, or another injury (the upper back isn't designed to twist much).

- **Shoulder pain:** Moving slightly outward from the back, the shoulders can be a source of pain for many people. The most common causes of shoulder pain are arthritis (see Chapter 11) or an overuse injury such as tendinitis or bursitis (see Chapter 12). Still, many of the tips outlined below can help you cope with shoulder pain.

- **Strains and sprains:** Most back, neck, and shoulder pain is caused by either strains involving trauma to muscles and tendons or sprains caused by pulled or stretched ligaments that attach bone to bone. Strains can develop from years of poor posture; sprains are more often caused by an injury or accident. A strain or sprain is characterized by stiffness and muscle spasms in which the pain is localized—that is, the pain doesn't radiate down your arms or legs.

- **Disk-related pain:** The disks that live between the bony vertebrae of the spine are oval-shaped, with a tough outer layer surrounding a soft center. Your disks act as shock absorbers for the spinal bones, but as a normal part of aging, they experience a lot of wear and tear. When the stress becomes too great, they can dry out and crack. If too much of a disk wears away, bone can rub on bone and cause pain. Or a disk can bulge or slip out of alignment and pinch a nerve. When low back pain is caused by bulging, slipped, or broken disks, the pain radiates down one or both legs (called sciatica). Disks can rupture in the neck area as well, but the radiating pain in this case would be felt down one or both arms. Because the upper back is stable and doesn't do a lot of moving, disk issues are rare in this region.

- **Arthritis:** Just like all the other joints in the body, the bones of the spine can become arthritic and this can cause narrowing of the spinal cord. (See Chapter 11 for more information on diagnosing and treating your arthritis-related pain.)

- **Fractured vertebrae:** A spinal fracture caused by an injury or accident will cause immediate and apparent back pain. But in other cases, such as when a person has osteoporosis, the fracture may occur gradually and cause no pain at all. If you have this condition, you should be under a doctor's supervision to make sure a fractured vertebra has not occurred. In some instances the fracture may evolve into chronic back pain or a subtle curvature of the spine.

- **Slipped vertebra (spondylolisthesis):** In this condition, a vertebra cracks or slips forward so that bone is touching bone. This can also cause a pinched nerve. Spondylolisthesis in children is often caused by a birth defect. In adults it's usually related to arthritis. Slipped vertebrae are fairly rare, occurring in about 3 to 6 percent of people,[9] and can impact the body anywhere along the spine from the neck to the low back. Symptoms often begin with low back pain and muscle aches or pain in your buttocks and down your leg.

When to Call the Doctor

Get medical help immediately if you or a loved one has any of the following symptoms.

- Back, neck, or shoulder pain after an injury or accident
- Pain accompanied by extreme numbness or loss of strength in the arms or hands
- Back pain accompanied by problems urinating or having bowel movements
- Inability to touch your chin to your chest
- Back, neck, or shoulder pain that is constant, intense, and interferes with your day-to-day routine
- Pain that intensifies when you lie down
- Back pain with weakness, numbness, or tingling that radiates down one or both legs, especially if the pain goes below your knee
- Back or neck pain that's accompanied by pain or throbbing in your belly
- Back, neck, or shoulder pain with a fever
- A first back pain incident that occurs after the age of 50
- Back, neck, or shoulder pain paired with a history of cancer, osteoporosis, steroid use, or drug or alcohol use

- **Spinal stenosis:** When the spinal column narrows as a result of damaged disks, arthritis, infection, spinal defects, an injury, or other reasons, the condition is known as spinal stenosis. Spinal stenosis does not always cause symptoms, but it can cause pain or numbness in the back and/or legs. Weakness or cramping in the legs may also occur. Rarely, bowel and/or bladder problems occur as well.

- **Scoliosis and kyphosis:** Skeletal abnormalities such as scoliosis (a curvature in the spine) and kyphosis (dowager's hump) can cause pain in the upper back.

Fast Relief Now

While it will take more extensive steps to gain long-term relief from neck, upper back, or shoulder pain, you have a number of options at your disposal for quelling the pain quickly in the short term. Here are some simple steps that can help.

1. **Take an over-the-counter pain reliever.** Ibuprofen, naproxen, or acetaminophen will all do the trick, so choose the one that works best for you. It's best to keep your use to fewer than 5 consecutive days to minimize the risk of side effects.

2. **Use an ice pack.** Wrap an ice pack (or a frozen bag of peas) in a towel or other cloth and place it under your neck as you lie on your back. Make sure your neck is also supported with pillows as necessary so that your head is not tilted up or down. Put a couple of additional pillows under your knees to support your back.

3. **Breathe and relax.** Stay put for 20 to 30 minutes and repeat every few hours. If you have trouble relaxing, try meditation or guided imagery. (See Chapter 5 for more details.)

When low back pain has you hurting, follow these strategies to get feeling better fast.

1. **As soon as you realize a flare-up is coming on, check your surroundings.** How are you sitting? What have you been doing? Keeping an eye on common triggers—poor posture, overzealous furniture rearranging, shoveling snow, too much time at the computer—can help you catch pain early. The earlier you pinpoint a trigger, the better your chances of stopping the pain before it has you on your back.

2. **If your pain is mild to moderate, take some acetaminophen or naproxen.** As discussed in Chapter 6, these two OTC pain relievers seem to have the fewest side effects. Follow the package directions and stick to the recommended dosage. (If you go lower, you may have breakthrough pain; if you go higher, you may have dangerous side effects.) Keep your use to fewer than 5 consecutive days to minimize the risk of side effects.

ThinkTwice:
Artificial Disks for the Lower Back

If surgery is required for your low back pain, you typically have two options: spinal fusion, in which two or more spinal disks are fused together, or an artificial disk replacement, in which the damaged disk is removed and replaced with an artificial one.

While artificial disks have their uses, particularly in the neck, Donald S. Corenman, MD, DC, a back and spine specialist with the Steadman Clinic in Vail, Colorado, says that fusion is the best option for lower back surgery. "An artificial disk replacement requires going in through the front, which is an extremely invasive surgery for the lower back," he says. Dr. Corenman says that the main concern here is that such a surgery requires moving the intestines and other critical organs out of the way to perform the surgery. This can be done, but is much more invasive than surgeries that start at the back of the body.

Another concern with disk replacement surgery is the lingering question about how long they'll last. "We don't really know their longevity," he says. "If you get into a situation where you have to replace them two, three, or four times, this becomes extremely problematic." Dr. Corenman adds that while artificial disks allow good range of motion, they are not very well suited to absorbing shock, which means you might still experience pain when performing any jarring activities.

However, a spinal fusion surgery is not without risk either, and a recent study showed that the complication risk for spinal fusion is actually higher than it is for a disk replacement.[10] The most common complications are that the pain experienced is not relieved, or that the fusion is not successful, requiring additional surgery. With most back pain, surgery should be viewed as a last resort and only undertaken after careful consideration and discussion with your doctor.

3. **Use an ice pack.** Wrap an ice pack (or a frozen bag of peas) in a towel or other cloth and place it wherever it hurts most. Soothe your aches for 15 to 20 minutes.

4. **Prop up your legs.** If you're at work, close your office door, turn your office chair around, and lie on the floor faceup while resting your calves on the seat of the chair for 10 minutes or so. If you're at home, a few pillows may do the trick. This is a modified yoga pose known to relieve strain in the back and soothe your aches. See Part Three for other yoga exercises that help relieve pain.

5. **As soon as you can, get up out of bed and walk.** First walk around your house, then around the block, then work up to 30 minutes of walking most days of the week. It's okay to walk with moderate back and neck pain as long as it doesn't make your pain worse afterward. Don't lie around for longer than 3 days. Staying in bed longer than this can cause you to lose muscle, which increases back pain risk.

Relief at Last

Whether you've got a screaming neck, an aching back, or a sharp pain in your shoulder, most of the following relief strategies will help all types of agony related to your spine. If your pain comes on less than once a month and responds well to the suggestions for fast relief listed above, then that may be all you need when the area affecting you becomes painfully inflamed. Still, many of the suggestions below can help keep your flare-ups to a minimum while you get the maximum benefit out of your life—living it!

Step 1: Keep bed rest to a minimum. While some bed rest is helpful for back pain, it shouldn't go on for longer than 3 days. And no, you shouldn't wait until you are pain free to start moving. Once you feel that you are able, get up and start walking. As your pain improves, strive for 30 minutes a day, 6 to 7 days a week, of gentle activity. Walking and swimming are two great ways to get started. See Part Three for some gentle workouts to get you started.

Step 2: Choose nondrug remedies whenever possible. The days of popping pills are over, or they should be. The results of what is now a plentiful wealth of research on the nondrug versus drug topic conclude that therapies such as acupuncture, massage, and/or chiropractic either trump meds by the absence of adverse side effects or equal them in their effectiveness at lowering pain. Better yet, nonmedicinal methods do a better job than drugs at providing pain relief over the long haul. For example, acupuncture successfully treats back pain about as effectively as medications but without adding any groggy, drug-induced side effects.[11, 12]

Step 3: Get a clean bill of mental health. Having high self-esteem, being self-assured, and developing a positive outlook for the future can all improve your chances of living life pain free. People who live with chronic pain are more likely to suffer from depression and anxiety.

Step 4: Choose nondrug combination treatments. Mixing and matching from a variety of healthy and nondrug treatments is in vogue. Chiropractic care, massage, and stretching can all be done as one treatment for reducing back and neck pain.

Step 5: Stop smoking, start moving. Smoking increases your risk of developing low back pain by blocking your body's ability to deliver nutrients to the disks in the lower back (and a smoker's cough doesn't help, either). It also increases the production of inflammatory chemicals that may prime you to feel more pain. Plus, smokers tend to be less physically active. Incorporate exercise that includes stretching (think yoga), strengthening, and heart-pumping walking.

Step 6: Try an acupuncture and physical therapy combo. According to recent research, doing physical therapy and acupuncture together may reduce pain more effectively than one or the other alone. This seems to work especially well for chronic computer users. In a pilot study of adults who either had acupuncture alone, physical therapy alone, or both in combination, the combo group reported the largest reduction in neck pain.[13]

Pain Prevention Strategies

Food and Supplements

ALPHA-LIPOIC ACID: Alpha-lipoic acid is found naturally in every cell in your body, where it protects against damage by free radicals, the destructive molecules produced in the body when you digest food. In supplement form, it may play a role in reducing back pain.

The evidence: This strong antioxidant helped ease back pain significantly for people who were also in an exercise program in one recent Italian study.[14] It has also been shown to ease pain and other symptoms of diabetes-related nerve damage, called *neuropathy*, say Dutch researchers who reviewed six studies investigating this supplement.[15]

»More Research Needed

Herbs and Supplements for Back, Neck, and Shoulder Pain

As of press time, the following herbs and supplements don't have enough research behind them to recommend their use.

White willow bark:[16] This herb has the same active ingredient as aspirin, but research using it for back pain has had inconclusive results.

Devil's claw:[17] This African herb has a long history of medicinal use. Some research shows that it can ease chronic back pain to some extent, but the herb can also cause stomach upset, nausea, and diarrhea.

Comfrey root: Comfrey root also has pain-relieving abilities but it is toxic when ingested orally. German researchers used the herb successfully in a topical formula. (The ointment used in the study is called Kytta Salbe, which is not available in the United States.) When 120 men and women either used a comfrey root cream or a placebo, the herbal group's pain intensity dropped 95.2 percent compared to 38 percent in the placebo group, but there were still some reports of stomach upset. Ointments containing comfrey may increase cell turnover, which speeds up healing, researchers speculate.[18]

Vitamin D: As discussed in Part One, vitamin D is controversial when it comes to pain relief. Although it is critically important for keeping bones and muscles healthy because it helps maintain the right levels of calcium in your body, it seems to help with back pain only if you are already deficient. It's worth checking out, though, especially if you live in a very rainy climate (just 10 minutes of sun will give you all the D you need). University of Maryland researchers found that women who are vitamin D deficient were twice as likely to have back pain as those who were not lacking in the sun-powered supplement. Their study analyzed the vitamin D levels and type of chronic pain in more than 1,000 men and women. Only back pain in women was related to vitamin D deficiency. The researchers speculate that deficiency of vitamin D may lead to osteomalacia, a disease-related softening of the bones. If you suspect that you are vitamin D deficient, ask your doctor to run a blood test to check.[19]

How it works: Researchers aren't exactly sure why alpha-lipoic acid is so effective for neck and back pain, but some evidence indicates that this super-antioxidant may help hasten the regeneration and healing of nerve tissues in the body.

What you need to know: Side effects are uncommon, but you should skip this drug if you're pregnant or breast-feeding. Talk to your doctor before taking alpha-lipoic acid if you have diabetes; it can lower blood sugar and could lead to dangerous blood sugar lows when combined with your medications.

OMEGA-3 FATTY ACIDS: A nonsteroidal anti-inflammatory drug (NSAID) such as ibuprofen or aspirin can reduce painful inflammation that's partly to blame for back, neck, and shoulder pain, but new research shows that omega-3 fatty acids, the healthy fat found in fish, work just as well.

The evidence: In a University of Pittsburgh study of people taking NSAIDs for long-term back and neck pain, researchers added a daily 2,400-milligram dose of omega-3s to the patients' diets for 2 weeks. The researchers then asked study participants to taper off their NSAID use and continue with a daily dose of 1,200 milligrams of omega-3s for another 2 weeks. After a month, nearly two-thirds reported a significant improvement in pain.[20] The actual content of the omega-3 fatty acids EPA and DHA varies greatly from product to product, so check the label of your fish oil capsule carefully before choosing one.

How it works: Omega-3 fatty acids impede the production of chemical messengers called *prostaglandins*; these trigger pain and swelling, researchers say.

What you need to know: Omega-3 fatty acids are found in many foods, including fatty fish like salmon and tuna, and many vegetables and nuts. Because it can be difficult to get enough omega-3 fatty acids from your diet alone, take 1,000 to 1,200 milligrams a day in a fish oil capsule for a month or two to get relief. Fish oils also break up blood platelets, so avoid this treatment if you're on blood thinners.

Exercise and Movement Therapies

AEROBIC EXERCISE: Moving can reduce back pain by 40 percent compared to doing the conventional "take two and go to bed" or other conservative measures. No matter how sympathetic your doctor is to your achy plight, if he knows what he's doing, he's going to tell you to get moving, even if you hurt.

The evidence: In a University of North Carolina study, researchers polled more than 650 men and women with chronic back or neck pain and found that only about 15 percent of them had received recommendations from their doctors to get active. Considering the overwhelming scientific evidence that exercise works, it's a bit shocking.[21]

Researchers in Greece also found that after a 3-month regimen of aerobic exercise (30 minutes, 3 times weekly), subjects reported 40 percent less pain, 31 percent less disability from the pain, and 35 percent fewer psychological issues, such as depression and anxiety, compared to a no-exercise group.[22, 23, 24] In another study from the University of California, Los Angeles, researchers followed 610 men and women with a history of chronic low back pain. After 1½ years, they found that patients who exercised regularly were 31 percent less likely to experience an increase in pain and disability than their sedentary counterparts.[25]

How it works: When you exercise, your brain releases natural painkillers and mood-enhancing hormones to make you feel better. Other research indicates that exercise actually creates new stem cells in the brain (something experts once thought was impossible). Stem cells have the unique ability to morph into whatever type of cell your body might need, so exercise, researchers speculate, may help create cells that can repair damaged areas that are causing you pain in your neck or back.

What you need to know: Choose a moderate aerobic activity such as walking, low-impact aerobics, or swimming. One caveat for neck pain sufferers: You may want to skip cycling. Some studies show that people with chronic neck pain have a higher incidence and recurrence of pain if biking is the form of exercise they choose. Not only do you have to hyperextend your neck on a bike, but you also have to do a lot of craning and twisting, which are not neck-friendly movements.[26]

STRENGTH TRAINING: Along with getting your recommended 30 minutes of moderate aerobic exercise most days of the week, adding basic strength training (as suggested in Chapter 3) will further reduce your pain and your chance of painful flare-ups.

The evidence: Doing twice-weekly strength-training workouts can reduce your back pain by up to 60 percent, according to Canadian researchers. A University of Alberta study found that those who followed a basic strength-training program for 4 months also lost 15 percent of their body fat, compared to no changes in those who did not undergo the training.[27] In another study, Danish researchers found that neck pain was reduced by 80 percent among women who did specific neck exercises three times a week for 10 weeks, compared to women who did no exercise.[28]

Exercises for Neck Pain

Three strength-building sessions a week can reduce neck pain by almost 80 percent in less than 3 months, say Danish researchers. Investigators from Denmark's National Research Centre for the Working Environment had women ages 36 to 52 do the moves below for 10 weeks. Keep your knees slightly bent and choose a weight that tires you out after 8 to 12 repetitions. Aim to do three sets three times a week on non-consecutive days. As always, stop if you feel any sharp pain while doing the exercises (a little soreness, though, is normal) and consult your doctor or physical therapist.

1. Shoulder shrugs: Hold your arms at your sides, palms facing in. Keeping your arms straight, pull your shoulders up toward your ears. Pause for a second, then lower your shoulders.

2. Reverse flies: Bend forward so your chest faces the floor. Let your arms hang down, palms facing in. With your elbows slightly bent, squeeze your shoulder blades and raise your arms toward your sides, parallel to the floor. Pause, then lower your arms.

3. Upright row: Start with your palms in front of your thighs and facing your legs. Bend your elbows out to the sides and pull the weights up to about the level of your collarbone. Pause, then lower.[22]

How it works: When your muscles get stronger, they offer more support to your spine and are less likely to get strained or stressed. Muscle also burns more calories than fat, so building strength can help you maintain a healthy weight, which lowers the strain on your back. Also, researchers speculate that strength training may help you generate new healthy muscle tissues where there once was injured tissue, which may reduce pain.

What you need to know: You have to strengthen all the major muscles in your body to see the benefit. Having strong chest, abdominal, and back muscles will help keep you from hunching forward, and leg strength will protect your back when you need to lift something heavy. Start with light weights and gradually build up. See the routine in Part Three. If you have neck pain, consider adding the neck exercises in the box above on the days you do your regular strength training.[22]

YOGA: Yoga helps all sorts of back, neck, and shoulder pain and is a healthy habit for anyone. This ancient practice has proven to be a powerful adjunct to other pain-relieving therapies.

The evidence: When West Virginia University researchers assigned 90 men and women to either a twice-weekly yoga class or no treatment, they found that those performing yoga reported significant reductions in pain as well as an increase in their day-to-day abilities.[29] In another study, 118 men and women with increased curving in the upper back (a painful condition called *kyphosis* or *dowager's hump*) either practiced yoga three times a week for an hour per session or were assigned to a control group that attended a monthly luncheon and received mailings about back health. At the end of 6 months, the yoga group had reduced the curves in the upper back by up to 6 percent; the control group's back curvature increased.[30]

Finally, University of Washington researchers found that of 101 adults with back pain, those who did gentle yoga recovered from their pain faster than those who attended a vigorous class or read a self-help book. The yoga group also was taking less medication for pain than the control group at the conclusion of the study.[31]

How it works: Yoga strengthens muscles that protect the spine, and those who practice it have lower levels of stress, improved immunity, greater flexibility, and a larger range of motion. That means less chance of injury or flare-ups.

What you need to know: As described in Chapter 3, there are many types of yoga, not all of which are suitable for people with injuries or pain. Turn to Part Three for a sample yoga routine designed to help improve pain or seek out a gentle yoga class with a certified teacher who can adjust and modify poses so they work for you.

ALEXANDER TECHNIQUE: This posture-improving method, developed in the 1890s, helps align your head, neck, and back muscles and is a proven back pain reducer.

The evidence: When a team of British researchers from the University of Southampton and the University of Bristol randomly assigned more than 500 men and women to a year of either Alexander Technique lessons, aerobic exercise, or massage, the group that practiced the Alexander Technique reported a 40 to 45 percent improvement in their ability to do daily activities. They also experienced 86 percent fewer days in pain than those who just exercised or had a massage.

How it works: Proponents of the Alexander Technique believe that until about age 5 we're untainted, balanced, and ready to move. In these classes, you learn how to release muscular tension and restore your posture.

What you need to know: The Alexander Technique is usually taught one-on-one; a session lasts from about 45 minutes to an hour.[32]

Touch Therapies

ACUPUNCTURE: Acupuncture can relieve pain, help you heal faster, and reduce your use of medication. You'll also have more energy and relieve stress.[33]

The evidence: When Seattle researchers had nearly 700 men and women with spine-related pain try sessions of either acupuncture, conventional painkillers, or physical therapy, they found that 60 percent of the "needled" group reported a good amount of relief compared to just 39 percent of those in the other groups.[34] Another study of 24 Norwegian women with neck and shoulder pain found that those who had gotten acupuncture treatments over 3 to 4 weeks had 50 percent less pain, slept better, and felt less anxious and depressed. What's more, these symptoms continued to improve over the next 3 years.[35]

How it works: Eastern practitioners of acupuncture believe that the needle points work by opening up channels of energy that are supposed to restore your body to a balanced state. Western doctors say that they aren't sure of the cause but they tend to believe that the needles stimulate some sort of positive reaction, perhaps by causing a release of mood-boosting and pain-relieving hormones.

What you need to know: Before you seek out acupuncture treatment, check with your insurance company. Many are now at least

On the Horizon

Acupressure

Want the benefits of acupuncture at home? Then you may want to look into acupressure, a touch therapy that researchers believe works much like acupuncture does. In fact, the latest research shows that acupressure might be more effective than physical therapy for quelling back pain. In a study of 129 Chinese patients who underwent physical therapy or acupressure therapy for 1 month, the patients in the acupressure group experienced greater pain reduction and function at the conclusion of the study and at a subsequent 6-month follow-up.[36]

"Most back pain is coming from muscle spasm and shortening that results in tender knots called trigger points," says Jacob Teitelbaum, MD, medical director of the Fibromyalgia & Fatigue Centers found across the United States. "Seventy percent of the common acupressure points correspond to the area of the trigger points. Putting 30 to 45 seconds of deep pressure on the points will make the muscles release and often leads to pain relief."

ThinkTwice:

Chiropractic Care

Some people swear by visits to the chiropractor during flare-ups. The theory behind chiropractic care is that you hurt because your spine is out of alignment, which causes stress and strain. Through spinal manipulations and various other treatments, the practitioner coaxes your spine back into alignment.

According to a recent Cochrane Collaboration review that analyzed 12 studies involving 2,887 adults with low back pain, it may work as well as over-the-counter medications, physical therapy, and exercise.[37] However, the researchers noted that pain in sufferers diminishes only about 10 percent (a relatively small number) in the first several weeks they are in pain compared to those who stick to traditional care. When the researchers turned their attention to long-term chronic low back pain, they didn't see any difference.

Treatments that include quick thrusting of the neck can potentially cause serious harm, including permanent injury or even death.[38] For these reasons, quick thrusting is not recommended for neck pain. In addition, some people are concerned that getting chiropractic care might increase their risk of developing a vertebrobasilar artery stroke, a very dangerous type of stroke that affects the brain and causes death or severe brain damage in many sufferers. Chiropractic care has been associated with this stroke in many recent news stories.

Several studies have looked at this association, including a large study that looked at every incident of vertebrobasilar artery stroke in Ontario, Canada, hospitals from 1993 to 2002. These researchers noted that those in a group that visited a chiropractor were three times more likely to experience a stroke than those in a control group. Still, the researchers noted that the stroke is incredibly rare, and the few chiropractic patients who did experience such a stroke likely had a high risk of developing the stroke whether they received chiropractic care or not.[39]

The bottom line? Chiropractic care may help if you just have occasional flare-ups of back, neck, or shoulder pain but side effects, while very rare, can be severe.

---

partially covering these visits. Make sure you go to a licensed acupuncturist; you can find more information on how to find one in Part Three.

SELF-MASSAGE: Research suggests that massage can help with back and shoulder pain, cancer pain, and tension headaches. It may also ease fibromyalgia and neck pain.[40]

The evidence: In a study of 40 men and women, researchers had adults either try a Thera Cane (a hooklike tool for self-massaging the back) or enter a control group that did not receive treatment. At the end of 5 days, the self-massage group reported half the pain intensity of the control group.[41]

A similar device to the Thera Cane, the Backnobber II has also proven effective in a recent study. In 28 patients with back pain, this device was able to reduce pain when used every other day for one week.[42]

How it works: Researchers suspect that this form of self-massage is similar to acupressure in that it targets trigger points in the back and neck to bring temporary relief to pain.

What you need to know: Massaging sore spots, whether with a tool like the Thera Cane (www.theracane.com) or Backnobber II (www.pressurepositive.com) or with your hands if you can reach them, will help you find relief for your pain. Studies show that using this sort of trigger point technique can cut your neck pain in half. Don't be bashful about asking a loved one for a gentle massage at the source of the pain if you need it.

ICE AND HEAT: What do heating pads and ice packs have in common? They're both the treatments of choice on the front lines of back, neck, and shoulder pain, and most people who've tried them say they work to relieve pain for the short term. Exactly how much relief they offer is still up for debate.

The evidence: A Johns Hopkins University study found that putting on a portable heat wrap 8 hours a day for 3 days reduced the intensity of back pain by 60 percent compared with going without one (both groups were also taking pain medication). The benefits lasted for up to 2 weeks.[43]

In another study conducted at the Stony Brook University Hospital in New York, a group of people with back pain was randomized to get either heat therapy or an ice pack for 30 minutes. The results looked good, with both groups reporting similar levels of pain relief (52 percent of patients found relief from heat; 62 percent found relief from cold) from the treatments.[44, 45]

How it works: There is certainly some evidence that heat and cold can play a role in relieving pain in a relatively noninvasive way. The cold sensation brings relief by taking your mind off the pain, while the heat allows the painful area to stretch out and become more limber.

What you need to know: If hot and cold treatments bring you relief, there is certainly not going to be much harm in trying them. A portable heat wrap is a convenient way to apply heat to your back.

Mind-Body Therapies

**MINDFULNESS MEDITATION AND PROGRESSIVE MUSCLE RELAX-
ATION:** Nearly 30 percent of people with low back pain find great benefit in relaxation techniques such as mindfulness meditation or progressive relaxation techniques. Not only can these practices lead to reduced pain, better attention, and more restful sleep, but they are completely free of adverse side effects.[46]

The evidence: More than 60 percent of adults with chronic low back pain reported that their concentration improved after completing an 8-week mindfulness meditation course, and nearly half reported that they were able to reduce their pain medications thanks to the exercise.[47] University of Massachusetts researchers reported that 60 percent of subjects said meditating helps them achieve a "moderate to great improvement" even after 4 years of practicing it,[48] while the Harvard researchers found that areas responsible for good moods in the brain become more active when you practice meditation.[49]

How it works: Many people who practice mindfulness meditation report that the exercise has a quieting effect that gives a sense of peace and allows you to deflect back pain and focus on other parts of your body.

What you need to know: Once you get the hang of it, mindfulness meditation is simple to do as needed. You may start by taking a local class once a week to gain guidance, then you can devote a few minutes on your own to it every day. The idea is that you continue to practice it as needed throughout your life. Try the simple progressive relaxation technique in Chapter 5, and see Part Three to find classes or other resources to help you learn these techniques.[50]

COGNITIVE-BEHAVIORAL THERAPY: Talking about your pain can help you feel twice as good as suffering from your back pain alone, according to a recent study in the journal *The Lancet*. In fact, just six sessions of group cognitive-behavioral therapy doubled the chances of recovering from back pain. ·

The evidence: Researchers from Warwick Medical School and the University of Oxford found that 60 percent of adults suffering from chronic low back pain (longer than 3 months) who participated in group sessions of cognitive-behavioral therapy reported that they'd recovered from their chronic low back pain, compared to 30 percent of people who did not have therapy. The study included 701 people from across areas of England who suffered from persistent low back pain. The group was randomly assigned to either six sessions of a group cognitive-behavioral therapy course or to a control group that received no treatment.

How it works: The United Kingdom researchers speculate that the cognitive behavioral therapy technique of helping you identify the way you feel about your pain and how you react to it can make your pain better.

What you need to know: While these studies looked at long-term low back pain, past research has indicated that this type of therapy (in groups or

The Skinny on Back Surgery

One of the most recent advances in low back pain research is the realization that surgery is often overprescribed. Often it's not needed to address the source of low back pain. What's more, many who receive surgery for their low back pain do not gain relief.

Of course, there are times when surgery is necessary. One of the most common instances when it is necessary is when there is a painful tear in a spinal disk or when a spinal disk is compressed, which causes pinching on a nerve and severe pain.

The bottom line: Surgery should always be viewed as the last resort for relieving low back pain. "Surgery should be considered only after conservative measures have failed to relieve the pain, the etiology of the pain can be identified, and surgical correction is felt to resolve the pain," says Edna Ma, MD, an anesthesiologist in Santa Monica, California.

If after careful consideration you and your doctor decide that surgery is the best course of treatment, the type of surgery is now an important consideration. A procedure known as a microdiskectomy can be the least invasive type with good outcomes, but it does not resolve some back problems. "A microdiskectomy is one of the most successful surgeries for pain related to nerve compression," says Dr. Ma. "The surgery involves removing part of the bone and/or disk over the impinged nerve root." The other surgery that's used for low back pain is a spinal fusion, which involves connecting the bones of the spine together.

Surgery has several pros and cons, and your doctor should have a frank, open discussion with you before performing any procedure. "Patients need to be realistic about their expectations," says Donald S. Corenman, MD, DC. "After a successful surgery, they will be able to resume function and live a normal life, but they probably won't be able to do extreme activities and sports like tennis, basketball, or skiing any more." He adds that the extent of the surgery also plays a role. If just two disks need to be fused, the outcome is likely to be better than a fusion involving three or more disks.

See Chapter 6 for tips on what to consider before deciding on surgery.

one-on-one) works on all types of chronic pain, including neck and upper back pain.[51]

Cognitive therapy groups typically meet for 1 hour a week and end after a specific period of time (often after 16 sessions). Many larger insurance companies and hospitals offer cognitive-behavioral therapy groups, so begin by asking your doctor and checking local hospitals. Also, see Part Three for help finding a therapist.[52]

BIOFEEDBACK: Biofeedback is a technique that teaches you to control bodily functions, such as your heart rate, by using your mind. Think of biofeedback as sort of a sixth sense: It allows you to "see" things that you wouldn't normally be able to see. When you are attached to a biofeedback machine, every time the offending muscles tighten up, you get a cue to relax. With practice, you'll learn to do this without the aid of the machine.

The evidence: In a review of 22 randomized controlled trials (the gold standard) that tested various alternative treatments on low back pain, the researchers found that all the different therapies were beneficial. The interventions included cognitive-behavioral therapy, biofeedback, relaxation, and hypnosis. Biofeedback, however, was near the top of the list of helpful treatments.[53] Another study from low back pain researchers in Germany found that among 42 men and women who had low back pain, those who received biofeedback reduced pain significantly more than those who received a placebo version of biofeedback.[54]

How it works: At a typical appointment, you are connected to electrical sensors that measure and provide information about your body. These machines show you how to make subtle changes—like relaxing certain muscles—that can reduce pain.

In a way, the process is almost like stepping on a scale. The machine gives you a number (feedback) so you are empowered to make a change. In a similar fashion, the biofeedback machine will beep or vibrate or give you a visual cue, then you'll know that you're tensing a certain area or that your heart rate is going up. Over time, this can help you learn to stay relaxed in the face of situations that might normally cause a flare-up.

What you need to know: It's important to see a qualified biofeedback therapist, so make sure that the specialist you see is licensed to practice the technique. In fact, it might be a good idea to ask a trusted health care provider (such as your doctor) for a referral. The sessions typically last 30 to 60 minutes, and the frequency and number of sessions needed can vary greatly from patient to patient. See Part Three for more information on how to find biofeedback centers.

Pain Medication and Medical Therapies

ANTIDEPRESSANTS:[56] We've already discussed how being in a better mood can reduce your pain. Now a growing volume of research is showing that mood-boosting medications such as antidepressants can pay dividends when it comes to back pain as well.

The evidence: In a retrospective study (looking at past data on patients), Johns Hopkins University researchers found that of 26 patients suffering from low back pain and spinal stenosis (narrowing of the spinal column) who were prescribed antidepressants, 20 reported a reduction in pain (about 76 percent).[57] In a Walter Reed Army Medical Center review of the mood-boosting drugs and back pain, the researchers found that antidepressants do decrease back pain but don't improve how well you are able to get around.

How it works: The researchers speculate that antidepressants may kick in personality traits that can help change perception of pain, including being more optimistic and empowered. These medications can also increase levels of serotonin in the body, which in turn influences chemicals that influence your perception of pain.[58]

What you need to know: Talk with your doctor if you feel you may be a candidate for antidepressants. These studies were done on patients with low back pain, but there's also evidence from a review by Singapore researchers that many antidepressants may be helpful with many varieties of chronic pain, so it's always a good thing to discuss with your doctor. Remember that all medications come with side effects.[58]

CAPSAICIN GEL OR CREAM:[60] This cream, made from the hottest part of hot peppers, soothes your pain by desensitizing nerves that detect pain near the skin. It also causes a mild tingling or burning sensation.

The evidence: Danish researchers gave 41 men with surgically repaired hernias either capsaicin powder or a placebo to apply to their wounds topically after surgery. During the first 3 days, men in the capsaicin group had significantly less pain.[61]

How it works: Capsaicin appears to work by depleting the pain-provoking nerve chemical substance P.

What you need to know: In general, these gels and creams seem to work best during flare-ups, not when your pain is at a low level. So keep some in your medicine cabinet. Capsaicin ointments and creams are sold in pharmacies and health stores. Try the 0.025 percent cream and take it according to the directions and see if it brings relief. Avoid the similar-sounding capsicum, which is also a pepper compound but can irritate the skin and isn't as potent.

Wear rubber gloves and use a cotton ball when applying capsaicin cream. Wash your hands thoroughly after you apply it, as the cream can burn. It's normal to feel a slight burning sensation where you apply the cream; part of the speculation about how this cream works is that it distracts you with another sensation.

Other Strategies

PERFECT YOUR POSTURE: Having good posture and taking frequent moving breaks reduces fatigue and stress on your back, which reduces pain and wards off a flare-up.

The evidence: Hong Kong researchers strapped accelerometers onto 33 employees who worked in a facility for severely handicapped people and had them go about their workday. Half of the workers had low back pain. After wearing the posture-tracking machine for 6 hours, the researchers found that those who had back pain spent more time with their backs in one position compared to those who were pain free. Those who were aching also spent more time with their backs bent and bent farther than those who had no pain.

How it works: In essence, having good posture puts your body in the position it's supposed to be in for the least amount of stress and strain. If you deviate from good posture, your body will eventually pay the price.

What you need to know: If you sit all day, make sure you get up for

5 minutes at the end of every hour. Stretch, walk around, and drink a glass of water. If you are on your feet all day, then once an hour make sure you stretch, sit down, and rotate each foot in a circle a few times to stretch it thoroughly.[62]

LUMBAR ROLL SUPPORT: A step as simple as using a lumbar support pillow while sitting in a chair helps your lower back. It can also help your neck. Yes, it goes behind your lower back, but it helps relieve neck pain because it causes you to sit up straighter and not jut out your head (which puts loads of strain on your neck and upper back).

The evidence: When researchers had 30 men sit in chairs with and without

When Back Pain Is a Symptom

Sometimes, back pain is a symptom of a more serious condition. Here are the odds of that, and what to look out for.

- **Cancer:** Your chance: 1 percent. Back pain can be caused by cancer that has started in your spine or that has spread there from somewhere else in your body.

- **Ankylosing spondylitis:** Your chance: 0.3 percent. This rare inflammatory disorder affects the ligaments and bones of your spine. It is more common among younger people with back pain. For more information on ankylosing spondylitis, see Chapter 11.

- **Spondylolisthesis:** Your chance: about 5 percent. In a small portion of the adult population there is a developmental crack in one of the vertebrae that may develop into a stress fracture. Because of the constant force the low back experiences, this fracture does not usually heal as normal bone. This type of fracture, called a *spondylolysis*, may cause no problem at all. However, sometimes the cracked vertebra slips forward over the vertebra below it, causing isthmic spondylolisthesis.

- **Scoliosis:** Your chance: 0.3 percent. This spinal curvature usually occurs in children during the growth spurt just before puberty. Regular checkups with a doctor are your best preventive. If she catches it early, she can usually correct scoliosis without surgery. If it progresses, surgery may be necessary.

- **Spinal infection:** Your chance: 0.01 percent. Very rarely, pain in your back is caused by an infection in that area. Usually it will have spread from another place, such as your urinary tract or your bloodstream. The pain can be accompanied by a fever at times.[63]

lumbar support pillows, they saw that without the pillow the men were more likely to stick their necks out in a manner that causes pain.[64]

How it works: The main effect of a lumbar support pillow on neck, back, and shoulder pain comes from improving your posture. Putting the pillow behind your back makes you sit up straighter, which helps your back, and hold your head in a more natural position, which helps your neck and shoulders.

What you need to know: Simply choose one of the many lumbar support pillows available or ask your doctor if he has a specific recommendation.

GET A NEW MATTRESS: If you suspect that your bed might be contributing to your back pain, you may be right. Having a mattress that's either too firm or too soft can make it more likely that you'll wake up with an aching back or neck.

The evidence: Danish researchers discovered that both overly firm and overly soft beds can hurt your back. The investigators from the Back Research Center in Denmark found that women with back pain who slept for 4 weeks on either a water bed or a body-conforming foam mattress hurt less and got more shut-eye than those on a firm futon mattress with no springs.[65]

How it works: A mattress that conforms correctly to the shape of your body will keep it in a more natural position as you sleep. What's more, it may help you sleep better, and lack of sleep is also a contributor to many types of pain.

What you need to know: Here's what to remember when looking for a new mattress.

- **Shop in the evening or late afternoon.** Your body is less sensitive to discomfort in the morning, so you'll want to try out mattresses after a normal day's activities when aches and pains are more likely to be evident.

- **Wear loose clothing.** It's important to take a mattress test-drive before buying, so wear clothes you could sleep in when you go shopping. When you find a bed that looks good, slip off your shoes and spend around 10 minutes lying on your sides, back, and tummy. The mattress should mold to the contours of your neck, back, waist, and knees while keeping your spine in a neutral position.

- **Skip bells and whistles.** Fancy fillers and special coverings have zero effect on warding off back pain. Just don't head home with the cheapest, oldest mattress in the store, and you'll be fine.

- **Get a good exchange policy.** Some companies will let you try out your new mattress for a few weeks and return it if you're unsatisfied.

- **Consider an orthopedic pillow.** Along with a more comfortable mattress, an orthopedic pillow may place your neck and shoulders in a more comfortable position to alleviate neck pain.

FORGIVE: Anger and resentment increase and intensify your perception of pain, especially if your anger is about what caused your pain in the first place. In fact, some past research indicates that anger and resentment actually excite nerves involved with sending pain messages to the brain.

The evidence: People who report the highest levels of forgiveness have lower levels of pain, anger, and emotional upset, according to a Duke University study. The researchers at Duke in the Pain Prevention and Treatment Research

Common Causes of Back Pain for Women

Although men and women are at risk of developing back pain, a few lifestyle events or experiences unique to women can put them at risk. Here's how to take these life challenges and prevent them from leading to the additional challenge of back pain.

- **Pregnancy:** Pregnant women may experience back pain not only because of the extra weight they are carrying, but also because the body produces hormones that relax the joints and ligaments and aggravate pain. Edna Ma, MD, an anesthesiologist in Santa Monica, California, suggests exercising; using massage, over-the-counter pain relief, and hot and cold compresses; and sleeping on your side. Using proper posture when bending and lifting will also help you avoid aggravating your back.

- **Heavy bags:** Toting around a heavy purse or bag can cause what is in essence an overuse injury. Gerard W. Clum, DC, the president of Life Chiropractic College West in Hayward, California, says that the best approach is to clean out your purse or briefcase frequently so that you are carrying a lighter load. Backpacks are also preferable to purses or briefcases as they distribute weight evenly on your back instead of over one shoulder.

- **Being well-endowed:** Women with large breasts may experience back pain resulting from altered posture and the pressure it puts directly on the upper back. Dr. Ma sees breast reduction surgery as a last resort. Losing weight will often have the added benefit of reducing your breast size to a more manageable level. Wearing a sports bra or strengthening your core with yoga and Pilates can also be helpful.

Program interviewed and tested 61 adults with chronic low back pain on their levels of resentment, anger, and forgiveness. Patients who reported an inability to forgive had the highest levels of pain.

How it works: Patients who have a greater ability to forgive feel less pain and are less likely to hold on to angry thoughts or act out in anger. When you learn to forgive, you let go of anger and distress, which lowers pain, possibly by affecting the messages pain nerves carry to your brain.

What you need to know: Although this study was done on low back pain, the researchers speculate that having a forgiving mind-set can help with any sort of pain.[66] If you have a grudge you feel you can't let go of, try this.

- **Get specific.** Write down what you want to forgive in clear and specific words. For example: "I want to forgive the man who rear-ended my car because I know it was truly an accident."

- **Understand how anger makes you feel.** The theory that most experts in this field agree on is that feeling angry somehow excites pain nerves involved with the messages that go to and from the brain. This means that feeling angry can physically make you feel depressed and anxious, and experience a higher intensity of pain. Researchers speculate that this has something to do with a chemical known as substance P, which is released when you experience pain and seems to cause aggressive feelings and behavior. The result can be a vicious cycle of anger and pain feeding off one another.[67]

- **Understand forgiveness.** Take time to understand that having a forgiving mind-set calms agitated nerves, which in turn can lower pain, depression, and anxiety. Forgiveness also makes you feel empowered, and other research has pointed out that the more in charge you feel about managing your condition, the less pain you'll have.

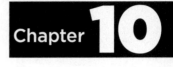

Chapter 10

Knee, Leg, and Foot Pain

Peripheral vascular disease and peripheral artery disease, Achilles tendinitis and other ankle pain, plantar fasciitis, gout, bunions and corns, flat feet and fallen arches, hammertoe, Morton's neuroma

Believe it or not, you and every other human were born to run. Recent research by biologists Dennis Bramble of the University of Utah and Daniel Lieberman of Harvard University has shown this to be the case. As humans first dropped out of the trees and began chasing animals across the plains, their bodies changed to outlast the wildebeests and antelopes they pursued. Humans developed large hip, knee, and ankle joints that acted like shock absorbers, short toes for running, and arched feet that worked like springs.[1] One result is a modern foot that's a true feat of engineering—26 bones, 33 joints, and more than 100 tendons, ligaments, and muscles that support your body for a lifetime.

Despite all this, the modern marvels that are our feet and legs still take a

Pain in the Knees

One joint in the leg that is particularly susceptible to pain or injury is the knee. It is a common victim of the joint deterioration that comes in the form of osteoarthritis. You can read all about how to tame osteoarthritis pain on page 214. Other times, the knee is victim to overuse or an injury in the form of tendinitis, bursitis, or patellofemoral pain. Treatments and remedies for those painful conditions can be found on pages 256 and 284.

serious beating. Some problems, like plantar fasciitis or Achilles tendinitis, can occur from overuse or injuries. Others, such as gout and peripheral vascular disease, are more chronic problems related to other issues in the body. But whatever pain your legs are experiencing, there are nonsurgical options that can help bring you relief.

The old thinking about leg and foot pain used to be this: If it hurts, stay off your feet until it no longer hurts. It was hardly a remedy that jelled with our busy modern lives. Luckily, strategies for dealing with foot and leg pain have come a long way. Today's foot solutions are geared at getting you moving as soon as possible.

The best remedy for feet seems to be exercise: creative moves and stretches that can keep feet happy.

Here's a rundown of some of the most common foot- and leg-related aches and pains and the best ways to keep them healthy and strong for the long haul.

Peripheral Vascular Disease and Peripheral Arterial Disease

When it comes to most types of leg pain, the muscles, tendons, and joints are often the culprits behind the pain. But one very serious type of leg pain stems from your veins. It's peripheral vascular disease, also known as PVD. The sometimes life-threatening condition affects 8 to 12 million people in the United States alone.

Most people think of vein blockages as occurring in and around the heart. But when a blockage occurs in the veins and arteries in other parts of the body, it's known as PVD. One subset of PVD is peripheral arterial disease, or PAD. The most common form of PVD, it only affects the arteries and not your other blood vessels.

PVD most commonly occurs in the legs. As cholesterol and fatty deposits begin to build up in the vein walls and form plaque, blood can no longer flow through as efficiently. This can lead to a painful squeezing sensation known as *claudication*, which often starts when you're walking as your veins fight for oxygen. The result is a cramping, aching sensation that can stop you in your tracks. After rest, the pain often subsides.

As you might expect, the constricted blood flow in the legs related to PVD and PAD can indicate circulatory problems elsewhere in the body, including the heart. It's also closely tied to deep vein thrombosis, which is the presence of a blood clot in the veins. This can be dangerous, especially if the blood clot breaks free and travels to other parts of the body like the lungs or heart.

Because of the seriousness of PVD, a combination of drugs to lower your cholesterol, control your blood pressure, prevent blood clots, manage your symptoms, and possibly lower your blood sugar is your first line of defense. However, the latest research has shown how diet, exercise, and other lifestyle changes like quitting smoking can play a dramatic role in reversing PVD before it becomes dangerous.

Is It PVD?

The concerning thing about PVD is that about two-thirds of those with the disease do not feel these symptoms. This puts them at great risk, as their veins might be narrowed by 60 percent or more by the time they do feel the pain. Here are the warning signs to look out for when it comes to PVD.

- Cramping, pain, numbness, or weakness in the muscles of your leg after activities like walking

- Sores on your legs, feet, or toes that don't seem to heal

- Slower growth of leg hair or toenails

- Shiny skin, or change of the color of the skin on your legs

- A weak pulse from your legs or feet

- Erectile dysfunction

PVD is a serious, potentially life-threatening condition and requires immediate consultation with your doctor. When you arrive at the office, the doctor will likely start with a physical examination of the affected leg. She might be able to identify the blockage by that method alone by the sound it makes through the stethoscope. Blood pressure readings on the leg can also indicate a blockage. Other tests that a doctor might use to diagnose PVD include an ankle-brachial index, ultrasound, and angiography.

Fast Relief Now

PVD can be quite serious and should certainly not be viewed as a condition that can be fixed quickly. Yet there are a few things you can try to bring some relief.

1. **Stay off your feet in the short term.** Although walking and exercise are keys to curing PVD, taking a rest can make the immediate pain subside.

2. **Try over-the-counter pain relievers.** Tylenol, Advil, and others might bring some temporary relief when used according to the manufacturers' instructions.

3. **Don't smoke.** Smoking immediately constricts the blood vessels, so avoid smoking; ultimately, kicking this habit is key.

4. **Avoid certain cold medicines.** Over-the-counter cold medicines that contain pseudoephedrine—such as Advil Cold & Sinus, Aleve Sinus & Headache, Claritin-D, Sudafed, Tylenol Cold, and Zyrtec-D—restrict blood flow.

Relief at Last

If you stop walking, that may make the pain go away in the short term, but it will hardly solve the problem. A combination of medications prescribed by your doctor and significant lifestyle changes is really the best way to manage PVD effectively. Here are the steps to pain-free legs.

Step 1: See your doctor about medication. Depending on the severity of your condition, drugs to manage cholesterol, blood pressure, blood sugar, clotting, and the symptoms of PVD may all be appropriate.

Step 2: Follow a heart-healthy lifestyle. When it comes to life changes, PVD should be addressed much like other blood vessel problems. Possible areas for improvement include eating a heart-healthy diet rich in fruits and vegetables and low in saturated fat, exercising regularly, and quitting smoking.

Step 3: Try ginkgo biloba. This herbal supplement has a mild blood-thinning effect and may be helpful to ease PVD pain.

Step 4: Consider more serious therapies. In more serious instances, an angioplasty, bypass surgery, or a clot-dissolving injection might be required to put a stop to your PVD.

Pain Prevention Strategies

Food and Supplements

HEART-HEALTHY DIET: When it comes to what you eat, PVD should be treated no differently than a heart problem.

The evidence: A number of studies have shown that eating a healthy diet with plentiful fruits and vegetables can reduce your risk of developing atherosclerosis (plaque buildup in the arteries), of which PVD is just one kind. One study showed a risk reduction of 38 percent.[2]

How it works: In countless studies, foods like fruits and vegetables, fatty fish, nuts in moderation, and fiber have shown a heart-protective effect. Red meat, whole dairy products, and other foods laden with saturated fat contribute to cholesterol and plaque buildup in the arteries.

What you need to know: Limit your fat intake to between 25 and 35 percent of your total calories, restrict saturated fat intake to under 7 percent by reducing red meat and whole dairy intake in favor of low-fat dairy products, healthy fish, and nuts, pump up fiber consumption to 25 to 30 grams a day with fruits, vegetables, and whole grains, and reduce the amount of salt in your foods.

GINKGO BILOBA: In some patients, the herbal supplement ginkgo biloba has allowed them to walk farther with less pain during their exercise programs.

The evidence: This was most recently tested in a group of 62 patients in 2008. In the test, 300 milligrams of ginkgo a day created a moderate increase in the amount of time the subjects were able to walk pain free over the course of 4 months. The researchers recommended studying the treatment over a longer period of time in future trials.[3]

How it works: Ginkgo biloba has a mild blood-thinning effect. This may help the blood circulate more efficiently as PAD patients are walking.

What you need to know: Ginkgo can be dangerous when paired with antiplatelet medications and aspirin, as well as other blood-thinning supplements like ginseng, garlic, ginger, and fish oil. Make sure to talk to your doctor before trying any supplement therapies on your own.

Exercise and Movement Therapies

WALKING: One of the most important steps on the road to recovery from PVD is starting a supervised exercise program. Ask your doctor to refer you to a physical therapist or exercise specialist who can begin a program tailored to your needs. At first, this program will begin with walking either on a treadmill or track. As your abilities grow, the specialist will gradually increase the distance you travel.

The evidence: People who start an exercise program for PVD will begin to show improvement within a month and continue to improve over the course of 6 months. In one recent study, sticking to this program increased walking times in the participants by 150 percent.[4]

How it works: Our appreciation of the importance of exercise is growing all the time, and PVD is a perfect example of this, since walking is now considered a first-line treatment for the disease. Regular exercise makes the heart and arteries pump blood more efficiently. For those with PVD, this can ultimately lead to better circulation and an end to their problems if they stick to walking.

What you need to know: The standard exercise program for PVD usually involves at least three sessions a week. At first, participants will continue for 8 to 10 minutes until the pain reaches moderate severity (a 3 on a scale of 1 to 5), and then they'll take a break and resume when the pain subsides. The goal is to walk for a total of 35 minutes in the first sessions, and ultimately reach a point where they can walk 50 minutes pain free.

These sessions can be challenging since they involve exercises that directly cause pain, but the rewards are well worth it to patients who stick with the program.

Pain Medications and Medical Treatments

DRUG COMBINATIONS: A combination of drugs such as cholesterol-lowering statins, blood pressure–lowering medication, antiplatelet drugs like clopidogrel (Plavix) that reduce blood clots (in some cases), cilostazol (Pletal) to reduce the pain, and medication to control blood sugar has been shown effective in reducing PVD and the related risks to the heart in many patients with PVD.

The evidence: In 2001, a landmark study called the PAD Awareness, Risk, and Treatment: New Resources for Survival (PARTNERS) program examined 6,979 patients at 350 offices across America. It found that even though patients with PVD had similar risk factors for atherosclerosis as those with cardiovascular disease, the patients with cardiovascular disease were treated with drugs for cholesterol, blood pressure, and blood clotting much more frequently than those with PVD.

The researchers saw this as a real problem among practitioners, and one that was potentially raising the future heart disease risks of those with PVD.[5] In many instances, these drugs are appropriate treatment for PVD symptoms, so be sure to ask your doctor if they might be right for you.

How it works: Since PVD is ultimately a circulatory problem that's closely tied to heart disease, researchers have concluded that the same drugs can be helpful for both. Cholesterol-lowering drugs keep not only your heart clean, but your arteries as well. The same goes for antiplatelet and blood sugar medications.

What you need to know: In some cases, PVD has not yet led to more serious heart problems. Since you certainly don't want to be on more medication than you have to, have a serious discussion with your doctor about what is appropriate for you. In many cases, eating better and sticking to a walking program can generate real and tangible results.

ANGIOPLASTY, BYPASS SURGERY, OR THROMBOLYTIC THERAPY: In more severe cases, doctors may have to address PVD with techniques similar to those used to open heart arteries.

The evidence: A recent review by the Society of Interventional Radiology has shown all three procedures to be fairly effective in the right situations. In particular, percutaneous transluminal angioplasty, the most commonly used type of angioplasty for treating PAD, has a success rate of 90 percent.[6]

How it works: Angioplasty involves using a balloon on the end of a catheter to clear the blockage and possibly installation of a stent. Bypass surgery, in which a vein from elsewhere in the body is used to bypass the blockage, also opens the veins. In thrombolytic therapy, a clot-dissolving drug is injected into the artery.

What you need to know: Candidates most likely in need of these types of therapies for PVD include patients who have not been successful at exercise therapy and other methods of stopping PVD, as well as those with severe PVD that threatens a limb or who present other nonhealing ulcers, infection, or gangrene.

Achilles Tendinitis and Other Ankle Pain

Your body has a lot of complex joints, but few are more critical to daily functioning than the elaborate composition of muscles, ligaments, tendons, and bones that make up your ankle. It seems that there's a very good reason for this, as the ankle is on the front lines of injury all the time. The National Institute of Arthritis and Musculoskeletal and Skin Diseases (NIAMS) estimates that one million ankle injuries occur each year, and 85 percent of those are sprains. Every day, 25,000 people in the United States experience an ankle sprain.[8]

Of course, an ankle sprain that's caused by an injury or overuse of the ankle is the most common type of ankle pain. Most of us have experienced this type of injury at one point or another in our lives. But ankle pain can be a symptom of other conditions that are not injury related. These include arthritis, gout, nerve compression, and others.

Then there's the Achilles tendon, the thick band of tissue that connects the heel to the calf. Injuries and pain to this area, known as Achilles tendinitis, are also quite common, with around a quarter of a million occurring each year.[9]

Though slightly apart from the ankle, these injuries can be addressed in many of the same ways as ankle pain.

Recently, a study brought to light the fact that tendon problems might be more common than previously realized. Approximately 40 percent of those who suffer an ankle sprain will experience chronic ankle pain even after being treated for their initial injury.

A review article published in May 2009 that reviewed the results of several previous studies on ankle injuries theorizes that unidentified injuries to the peroneal tendons (the tendons behind the outside portion of the anklebone, or fibula) may be the cause of this chronic pain in many instances. These injuries are often untreated or overlooked, which contributes to the chronic pain. Addressing the tendons as part of ankle pain should help doctors come a long way in dealing with this type of chronic pain.[10]

Is It Achilles Tendinitis or Another Ankle Pain?

As you can imagine, ankle pain is pretty easy to identify. The key is to locate the source of the pain, so you can determine whether it's related specifically to the ankle or to the Achilles tendon. The types of pain fall into the following categories:

- Dull, aching pain that seems to emanate from inside the ankle
- Pain directly felt along the outside of the ankle
- Soreness, stiffness, or pain of the Achilles tendon

When to Call the Doctor

Seek emergency medical help if:

- You hear a popping sound and immediately can't put weight on your ankle
- The ankle appears deformed or broken
- The pain occurs even when no weight is put on the ankle

See your doctor if:

- Your ankle pain is severe and disrupts your ability to walk
- The ankle is red and warm, or you contract a fever, both signs of infection
- You have swelling that does not go down within 2 to 3 days
- You have mild pain that doesn't go away after 2 weeks

Determining if you have Achilles tendinitis or another type of ankle pain starts with a physical examination of the foot to determine the type and intensity of the pain. The doctor will also test the range of motion and reflexes of your foot and ankle. Other tests that can help the doctor hone in on the true source of your pain include x-rays, ultrasounds, or magnetic resonance imaging (MRI).

Fast Relief Now

As soon as you feel pain in your ankle, the tried-and-true strategy of RICE (rest, ice, compression, and elevation) is the best approach to treating the short-term pain. The primary objective here is to reduce the pain and swelling in the short term so you can work on healing the cause of the pain in the long term. After the pain subsides, you can begin to work on healing with the help of your doctor and physical therapist. This includes stretching exercises and possibly medical treatment.

1. **Ice the area for about 20 minutes.** Do this several times a day to reduce pain and swelling.

2. **Use elastic bandages or compression wraps.** This will keep down swelling of the area around the tendon.

3. **Rest when you can.** Stick to less intense activities that won't aggravate the injury. While resting, elevate the ankle to reduce the swelling, especially at night.

4. **Try low-impact activities.** Too much inactivity can cause stiffness. Cycling is often a good choice because of its low impact on the ankle.

5. **Use an over-the-counter pain reliever as needed.** No one particular OTC pain reliever is better than the others for ankle pain. Just use it according to the manufacturer's directions and avoid taking it for more than 5 consecutive days, as this can increase your risk of liver damage.

Relief at Last

Once you get through the immediate steps of reducing pain and swelling, the process of healing can begin. As with many foot and leg problems, exercises play a critical role here. This sequence will lead you to healthy ankles again.

Step 1: RICE. As outlined above, the simple sequence of rest, ice, compression, elevation is the first step in treating the mild to moderate ankle injury.

Step 2: Start exercising. A variety of simple stretching exercises paired with low-impact aerobic activities like cycling and walking can get you back on the track to good health.

Step 3: Rethink your footwear. Orthotics such as wraps and shoe inserts will keep your ankle or tendon in a good position during and after healing.

Step 4: Ask your doctor about surgery. As with most foot problems, surgery is the last resort but can help many when other approaches fail. A common procedure is the tenotomy, which involves the release of the tendon, or more extensive procedures to repair damaged tissue.

Pain Prevention Strategies

Exercise and Movement Therapies

SIMPLE STRETCHES: Once your doctor clears you for treatment, you can work with a physical therapist on a few simple exercises to strengthen the Achilles tendon. One type of exercise that has been shown to be effective is "eccentric" strengthening. These are exercises that lengthen the muscle.

The evidence: Studies indicate that eccentric, muscle-lengthening exercises may be more effective than other stretches at healing Achilles tendinitis, although study results have been mixed, and athletic patients see greater results than sedentary patients. In a study of 45 athletic patients in 2008, about 60 percent improved their Achilles tendinitis with eccentric strengthening alone.[11]

How it works: The standard "heel drop," the mainstay of eccentric strengthening for Achilles tendinitis, is done by standing with the balls of your feet on a step and your heels over the edge. While supporting your body, you gradually lower the heels, pause at the bottom, and return them to a straight position. You can also hold light dumbbells in one hand to add resistance as your condition improves.

What you need to know: If your ankle or Achilles tendon pain is fairly mild, this move is safe to try on your own, but if you experience any pain, it's probably a good idea to stop and consult a physical therapist to make sure you're doing it safely. For more severe ankle pain, the physical therapist is your expert for guidance on how to do this exercise properly.

Touch Therapies

MASSAGE: A light soft-tissue massage right at the source of the tendon pain can help bring relief and remove scar tissue related to tendinitis.

The evidence: Massage's effectiveness is tough to measure, but it's hard to argue with how good it feels. Doctors theorize that the massage keeps the tendon loose and also helps remove scar tissue from the area.

How it works: The cross-friction massage may be most effective for relieving Achilles tendinitis or ankle pain. Sit in a chair with your leg elevated and your foot pointed up in a stretched position. Have a family member or friend gently rub across your tendons (rather than along their length, to create cross friction) with one finger, and work his or her way toward the sprained area. Rub for about 5 to 10 minutes every other day.

What you need to know: Wait about 48 to 72 hours before trying massage to give the sprain time to heal. If the pain is still severe or other complications such as broken bones exist, do not attempt a massage at home. Ask your doctor if a massage by a qualified physical or massage therapist might be appropriate.

ACUPUNCTURE: Acupuncture treatment that focuses directly on the Achilles tendon may have an impact on the speed with which tendinitis heals, preliminary evidence suggests.

ThinkTwice:
Injections for Your Achilles

Injections are considered one of the treatment options for Achilles tendinitis, but a series of recent studies is making people rethink that notion. First is the corticosteroid injection, a mainstay of treatment for many foot and leg problems, including tendinitis. However, several studies have shown an increased risk of rupture to the Achilles tendon from these injections. As a result, many doctors have begun to see this as more of a last resort.[12]

Then there are platelet-rich plasma, or PRP, injections, the trendy tendinitis treatment of just a few years ago. The theory was that injecting your own blood plasma into the inflamed tendon would speed healing. However, a 2010 study published in the *Journal of the American Medical Association* has largely debunked this treatment. In a study of 54 patients with Achilles tendinitis, those who received the PRP injections did not fare better than those who received a placebo.[13]

The evidence: A 2010 study of nine healthy males showed that inserting needles into the Achilles tendon increased blood flow and oxygen saturation not only during the treatment, but afterward.

How it works: The researchers theorized that this boost of blood and oxygen to the Achilles tendon could speed healing, giving acupuncture a significant role in treating tendinitis.[14]

What you need to know: See Part Three for resources on finding a licensed acupuncturist in your area. The number of treatments needed will vary based on the severity of your pain.

Pain Medications and Other Medical Treatments

SURGERY: If the tendon doesn't heal after several months of treatment, or is partially or completely ruptured, then your doctor might consider surgery to repair the damage.

The evidence: A 2010 study showed that surgery was highly effective at healing an Achilles tendon rupture. In 29 patients studied, all 29 of them showed good function, few limitations in their activities, and high satisfaction even 3 years after the surgery.[15]

How it works: Recent advances in the techniques used for Achilles tendon surgery have created less invasive treatments and speedier recovery times. Some of these include radio frequency treatments, new arthroscopic procedures, bone anchors, and tissue grafts.

What you need to know: Despite the advancements, recovery from Achilles tendon surgery can take up to 6 months. Have a serious discussion with your doctor about whether this is the right step for you, then take your recovery seriously.

Other Strategies

SHOE INSERTS: Doctors will often recommend shoe inserts or wedges for Achilles tendinitis.

The evidence: Shoe inserts have been shown to be particularly effective for runners. Studies have shown that they have a 75 percent success rate in preventing injuries.[16] But experts agree that they can certainly be effective for others suffering from the injury as well.

How it works: Shoe inserts elevate the heel slightly, which takes pressure off the tendon to relieve pain and speed healing.

What you need to know: Talk to your doctor about which type of insert would be right for you. There are custom-made, flexible orthotics for all parts of the feet depending on where you need the most support.

Plantar Fasciitis

Heel pain plagues around two million Americans every year, making it the most common foot pain complaint.[17] Among heel complaints, plantar fasciitis is the most common of all. The condition occurs when the long fibrous ligament, the plantar fascia, along the bottom of the foot develops tears in the tissue, resulting in pain and inflammation. If you suffer from plantar fasciitis then you know that the sharp pain is usually felt where the ligament attaches to the heel bone.

Often, plantar fasciitis is caused by high-impact activities, either by athletes or overzealous beginning exercisers. But this condition can also result from poor shoes, high or low arches, and arthritis.

In the past, plantar fasciitis caused plenty of consternation among athletes who feared that the condition meant turning in their running shoes for good. But the good news is that about 90 percent of plantar fasciitis cases will resolve with basic treatments within a few months.[18] Most athletes can even resume their previous activities without complications.

The basic treatments for plantar fasciitis are pretty cut-and-dried: Keep off your feet when you can, use ice and stretches to relieve the pain, and take over-the-counter pain relievers. But other things you can now add to your heel pain arsenal include greatly improved footwear and shoe inserts, acupuncture, and even shockwave therapy in some instances.

Is It Plantar Fasciitis?

Some of the indicators that your heel pain is plantar fasciitis include:

- Pain develops gradually over time, and usually just in one foot
- The pain is often the worst right when you get out of bed, although it can also flare up after long periods of being off your feet, such as after a car ride or after sitting in your office chair for a while
- At this point, it often feels like a sharp, piercing pain
- By the end of the day, the pain may be replaced by a dull aching that improves with rest
- Most people complain of increased heel pain after walking for a long period of time

If you have heel pain, the first thing your doctor will do is take a closer look at your foot. The warning signs he is looking for are high arches, an area just in front of the heel bone that is particularly tender, pain that is worst right on the plantar fascia and improves when you point your heels down, or a limited range of motion in your ankle. Your doctor might also recommend x-rays or other imaging tests to identify the pain more precisely.

Fast Relief Now

If you think you have plantar fasciitis, these tried-and-true steps will help bring immediate relief and speed healing.

1. **Apply ice to reduce pain and swelling.** Do this just after an activity that aggravates your pain. Place the painful heel on a cold pack, a bag of frozen vegetables, or a plastic bag filled with ice.

2. **Elevate your painful foot.** Do this as much as possible, and while icing the heel for extra benefit.

3. **Reduce activity until the problem improves.** Rest is really the best medicine to allow the heel to heal.

4. **Wear foot pads.** They will prevent rubbing and irritation. When you do have to move with painful plantar fasciitis, this can help reduce the pain.

5. **Take over-the-counter pain medicine.** Ibuprofen or acetaminophen will help, and neither one is proven to be more effective than the other. Just take the one that's helpful for you, according to the manufacturer's directions.[19]

Plantar fasciitis is rarely a serious health concern, so the basic steps of rest, ice, stretching, and pain relievers will usually do the trick in the short term while the pain improves. Of course, there are cases when the pain is severe and more drastic treatment is needed.

Relief at Last

A variety of treatment options is available for plantar fasciitis, ranging from simple range-of-motion exercises to surgery. Here is the order in which these treatments should be employed, based on the severity of your heel pain:

Step 1: Try over-the-counter pain relief, stretching, and taking it easy. These are the mainstays of plantar fasciitis treatment and will bring relief to the most people.

Step 2: Ask your doctor about night splints and new shoes or insoles. Night splints hold your foot in a lengthened position overnight to help it stretch more effectively. Several shoes and insoles can also relieve pain and speed healing.

Step 3: See a physical therapist. A more regimented, detailed stretching and exercise routine is helpful for many.

Step 4: Try acupuncture. This ancient practice has shown real results in relieving plantar fasciitis pain.

Step 5: Ask your doctor about corticosteroids, shockwave therapy, or surgery. For severe and serious plantar fasciitis, these treatments have helped people when other treatments have failed.

Pain-Relief Strategies

Food and Supplements

WEIGHT LOSS: We all know about stressors such as badly fitting shoes and high heels. But did you know that excess weight is also tough on your feet? A study of people who lost an average of 90 pounds after bariatric surgery found that their foot pain complaints dropped 83 percent.[20]

The evidence: Obese children have more leg, foot, and ankle injuries than similarly aged children of a healthy weight, according to a study in the April 2010 issue of *Pediatrics*. The study measured 23,000 children, ages 3 to 14 years, about one in six of whom was considered obese.[21]

How it works: Extra weight is hard on our bodies in many ways, but it puts a ton of extra pressure on our feet. Losing that weight relieves the pressure and minimizes the chances of pain occurring.

What you need to know: Reducing calorie consumption by eating a healthy diet and exercising regularly are the keys to weight loss. If you need help, join a local support group or find a registered dietitian in your area.

Exercise and Movement Therapies

STRETCH: When it comes to the pain and stiffness of plantar fasciitis, simple stretches are part of the equation to speed healing.

The evidence: The American Academy of Orthopaedic Surgeons calls the following two stretches "the most effective way to relieve the pain that comes with this condition."[22]

How it works: Try the following stretches.

Calf stretch: Stand slightly away from a wall, place your hands on it, put one foot in front of the other, and bend the front knee slightly. You should feel a pull in the calf of your rear leg. Hold it for 10 seconds and relax. Repeat the exercise 20 times for each foot.

Plantar fascia stretch: Before you get out of bed in the morning, take a seated position on the edge of the bed and cross the affected foot over the other knee. Grab the toes with one hand (use a towel if you can't reach), and support the plantar fascia with your other hand. Then pull the foot slowly and easily toward your body. Hold it for 10 seconds and relax. Repeat the exercise 20 times for each foot.

What you need to know: These stretches can help many with plantar fasciitis, but more severe plantar fascia pain might call for additional guidance and stretches from a physical therapist. Don't be afraid to ask your doctor for a referral if the pain isn't going away on its own.

Touch Therapies

ACUPUNCTURE: This ancient Chinese practice of inserting needles into the body has shown real results in relieving plantar fascia pain.

The evidence: Sixty men and women were given either acupuncture or a sham acupuncture treatment (the needle is put in a nonheel spot) for plantar fasciitis. At the end of the study, the acupuncture group reported lower levels of morning pain and lower levels of pain during exercise or other activities than the sham group.[23]

How it works: As in other acupuncture treatments, the practitioners believe that using needles helps unblock channels of energy in the body. Western doctors think that possibly some stimulation goes on at the needling site that may help reduce pain.

What you need to know: If you're interested in trying acupuncture, start by checking your medical insurance. Many companies are now covering, at least partially, acupuncture treatments for pain. See Part Three to find a licensed acupuncturist near you.

Pain Medications and Medical Therapies

NIGHT SPLINTS: Meant to be worn while sleeping, night splints have shown real results in helping people with plantar fasciitis heal faster.

The evidence: In a 2010 study, 60 patients were given the usual treatments for plantar fasciitis (pain relievers, new footwear, and corticosteroids as needed), but 30 of the patients were also treated with night splints. The night splints improved the outcomes so significantly that the study authors recommend that the splints should be part of the standard of care for treating plantar fasciitis.[24]

How it works: The night splint holds your plantar fascia and Achilles tendon in a lengthened position while you sleep to stretch them more effectively.

What you need to know: One popular and well studied over-the-counter night splint is the Strassburg Sock. It's available at many running stores or online at www.thesock.com. In a 2002 study of 160 patients with plantar fasciitis, the group that used the Strassburg Sock healed their plantar fasciitis in 18.5 days on average, much faster than a group that used stretching as treatment. What's more, all the patients who used the flexible Strassburg Sock were able to sleep comfortably through the night wearing the splint.[25]

SHOCKWAVE THERAPY: If your plantar heel pain hasn't responded to other forms of treatment, you might consider radial extracorporeal shockwave therapy (ESWT). This therapy isn't as invasive as surgery, it doesn't have long recovery times, and it appears to work about twice as well as a sham treatment, according to recent research.

The evidence: German researchers randomly assigned 245 patients with chronic plantar fasciitis to undergo three shockwave treatments 2 weeks apart, or a sham procedure with a device that did not transmit shockwaves. At the end of 12 weeks, the shockwave group had reduced their pain more than 70 percent, while the placebo group averaged 45 percent. A year later, the pain scores in the shockwave group were 85 percent lower than at the beginning of the study, while the sham group was at 43 percent.[26]

> ## Quick Tip
> Researchers in Brazil had men and women wear both inexpensive, store-bought gel inserts and expensive, custom-made inserts to manage their plantar fasciitis pain. They found that both were equally effective at relieving pain.[30]

How it works: Experts aren't exactly sure how this therapy works, but one prevailing theory is that the shockwaves trick the body into thinking that a new injury has occurred, and it rushes in with increased blood flow to help with healing. As a result, the injury that is already present gets treated.

What you need to know: Shockwave therapy is relatively new on the scene, but emerging studies are now backing up the initial results of the German study mentioned above.[27] You may want to consider asking your physician about it if you haven't had success with other treatments.

Other Strategies

GET NEW SHOES: Take a simple step: Choose footwear or insoles that can help relieve plantar fasciitis. More than 60 percent of Americans confess that they wear shoes that hurt their feet, according to a poll conducted by the American Podiatric Medical Association, and about 12 percent wear the hurtful footwear on a daily basis.[28]

The evidence: Boston researchers interviewed thousands of women who were part of the landmark Framingham Heart Study. They determined that women who wore athletic shoes or sneakers were two-thirds less likely to have foot pain than women who wore high heels or other less comfortable choices.[29]

How it works: High heels and other types of dress shoes may look stylish but they don't offer much in terms of support for your heel. As your feet take a pounding day after day, these uncomfortable shoes can ultimately lead you down the road to plantar fasciitis pain.

What you need to know: Tennis shoes, running shoes, and other athletic sneakers seem to have better cushioning for preserving your heels. If you can, make these your everyday footwear choice. The shoes you choose should have good arch support and a slightly raised heel. Sandals are not the best choice for plantar fasciitis, as they don't provide much in terms of heel support. But a number of stylish shoes, even dress shoes, are available for people with plantar fasciitis pain. Ask a sales clerk if she has any shoes that would be right for you.

Gout

As you'll see throughout this chapter, toes can cause people a lot of problems, and usually your shoe selection plays at least some role.

In one particular instance, however, the joint of your toe can break out in stabbing, unbearable pain, regardless of your shoe selection. At times, often in the middle of the night, the piercing pain—it feels like shards of glass stabbing the toe—is so severe that it will wake you up and make you want to throw off the covers. That pain is known as gout.

Gout is actually a form of arthritis that usually affects the joint at the base of the big toe. Men are more likely to get gout but it affects women, too, especially after menopause. The cause is uric acid—mineral deposits that accumulate around the big toe joint. Uric acid is naturally found in the body, but foods high in purines (liver, dried beans, asparagus, mushrooms, and others) can also boost levels. Gout is often caused by genetics, but heavy alcohol drinkers also run a greater risk of developing it.

Gout can be debilitating, but there is some good news. In recent years, breakthrough developments in the field of gout treatment have made the disease much easier to manage. The most promising recent drug is probenecid (Probalan), which helps the body break down and remove uric acid.

The other important gout-related breakthrough is the critical role experts now acknowledge that diet and nutrition can play. There's a real chance that you can control gout symptoms with the foods you choose, such as coffee, cherries, or oranges.

Is It Gout?

Gout is distinct from other types of foot pain and usually easy to identify. Here's what to look for.

● Sudden, intense pain occurs in the joint at the base of the big toe.

● The pain is accompanied by swelling, tenderness, or redness.

● Discomfort in the joint continues after the episode of intense pain.

- In rarer instances, gout can affect the joints elsewhere in your feet, or also in your ankles, knees, hands, and wrists.

Gout is typically easy to diagnose based on the symptoms, but your doctor may also perform a joint fluid test to determine your levels of uric acid or a blood test.

Fast Relief Now

A bout of gout pain starts out subtly, then builds up to roaring pain, often within 12 to 24 hours. With exercise and rehydration, you might be able to minimize its severity. If not, drugs and other ways to cope with the pain are your best options.

1. **Try some walking or other light exercises.** If pain is not severe, stretch the toes or the lower body to make the pain go away.

2. **Drink plenty of water.** Dehydration can cause a gout flare-up. Drinking an adequate amount of water can dilute uric acid levels in the blood and make this less likely to occur.

3. **Take over-the-counter pain medication.** If the pain is severe, Tylenol, Advil, Aleve, and others are all effective when used according to the manufacturer's directions. In some cases, your doctor can prescribe something stronger if these are ineffective.

Relief at Last

Gout is one condition where a combination of medical and lifestyle strategies can be highly effective. Here are your steps to success.

Step 1: Reset your diet. Simple steps like drinking plenty of water (8 to 16 glasses a day), avoiding alcohol intake, limiting protein to healthy

Quick Tip

The pain of gout can be severe at times, and studies have shown that meditation and breathing techniques can help people cope with it. Margaret Lewin, MD, the medical director of Cinergy Health in Aventura, Florida, says that deep breathing can be as simple as closing your eyes and taking long, deep breaths. While breathing, visualize a relaxing scene, or simply count backward from 10 to 1 until the fierce pain subsides.

levels, and avoiding foods high in purine (organ meats, dried beans, asparagus, mushrooms, herring, and anchovies) can play a major role in reducing the incidence of gout.

Step 2: Get the right prescription. Drugs definitely play a role in the management of gout pain, particularly with new drugs on the scene such as probenecid, which can actually remove uric acid from the body and eliminate the pain more effectively than ever before.

Step 3: Try the gout superfoods. A few specific foods have shown promise in managing gout symptoms, such as coffee, cherries, and berries, and vitamin C-rich fruits and vegetables.

Step 4: Try other lifestyle treatments. Exercise, meditation, breathing techniques, massage, and acupuncture can also play a role in gout pain management. Read on to see how it can all work together.

Food and Supplements

AVOID PURINES: Avoiding foods rich in amino acids known as purines should reduce the incidence of gout.

The evidence: This has been well studied. A recent review of the literature on the topic showed that several studies indicated the efficacy of a low-purine diet in reducing gout. One study indicated that consuming a low-purine diet can reduce uric acid levels in as few as 10 days.[31]

How it works: Purines directly create uric acid as their end product. Since uric acid in the blood is the direct cause of gout flare-ups, avoiding these purine-rich foods can go a long way toward reducing the incidence of gout.

What you need to know: Foods high in purines include red meats (especially organ meats), seafood, dried beans, asparagus, and mushrooms. If you have gout, limit intake of these or replace them with alternatives in your diet.

STAY HYDRATED: One of the simplest ways to prevent gout outbreaks is to drink plenty of water.

The evidence: In a 2009 study of 535 people with gout, those who drank five to eight glasses of water a day experienced a 43 percent reduction in gout attacks. Those who drank eight or more experienced a 48 percent reduction.[32]

How it works: When you're dehydrated, the uric acid levels in your blood are at a higher concentration and more likely to lead to gout pain. Staying properly hydrated can dilute those levels and possibly fight off a flare-up.

What you need to know: Strive for eight glasses of water or more day, but listen to your body. Generally drinking water whenever you feel thirsty is the best approach. Nothing is as efficient at hydrating you effectively as plain old water.

BANISH BOOZE: Alcohol consumption is directly tied to gout and seen as a major risk factor for the disease.

The evidence: In a 2008 study of 228 healthy men, those who drank more than 15 grams of alcohol a day had a 93 percent greater risk of developing gout than those who abstained from alcohol consumption.[38]

How it works: The main effect here is that drinking alcohol dehydrates you. Thus it has the opposite effect on uric acid levels that drinking water would have.

What you need to know: Though two drinks a day are considered safe for most men, you may want to consider abstaining entirely if you have gout.

PICK YOUR PROTEINS WISELY: Several studies have shown that high meat consumption increases gout risk. Conversely, dairy and plant-based proteins reduce gout risk.

The evidence: In a landmark 2004 study of over 47,000 men, those who ate the most meat and seafood increased their risk of getting gout by about

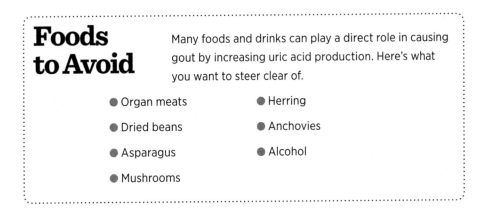

Foods to Avoid

Many foods and drinks can play a direct role in causing gout by increasing uric acid production. Here's what you want to steer clear of.

- Organ meats
- Dried beans
- Asparagus
- Mushrooms
- Herring
- Anchovies
- Alcohol

50 percent. Conversely, those who consumed the most dairy products cut their risk in half.[33]

How it works: Meats are more likely to contain purines, which turn into uric acid once they reach the bloodstream. Dairy products and most plant foods (asparagus is an exception) do not contain purines.

What you need to know: Limit your daily intake of meat, fish, and poultry to 4 to 6 ounces. Replace those sources of protein in your diet with low-fat dairy products, eggs, tofu, and nut butters.

CHEW ON CHERRIES AND BERRIES: Researchers aren't exactly sure why, but study after study has shown that consumption of different kinds of cherries or cherry juice reduces uric acid levels and the occurrence of gout pain.

The evidence: A 2003 United States Department of Agriculture study of 10 healthy women showed that they excreted more urate crystals in their urine and their blood levels of urate dropped significantly after consuming 2 servings of cherries. Urate crystals are one of the major contributors to gout pain, so this seems to support the notion that cherries help relieve gout.[34]

How it works: A 2009 study reported that anthocyanins, a bioactive antioxidant with anti-inflammatory properties that are present in cherries in large quantities, might be the catalyst behind cherries' gout-relieving properties.[35]

What you need to know: Adding cherries and other dark-colored berries that also contain anthocyanins is certainly a healthy supplement to your daily fruit and vegetable intake.

GET MORE VITAMIN C: A growing amount of research is showing that vitamin C supplementation might reduce the risk of gout.

The evidence: A 2009 study of almost 47,000 men showed that men who took 1,500 milligrams of vitamin C a day cut their risk of developing gout in half.[36]

How it works: Vitamin C reduces blood uric acid levels, the primary cause of gout. In addition, vitamin C-rich fruits like oranges contain a phytonutrient known as betacryptoxanthin, a powerful antioxidant that seems to shut off pain by reducing oxidative stress within the body.

What you need to know: Taking vitamin C in such high doses can present some risks, so ask your doctor about it before starting vitamin C supplementation on your own. In the meantime, there is certainly no risk in filling up your diet with vitamin C–rich fruits and vegetables like citrus fruits and tomatoes.

DRINK YOUR MORNING COFFEE: Studies show that drinkers of coffee (even decaffeinated) may be protecting themselves from gout.

The evidence: A 2007 study of almost 46,000 men showed that the more coffee they drank, the more they lowered their risk of gout.[37]

How it works: Another recent study showed that coffee lowers blood levels of uric acid, a direct contributor to gout pain.[38]

What you need to know: Drinking too much coffee can cause other adverse health effects, such as restlessness, anxiety, irritability, and sleeplessness, so most healthy people should limit intake to 2 to 4 cups a day.

Pain Prevention Strategies

Exercise and Movement Therapies

EXERCISE: Gout and exercise have had an interesting relationship. Once believed to elevate uric acid levels and contribute to gout, moderate exercise has now been shown to prevent gout and relieve symptoms.

The evidence: In a 2008 study of 228 men in California, those that were the most physically active had the lowest risk of developing gout.[39]

How it works: Regular exercise improves blood circulation and reduces uric acid levels.

What you need to know: If you already have gout, stick to low-impact, moderate activity. There is some evidence that vigorous activity can elevate uric acid levels.

Touch Therapies

ACUPUNCTURE: Traditional Chinese acupuncture is well studied and seems to be effective in treating gout-related pain.

The evidence: A 2006 study of 130 patients with gout divided them into an acupuncture group and a group that received medication. Both therapies were effective at treating gout, but those in the acupuncture group had a greater cure rate.[40]

How it works: Doctors aren't exactly sure how acupuncture works, but some believe that it may increase circulation and bring a greater flow of blood to the treated area, which could help alleviate gout pain.

What you need to know: See Part Three to learn how to find a licensed, qualified acupuncturist in your area.

XANTHINE OXIDASE INHIBITORS: This class of drugs, which includes allopurinol (Zyloprim, Aloprim) and febuxostat (Uloric), has been shown to be effective at reducing the incidence of gout flare-ups.

The evidence: The most recently approved drug is febuxostat (Uloric), which reduced uric acid levels significantly in 67 percent of patients in a 2009 study.[41]

How it works: These drugs actually block your body's production of uric acid. This then lowers the levels of uric acid found in the blood and reduces the incidence of gout.

What you need to know: Xanthine oxidase inhibitors have side effects that include rash, low white blood cell counts, nausea, and reduced liver function. You need to make sure a recent gout attack is totally resolved before taking them, as the drug could trigger another attack if not. Talk to your doctor about what medication might be right for your gout treatment.

PROBENECID (PROBALAN): This relatively new drug has also shown promise in reducing gout attacks.

The evidence: A 2008 study showed that the reason probenecid works well for gout pain is that it increases the ability of the kidneys to remove uric acid from the body.[42]

How it works: If your body removes uric acid more efficiently, it is less likely to make its way to the feet via the bloodstream and cause gout-related pain.

What you need to know: Side effects of probenecid include rash, stomach pain, and kidney stones. Talk to your doctor about what medication might be right for your gout treatment.

Bunions

If you feel a painful, bony bump at the base of your big toe, then you might have a bunion. As the bunion grows, it pushes the big toe against the others. Over time, this can cause swelling, soreness, and thickening of the skin, not to mention limited movement. Genetics also plays a role in bunions, but one of the main causes is usually tight-fitting shoes such as high heels.

Though you can develop a bunion at any age if you're genetically predisposed or if you've really abused your feet, they are more common as you get older. One study found that women in their forties were $1\frac{1}{2}$ times more likely to have bunions than thirty-somethings. Those in their fifties were three and a half times more likely. From 60 to 69, the likelihood rose to six times.

Bunions form when the normal forces exerted on the joints and tendons of your feet change, usually a result of ill-fitting shoes or strenuous activities. This leads to instability in the big toe joint and can cause it to deform.

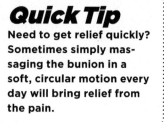

Quick Tip
Need to get relief quickly? Sometimes simply massaging the bunion in a soft, circular motion every day will bring relief from the pain.

Sometimes arthritis can contribute to the formation of a bunion. Other times, a job that puts stress on your feet or requires you to wear ill-fitting shoes might play a role. Cowboys (and cowgirls) and professional dancers are two groups that have a higher risk of developing bunions.

Most of the standard recommendations for bunions involve over-the-counter pain relievers and wearing more comfortable shoes. While those steps will definitely help, some new exercises can actually reverse a bunion and bring your toes back to their more normal position.

Is It a Bunion?

If you think you might have a bunion, look out for the following.

- A bump on the outside of your big toe, near the base

- Thicker skin at the base of your big toe

- Corns or calluses, usually where the first and second toes overlap

- Swelling, redness, or soreness at the big toe joint

- Pain or restricted movement of your big toe

Unlike other types of foot and leg pain, your doctor likely can detect a bunion just by looking at it, though he may deem an x-ray necessary to determine its severity. He might also test your range of motion and pain, ask you about the types of shoes you wear, and determine your family history of foot problems.

Fast Relief Now

Often the pain of a bunion can be managed with these simple steps alone. But if the pain persists, you can talk to your doctor about other strategies like surgery.

1. **Apply a cold pack to the bunion.** This will reduce any immediate pain. Use a bag of frozen vegetables, a cold pack, or a plastic bag filled with ice cubes. Just elevate the leg slightly and use a band or wrap to secure the bag to the foot if necessary. You may want to wrap the bag in a thin towel if the cold is too much to bear.

2. **Try bunion pads.** These cushion the bunion and relieve pain. A number of bunion pads are available over-the-counter at drug and grocery stores, including those made by Dr. Scholl's and PediFix.

3. **Switch to shoes that give your toes more room.** Avoid high heels, which put undue pressure on the feet and exert the force that leads to the development of bunions in the first place. We'll provide more detail on choosing the right pair of shoes on page 203.

Relief at Last

A bunion is undoubtedly painful, but most can be resolved without resorting to extreme measures. Here are the steps to take to banish those bunions.

Step 1: Buy new shoes. Since shoes are often the cause of bunions, choosing a comfortable pair is your first step toward relief. Don't be afraid to spend a little time barefoot each day to give your feet a break! In severe cases, you may want to talk to your doctor about custom footwear to help relieve your bunion pain. Bunion pads and splints (which position the foot in a way that effectively relieves the pain) may also be helpful, along with the right pair of shoes.

Step 2: Try cutting-edge exercises. Our experts say that doing the right exercises can not only relieve bunions, it can actually reverse the foot damage!

Step 3: Give surgery a go. In extreme cases, surgery might be necessary to relieve your bunions.

Pain Prevention Strategies

Exercise and Movement Therapies

TOE-STRETCHING EXERCISES: A few simple foot exercises are great for relieving the pain and pressure of bunions. Some research indicates that they may even be able to reverse the damage to your feet.

The evidence: Hylton B. Menz, PhD, the editor in chief of the *Journal of Foot and Ankle Research*, has actually helped patients coax their big toe back to its original position when it started drifting inward.

How it works: Sit down, place your feet side by side, and loop a thick elastic band (such as Thera-Band Exercise Tubing, www.thera-band.com, and similar

Curing Corns

One unfortunate side effect to bunions and other foot problems is a corn, a pesky little growth with a hard center that often forms on the tops or sides of toes. Corns can sometimes be painful, but they are easy to treat. Here's the quick cure.

- Soak your foot in warm, soapy water. This softens the skin and makes it easier to remove.

- Try an over-the-counter medicated corn pad. These contain salicylic acid to remove the corn. If you have diabetes or poor circulation, talk to a doctor first.

- Keep the affected area clean and dry. After removal, it's important to treat the skin to avoid infection.

- Buy comfortable shoes and socks. This will prevent irritation that could make the corn come back.

- See your doctor if the corn is painful or inflamed.

On the Horizon

Botox for Bunions

Most of us have heard of Botox as a method for fighting wrinkles, but could it help for bunions, too? In a 2008 study, doctors relieved the pain and reduced the physical deformity of the bunion with an injection of botulinum toxin A, otherwise known as Botox. Although this is not a commonly prescribed solution, and clearly more research is needed, it does show an intriguing possibility for the future of bunion treatment.[43]

products) around your big toes. Slowly pull your feet apart to tighten the elastic. Hold for 20 seconds. Repeat 10 times. Do three sets once a day every day to maintain the improvement.

Another simple exercise that can bring relief is the toe spread. Simply put the band around all the toes of one foot and spread them to stretch them out.

Pain Medications and Medical Treatments

FLEXIBLE SPLINT: A flexible splint can reduce mild displacement of the big toe. Dr. Menz says that such devices do not cure bunions but reduce pain while they're being used.

The evidence: In a 2008 study of 30 women, wearing flexible splints did nothing to cure the bunion but it did help the patients greatly with the pain while wearing them.[44]

How it works: The splint typically fits over the toe and part of the foot and is held tightly in place with a hook and loop (Velcro) strap. It pulls the toes apart and positions them in a way that relieves pain.

What you need to know: Try the Bunion Aid, available from Alpha Orthotics (www.alphaorthotics.com).

SURGERY: If steps like new shoes, splints, and exercises aren't doing anything to help your bunion, then surgery might be the way to go. However, it's not recommended unless the pain is severe and interfering with your daily activities.

The evidence: A number of studies have been conducted on the efficacy of bunion surgery. After reviewing those studies, the American Academy of Orthopaedic Surgeons has concluded that 85 to 90 percent of people are satisfied with the results of the surgery.[45]

How it works: Most bunion surgeries include a "bunionectomy," which involves removing the swollen tissue that makes up the bunion, as well as some removal, realignment, and joining of bones to reform your foot properly.

What you need to know: As with any surgery, there are risks involved. These include recurrence of the bunion if proper steps are not taken after the surgery, such as wearing appropriate footwear. Full recovery from bunion surgery can take up to 8 weeks.

Other Strategies

CHOOSE THE RIGHT SHOES: Sometimes the simplest solution is the best, and this is definitely the case with bunions. Almost all cases of bunions can be managed by choosing properly fitting shoes for your feet.

The evidence: Studies have shown that bunions are nine times more common among women than men. What's more, a whopping 88 percent of women in the United States wear shoes that are too small for them. Not surprisingly, 55 percent of all women in this country have bunions.[46]

How it works: Considering that most people wear shoes that don't fit them properly, just giving your toes the room they need to rest comfortably is a simple step to bunion prevention and to relieving bunion-related pain.

What you need to know: When shoe shopping, make sure your toes have plenty of room to stretch out in the front of the shoe. It may help to go later in the day when your feet are swollen to get a true sense of how much room your toes will truly need. Don't be afraid to ask a salesperson for assistance. Once the shoes are on, place your finger above the toe box to make sure there is room in front of your toes—you should have between three-eighths and one-half inch of space between your shoes and the front of the toe box. Walk around the store and make sure your heels stay in place. (This doesn't apply to open-heeled sandals, obviously.) The shoes need to be wide enough as well. You shouldn't feel pinching or tightness in any part of the foot.

Hammertoe

For anyone with a carpentry background, hammertoe certainly doesn't sound pleasant. And though the condition has nothing to do with hitting your toes with a hammer, it can be quite painful in its own right.

In reality, the condition derives its name from the shape your toes begin to take. Thanks to shoes that are too tight, heels that are too high, or muscular imbalances, your toes begin to curl into a clawlike shape (it is also sometimes called *claw toe*). Over time, they stay that way, causing pain and difficulty moving.

Flatfeet and Fallen Arches

Some people never develop an arch in their foot at all. Often this is painless and presents very few problems. This is known as flatfeet syndrome.

In others, the posterior tibial tendon fails and the arch gradually collapses, creating flatfeet later on in life (usually between the ages of 60 and 70). In other cases, carrying too much weight or doing high-impact exercises like running can cause the collapse. This is known as *fallen arches* and can often be painful. Another name for the condition is *overpronation*.

When painful, flatfeet and fallen arches can usually be managed with self-care strategies like rest, arch supports, and exercise. Recent research also shows the vital role of massage and acupuncture in pain management. And some shoes now available can even return those with flatfeet to their favorite activities. Surgery is required in the rare case of a tendon tear but is usually not necessary to manage the condition.

One of the simplest exercises to try at home is to stand with your hands on a wall and put one foot in front of the other. Keep the back heel planted firmly on the floor and begin bending your front knee until you feel a pull through your back calf. Hold it for about 15 to 30 seconds, and repeat 2 to 4 times for each leg. Do this three or four times a day.

Massage is also useful to ease muscle tension and bring blood flow to the foot. A 2008 study that analyzed treatment for flatfeet incorporated a 5-minute massage among other methods of treatment. After 6 months, the patients experienced a significant reduction in pain and no recurrence.[47]

In addition, over-the-counter arch supports can relieve the pain of flatfeet for many. A study published in 2008 supported the notion that orthotics can be an effective method for managing the pain related to flatfeet, though it does not help reverse the condition.[48]

If you're a runner, look for one of the cutting-edge running shoes designed specifically for people with flatfeet. Some of the key words to look for when shoe shopping are *stability*, *support*, and *motion control*. Go to a shoe store that focuses on running so they can help you choose the proper shoes. If you can, try some runs barefoot on a soft surface! The Nike Free is a popular running shoe that closely simulates barefoot running. Some experts believe that running barefoot keeps your foot in a more natural position and makes it less likely that you'll experience a foot injury.

In recent years, some basic toe and foot exercises (things as simple as scrunching up a towel with your toes, or picking up marbles with your toes) have proven remarkably effective at reversing mild or moderate hammertoe (see details below). For severe hammertoe, a breakthrough implant called the Smart Toe has eased the recovery process.

Is It Hammertoe?

If you have hammertoe, it's readily apparent because of the curled, clawlike shape of the toe (or toes). Other symptoms include:

- Difficulty moving the toe

- Pain in the toes and foot

- Development of corns and calluses

A doctor will likely be able to see right away if you have hammertoe. He may test the range of motion of your toes to determine the extent of the pain and the severity of the condition; x-rays can also be useful for this.

Fast Relief Now

Hammertoe won't go away on its own, but you can do plenty of things to reduce the pain and prevent its progression.

1. **Try some simple stretches.** Spend a few minutes crumpling a towel with your toes or using your toes to pick up marbles or other small objects. These are long-term exercises that you should do every day for hammertoe, but they also stretch the toes for short-term relief.

2. **Wear corn pads or straps.** These won't cure hammertoe, but they will cushion and position the toes properly to relieve the pain.

When to Call the Doctor

You might be able to avoid surgery if you catch the symptoms of hammertoe early enough, so call your doctor if you have any of these symptoms.

- You notice any signs of a curling toe.

- You have a toe that is painful.

- The toe affects your ability to walk or use your feet in other ways.

3. Treat your feet right. Go barefoot or put on your most comfortable pair of tennis shoes with plenty of room in the toe box.

Relief at Last

Treatments for hammertoe range from simple home solutions for mild hammertoe to serious surgery for severe hammertoe. Here's the sequence to try.

Step 1: Try exercises and new shoes. These are the first steps toward relief and reversal of symptoms if you have mild or moderate hammertoe.

Step 2: Put in pads, splints, or straps. A few commercially available and custom orthotics might be the answer for coping with hammertoe.

Step 3: Try surgery. For serious cases of hammertoe, surgery is the answer for correcting the problem.

Pain Prevention Strategies

Exercise and Movement Therapies

TOE EXERCISES: Depending on its severity, some simple toe-stretching exercises can strengthen your toe muscles, prevent the progression of the disease, and possibly even reverse it in moderate cases.

The evidence: Stretching exercises can help anyone with hammertoe, but they seem to have the greatest impact on reversal in children. In a 2009 study of 122 pediatric patients, toe-stretching exercises played a critical role in reversing the symptoms as part of a treatment program.[49]

How it works: Some common exercises you can try yourself include picking up marbles or small items with your toes while in a seated position, placing a towel on the floor and scrunching it up with your toes, or simply stretching out your toes while sitting.

What you need to know: Work with a physical therapist on the correct toe-stretching exercises for you.

Pain Medications and Medical Treatments

SURGERY: When it comes to actually reversing the symptoms of hammertoe, surgery is the most effective option.

The evidence: Hammertoe surgery is generally regarded as a fairly safe and highly effective treatment, with recent studies claiming success rates ranging from 82 to 95 percent.[50]

How it works: Moderate hammertoe can often be relieved with a surgery that realigns the foot tendons to relieve the pain and pressure in the toes. More severe hammertoe may require realignment of both the bones and tendons, as well as the use of pins to hold the toes in place while they heal.

What you need to know: Hammertoe surgery is minimally invasive and typically done with local anesthesia. Patients can often go home the day of the surgery.

Other Strategies

ORTHOTICS: A variety of different custom or commercially available footwear may help to prevent the progression or alleviate the pain associated with hammertoe.

The evidence: Unfortunately, very little research has been done in this area, but a 2007 case study looked at the effectiveness of splinting for a 52-year-old woman with severe pain related to hammertoe. After a 10-week splinting regimen, she had significantly reduced pain and improved function in her foot.[52]

How it works: Straps and splints can sometimes hold the toes in the correct position to help correct or slow the progression of hammertoe. If the condition has caused corns, bunions, or other toe pain, foot pads and shoe inserts might be helpful to alleviate this pain.

What you need to know: If you have diabetes or poor circulation, consult a doctor before trying an over-the-counter remedy. Some may do more harm to your feet than good.

NEW SHOES: Since shoes that don't fit are the most frequent cause of hammertoe, choosing comfortable, roomy shoes is a critical part of preventing the condition or slowing its progression.

The evidence: A 2005 study of 176 elderly patients with foot deformities affirmed what many experts had believed for years: Poorly fitting shoes are a strong contributor to these problems.[53]

On the Horizon

Smart Toe

The traditional method for holding toes in place as they heal from surgery is to use implanted pins that actually stick out through the front of the toes. This is often as painful as it sounds. A smaller, less invasive implant called the Smart Toe has shown success in healing hammertoe without the associated pain. A 2008 review touted its ease of installation and stated that it had several potential advantages over traditional pins.[51]

How it works: Shoes that don't have enough room for the toes force them into unnatural positions. As the years go by, the toes tend to stay that way. Hammertoe is one of many unfortunate results of this phenomenon.

What you need to know: Avoid high heels, or choose roomy, comfortable athletic shoes with at least a half-inch of space in front of your big toe. Go with wide shoes if needed to give the toes plenty of space. Sandals can also be a good choice because of the open space they give to your toes.

Morton's Neuroma

Nobody likes the sensation of having a rock or a bunched-up sock in their shoe. Now imagine if you had that sensation all the time. This is the unfortunate plight of those with Morton's neuroma, a condition in which the tissue surrounding a nerve near the base of the toes thickens, causing tingling, numbness, or pain that radiates to surrounding areas.

Morton's neuroma frequently develops between the base of the third and fourth toes. It's up to 10 times more common in women than men, possibly because women's feet are structured differently and because they tend to wear narrow, high shoes or very flat ones. "If you have Morton's neuroma, walking can irritate it," says Phillip Ward, a podiatrist in Pinehurst, North Carolina.

As with many foot problems, conservative strategies are the first line of treatment for Morton's neuroma. These include over-the-counter pain relievers, ice, rest, and new shoes. But there are promising new treatments that might help. For example, two studies in 2007 showed that diluted alcohol injections were very effective in reducing the size of the neuroma and relieving the pain.

Is It Morton's Neuroma?

Symptoms of Morton's neuroma may include one or more of the following:

- A tingling, burning, numb, or painful sensation in your toes

- The unusual feeling that there is actually something inside the ball of your foot, like you have a rock or a bunched-up sock in your shoe

- A gradual progression of these symptoms, starting while wearing tight-fitting shoes or doing aggravating activities, then worsening over time

Morton's neuroma often isn't visible on the outside of your foot, so the doctor may need to feel around for a tender mass on the base of your foot. Your doctor will also ask about your symptoms and may order an x-ray to rule out other foot problems.

Fast Relief Now

The feeling of a rock under your heel that you get with Morton's neuroma is certainly unpleasant but there are a few simple steps you can take to make things better. Consider this your immediate relief action plan.

1. **Avoid any aggravating activities.** This can include jogging and other intense aerobic activities. In the short term, it might be best to stay off your feet as much as possible.

2. **Try an ice massage.** Although ice can relieve many foot problems, an ice massage is especially nice for Morton's neuroma. Simply freeze a round container full of water (a cup works great) and roll it over the painful area a few times a day for relief.

3. **Take over-the-counter pain relievers.** No particular one is recommended specifically for Morton's neuroma. Try Advil, Tylenol, or Aleve, or any other that you've had success with, and take it according to the manufacturer's directions.

4. **Buy more comfortable shoes.** They should fit well and, most important, have plenty of room for your toes.

Relief at Last

Like many foot problems, treatment of Morton's neuroma starts with conservative self-care strategies but can be resolved with surgical procedures if necessary. Here is the order in which you should try to find relief.

When to Call the Doctor

Morton's neuroma is a condition that responds much better to treatment if you catch it early. Considering this, head to the doctor if:

- You feel any tingling, numbing, burning, or pain at the base of your toes

- This especially occurs while wearing tight shoes or doing a strenuous activity

- The sensation feels like something is inside your heel, or like you have something in your shoe, or your sock is bunched up in your shoe

Step 1: Get off your feet, get relief, and get new shoes. Pain relievers, ice, rest, and new shoes are the first line of defense against Morton's neuroma.

Step 2: Try arch supports or pads. A number of over-the-counter arch supports or pads can provide relief.

Step 3: Ask your doctor about injections. Corticosteroid injections are the mainstay of Morton's neuroma treatment, but new injections of diluted alcohol are also showing promise. You'll find more on this in the "Pain Prevention Strategies" below.

Step 4: Go with the surgical option. Surgery is the last resort for Morton's neuroma, but it helps many for whom the other approaches have not worked.

Pain Prevention Strategies

Exercise and Movement Therapies

EXERCISE AVOIDANCE: While it's hard for many to hear, the best approach to relieving Morton's neuroma is to avoid aggravating exercise.

The evidence: Runners are one group often affected by Morton's neuroma, but others who might need to take it easy are athletes who "spin on the balls of their feet," according to studies.[54] This can include golfers, bowlers, tennis players, baseball players, and dancers.

How it works: Taking a break gives your foot a rest, allowing the growth to heal on its own in some cases, or at least to subside. This is effective when the Morton's neuroma is mild to moderate.

What you need to know: Give your painful toe at least 2 or 3 weeks to get better and for the pain to subside to improve your foot condition generally and to avoid painful complications like bunions, flatfeet, or hammertoe. Then start with low-impact activities like walking, and work your way back into your favorite activities. If the activities are still painful, see your doctor for further advice.

Pain Medications and Medical Treatments

ALCOHOL INJECTIONS: This cutting-edge treatment has shown the most promise recently in treating Morton's neuroma. It involves injecting diluted alcohol directly at the site of the neuroma.

The evidence: Two studies published in 2007 examined the effectiveness of diluted alcohol injections. One of the studies looked at 101 patients who received an average of four injections. The results were incredibly promising, with 94 percent of patients reporting improvement and 84 percent becoming totally pain free.[55] The other study was slightly less successful but still showed a 61 percent success rate.[56]

How it works: The alcohol seems to dissolve the painful growth and improve pain and function in people who receive it.

What you need to know: Researchers noted very few side effects or complications, but they did note that it might take up to five injections for true effectiveness. Many health care providers do not offer this treatment just yet, but it certainly couldn't hurt to ask your doctor about it.

SURGERY: If more conservative treatments are unsuccessful, surgery might be appropriate for Morton's neuroma. This procedure involves the physical removal of the growth.

The evidence: Complications exist, but some studies have shown a success rate ranging from 80 to 96 percent for surgery.[18]

How it works: During a surgery for Morton's neuroma, the surgeon removes the growth as well as the nerve it affects. This can bring relief to the previously painful area.

What you need to know: Doctors usually view surgery as a last resort for Morton's neuroma. Though it is often successful, the potential complications include permanent numbness in the affected toes.

Other Treatments

METATARSAL PADS: The foot pad that is recommended for Morton's neuroma is called a metatarsal pad.

The evidence: Study reviews have been mixed, but most research participants have received some pain relief from the pads, and about 50 percent of participants gain greater than 50 percent relief.[57] The major problem with the studies is that they have not been properly controlled, so the placebo effect may be significant. Still, even if a degree of efficacy is related to belief, it doesn't make the insoles any less effective.

How it works: A metatarsal pad rests under the ball of the foot so it provides relief directly to the area affected by the pain.

What you need to know: A number of metatarsal pads are available over-the-counter and online. These are sold as "metatarsal pads" or "metatarsal arch

Quick Tip

The shoe company New Balance, which manufactures all its shoes in the United States, has shoes specifically designed for people with Morton's neuroma. To browse the company's selection, visit http://www.nbannapolis.com/new_balance/mortons-neuroma-c-43_45_65.html.

supports." Or talk to your doctor about which one you should choose. He might be able to prescribe a custom pad that is precisely fitted to your foot.

COMFORTABLE SHOES: Here again, comfortable shoes are your first line of defense against Morton's neuroma.

The evidence: Surveys show that women are 8 to 10 times more likely to suffer from the condition, which is directly related to the uncomfortable shoes (such as high heels) women often wear.

How it works: Ultimately, Morton's neuroma often stems from scrunched-up toes, and it's also closely tied to other shoe-related conditions like bunions and hammertoe. This makes choosing the right shoes a major player in the fight against Morton's neuroma.

What you need to know: Choose a comfortable shoe with plenty of room in the toe box (about three-eighths to one-half inch in front of the toes). Also make sure they offer plenty of support and are wide enough for your feet.

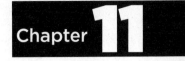

Chapter 11

Arthritis and Joint Pain

Osteoarthritis, cysts, lupus, rheumatoid arthritis and psoriatic arthritis, adult Still's disease, ankylosing spondylitis

The first type of pain that comes to mind when one thinks of joint pain is arthritis. Arthritis actually encompasses two medical conditions that are completely different, though the pain at times can feel similar.

"The pain from rheumatoid arthritis arises as a result of chronic autoimmune-driven inflammation," says Nathan Wei, MD, director of the Arthritis Treatment Center in Frederick, Maryland. "This inflammation affects not only joints but is a systemic process that also affects internal organs. On the other hand, osteoarthritis is primarily a disorder of cartilage, the gristle that caps the ends of long bones. Osteoarthritis affects primarily weight-bearing joints, and the pain is due to the mechanical dysfunction caused by the wearing away of cartilage and the subsequent irritation of the surrounding joint capsule."

Rheumatoid arthritis isn't the only autoimmune disorder that affects the joints. Diseases like lupus, ankylosing spondylitis, and Still's disease are also conditions that result in painful and aching joints for those who suffer from them.

Fortunately, if you're one of the 50 million Americans who have to deal with joint pain, you don't have to cope alone. Researchers are making new advances in joint pain research every day. Conventional medicine has advanced to the point that certain autoimmune disorders can be put into remission with the right combination of drugs. A variety of cutting-edge therapies ranging from stem cell treatments to laser therapies are showing new promise previously unseen in the area of joint pain.

You don't have to rely totally on your doctor to treat arthritis. Exercise, nutrition, and other at-home therapies have shown more promise than ever before. These breakthroughs have empowered people to take charge of their own health and put a stop to the pain. "Altering your diet by increasing fatty fish such as tuna or salmon, switching from grain-fed to grass-fed meats, and decreasing excess sugar intake can all be very helpful," says Jacob Teitelbaum, MD, medical director of the Fibromyalgia & Fatigue Centers found across the United States.

Read on for your individual action plans for every type of joint pain.

Osteoarthritis

Far and away the most common form of joint-related pain, osteoarthritis affects more than 27 million Americans. Unlike many other causes of joint pain, which are autoimmune disorders within the body, the cause of osteoarthritis is more direct and better understood.

Where bone meets bone inside your body, the joint is protected by a soft, rubbery cushion known as cartilage. Age, wear, and other factors, however, can wear down this cartilage over time. The result is bone rubbing against bone, a situation that can be extremely painful. Osteoarthritis can occur in joints throughout the body, but the most common joints affected are the spine, hips, knees, and hands.

Osteoarthritis can be painful and debilitating, but there are now more ways than ever to take charge of your health and get back on your feet. It's a classic case of using combinations of traditional and alternative therapies to manage the condition. In addition to drugs, some of the treatments that can help you manage osteoarthritis include diet, supplements, exercises, support groups, yoga, and acupuncture. Cutting-edge therapies like laser therapy and stem cell treatment are also showing promise in putting a stop to pain.

Is It Osteoarthritis?

If you think that you might have osteoarthritis, here are some of the signs and symptoms to look for.

- You feel a sharp pain, dull ache or burning in a joint during or after movement.

- The area feels tender when you touch it lightly.

- Occasionally, you may actually be able to hear or feel the grating sensation of bone on bone within the joint.

- You gradually lose flexibility and cannot move the joint through its full range of motion.

- You may feel stiff and sore, often first thing in the morning or when you are inactive for a while.

- You may experience swelling of the joint.

A thorough physical examination is your doctor's first step toward diagnosing osteoarthritis, though x-rays or MRIs can also be useful in seeing the severity of the disease and the actual loss of cartilage. A blood test can also help the doctor rule out autoimmune disorders such as rheumatoid arthritis, and a joint fluid test will help determine whether there is an infection at play.

When to Call the Doctor

If you experience any of these situations, it's critical to get an appointment with your doctor as soon as possible. The sooner you can begin treatment and start effectively managing your arthritis pain, the better the outcome will be.

- You have pain, soreness, or stiffness in any joints, particularly the spine, hip, knees, or hands.

- The joint has swelling or stiffness that persists for 2 weeks.

- The sensation in the joint makes it difficult to live your daily life and carry out your daily functions.

- If the pain is severe, makes it almost impossible to move, or the joint is red or hot to the touch or accompanied by a fever, seek emergency medical help.

Fast Relief Now

Though more extensive steps are necessary to manage arthritis pain, these simple steps can bring relief to immediate pain quickly.

1. **Rest the joint completely if possible.** If it's necessary to continue to move the joint, keep the motions gentle and take at least a 10-minute break every hour if complete rest is not possible.

2. **Take an over-the-counter pain reliever.** Advil, Tylenol, Aleve, and other over-the-counter medicines are all suitable choices for mild arthritis pain. Use according to the manufacturer's directions and avoid taking the medication for 5 consecutive days.

3. **Alternate between warm and cold treatments.** Use each for 20 minutes several times a day, alternating between hot and cold. For the warm treatments, use a heating pad, a hot water bottle, or a warm bath. The cold treatment can be an ice pack or a bag of frozen vegetables.

4. **Try an over-the-counter cream that's used to reduce pain right at the joint.** Zostrix, Bengay, Aspercreme, IcyHot, and others all seem to be effective for short-term pain relief.

Relief at Last

Osteoarthritis requires a concerted effort and a combination of approaches to successfully manage the pain. Here are your steps to success.

Step 1: See your doctor. Depending on the severity of your arthritis, drug treatment might be the first-line defense. And the best way to find out is with the help of your doctor.

Step 2: Try classes and therapy. Physical therapists can recommend the right exercises, occupational therapists will show you how to do your daily tasks in a pain-free way, and arthritis and pain management classes can teach you good techniques and provide support from your peers. These classes don't just focus on movement. They provide you with insight and support to learn to cope with what can often be a painful condition.

Step 3: Do the right exercises. Sticking to your approved exercise routine can strengthen joints and muscles to reduce pain. Yoga and tai chi are also great choices for people with arthritis.

Step 4: Try diet and supplement strategies. A number of dietary changes, including supplements, have shown effectiveness in managing arthritis pain. These strategies include eating more healthy fish like salmon, plentiful fruits and vegetables, and trying supplements like fish oil, ginger extract, and others.

Step 5: Try hands-on solutions. Both acupuncture and chiropractic care have helped those with arthritis.

Pain-Relief Strategies

Food and Supplements

ANTI-INFLAMMATORY DIET: According to Dr. Teitelbaum, many of the components of the modern diet contribute to inflammation. These include sugar as well as saturated fats and trans fats. Decreasing sugar intake and focusing on getting more omega-3 fats can help reduce the inflammation that contributes to osteoarthritis.

The evidence: A 2006 review article that looked at a number of studies showed that there is evidence that a diet high in fruits, vegetables, whole grains, and omega-3 fats can indeed reduce inflammation.[1]

How it works: Since inflammation plays a direct role in arthritis pain, replacing pro-inflammatory foods like red meat and sugar with anti-inflammatory fruit, vegetables, fish, and whole grain is helpful. What's more, eating better often leads to weight loss, and excess weight is one of the major risk factors of developing osteoarthritis. In a recent study of 192 osteoarthritis patients that followed either a very low-calorie diet or a low-calorie diet for 16 weeks, both groups lost weight and had a similar reduction in osteoarthritis-related pain.[2]

What you need to know: Replace red meat with fatty fish like salmon and plant-based sources of protein like beans, seeds, and nuts. Choose grass-fed beef over grain-fed. And fill up on carbohydrates from fruits, vegetables, and whole grains instead of sugary substitutes.

EGGSHELL MEMBRANE: A number of supplements have been tried over the years with varying degrees of success for osteoarthritis. One of the most recent that has garnered a lot of attention is eggshell membrane.

The evidence: In a 2009 study of supplements, 67 osteoarthritis patients received either 500 milligrams of eggshell membrane daily or a placebo for 8 weeks. The patients taking the eggshell membrane experienced a significant reduction in pain and improvement in function over the placebo group. These positive benefits were seen in as few as 10 days and continued into the 60th day of the study.[3]

How it works: Eggshell membrane contains glucosamine and chondroitin, two compounds that have traditionally been seen to be helpful in curbing pain related to osteoarthritis. It also seems to have general anti-inflammatory properties that quell the inflammation related to many types of pain.

What you need to know: The eggshell membrane supplement available in the United States is known as Fast Joint Care+. In this study of eggshell membrane, the patients tolerated it well and showed few side effects.

FISH OIL: The long-chain fatty acids EPA and DHA that are found in oily fish like salmon have been shown to be helpful for a number of health conditions. The same may also be true for the pain and stiffness of osteoarthritis.

The evidence: Several studies have shown fish oil supplements to be helpful in reducing osteoarthritis pain. A 2009 study of 81 patients showed that those who took a fish oil supplement regularly were able to reduce their use of nonsteroidal anti-inflammatory drugs and analgesics.[4]

How it works: Fish oil has been well studied, and the fatty acids found within the oil have proven to have powerful anti-inflammatory properties. This makes them useful for addressing the symptoms of a number of pain-related conditions.

What you need to know: Fish oil supplements vary greatly in quality, so you'll want to take care when choosing the right supplement. You'll want to read the label and check the content of DHA and EPA in the supplement. Our experts recommend about 1 to 2 grams of these fatty acids daily. Don't be afraid to ask your doctor if he has any specific recommendations about what kind of fish oil to take.

AVOCADO SOYBEAN UNSAPONIFIABLES (ASUS): Another up-and-coming supplement in the fight against osteoarthritis is a bit of a mouthful, but seems to be effective: avocado soybean unsaponifiables, or ASUs, which are made from a mixture of avocado oil and soybean oil.

The evidence: ASUs have looked quite intriguing in recent research. Some studies suggest that the supplement may even slow cartilage degradation and promote its repair in hip and knee joints.[5]

How it works: Researchers aren't exactly sure why they work so well, but the concentrated oils seem to have strong anti-inflammatory properties that directly address osteoarthritis-related pain.

What you need to know: It usually takes about 2 months of use to begin feeling relief from ASU supplements, so don't expect immediate results. However, the supplement seems to be relatively free of side effects compared to some other osteoarthritis treatments.

Exercise and Movement Therapies

PHYSICAL THERAPY: If you already have osteoarthritis, the best exercises are done with the instruction and guidance of a physical therapist. This expert can work up a specific exercise regimen that will help you strengthen your joints and muscles and relieve pain right at the source.

The evidence: A study of 83 patients with osteoarthritis of the knee showed that those who underwent a standardized exercise program for their pain increased the distance they were able to walk in 6 minutes by 13 percent after 8 weeks and their overall pain and stiffness by 55 percent over a placebo group. After one year, 20 percent of the patients in the placebo group had to undergo knee surgery. This was required in only 5 percent of the physical therapy group.[7]

How it works: Although your joints are under attack when you have osteoarthritis, keeping them strong and limber through safe stretches and strength training is the best way to prevent further damage and even improve your symptoms.

What you need to know: Find a qualified physical therapist in your area to get you started on an osteoarthritis exercise program. In Part Three, you'll find some gentle exercise routines you can start with, along with resources on finding physical therapists and appropriate exercise classes in your area. Eventually these individualized exercises can give way to enjoyable low-impact exercises you can do on your own, such as walking, biking, and swimming, as well as stretches and strength training.

YOGA AND TAI CHI: Both are ancient exercises that involve gentle movements and stretching, and both have proven helpful in reducing osteoarthritis pain in studies.

The evidence: While few studies have tried to measure the actual effect of exercises like yoga and tai chi, a 2009 review article looked at the results of eight studies involving 267 participants in yoga or tai chi. All eight showed clear benefits for people with osteoarthritis in terms of pain management and overall quality of life.[8]

How it works: Though they weren't originally intended to be osteoarthritis treatments, the slow, controlled movements of yoga and tai chi are perfectly tailored to people with joint pain. They provide the needed exercise without overtaxing the joints and muscles.

What you need to know: Because of the risk of injury, it's best to start a yoga or tai chi program with a qualified instructor and to let her know about your condition. Once you gain more confidence, you can branch out and try more moves on your own.

HYDROTHERAPY: By moving the exercise program to the water, patients can still gain the joint- and muscle-strengthening benefits without the high impact of exercises on dry land.

The evidence: Sixty-four patients with osteoarthritis of the knee were placed in either a water-based exercise group or a land-based exercise group for the 18-week study. At the end of the trial, both groups had positive results, but the water-based group experienced a greater decrease in pain.[9]

How it works: Put simply, exercising in the water decreases the impact on your body. This makes it a great choice for people who are suffering from joint pain.

What you need to know: If you have mild to moderate osteoarthritis pain, slow swimming or water aerobics classes are a great option. Many cities offer water aerobics classes specifically for those with arthritis. See Part Three for an easy routine and resources on finding a class near you.

OCCUPATIONAL THERAPY: A physical therapist can help you with exercise, while an occupational therapist will help you go through your work and daily activities in a manner that is as pain free as possible.

The evidence: In a 2009 study of 54 elderly patients, those who received both physical therapy and occupational therapy had larger pain decreases and an overall increase in physical activity compared to subjects who received just physical therapy and education. These results held true after the 4 weeks of therapy and after a 6-month follow-up.[10]

How it works: In a nutshell, an occupational therapist will help you look at the activities in your daily life, isolate the ones that are causing you pain, and provide strategies for performing these activities in a way that reduces the pain. These can be as simple as getting in and out of a car or chair differently, or as complex as teaching you new methods for grabbing and holding items to reduce arthritis pain in the hands.

What you need to know: Occupational therapists teach group classes in many areas to provide general advice for osteoarthritis sufferers. You can also take individual classes to get a more personalized program tailored to your own situation. The number of times you'll need to meet with the occupational therapist varies based on the severity of your pain. The programs taught by occupational therapists that can help those with osteoarthritis are often referred to as "activity strategy training." See Part Three to find a qualified occupational therapist in your area or ask your doctor for a referral.

Touch Therapies

MASSAGE: Like many alternative treatments, massage is gaining ground as a treatment for osteoarthritis and scientific research is now backing up the results.

The evidence: A 2006 study of 68 adults with osteoarthritis of the knee received either 8 weeks of massage therapy or a placebo. Those who received the massage therapy showed a significant improvement in pain and function.[11]

How it works: A qualified massage therapist will know how to work the joints of arthritis sufferers gently and properly in order to provide soothing relief right at the source of the pain. It seems that both the relaxing aspect of the massage itself as well as its direct treatment of the affected area play a dual role in pain management.

What you need to know: Great care must be taken with the inflamed and damaged joints present with osteoarthritis, so it's very important that you see a qualified massage therapist and clearly explain your pain so that the therapist can treat it properly. Possible side effects include temporary pain or discomfort, bruising, or swelling.

Pain Medications and Medical Treatments

PAIN RELIEVERS: The pain relievers prescribed for osteoarthritis pain range from acetaminophen (Tylenol) and other nonsteroidal anti-inflammatory drugs for mild pain to stronger painkillers like codeine and propoxyphene (Darvon) for more severe pain.

The evidence: A review of 15 studies that included almost 6,000 people who took Tylenol for their osteoarthritis pain showed that the drug was significantly more effective than a placebo at reducing pain and stiffness and improving function.[13]

How it works: Most of these drugs directly affect the body's inflammatory response to provide fast pain relief.

What you need to know: Obviously, as the intensity of the drug used increases, so does the risk of side effects from using that drug. These can range from liver damage from acetaminophen to nausea, constipation, and sleepiness from strong painkillers like codeine. Be sure to work closely with your doctor when determining the right course of action for your pain, and make sure to inform her of any over-the-counter pain medication you are taking.

VISCOSUPPLEMENTATION: This cutting-edge treatment involves injecting a fluid called hyaluronic acid into the knee to provide some cushioning and relief. The acid is made from rooster combs and is similar to a component normally found in joint fluid.

The evidence: A 2007 review of five studies of the use of viscosupplementation for knee osteoarthritis showed that it was found to be helpful in all five studies.[14]

How it works: Injecting this fluid directly into the affected joint provides some cushioning and comfort that has been lost as a result of the damage related to osteoarthritis.

What you need to know: Viscosupplementation is only approved for use in the United States for osteoarthritis of the knee, but it is being studied for uses in other forms of osteoarthritis as well. Studies have shown that it is generally well tolerated with minimal side effects. Stay tuned for more news on this exciting treatment.

SURGERY: For the most severe, debilitating forms of osteoarthritis, surgery is an option.

The evidence: Studies of the use of surgery for osteoarthritis pain and symptoms have been mixed. A 2008 study of 86 patients who had arthroscopic surgery for knee osteoarthritis showed that it did not provide much benefit over a control group.[15] In a 2008 study of elderly patients who received joint replacement surgery of the hip or knee, the long-term outcomes were generally excellent.[16]

How it works: The three main types of surgery typically recommended for osteoarthritis are a joint replacement with an artificial joint, bone realignment to reposition the bones to generate less pain, or a bone fusion that joins two bones together to increase stability and reduce pain.

What you need to know: Surgery has benefits for some, but also many inherent risks.

On the Horizon

Laser Therapy

Though he acknowledges that more study is needed, Marvin Kunikiyo, a chiropractic physician and author of *Revolutionizing Your Health,* has been impressed with the impact of low-level laser therapy (LLLT) on osteoarthritis. "It appears that low-level laser therapy reduces the excitability of the nerve cells by an interruption of the fast pain fibers with a resultant reduction in pain," he says. "Although not many studies have been done . . . I would think significant pain relief would be had from nearly all types of arthritis. LLLT is relatively safe, since due to its nonthermal nature it does not cause cellular destruction but simply alters cellular function."

Indeed, a recent study showed that participants experienced an 80 percent improvement in pain after twice-weekly treatment with laser therapy for 2 months.[17] Low-level laser therapy is currently not available in the United States, but stay tuned for more news on this promising treatment for osteoarthritis.

Stem Cell Treatment

The reality is that most osteoarthritis treatment involves managing the pain. The only way to eliminate the condition is through surgery. But a number of new studies on the impact of stem cells on osteoarthritis might be changing that notion. In a recent study performed by Christopher Centeno, MD, a rehabilitation doctor in private practice in Broomfield, Colorado, and his colleagues, the patients' own stem cells injected into joints dramatically reduced pain in two of three people who were told they needed a total joint replacement. Dr. Centeno has also seen good results in treating isolated knee cartilage lesions, partial shoulder rotator cuff tears, and meniscus tears with stem cell injections, helping many patients avoid more invasive surgery.

That being said, often it is an option that is successful for those with debilitating arthritis when other treatments have failed. Have a long talk with your doctor to make sure surgery is the correct choice for you.

Other Strategies

PAIN MANAGEMENT CLASSES: Take a class for those with chronic pain and osteoarthritis offered by the Arthritis Foundation or another medical center. These classes not only teach you coping skills and strategies, but they can also act as a support group by connecting you with others with your condition.

The evidence: These classes incorporate a number of strategies that have been proven to be effective in other studies, such as hydrotherapy, yoga, and tai chi. *The Journal of Family Practice*'s 2009 guidelines recommend that physicians refer their osteoarthritis patients to these classes.[18]

How it works: By incorporating a variety of techniques, both exercise and support related, that have been proven to be helpful for people with osteoarthritis, these classes offer a broad spectrum of supportive strategies and activities.

What you need to know: The Arthritis Foundation's program is known as the "Life Improvement Series" and includes a variety of techniques that have been proven to help those with osteoarthritis pain, including exercise, aquatics, tai chi, self-help, and walking. Support groups and discussion sessions with other people with osteoarthritis are also an important part of the series. To find a class in your area, visit the Arthritis Foundation's Web site at www.arthritis.org. Then enter your zip code, and contact your local office for more information.

Cysts

One occasional complication of arthritis (usually osteoarthritis) is a cyst, a fluid-filled lump that gradually grows along the tendons or joints. If you have osteoarthritis of the hand or wrist, you may develop what is known as a ganglionic cyst. In the knee, it's known as a Baker's cyst. These cysts can also occur in other joints throughout the body in rare instances.

Sometimes the cyst will cause you no pain whatsoever and may even go away on its own over time. In those cases, no treatment is needed. Other times, though, the cyst can create discomfort and even pain. It may disrupt your ability to move the joint properly. In these instances, you'll want to get the cyst treated, either by draining the fluid from it (aspiration) or by removing it surgically. For a Baker's cyst in the knee, however, these procedures can be more invasive. That's why the latest line of treatment is to use less intrusive techniques like ice, compression wraps, and exercise to shrink the cyst and regain mobility in the knee. Cysts are often related to arthritis of the joints, so treating arthritis symptoms can prevent the recurrence of cysts. You can learn how to manage arthritis in this chapter.

Is It a Cyst?

When a cyst is visible, it's pretty easy to tell what it is. There are times, however, when a cyst is hidden beneath the surface of the skin and lets its presence be known only by the pain and discomfort it produces. Here are the signs and symptoms of cysts.

- A round, firm, and fluid-filled lump that's visible on your wrist or finger joints

- Pain, weakness, numbness, or tightness at the joint

- Growth of the cyst when the joint is in use and shrinkage when it's at rest

- Swelling in your knee or leg

Your doctor may poke and prod at a visible cyst a bit to determine the extent of the pain it produces. If he can't see the cyst, an x-ray, MRI, or ultrasound can be used to find it and determine its shape and size. These tests are also useful to determine if the cyst is causing your pain or whether another joint problem like arthritis is the culprit. Finally, your doctor may want to draw fluid from the cyst and test it to make sure it is indeed a cyst and not something more dangerous like a cancerous tumor.

Fast Relief Now

These steps will help reduce the pain, but a doctor's guidance will be needed for more complete relief from cyst-related problems.

1. **Quit using the painful, affected area.** Give your hand, wrist, or knee as much rest as possible. Complete rest usually isn't required, but do your best to avoid jarring motions and activity.

2. **Apply ice for about 20 minutes.** This will soothe the ache and take your mind off the pain. You can use a bag of peas, a cold pack, or a plastic bag filled with ice cubes.

3. **Try an over-the-counter pain reliever.** No one particular pain reliever is specifically recommended for cysts. Just use your pain reliever of choice according to the manufacturer's directions, and don't use it for more than 5 consecutive days.

4. **If the pain is in your knee, put on a compression wrap.** This will restrict the movement of the knee and keep it in a more comfortable position to avoid painful flare-ups.

5. **Rest until the pain subsides.** Once it does, try to take it easy even after the pain stops.

Relief at Last

A cyst usually isn't a serious problem, but it's worth a trip to your doctor to find the right approach for treating it. Here's a step-by-step way to stop cyst pain.

When to Call the Doctor

Even if a cyst isn't painful, it's worth having your doctor take a look to make sure it isn't something more serious like a blood clot or a tumor.

- You notice the presence of a round, smooth bump on your hand, wrist, or knee.
- You have persistent pain in your hand, wrist, or knee.
- Movement in your hand, wrist, or knee is limited and affecting your daily activities.

Step 1: Get the doctor's diagnosis. Your doctor will help you determine that it is indeed a cyst and not a cancerous tumor or a more dangerous growth.

Step 2: Use ice, compression, and exercise. Particularly for Baker's cysts of the knee, these simple steps can help you regain mobility and shrink the cyst.

Step 3: Ask about aspiration. In most cases, your doctor can easily drain the cyst during a routine office visit to relieve the pain and swelling.

Step 4: Contemplate surgery. Though more extensive, surgery is the most surefire way to remove the cyst and its related pain completely.

Step 5: Use other arthritis pain prevention strategies. Cysts are often complications of arthritis, so managing arthritis is a good way to prevent cysts from coming back (see the rest of this chapter).

Pain Prevention Strategies

Exercise and Movement Therapies

SIMPLE STRETCHES: Some simple, gentle exercises have been shown to be helpful in regaining knee function and reducing pain related to a Baker's cyst in the knee.

The evidence: The most commonly recommended exercises for the knee are range-of-motion exercises.

How it works: One simple strategy you can try is a heel slide. While lying on your back, simply slide one heel along the floor toward your buttocks. Keep sliding until you feel mild tension in your leg. Hold it for 1 to 2 minutes, and repeat the exercise 10 times.

While lying flat, you can also do supine leg hangs. Simply raise the injured leg, grab your thigh with your hands, and pull the leg toward you. Leave the knee bent above your hands. Hold for 2 to 3 minutes, then straighten the leg. Repeat 5 times.

What you need to know: These are just two of many range-of-motion exercises to try. It's best to work with a physical therapist to come up with the right routine for you and learn how to do each exercise safely.

Pain Medications and Other Medical Treatments

ASPIRATION: The mainstay of painful cyst treatment is to remove the fluid from the cyst with a needle in a technique called *aspiration*. For cysts inside the body, doctors can even guide their needle via ultrasound to drain a cyst successfully.

The evidence: Though the procedure is successful for short-term pain elimination, research has shown that about 60 percent of cysts drained by aspiration will recur.[19]

How it works: Most of the pain from a cyst is related to the pressure it puts on the body parts around it, especially during movement. Draining fluid from the cyst removes this pressure, thus relieving the pain.

What you need to know: Aspiration is a relatively simple procedure that can bring at least short-term relief in most cases. It is most useful for cysts that are particularly painful or significantly limit your range of motion. There are few side effects, but you should be aware that cysts often recur after draining.

SURGERY: Surgery is usually reserved for significant pain or joint problems related to the cyst. The procedure is often done on an outpatient basis, but it still is a significant operation that may require some recovery time to heal fully.

The evidence: A number of individual case studies have shown the dramatic impact of surgery for patients with particularly large and debilitating cysts. In one 2008 case study, a man had a ganglionic cyst on his spine that was so severe he was unable to walk. Two days after the surgical removal of the cyst, he was walking on his own without problem.[20]

How it works: By physically removing the cyst from your body, surgery is the most surefire way of eliminating the pain associated with it.

What you need to know: Most cyst operations require a 2- to 6-week recovery period, so you'll need to rest and keep the area clean during that time. Some people need physical therapy to rehabilitate fully after the surgery, though this is the exception rather than the rule.

Lupus

Lupus can make your joints hurt much like arthritis does. And just like rheumatoid arthritis, lupus is an autoimmune disorder, which means it occurs when the body essentially attacks itself. The immune system gets confused, and parts of your body are the victims of these attacks.

But although the joints are the main victims of these attacks in people with rheumatoid arthritis, those with lupus aren't so lucky. In lupus, the immune system focuses its attacks on internal tissues and organs. For the 1.5 million people in America who have lupus, the condition can create a lot more problems than just joint pain.[21]

The outlook for lupus patients used to be pretty grim, but breakthroughs in drugs for autoimmune disorders have made it look much brighter. Of course, using those drugs in combination with effective alternative therapies like exercise and diet modification can make the outcome for lupus even more successful.

Is It Lupus?

The good news about lupus is that most cases of the condition are mild. Like rheumatoid arthritis, they can be characterized by flares, or periods of time where the symptoms get much worse and then subside.

The bad news about lupus is that it can present a veritable laundry list of different signs and symptoms, many of which overlap with other conditions. Here are just a few of the indicators that you might have lupus.

- Arthritis-like joint pain, swelling, or stiffness
- Rash on the cheeks and bridge of the nose, often in the shape of a butterfly
- Sores that appear or get worse with sun exposure
- Mouth sores
- Hair loss
- Fever and fatigue
- Unexpected weight loss or weight gain
- Anxiety, depression, or memory loss
- Shortness of breath
- Dry eyes

- Easy bruising

- Fingers or toes that turn white or blue when you are stressed or cold (Raynaud's disease)

- Seizures, psychosis, or another neurological disorder

Lupus can be so difficult to pinpoint, in fact, that the American College of Rheumatology developed a checklist of 11 items to help your doctor make the diagnosis. If you meet 4 of the 11 criteria, you are likely to have lupus. They are:

- The face rash discussed above

- A raised, scaly, patchy rash known as a discoid rash

- Lesions or rash from sun exposure

- Mouth sores

- Joint pain or swelling

- Swelling of the lining around the lungs or heart (Your doctor will need to perform tests to determine this.)

- Seizures, psychosis, or another neurological disorder

- Kidney disease

- Low blood counts

- Positive antinuclear antibody blood test

- Positive blood tests for other autoimmune diseases

Relief at Last

Lupus is a serious diagnosis and it's not one that you should try to take on by yourself. Your doctor needs to play a role in getting you the medication and treatment you need to manage the condition properly.

However, that's not to say that alternative medicine isn't important in the process. Exercise can help you feel your best and keep the fatigue and pain associated with lupus at bay. And dietary therapies and supplements have shown real promise in counteracting some of the signs and symptoms of lupus.

Step 1: See your doctor about medication. Nonsteroidal anti-inflammatory drugs and corticosteroids are the typical treatments for lupus, but some immunosuppressive drugs and the biologic therapies now being used to treat arthritis have also shown promise for lupus. The hormone DHEA has also helped many with lupus.

Step 2: Exercise regularly. It's hard to psych yourself up for exercise when you feel achy and exhausted, but staying active is one of your body's best defenses. There are many ways to do it safely despite the symptoms you might be experiencing.

Step 3: Change your diet. Many people with lupus have had success by changing their diet to include more fruits and vegetables, heart-healthy fish, and whole grains and incorporating a few safe supplements like fish oil into their regimen. We have a few simple suggestions that can help.

Pain Prevention Strategies

Food and Supplements

HEART-HEALTHY DIET: Considering the widespread effect of lupus on joints, organs, and systems throughout the body, it would make sense that the whole-body preventive medicine of a healthy diet would be an excellent treatment approach. Fruits and vegetables, dietary vitamin C, and fiber may be

---

When to Call the Doctor

If you develop any of the potential signs and symptoms of lupus listed on the previous page, it's worth scheduling a doctor's visit to discuss your concerns. If you have already been diagnosed with lupus you should be seeing your doctor regularly for treatment and management of the condition. Here are a few potential lupus complications that require medical attention.

- You experience a seizure.
- You develop a severe rash or blister, or an existing rash worsens.
- You have chest pain or difficulty breathing.
- You have persistent joint pain or swelling.
- You develop a fever that doesn't break after 48 hours.
- You have persistent aching and fatigue.

protective against progression, while excess inflammation-promoting vegetable oils as a fat source may promote progression.

The evidence: A Japanese study of 216 female patients with lupus showed that those with higher vitamin C and fiber intake were less likely to see the symptoms of their lupus become active.[22]

How it works: Foods like fatty fish, whole grains, fruits and vegetables, and other components of a heart-healthy diet have an anti-inflammatory effect on the body and seem to play a critical role in reducing the incidence of inflammatory diseases like lupus.

What you need to know: Eating a healthy diet can not only reduce the symptoms of lupus itself, but since heart disease can be a complication of lupus, following a heart-healthy diet is a good approach for that reason, too. This includes replacing red meat proteins with fatty fish like salmon a couple times a week, eating plentiful fruits and vegetables, and shunning overly processed foods in favor of whole grains.

OMEGA-3 FATTY ACIDS: As with other arthritis-related conditions, the anti-inflammatory effects of fish oil supplements seem to show real results for those with lupus.

The evidence: Sixty patients with lupus took either a placebo or 3 grams of the EPA and DHA fatty acids found in a fish oil supplement daily for 24 weeks. The fish oil group showed significant cardiovascular benefits, including improved blood flow and reduced oxidative stress on their heart and veins.[24] Several other studies have also shown the value of fish oil as a treatment for lupus.[25, 26]

How it works: The long-chain omega-3 fatty acids found in fish oil, DHA and EPA, have natural anti-inflammatory properties. In the concentrated form of a fish oil supplement, they seem to play a role in managing lupus symptoms.

What you need to know: Most experts recommend taking 1 to 2 grams of fish oil daily, so you should speak with your doctor before taking more than that. People with diabetes, liver disease, a pancreatic disorder, or an underactive thyroid should also speak to their doctor before taking it on their own. For those who can take it safely, fish oil is generally viewed as a daily supplement to take for overall health support.

Exercise and Movement Therapies

LOW-IMPACT EXERCISES: You often may not feel up to exercise when you have lupus, and it's okay to rest when your body tells you to. But when you're feeling better, getting regular exercise is a great way to improve your overall mood and well-being, as well as to protect yourself from some of the complications of lupus, like an increased risk of heart disease.

The evidence: A 2010 study of 41 adults with lupus showed that those who exercised regularly had significantly less stiffness in their arteries, an early sign of heart disease.[27] Since heart disease is a fairly common complication from lupus, this protection is critically important.

How it works: "Exercise can certainly play a big therapeutic part in lupus, increasing blood flow and nutrients to the joints, as well as the elimination of waste products from the joint," says Dr. Kunikiyo.

What you need to know: Since joint pain and inflammation are common symptoms of lupus, choosing a low-impact exercise to try for around 30 to 60 minutes on most days is a good idea. "Excellent exercises are swimming, walking, and other low-impact exercises that put the body through a full range of motion without overstressing it," says Dr. Kunikiyo.

Pain Medications and Other Medical Treatments

DRUG COMBINATIONS: Nonsteroidal anti-inflammatory drugs (Advil, Motrin, Aleve), antimalarial drugs, and corticosteroids have all shown effectiveness in treating lupus symptoms. Immunosuppressive drugs are also sometimes used but can have serious side effects. Often these drugs are used in combination, especially immunosuppressive drugs and corticosteroids for more severe cases of lupus.

The evidence: A recent study of 154 patients with lupus, many of whom were on immunosuppressive drugs to control their symptoms, showed that the corticosteroid prednisone was particularly effective at preventing severe flares of pain and symptoms.[28]

How it works: As the name suggests, immunosuppressive drugs keep the immune system from overreacting. And since the symptoms of lupus stem from the immune system attacking itself, this is an important part of the treatment process for people with severe lupus. When occasionally severe flare-ups occur, steroids counteract those symptoms quickly.

What you need to know: All these drugs have side effects and risk factors so you need to discuss your options carefully with your doctor to weigh the risks and benefits of each. Side effects of prolonged steroid use can include infections, mood swings, osteoporosis, and high blood pressure. Immunosuppressive drugs also leave you at a greater risk of an infection and can even increase your risk of liver damage, cancer, or infertility.

DHEA: "Taking the hormone DHEA (dehydroepiandrosterone) at a dose of 200 milligrams a day (a quite high dose) has been shown in repeated studies to improve the outcome of lupus patients," says Dr. Teitelbaum.

The evidence: A 2009 review of 842 participants in seven studies who received DHEA showed mixed results, but there was an overall significant improvement in quality of life (11.5 percent) experienced by the study participants.[30]

How it works: Your body uses DHEA to make sex hormones. In lupus, it appears that the hormone might have muscle-building and immune-boosting properties that help, though more research is clearly needed.

What you need to know: "This should be done under the supervision of a doctor, even though it is over-the-counter, because higher dosing can cause acne or darkening of facial hair," says Dr. Teitelbaum. "For unknown reasons, this is less likely to be seen in people taking it for lupus, where the side effect is rare."

RITUXIMAB: Rituximab (Rituxan), a drug that inhibits the number of B-cells (a type of white blood cell) your body produces, has shown effectiveness in treating lupus.

The evidence: Study results have been mixed, but a 2007 study of seven female patients taking rituximab for their lupus symptoms had very positive outcomes for all the patients.[31]

How it works: Rituximab decreases your body's B-cell count, which is one of the white blood cells involved in the autoimmune response during a flare-up of lupus symptoms.

What you need to know: Rituximab is still a fairly new lupus treatment, but it may play a role if other treatments are unsuccessful. It does have several severe side effects, including irregular heartbeat, chest pain, and breathing trouble after injections, so be sure to weigh these risks and discuss your concerns with your doctor.

Rheumatoid Arthritis

Though they share a name, it's amazing how different osteoarthritis and rheumatoid arthritis really are. The one thing they have in common is the inflammation that leads to the throbbing, aching pain they inflict on the joints of the body. But according to experts, even these sensations of pain can exhibit subtle differences.

"The pain related to osteoarthritis is produced primarily from nerve irritation, and can be sharp, dull, or occasionally burning," says Dr. Kunikiyo. "The pain from rheumatoid arthritis is coming primarily from inflammation of the joint, and consequently feels hot and inflamed, or with a deep, throbbing ache, and tends to be more unrelenting."

The main distinction, though, is between the causes of osteoarthritis and rheumatoid arthritis. Although it's unpleasant, osteoarthritis is at least easy to understand: The pain comes from wear and tear on your joints, which damages the cartilage between them over time. Rheumatoid arthritis is an autoimmune disorder, which means the body literally attacks itself. Your immune system mistakenly thinks something is going wrong in the body and its first perceived enemy is the synovium, the lining of the membrane that surrounds your joints.

Doctors aren't quite sure what initially causes rheumatoid arthritis, but it tends to run in families. It also occurs much more often in women than men (by about a 3:1 ratio), typically starts between the ages of 40 and 60, and commonly affects small joints in the hands and feet, though it can happen elsewhere in the body, too.

The bad news is that no cure exists for rheumatoid arthritis. The good news is that people who suffer from rheumatoid arthritis have more weapons than ever before at their disposal to manage their pain and live a healthy, fruitful life. Cutting-edge medications like antirheumatic drugs and tumor necrosis factor (TNF)–alpha inhibitors are showing increased promise in treating arthritis pain in clinical studies. Exercises like yoga, tai chi, swimming, and stretching—paired with guidance and advice from an occupational therapist—are making life more rewarding and fulfilling for rheumatoid arthritis sufferers. Finally, let's not forget all the great ways to cope with pain in a relaxing, fulfilling manner, such as guided imagery, deep breathing, and muscle relaxation. All these can play a role in your pain-free life program.

Is It Rheumatoid Arthritis?

At first, it may be difficult for you and your doctor to tell the difference between rheumatoid arthritis and osteoarthritis. But rheumatoid arthritis does offer a few subtle differences in its signs and symptoms that let you know it's the source of the pain. Here's what to look for.

● You feel pain, swelling, or tenderness that affects the small joints in your hands, wrists, ankles, or feet.

● The symptoms are felt in the same joints on both sides of the body.

● Your hands become red and puffy.

● You develop rheumatoid nodules, firm bumps under the skin of your arms.

● You also experience fatigue, fever, or weight loss along with the pain symptoms.

● The symptoms tend to flare up and become severe for a few hours or days, then go into remission for a while.

● As the pain progresses, it can also affect the jaw, neck, elbows, hips, and knees.

In its early stages, rheumatoid arthritis can be difficult to diagnose since it can present symptoms that are a lot like those of osteoarthritis. The key is to

When to Call the Doctor

Though it's difficult to diagnose right away, the sooner you can catch rheumatoid arthritis in action, the better. If you experience any of the following complications, make sure to seek emergency medical help immediately.

● The pain flares up in great intensity, to the point that it impacts your ability to function.

● The pain is accompanied by fever, fatigue, or weight loss.

● The pain has moved beyond the hands and feet to other parts of the body like the jaw, neck, shoulder, hip, or knees.

look for any signs and symptoms of rheumatoid arthritis that are unique, such as similar pain in both hands or feet, the flare-ups, or the presence of fatigue, fever, and weight loss along with the pain. Make sure to tell your doctor about these symptoms.

A few blood tests can yield clues that rheumatoid arthritis might be the cause of your pain. For example, your doctor might check your erythrocyte sedimentation rate (or "sed" rate), which essentially looks at how fast your red blood cells sink in a test tube of fluid. If they fall rapidly, that indicates the presence of inflammation in the body. The doctor can also check your blood for rheumatoid factor and other antibodies that indicate the presence of rheumatoid arthritis. X-rays are useful for determining the progression of the joint damage.

Fast Relief Now

Experts are gradually coming around to the value of pain management techniques like visualization and deep breathing for flare-ups. Conventional over-the-counter pain relievers, as well as the tried-and-true technique of using hot and cold treatments for your aching joints, is also quite helpful.

1. **Push back the pain with hot and cold therapy.** Try soaking the aching joint in a tub of warm water for 4 minutes, and then cool water for 1 minute. Repeat for 30 minutes, ending the sequence with warm water.

2. **Practice deep-breathing techniques.** Breathe in deeply and slowly through your nose, taking 5 seconds to fill up the lungs and then the diaphragm. Then breathe out slowly through the mouth with your lips pursed like you're blowing out a candle. Repeat the process 5 to 10 times.

3. **Try visualization.** Close your eyes, relax, and picture something that puts you at peace. This can be your favorite vacation setting, the sun setting over an expanse of ocean, or a soothing, calming ball of light.

4. **When the pain subsides, try to go on a walk.** Any gentle activity will help.

5. **Take an over-the-counter pain reliever.** Standard OTC pain relievers like Tylenol, Advil, Aleve, and others can help with immediate pain from symptoms.

Relief at Last

You have a whole host of options for managing the pain and symptoms of rheumatoid arthritis, ranging from medication to exercise to diet and supplements.

Ultimately, some combination of strategies that have worked for others will be best for you.

Step 1: Manage the immediate pain. Before you can start to look at a long-term solution to rheumatoid arthritis, you have to get a handle on the immediate pain from the flare-ups. A combination of hot and cold treatment, relaxation therapies, and OTC pain relievers can work best for this.

Step 2: Ask your doctor about medication. Some cutting-edge medications can help manage rheumatoid arthritis pain without serious side effects. Drugs known as antirheumatics and biologic therapies can offer specifically tailored treatments to help reduce the painful symptoms and complications of rheumatoid arthritis.

Step 3: Get on the right exercise program. Staying active is a critical step in keeping rheumatoid arthritis pain from taking over your life. Walking, swimming, yoga, tai chi, and stretching exercises are all well tolerated and can help keep you strong and functional.

Step 4: See an occupational therapist. An occupational therapist will help you determine exactly what activities in your daily life are contributing the most to your pain. Then this expert will provide you with specific strategies and techniques for doing these activities in a manner that is less likely to contribute to pain.

Step 5: Try massage. Massage has shown some value in managing rheumatoid arthritis pain. The gentle technique relaxes your body and also provides useful support by activating trigger points right at the source: your achy joints and muscles.

Step 6: Change your diet. Ridding your diet of inflammation promoters and feeding on fatty fish like salmon and other anti-inflammatory foods are important in staying free of pain. Several supplements have shown great promise as well.

Pain-Relief Strategies

Food and Supplements

ANTI-INFLAMMATORY DIET: Many people with rheumatoid arthritis have felt their pain and stiffness get worse after eating certain meals and certain foods. Science has often turned a blind eye to these reactions, but now research shows that the food–rheumatoid arthritis connection is very real. Certain foods promote inflammation and create what seems to be an allergic reaction within the body, triggering rheumatoid arthritis symptoms. Other foods are anti-inflammatory, creating a soothing effect and quelling symptoms when consumed regularly.

The evidence: A 2006 study in Oslo, Norway, looked at the antibodies (the proteins your body produces when it is under attack) produced by 14 rheumatoid arthritis patients and 20 healthy subjects when fed cow's milk, cereals, eggs, codfish, and pork. Across the board, the rheumatoid arthritis patients produced significantly more antibodies in reaction to these foods after each feeding than the healthy group.[32]

How it works: Dr. Teitelbaum believes that the role of diet in rheumatoid arthritis does not get the attention it deserves. Some of the steps he recommends for diet modification include replacing inflammatory-promoting grain-fed meats with grass-fed options, eating fatty fish like salmon, and cutting out most refined carbohydrates and sugar-laden foods in favor of bountiful fruits and vegetables.

What you need to know: In general, adherence to a Mediterranean-style diet might be most effective, according to a recent study. This diet includes a lot of fish and seafood, fruits and vegetables, whole grains, nuts and seeds, olive oil, and grapes.[33]

FISH OIL: A daily fish oil supplement has proven extremely effective in managing the symptoms of rheumatoid arthritis.

The evidence: A 2010 study of rheumatoid arthritis sufferers showed that a daily fish oil supplement was more effective than nonsteroidal anti-inflammatory drugs like Advil, Motrin, and Aleve in reducing arthritis pain. The researchers recommended viewing fish oil as a first-line treatment for the disease.[34]

How it works: One of the long-chain fatty acids found in fish oil, EPA, has shown specific anti-inflammatory properties that are beneficial to people with rheumatoid arthritis.

What you need to know: Find a high-quality fish oil supplement that contains EPA. Studies have shown that around 2 grams daily provide the greatest benefit.

CURCUMIN: Curcumin, a substance found in the spice turmeric typically used in Asian cuisine, has shown new promise in fighting the symptoms of rheumatoid arthritis.

The evidence: A 2007 lab study showed that curcumin was specifically able to inhibit the degradation of the joints that typically occurs in rheumatoid arthritis.[35]

How it works: Curcumin seems to have anti-inflammatory properties. It may block specific enzymes—COX-2 and lipoxygenase—that contribute directly to the inflammation that causes rheumatoid arthritis.

What you need to know: Dr. Teitelbaum recommends the supplement Curamin, which contains a combination of curcumin, DLPA (DL-phenylalanine), and the herb boswellia. Talk to your doctor first if you plan to take the supplement and use it according to the manufacturer's directions.

Exercise and Movement Therapies

SWIMMING: If you can gain access to a pool, the latest research clearly shows that the relaxing, low-impact exercises of swimming or water aerobics are the way to go for rheumatoid arthritis sufferers.

The evidence: A 2007 study of 115 rheumatoid arthritis patients placed half of them in a hydrotherapy exercise program and the other half in a land-based exercise program. The program met 30 minutes a week for 6 weeks. At the end of the class, 87 percent of those in the water class felt better or very much better based on the researchers' test results. Only 47.5 percent of people in the land-based class felt better. What's more, 11 patients dropped out of the land-based class compared to only 4 in the water-based class.[36]

How it works: Simply put, exercising in the water has less impact on the joints and bones while still providing a great opportunity to strengthen these parts of the body. It's a perfect routine for those with rheumatoid arthritis.

What you need to know: Swimming and water aerobics are fine to do on your own as long as you don't overdo it, but you might want to find a local class for arthritis sufferers if one is available. These classes have water exercises specifically tailored to treat your arthritis pain. See Part Three for an easy routine to start with and for information on finding a class in your area.

PHYSICAL THERAPY: By working closely with a physical therapist to stretch and strengthen the joints and muscles of the body, many people with rheumatoid arthritis have found relief.

The evidence: In a study of 127 patients with rheumatoid arthritis, those who completed a 6-week physical therapy course showed significantly improved ability to function and also had much less morning stiffness.[37]

How it works: There are some risks involved with exercising when you have rheumatoid arthritis, so starting out with the guidance and input of a physical therapist is a good way to get a stretching and strengthening program that's tailored to your special needs.

What you need to know: Your doctor can likely refer you to a qualified physical therapist in your area. You can meet with a physical therapist one-on-one, or as part of a physical therapy class. The number of sessions will vary based on your individual needs.

YOGA AND TAI CHI: People with chronic pain have been gaining relief from these ancient, gentle exercise routines for centuries. Now science is slowly coming along and realizing the benefits of the techniques in several recent studies.

The evidence: A number of studies have shown the significant benefits of both yoga and tai chi. The most recent occurred in March 2010, when 15 rheumatoid arthritis patients took tai chi classes twice weekly for 12 weeks. At the end of the 12-week session, and then during a follow-up 12 weeks after that, the patients experienced greatly improved lower limb function, as well as stress reduction, improved physical condition, and more confidence moving than before the class.[39]

How it works: Both yoga and tai chi are based on gentle stretches and movements. Though they were not originally intended for this purpose, they seem to be almost tailor-made to match the exercise needs of those with rheumatoid arthritis.

What you need to know: Look around locally to see if there are any yoga and tai chi classes specifically for arthritis sufferers. That way you will know that the movements and exercises will be tailored to your abilities. Many local hospitals and medical centers offer them. If you can't find one, seek out a local instructor, explain your condition, and see if she has a routine that will work for you. As you gain confidence, you may be able to branch out and perform the exercises on your own.

OCCUPATIONAL THERAPY: An occupational therapist conjures up images of work, but in reality, the therapist's role in rheumatoid arthritis is retraining

On the Horizon

Thunder God Vine

It sure sounds impressive, and the research seems to be backing up the imposing name of this traditional Chinese remedy when it comes to rheumatoid arthritis. Supplements made from the peeled root of this plant seem to have natural anti-inflammatory properties. In a 2009 study, 121 patients took either 60 milligrams of a thunder god vine root extract three times daily or the drug sulfasalazine. After 24 weeks, those taking the supplement showed a greater improvement in joint pain symptoms.[38]

you how to do your daily activities in a way that doesn't cause pain, whether you are at work or at home. This training has proven highly effective for many with rheumatoid arthritis.

The evidence: In a 2009 study in Australia, 32 employed patients with rheumatoid arthritis were placed in either a group to receive occupational therapy or a group to receive standard rheumatoid arthritis care for 6 months. At the end of the period, the group who received occupational therapy experienced significant improvements in their pain and functioning as well as in their ability to carry out their daily duties.[40]

How it works: Whether it's a repetitive task at work, washing the dishes, or getting in and out of the bathtub, if you can learn to do these activities in a way that minimizes pain, your quality of life will improve. That's exactly the idea behind occupational therapy. These experts work closely with you to help you learn to lead your life pain free.

What you need to know: An occupational therapist will begin by assessing your daily life and helping you come up with the activities or items in your life that might be contributing to your pain. Then the therapist helps you arrive at solutions to these problems, whether it's changing how you grip and grasp things, or introducing devices into your life that will reduce pain, like a large-button telephone or a one-handed can opener. The number of times you'll meet with the occupational therapist will vary based on your individual needs.

Touch Therapies

MASSAGE: Some studies have shown the effectiveness of massage therapy for relieving stress and even reducing pain for rheumatoid arthritis sufferers.

The evidence: A 2007 study divided 22 adults with rheumatoid arthritis of the hand into a massage group and a control group for 4 weeks. The members of the massage group received a professional massage as well as tips for giving themselves a hand massage daily. At the end of the 4-week session, members of the massage group not only experienced less depression and anxiety, but they also had less pain and greater grip strength.[41]

How it works: Massage provides an overall whole-body relaxing effect that makes people generally feel better about themselves and their condition, but the specifically targeted touches also may provide some specific benefit to the afflicted bones and joints.

What you need to know: See a qualified massage therapist in your area. The positive benefits of massage are helpful but short lived, so if you are deriving benefit, you may want to get one every 1 to 2 weeks. You can also try gently massaging the joints of the wrist and hand for 1 to 3 minutes with your thumb. Side effects of massage include temporary pain or discomfort, bruising, or swelling.

Mind-Body Therapies

RELAXATION TECHNIQUES: Deep-breathing exercises, visualization techniques, meditation, and other methods of relaxation can help patients cope with the stress and pain related to rheumatoid arthritis.

The evidence: A 2006 study looked at the effects of the Benson Relaxation Technique, a deep-breathing relaxation technique, on 50 patients who were already on medication for rheumatoid arthritis. Half of the patients took medication alone, while the other half received medication and guidance in the Benson technique. At the end of the trial, both groups showed improvements in symptoms, but the relaxation group showed a much greater reduction in feelings of anxiety and depression, as well as a vast improvement in overall feelings of well-being.[42]

How it works: Anybody can do the Benson Relaxation Technique. Just sit quietly in a comfortable position, close your eyes, and relax every muscle in your body, starting at your toes and working toward your face. Then breathe in and out slowly through your nose, and say "one" silently to yourself after each breath out. Do this for 10 to 20 minutes. You can check the time, but don't use an alarm. Then sit quietly for a few minutes afterward, first with your eyes closed, and then with them open.

What you need to know: Other relaxation techniques include progressive muscle relaxation, meditation, and guided imagery. See Chapter 5 (page 46) for

»More Research Needed

Acupuncture for Rheumatoid Arthritis

Acupuncture is quite effective at treating a number of pain-related conditions throughout the body, but rheumatoid arthritis sufferers should not expect immediate relief from acupuncture. "Treating rheumatoid arthritis, and getting sustained relief, usually requires a much longer treatment regime, and it may take several years to reach a level of sustained pain reduction," says Rodney Dunetz, a licensed acupuncture physician and doctor of oriental medicine in Florida.

details on a progressive muscle relaxation exercise and Part Three for more information on other relaxation techniques.

Pain Medications and Other Medical Treatments

ANTIRHEUMATICS AND BIOLOGIC THERAPIES: Though a whole host of alternative therapies have gained ground in the treatment of rheumatoid arthritis, it's important not to overlook how effective modern medicine has become as well. "Approximately 90 to 95 percent of patients with rheumatoid arthritis can be put into remission with the combination of disease-modifying antirheumatic drugs such as methotrexate, along with newer biologic therapies," says Dr. Wei. "These medicines act like laser beams that focus on specific autoimmune abnormalities that are the cause of rheumatoid arthritis."

The evidence: Countless studies have been done on these drugs. One group of drugs used for rheumatoid arthritis, TNF-alpha blockers, was part of a review article published in the *New England Journal of Medicine* in 2010. After looking at studies that included more than 6,000 rheumatoid arthritis patients, the researchers concluded that TNF-alpha blockers when paired with methotrexate were an effective combination in reducing the joint damage caused by rheumatoid arthritis.[43]

How it works: Disease-modifying antirheumatic drugs seem to slow down the body's immune response, which slows the progression of the disease and rescues your joints and other body parts from further damage. At the same time, biologic therapies block specific inflammatory substances, like TNF, within the body that contribute to rheumatoid arthritis. As mentioned above, they seem to work best in combination.

Psoriatic Arthritis

People with the skin condition psoriasis run the risk of developing psoriatic arthritis, which exhibits many of the same painful symptoms as rheumatoid arthritis, such as joint pain, swelling, and stiffness. Just as with rheumatoid arthritis, these symptoms can flare up and become severe at times, then go into remission.

If you have psoriasis, especially if you develop lesions on your nails, you are at risk of developing this painful complication, so it is advisable to incorporate some of the arthritis prevention and relief strategies presented in this chapter into your daily life.

What you need to know: A few of the drugs that have shown efficacy in treating rheumatoid arthritis include the antirheumatic drug methotrexate; the TNF-alpha blockers etanercept (Enbrel), infliximab (Remicade), adalimumab (Humira), and golimumab (Simponi); T-cell drugs like abatacept (Orencia); B-cell drugs like rituximab (Rituxan); and the anti-interleukin medicine tocilizumab (Actemra). These drugs have a number of side effects, including an increased risk of infection and disease, congestive heart failure, lymphoma, and others. Work with your doctor on the right combination for your rheumatoid arthritis symptoms.

Adult Still's Disease

One rare form of rheumatoid arthritis is adult Still's disease, named after the English doctor who discovered the condition in 1896. Still's disease commonly occurs in children and is now known as systemic onset juvenile rheumatoid arthritis. But a quite similar condition can also occur in people when they reach adulthood, hence the word "adult" as part of the disease moniker.

Adult Still's disease cannot be cured, but it can be managed with a combination of medical treatments and lifestyle modifications. The good news is that the symptoms go away after a year in about 20 percent of people who have it and in a few years in about 30 percent.[44]

Is It Still's Disease?

Adult Still's disease often presents pain like arthritis pain, but a few other symptoms crop up that let you know that something else is going on. Here's what to look for.

- You have a high fever (usually around 102°) that persists for a week or longer.

- The peak of the fever is in the late afternoon or early evening.

- You experience pain and swelling in the joints that lasts for 2 weeks.

- A pink, bumpy rash appears on the trunk, arms, or legs.

- You may also have a sore throat, swollen lymph nodes, or other internal symptoms like an enlarged liver or spleen or heart and lung inflammation.

The symptoms of adult Still's disease can often mimic those of other conditions, especially rheumatoid arthritis, so it can be difficult for the doctor to pinpoint it. A bevy of tests can help your doctor figure out just what's wrong, including:

- An echocardiogram to look for inflammation in the heart and lungs

- X-rays of the bones and joints to look for telltale changes

- A CT scan or ultrasound to look for enlargement of the liver or spleen

- A blood test to look for high white blood cell and platelet counts and low red blood cell count

- A "sed" rate test, which looks at how quickly your red blood cells settle in a test tube (If you have Still's, the rate is rapid.)

- Blood tests to look for increased levels of C-reactive protein and ferritin

- Blood tests for rheumatoid factor and antinuclear bodies, which are usually negative in people with Still's disease

- Liver function tests

Because of the difficulty in diagnosing adult Still's disease, you can help your doctor by being as specific as possible about the symptoms you are experiencing. Write them all down, and be sure to point out any symptoms that might differentiate what you are experiencing from rheumatoid arthritis, such as the pink and bumpy rash.

Relief at Last

Medical treatment is the first-line defense against this serious condition, but lifestyle modifications can also play a role.

Step 1: See your doctor for treatment. Typical treatments for adult Still's disease include pain relievers, glucocorticoids to suppress the immune response, and anti-inflammatory medications. Other drugs known as biologic response modifiers have proven successful in some people in regulating their response to Still's disease.

Step 2: Bolster your body. A good diet and regular exercise can help your body respond better to treatment and help you manage the symptoms of Still's disease.

Step 3: Try supplements. Some of the drugs prescribed for adult Still's disease can put you at a greater risk of developing osteoporosis, so supporting your body with vitamin D and calcium supplementation, according to your doctor's guidance, might be advised.

Pain Prevention Strategies

Food and Supplements

ELIMINATE FOOD SENSITIVITIES: There's some evidence that certain food sensitivities and intolerances can contribute to the symptoms people experience from adult Still's disease. Many naturopathic physicians, including S. A. Decker Weiss, NMD, a naturopathic cardiologist in Scottsdale, Arizona, have had success treating adult Still's disease by eliminating some of the foods that cause sensitivities.

The evidence: Several studies, including one published in *The Lancet* in 2000, have shown that foods such as wheat and dairy products can elevate the body's inflammatory response, particularly in sensitive individuals, including those with adult Still's disease.[45]

How it works: Dr. Decker Weiss typically prescribes probiotics and restricts wheat and gluten products, as well as corn, dairy products, and soy. After 2 weeks, he usually sees a dramatic improvement in symptoms.

What you need to know: If you're interested in trying to eliminate potential food sensitivities that might be contributing to your pain symptoms, it's best to work closely with your doctor, a registered dietitian, or a naturopathic physician to determine the proper course of action. This will ensure that you safely eliminate foods from your diet while still getting proper nutrition.

Exercise and Movement Therapies

EXERCISE: Regular exercise can reduce pain and stiffness and give you a healthier attitude overall in the face of adult Still's disease.

The evidence: A recent study in the *European Heart Journal* showed that moderate exercise reduces levels of C-reactive protein in the blood, a chemical that contributes to inflammation. Since inflammation plays a role in adult Still's disease and many other conditions, this would suggest that exercise is helpful.[46]

How it works: As the study referenced above indicates, exercise plays a direct role in reducing inflammation and thus the symptoms of inflammatory illnesses.

What you need to know: Most experts recommend light-impact activities to reduce the adverse effect high-impact exercise can have on the joints. Dr. Kunikiyo suggests swimming as the ideal exercise for adult Still's disease sufferers. Walking is also quite useful if a swimming pool is difficult to gain access to.

Mind-Body Therapies

STRESS REDUCTION: Research indicates that stress plays a role in adult Still's disease, so reducing your stress can lower your chance of getting the disease and the symptoms that accompany it.

The evidence: In a study of 60 patients with adult Still's disease and 60 of their same-sex siblings without the disease, those who had experienced a stressful life event in the previous year were 2.5 times more likely to develop the disease.[47]

How it works: Though you can't control the occurrence of a stressful life event, you can control your reaction to it with the use of relaxation techniques like mindful meditation, relaxing breathing techniques, and low-impact exercise like yoga and tai chi.

What you need to know: One easy thing to try on your own is a deep-breathing technique. Breathe slowly through your nose, taking 5 seconds to fill up the lungs and then the diaphragm. Then breathe out slowly through the mouth with your lips pursed like you're blowing out a candle. Repeat the process 5 to 10 times.

Pain Medications and Other Medical Treatments

OVER-THE-COUNTER PAIN RELIEVERS: Many OTC pain relievers, such as Tylenol, Advil, and Aleve, are useful for managing the mild pain symptoms related to adult Still's disease.

The evidence: Several studies have shown that these drugs are a useful tool in the fight against inflammatory conditions like arthritis and adult Still's disease.

How it works: These drugs specifically block chemicals that contribute to inflammation, giving them a direct role in curbing pain.

What you need to know: Follow the manufacturer's directions. You generally don't want to take OTC pain relievers for more than 5 consecutive days. If you do have to use them frequently, your doctor should monitor your liver function, as they can damage your liver.

GLUCOCORTICOIDS: Glucocorticoids, most commonly prednisone, can reduce your body's immune response, lessening the symptoms of high fever, joint pain, and organ damage related to adult Still's disease.

The evidence: Glucocorticoids have been extensively studied for Still's disease. One study showed that the drugs were 76 percent effective at reducing the associated joint pain in a group of patients.[48]

How it works: Glucocorticoids suppress your immune function. Many of the symptoms of adult Still's disease come from your immune system attacking the body, and they lessen this response.

What you need to know: Glucocorticoids can increase your risk of infection and of developing osteoporosis. If you have to use this treatment, you may want to ask your doctor if you also need calcium and vitamin D supplementation to offset the risks of osteoporosis.

METHOTREXATE: In some people, the drug methotrexate (Rheumatrex, Trexall) helps people gain relief from adult Still's disease while taking fewer glucocorticoids, which minimizes some of the side effects related to those drugs.

The evidence: A study of 13 patients with adult Still's disease showed that methotrexate was a useful treatment, particularly when patients couldn't take glucocorticoids for various reasons. Eight of the 13 patients had at least some positive outcome from the treatment.[49]

How it works: Methotrexate works like glucocorticoids by suppressing the immune system, but it may work for some people when glucocorticoids do not.

What you need to know: Some serious side effects including lung damage, liver damage, severe nausea, and an increased risk of infection are related to methotrexate, so be sure to discuss any concerns you have with your doctor.

BIOLOGICAL THERAPIES: A growing volume of research has looked at biologic response modifiers, drugs that are specifically tailored to alter the body's reaction to autoimmune disorders like Still's disease.

The evidence: This is an emerging treatment for adult Still's disease, but it is showing real promise. A 2010 case study of a 38-year-old man with adult Still's disease showed his symptoms were totally resolved with the treatment.[50]

How it works: Methotrexate works similarly to glucocorticoids by suppressing the immune system, but it may work for people when glucocorticoids do not.

What you need to know: The specific biologic response modifier drugs that have shown promise in treating adult Still's disease in studies include infliximab (Remicade), adalimumab (Humira), etanercept (Enbrel), cyclosporine (Sandimmune), and anakinra (Kineret). Ask your doctor if any of these medications might be helpful in treating your condition.

Ankylosing Spondylitis

Rheumatoid arthritis might get most of the attention, but it's not the only inflammatory condition that can cause pain in the body. A similar condition, known as ankylosing spondylitis, affects about 600,000 Americans, mostly men. (Men are three times more likely to get it.[51]) And just like rheumatoid arthritis and other autoimmune pain disorders, its cause is poorly understood.

While rheumatoid arthritis has an impact on joints throughout the body, ankylosing spondylitis focuses on the lower back and hips, at least at first. As the disease progresses, it can lead to some frightening complications, such as restricted movement of the chest, a stiff, inflexible spine that causes you to stoop, and even eye pain and inflammation. "If left untreated, it eventually can cause the affected spinal bones to fuse together," says Dr. Decker Weiss.

The challenge with diagnosing ankylosing spondylitis is that at first it may feel like the symptoms typical of much more common low back pain. The key is to watch your symptoms closely and notify your doctor if any unusual complications arise that might pinpoint ankylosing spondylitis as the cause of the pain.

There is no cure for ankylosing spondylitis, but the good news is that the pain can be managed and the complications avoided with a cutting-edge combination of medications and physical therapy. Because of the potential risks involved with ankylosing spondylitis, you'll want to start your routine with the help of a physical therapist before doing exercises on your own.

Is It Ankylosing Spondylitis?

At first, ankylosing spondylitis will feel like low back pain. You may experience:

● General stiffness in the lower back or hips

● Pain and stiffness that is worst in the morning or after periods of inactivity

Over time, the symptoms can progress to include:

- Pain in your shoulders, knees, feet, ribs, or eyes
- Restricted expansion of the chest
- Fatigue, loss of appetite, or weight loss
- Bowel inflammation
- Eye inflammation

> ## *Quick Tip*
> Ankylosing spondylitis has a strong genetic component, so if a member of your family has it, your risk of developing the disease is much greater. Researchers have also isolated ankylosing spondylitis to a specific gene, HLA-B27. Though having this gene is no guarantee that you'll get ankylosing spondylitis, it does raise your risk significantly.

At first, your doctor might think you have low back pain, since that is a much more prevalent condition. Making matters worse is that early on in the condition, x-rays and other scanning techniques probably won't show the distinct signs of ankylosing spondylitis in your spine.

Other blood tests can help lend clues as to whether you have the disease. You may also want to ask your doctor about checking your blood for the HLA-B27 gene. If you have this gene, you have a much greater chance of developing ankylosing spondylitis.

Relief at Last

Ankylosing spondylitis must be treated with medication from your doctor. The good news about the condition is that with a combination of the right medicine and a dedicated commitment to physical therapy, most patients can live a healthy, normal life and keep their symptoms under control.

Step 1: Talk to your doctor about the right medications. Some of the medications commonly prescribed to manage ankylosing spondylitis include nonsteroidal anti-inflammatory drugs (NSAIDs), antirheumatic drugs, corticosteroids, and TNF-alpha blockers.

Step 2: Work with a physical therapist on the proper exercise program. The right exercises can greatly lessen your pain as well as improve your flexibility. These can include stretches, as well as breathing exercises to enhance your lung capacity.

Step 3: Quit smoking. Since restricted chest movement and rib pain are potential complications of ankylosing spondylitis, continuing to smoke is one of the worst things you can do.

When to Call the Doctor

Since your best bet with ankylosing spondylitis is to catch it and treat it early, be sure to see your doctor even if you only show some of the following early signs and symptoms. Don't be afraid to ask him if you might be at risk for the disease.

- You experience a persistent aching back or hips.

- You have a family history of ankylosing spondylitis.

If you already have ankylosing spondylitis, here are the complications to look out for that require a trip to the doctor or emergency treatment.

- You have pain in your back and hips that seems to be moving to other parts of the body, such as the ribs, shoulders, knees, feet, and especially the eyes.

- You feel chest tightness.

- Your spine is getting progressively stiffer.

Pain Prevention Strategies

Exercise and Movement Therapies

EXERCISE: Exercising can increase strength and flexibility to manage pain and prevent the progression of the disease into more serious complications like stooping. It can even help you breathe better if you experience restriction of your chest.

The evidence: In May 2008, several doctors reviewed past studies on the use of physical therapy for treating ankylosing spondylitis. They concluded that though there have been many breakthroughs in medical treatment, physical therapy still plays a critical part in the overall treatment of the disease. They particularly recommended water exercises because of their low impact on the body.[52]

How it works: You can't cure ankylosing spondylitis, but the stiffness and pain that accompany the condition can be minimized by staying active and keeping your muscles toned and limber.

What you need to know: Hydrotherapy, or water workouts, is particularly helpful. See Part Three for a simple routine and resources to find classes in your area. You'll also want to incorporate some land-based exercises that include range-of-motion, strengthening, and overall fitness exercises. Because of the potential complications from ankylosing spondylitis, it's best to start with the help of a physical therapist before doing exercises at home.

Diet and Supplement Therapies

FISH OIL SUPPLEMENTS: The omega-3 fatty acids DHA and EPA have anti-inflammatory properties that help with many types of pain. Research indicates that they can help for ankylosing spondylitis, too.

The evidence: A Scandinavian study divided 24 patients with ankylosing spondylitis between a low-dose group (roughly 2 grams) and a high-dose group (roughly 4.5 grams) of an omega-3 fatty acid supplement daily. The high-dose group showed a significant improvement in pain and function.[53]

How it works: Omega-3 fatty acids specifically target and block the chemicals in the body that cause inflammation. Fish oil supplements offer a high dose of these fatty acids.

What you need to know: Doctors typically recommend 1 to 2 grams of fish oil daily, so 4.5 grams is a fairly high dose. You may want to talk to your doctor about her recommendation. You may still derive some benefit from even a low dose of fish oil.

Pain Medications and Other Medical Treatments

DISEASE-MODIFYING ANTIRHEUMATIC DRUGS (DMARDS): Known as disease-modifying antirheumatic drugs (DMARDs), medications like sulfasalazine (Azulfidine) or methotrexate (Rheumatrex, Trexall) can treat the joints and limit the amount of damage that occurs in them. They are commonly prescribed for rheumatoid arthritis but are useful in the treatment of ankylosing spondylitis as well.

The evidence: A 2006 study of 230 patients with ankylosing spondylitis showed that those treated with sulfasalazine had significantly lower spinal pain and morning stiffness than those treated with a placebo.[54]

How it works: These drugs specifically target the chemicals involved in attacking the joints in diseases like rheumatoid arthritis and ankylosing spondylitis.

What you need to know: Ask your doctor if a disease-modifying antirheumatic drug might be the appropriate treatment for your ankylosing spondylitis symptoms. They are often most helpful when you catch the condition early on in the process, and they often need to be prescribed for several weeks in order to be effective. They are often prescribed in concert with nonsteroidal anti-inflammatory drugs (NSAIDs).

TNF-ALPHA BLOCKERS: A relatively new class of drugs known as tumor necrosis factor (TNF)-alpha blockers has shown great promise in treating the pain, stiffness, and swelling of the joints that can accompany ankylosing spondylitis.

The evidence: One TNF-alpha blocker called adalimumab (Humira) tested quite well in a 2006 study of 208 patients. Over the course of 24 weeks, those who took the adalimumab improved their scores by three times as much as the placebo group in one test of ankylosing spondylitis pain and function.[55]

How it works: As their name suggests, TNF-alpha blockers work by blocking TNF, a protein that acts as an inflammatory agent in the body.

What you need to know: Adalimumab (Humira), etanercept (Enbrel), and infliximab (Remicade) are just a few of the TNF-alpha blockers available. Though the benefits outweigh the risks, there are some serious side effects involved with these treatments, including nausea, headache, an increased risk of infection (particularly in people with a compromised immune system), and reactions at the site of the injection. Ask your doctor if any of these drugs might be right for you.

Other Strategies

QUIT SMOKING: We all know by now just how important it is to quit smoking for various health reasons. This is especially true if you have ankylosing spondylitis.

The evidence: Three different cross-sectional studies have shown that those who smoke are more likely to develop severe complications and have a worse outcome when it comes to functioning with ankylosing spondylitis.[56]

How it works: Restricted movement of the chest is a possible complication of ankylosing spondylitis, and quitting smoking can minimize the risk and severity of this complication.

What you need to know: Don't be afraid to try an over-the-counter smoking cessation aid or talk to your doctor if you need help in this often challenging effort. People have used nicotine replacement gum or patches or prescription drugs such as Zyban or Chantix in their efforts to quit, as well.

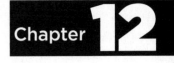

Sports and Overuse Injuries

Bursitis and tendinitis, carpal tunnel syndrome, stress fractures and metatarsal injuries, rotator cuff injuries and impingement syndrome, myofascial pain, patellofemoral pain syndrome

An overuse injury usually brings to mind a football player with turf toe, or a baseball pitcher with a torn rotator cuff. But you don't have to be a professional athlete to get an overuse injury. In fact, they are affecting more and more average, ordinary people every day.

Part of this is a result of the "weekend warrior" phenomenon. Now more than ever, people are drawn to intense physical pursuits—not just running, but training to run a marathon in the fall! In fact, marathon participation seems to grow year after year, gaining over 100,000 finishers since 2000.[1] This is just one example of Americans taking it to the extreme.

The only problem is, we average Joes and Janes lack the personal trainers, dietitians, and strength and conditioning coaches of professional and Olympic athletes. The result is that we tend to do more than we should—too much, too fast—and injuries are the unfortunate result.

"Because older individuals are more often involved in endurance sports such as running, cycling, or triathlon, chronic repetitive motion injury of hinge joints is common, particularly injuries of the lower back and knee," says Ben Greenfield, a certified personal trainer and strength and conditioning coach in Spokane, Washington. "Improper form or impact is a typical cause of acute injuries, while chronic problems are typically the result of muscular imbalances and inflexibility."

Of course, while our athletic endeavors have increased, our typical day-to-day activities at home and in the workplace have become more sedentary. And it's not just true of older folks. Many of us spend a good portion of our day looking at a computer screen and typing. In an ironic twist, this has led to the rise of another chronic overuse injury: carpal tunnel syndrome, a pain in the hands or wrists that's usually associated with computer and office work.

Luckily, whether your overuse injury is related to work or play, you have a number of tools at your disposal to get back in the game. Often, the age-old advice to use RICE—rest, ice, compression, and elevation—is step one in gaining immediate relief. Then a combination of cutting-edge exercise therapies and medical treatments can handle the rest.

Bursitis and Tendinitis

The overuse injuries bursitis and tendinitis affect two different parts of the body, but their symptoms and the way they are treated are virtually the same. If you're unfamiliar with either term, you have no doubt heard of some of the common conditions that fit under their heading: tennis elbow, golfer's elbow, pitcher's shoulder, swimmer's shoulder, and jumper's knee.

Both bursitis and tendinitis present the symptoms of pain, swelling, or stiffness in the joints, much like osteoarthritis. With bursitis, though, the pain comes from the bursae, which are fluid-filled sacks that act like padding between your bones, tendons, and muscles at the joints. Tendons, on the other hand, are stretchy bands of tissue that connect bones to muscles and allow movement.

You may not know which one you have, but you will know that something is wrong when you experience the pain of bursitis or tendinitis. One way to distinguish between the two is the cause. Bursitis often occurs when you put pressure on a joint, such as leaning on your elbows frequently. Construction workers who spend a lot of time on their knees laying tile or carpet tend to develop bursitis, for example. Tendinitis, on the other hand, is usually the result of repetitive motion—swinging a tennis racket, throwing a baseball, or running.

The typical treatments for bursitis and tendinitis won't surprise you: Rest the joint as much as possible, apply ice, and take an over-the-counter pain reliever as needed. But there have been some positive developments that can return you to action faster than ever. New exercises and stretches can specifically target your joint pain and heal it faster. Doctors are also using cutting-edge therapies like ultrasound to direct medication more efficiently to the source of your pain. Massage and acupuncture are other treatments that have shown real results for people with bursitis and tendinitis.

Is It Bursitis or Tendinitis?

The outcome for both bursitis and tendinitis is better if you can treat them before they become severe. Here are some of the signs and symptoms to look out for:

- You have dull achiness, stiffness, tenderness, or mild swelling in the joints.

- This can affect any joint, but some of the commonly affected ones include the elbows, shoulders, knees, or ankles.

- You'll occasionally see redness at the joint.

- The pain grows worse during activity, and then subsides at rest.

By performing a physical exam and asking a few questions, your doctor can usually identify the source of the injury without ordering any additional tests. If you can be as specific about your symptoms as possible, or come up with a list of daily activities or specific instances that might have contributed to your pain, that will help the doctor even more.

When to Call the Doctor

Many cases of bursitis and tendinitis are mild and can be self-treated. But if they get severe, it's best to address them with the help of a physician. Here's what to look for.

- Intense, almost unbearable pain at the joint
- Pain that prevents you from performing your day-to-day activities
- Pain accompanied by a rash or excess swelling, bruising, or redness
- Pain accompanied by fever
- Pain that does not subside with self-treatment methods after 3 or more days

Still, these conditions can mimic the symptoms of other, more chronic conditions like rheumatoid arthritis and osteoarthritis, so the doctor may want to perform an x-ray or additional lab tests just to make sure there isn't something more serious going on.

Fast Relief Now

Many people with bursitis and tendinitis want to return to their activities as quickly as possible, but it's important for you to wait until the worst of the pain subsides. Then you can start with stretching and gentle exercises to rehabilitate the joint.

1. **As much as possible, refrain from using the affected joint.** When you do have to use it, take care to make the movements gentle.

2. **Apply ice packs for 15 to 20 minutes at a time.** Do this every 4 to 6 hours as needed. You can use a cold pack, a plastic bag filled with ice, or a bag of frozen vegetables.

3. **Take an over-the-counter pain reliever according to the manufacturer's directions.** Medications like Tylenol, Advil, or Aleve all seem to help for short-term pain relief. Just avoid taking them for more than 5 consecutive days, as this can increase your risk of side effects.

Relief at Last

Most forms of bursitis and tendinitis are relatively mild and the people who experience them can return to normal activity in anywhere from a few weeks to a few months. In other cases, the pain is chronic and more serious medical treatment is required. In either case, here are the steps to take toward relief.

Step 1: Stop as soon as you feel pain. Addressing any pain immediately with ice, rest, and OTC pain relievers is a great early step to prevent making the injury worse. Don't try to power through, since you could make it harder for your body to heal in the long term.

Step 2: Try gentle exercises. When your body is ready, some gentle stretches and exercises will help you transition back into going full tilt. We provide some examples of simple stretches you can do for common types of tendinitis below.

Step 3: Buy braces, pads, or splints. In some cases, over-the-counter or prescribed insoles for your shoes, splints for your wrists, or braces for your elbows or knees can give the area the support it needs while you recover.

Step 4: See your doctor for treatment. Corticosteroids may be needed for more serious joint pain. Some doctors are using a cutting-edge ultrasound technique for this. The only instances where surgery is often used are for severe tendon injuries or possibly to drain fluid from an intensely painful bursa.

Pain Prevention Strategies

Exercise and Movement Therapies

ECCENTRIC STRETCHES: The latest research has shown that "eccentric" stretches, which lengthen the affected joint and muscles, might be the most effective stretches for healing an injured joint. "Eccentric muscle training has been shown to remodel and repair injured tissue," says Chantal Donnelly, a massage therapist, Pilates instructor, and professor of physical therapy in Los Angeles.

The evidence: A 2007 study looked at the impact of eccentric strength training on 92 patients with tennis elbow. The patients were divided into one group that received a standard, passive form of rehabilitation and one that received an eccentric-focused program. After one month, the group on the eccentric program showed a significant reduction in pain, increased strength in the affected elbow, a visible improvement in the tendons in examinations, and an increase in function and ability both for work and for other activities.[2]

The Science of Eccentric Stretching

A growing volume of research is showing just how valuable eccentric stretching is to recovery from injuries like tendinitis. Essentially, eccentric stretches are like strength training for the tendons. They help in three distinct ways.

1. **Lengthening:** Stretching the tendon with eccentric stretches will eventually make them longer even at rest. This reduces the chance of injury.

2. **Strengthening:** Gradually increasing the load supported by the tendons makes them stronger and less susceptible to future damage.

3. **Speed:** Stronger, longer tendons are also faster tendons. That means they can handle the motion of activity without getting pulled or torn.[3]

How it works: One simple stretch you can try yourself is to lengthen the affected joint slowly and keep it extended for 15 to 30 seconds. Repeat this movement 3 to 5 times. After a few days, you can gradually increase the speed and number of times you perform the exercise, then add weights.

What you need to know: Because of the nature of many joint injuries, it might be best to work with a physical therapist to come up with a specific routine for you.

Touch Therapies

MASSAGE AND ACUPUNCTURE: A gentle massage of the affected area has helped bring relief to many people with tendinitis and bursitis pain. A recent study has shown the effectiveness of a combination of acupuncture and tuina therapy, a traditional Chinese massage method, in treating tendinitis.

The evidence: The 2009 study took 50 patients with shoulder tendinitis and divided them into groups that received just acupuncture therapy or acupuncture plus tuina therapy. The therapies were given once daily for 10 days. Afterward, 74 percent of people in the acupuncture group found relief from pain, but a whopping 96 percent of patients gained relief from the combination of acupuncture and tuina therapy.[4]

Studies on massage alone for tendinitis have shown mixed results. A recent review of five studies of massage for tendinitis showed little significant improvement in pain and function.[5]

How it works: Acupuncture's effectiveness remains a mystery, but one prevailing theory is that the needle therapy enhances blood flow to the injured areas to speed relief and healing. The study mentioned above indicates that doing it in combination with massage therapy may provide additional benefit.

What you need to know: For relaxing relief, a gentle at-home self-massage or massage by a loved one is just fine. But for real results, a combination of acupuncture and massage performed by professionals might be the way to go. See Part Three to find licensed acupuncturists and massage therapists in your area. The number of visits will vary based on the extent of your injury.

Pain Medications and Medical Treatments

NONSTEROIDAL ANTI-INFLAMMATORY DRUGS (NSAIDS): In mild or moderate instances of tendinitis or bursitis, NSAIDs (nonsteroidal anti-inflammatory drugs), a class of medications that include over-the-counter pain relievers as well as stronger drugs prescribed by a doctor, may be sufficient for managing the pain.

The evidence: A 2009 review article that looked at 20 studies and 744 patients showed that NSAIDs were nearly as effective as more invasive corticosteroid injections at curbing short-term pain.[6]

How it works: Pain is related to inflammation, and these types of drugs are specifically targeted at reducing inflammation and making you feel better.

What you need to know: You can take most NSAIDs safely according to the manufacturer's directions. Just try to avoid taking them for more than 5 consecutive days, as that could increase your chance of liver damage. If an over-the-counter pain reliever is not doing the trick, you may want to consider seeing your doctor about stronger medication.

CORTICOSTEROID INJECTIONS: For severe cases of tendinitis or bursitis, your doctor may recommend a corticosteroid injection directly into the inflamed area to relieve the pain and pressure.

The evidence: A 2009 review article that looked at 20 studies and 744 patients showed that corticosteroid injections were relatively safe and more effective at curbing short-term pain than physical therapy for tendinitis.[7]

How it works: While NSAIDs are more of a whole-body anti-inflammatory medication, an injection of corticosteroids delivers this medication directly to the source of the pain for faster relief.

What you need to know: Corticosteroids certainly have some risks, including pain and infection at the site of the injection. Also, be wary of repeated injections, as these could potentially rupture the tendon. Still, corticosteroid injections are a relatively safe method for relieving pain quickly. Speak with your doctor about any concerns you have before receiving one.

ULTRASOUND THERAPY: Studies have shown that this cutting-edge treatment can be effective for treating the pain of tendinitis and bursitis.

The evidence: A 2008 study that compared the effects of ultrasound and exercise, low-level laser therapy and exercise, or an elbow brace and exercise for 58 patients with tennis elbow showed all three methods were effective at relieving pain and improving symptoms. Ultrasound and laser therapy were the most effective.[8]

How it works: Ultrasound therapy involves guiding high-energy sound waves directly into the joint to ease the pain.

What you need to know: If other approaches aren't helping your tendinitis or bursitis, you may want to speak to a physical therapist or occupational therapist to see if ultrasound treatment could work for you. The number of sessions you need will vary based on the severity and nature of your pain.

Other Treatments

BRACES, PADS, AND SPLINTS: Depending on where your bursitis or tendinitis is acting up, a knee or elbow brace, a wrist splint, or foot pads might be appropriate to support the joint while it heals.

The evidence: The recent study cited above compared the effects of ultrasound, low-level laser therapy, and an elbow brace for tendinitis treatment. Although the ultrasound and laser therapy were the most effective treatments, the elbow brace wasn't far behind.[9] Considering this, it certainly couldn't hurt to add a brace or another joint support method to your overall treatment.

How it works: In essence, a brace, pad, or splint supports the affected body part and restricts its range of motion. This allows the injury to heal properly and prevents further injury.

What you need to know: Try an over-the-counter product designed for your particular type of joint pain, or talk to a physical therapist about what the right option might be for you. In some instances, a custom brace might be appropriate. The time that the device needs to be worn will vary, but it's usually not for longer than a month.

Carpal Tunnel Syndrome

Most overuse injuries are the unfortunate by-product of an active lifestyle. One in particular, however, has risen in prevalence as Americans have become more and more sedentary. The repetitive motion of typing on a computer, assembling items on an assembly line, or otherwise using your hands and forearms to perform repetitive motions can put pressure on your median nerve, a large nerve that passes through your wrist into your hand through an opening called the carpal tunnel. Over time, this pressure can lead to the pain and numbness known as carpal tunnel syndrome.

Carpal tunnel syndrome's impact, particularly on the American workforce, is significant. It causes more lost workdays than any other injury. About 1 percent of Americans will experience carpal tunnel syndrome at one point or another, but among workers who repeatedly use their wrists and hands, the rate is 5 percent.[10]

The good news is that most people with carpal tunnel syndrome can return to daily function with a good outcome. Simple self-care strategies like physical therapy, occupational therapy, and ergonomics have come a long way in reducing the incidence of carpal tunnel syndrome and preventing its return. Wearing a splint is also quite helpful. In rare instances, surgery might be necessary to correct your carpal tunnel syndrome, but this should be viewed as a last resort.

Is It Carpal Tunnel Syndrome?

The symptoms of carpal tunnel syndrome will start subtly. Then their severity will gradually increase, and even extend beyond the hands and wrist. Here's what to look for.

- A very subtle achiness that starts in the wrist
- Numbness and a tingling sensation, particularly in your thumb, index, middle, or ring finger
- A feeling of weakness in your hand that may cause you to drop objects more frequently than usual
- Pain that radiates from the wrist up your arm after repetitive motion
- Symptoms that might be worse first thing in the morning, or even wake you up in the middle of the night

Since carpal tunnel syndrome is more likely to rear its ugly head while you perform certain activities, your doctor will probably ask you a series of questions to find out when the pain occurs. For example, she might ask you what type of activities you perform at your job, and when the pain occurs during these activities. The more specific you can be with her, the better. She also might check the feeling in your fingers or press on the median nerve to see if it brings on your symptoms.

If more extensive testing is needed, the doctor might test the nerve conduction in your muscles with a test called an electromyogram. A nerve conduction study is a slight variation on this test.

Fast Relief Now

These strategies might help to alleviate numbness and tingling temporarily. More extensive steps are needed to put a permanent stop to carpal tunnel pain.

1. **Wear a wrist splint at night.** You can try an over-the-counter splint or ask your doctor if a custom splint is right for you.

2. **Avoid sleeping on your hands.** This not only puts your hand in a position that can aggravate the injury, it also reduces blood flow to the impacted area.

3. **Take frequent breaks from painful activity.** While you take these breaks, gently stretch your wrist and hands.

4. **Try over-the-counter pain relief.** This can be Tylenol, Advil, Aleve, or other pain relievers, but avoid taking them for more than 5 consecutive days.

Relief at Last

If you catch carpal tunnel syndrome early and take the necessary steps to address the problems that led to it, your prognosis is good. Here's what to try.

Step 1: Change the offending activity. Occupational therapy can teach you how to perform your daily activities in a way that doesn't aggravate your pain. An ergonomic approach to your home or office can help you set up your workspace in the best manner for your body.

Step 2: Strengthen your wrist and hands. Wearing a splint at night and doing the appropriate stretching and strengthening exercises will pump up your wrist and hands to prevent carpal tunnel syndrome.

Step 3: Try alternative pain relief techniques. Massage, acupuncture, and chiropractic care all seem to have a viable role in treating carpal tunnel syndrome.

Step 4: Talk to your doctor. Medical options to relieve carpal tunnel syndrome pain include over-the-counter pain relievers, steroid injections, and surgery.

Pain Prevention Strategies

Food and Supplements

VITAMIN B$_6$: Jacob Teitelbaum, MD, author of *From Fatigued to Fantastic!*, recommends vitamin B$_6$ supplementation to help with carpal tunnel syndrome symptoms.

The evidence: Studies have been mixed, but they have noted that taking less than 100 milligrams a day seems to be relatively safe.[11] Most multivitamins provide a small amount of vitamin B$_6$ (the Recommended Daily Intake is only 1.3 milligrams), and you can also get B$_6$ from a variety of foods, including potatoes, bananas, beans, seeds, nuts, most meats, eggs, spinach, and cereals. You are unlikely to exceed a safe level of vitamin B$_6$ unless you take large amounts.

How it works: Doctors aren't exactly sure, but some believe that the stiffness and swelling related to carpal tunnel syndrome are related to a vitamin B$_6$ deficiency. Others believe that B$_6$ acts as a natural diuretic and helps you relieve excess fluid, which contributes to the disorder.

What you need to know: Tell your doctor if you'd like to take a vitamin B$_6$ supplement so that she can monitor your symptoms and make sure that you don't have any adverse side effects, such as chest pain, skin rashes, fatigue, or breathing problems.

ALPHA-LIPOIC ACID AND GAMMA-LINOLENIC ACID: Recent research indicates that a supplement that contains both alpha-lipoic acid (ALA) and gamma-linolenic acid (GLA) might also help reduce carpal tunnel syndrome–related pain.

The evidence: A 2009 study put 112 carpal tunnel syndrome patients on a supplement regimen that included either the ALA/GLA preparation or a vitamin B complex supplement for 90 days. The acid preparation improved pain and function by a greater margin than the vitamin B complex.[12]

How it works: Both ALA and GLA are essential fatty acids with natural anti-inflammatory properties. As this study indicates, these properties may help a concentrated supplement reduce carpal tunnel syndrome pain and improve function.

What you need to know: Alpha-lipoic acid is available as a supplement by that name or as ALA. Those in the study took 600 milligrams a day, generally regarded as safe. Possible side effects include rash or low blood sugar levels.

Gamma-linolenic acid is found in the supplements borage oil and evening primrose oil, as well as other plant oils. The dosage used in the study was 360 milligrams a day, which is thought to be a safe amount for most people. Side effects include diarrhea, soft stools, belching, and intestinal gas. It is not recommended while pregnant or breast-feeding.

Exercise and Movement Therapies

WRIST STRETCHING AND STRENGTHENING EXERCISES: A variety of different stretching and strengthening exercises for the hands, wrists, and other parts of the body add strength to put a stop to carpal tunnel syndrome.

The evidence: Tendon- and nerve-gliding exercises, which are stretches designed to move the tendons and nerves, seem to be particularly effective in reducing the pain associated with carpal tunnel syndrome. A 2006 study showed the effectiveness of these exercises in improving pain and function in 28 patients. The exercises seemed most effective when used in combination with other therapies, such as splints (see page 269).[13]

How it works: One simple exercise you can try yourself to prevent or relieve carpal tunnel syndrome is to hold both arms out in front of you. Then tilt your fingers up like you're telling somebody to stop, and hold for 5 seconds. Now make a fist, and hold again for 5 seconds. Finally, tilt the fist down, and hold one more time for 5 seconds. Repeat this 10 times.

What you need to know: Work closely with a physical therapist on the best exercises to treat your carpal tunnel syndrome. As your pain improves, you will likely be able to reduce the frequency of these exercises. The physical therapist can also help you determine which activities to avoid, such as exercises that are particularly jarring to the wrists and hands.

OCCUPATIONAL THERAPY: Occupational therapists teach people how to carry out their daily functions in a manner that doesn't aggravate pain.

The evidence: In a 2008 case study of three workers with carpal tunnel pain related to typing, all gained significant improvement through treatment with an occupational therapist.[14]

How it works: The role of an occupational therapist is to help you lead a pain-free life. The therapist will work closely with you to determine what aspects of your life are causing your pain, and then help you come up with strategies and techniques for conducting these activities in a new way.

What you need to know: Usually, the occupational therapist will spend the first session asking you questions to determine what activities in your life are the source of your pain. Subsequent sessions are often used to come up with strategies to alleviate that pain with specific techniques, changes in routine, or the use of accessories to relieve the pain in your hands. The number of sessions will vary based on your needs. Once the source of the pain is established and corrected, the positive results can be fairly immediate. Ask your doctor for a referral to an occupational therapist in your area, or see Part Three.

Touch Therapies

MASSAGE: Massage that is targeted directly to your wrist or hands seems to be helpful for patients with carpal tunnel syndrome.

The evidence: A 2008 study looked at the effects of twice-weekly general massage or targeted massage on 27 patients with carpal tunnel syndrome. Both groups gained benefit after 6 weeks, but the targeted massage group also showed increased grip strength.[15]

How it works: Massage produces a general relaxing effect that makes pain sufferers feel better, but there is also some evidence that the specific manipulation it provides to the affected area might increase blood flow and promote healing.

What you need to know: The people in the study received professional massages twice a week, but getting a massage whenever you can might still provide some relief. If you see a massage therapist, explain the nature of your pain and make sure that the therapist is comfortable massaging you to treat it. You can also massage the painful wrist or hand yourself by gently using a circular motion for a few minutes to bring some relief.

ACUPUNCTURE: The ancient art of acupuncture is used for many conditions, and carpal tunnel syndrome is certainly one in which acupuncture seems to play a role.

The evidence: Many studies have looked at the positive impact of acupuncture. The researchers in one study found it to be as effective as steroids in managing the pain of carpal tunnel syndrome in the short term.[16]

Using sophisticated brain imaging, researchers in one 2007 study found that the brains of people with carpal tunnel syndrome actually responded differently to acupuncture than the brains of healthy controls.[17]

How it works: The researchers speculate that acupuncture may turn down the dial on the hyperactivity of brain areas associated with the emotional processing of pain.

What you need to know: In studies, acupuncture has brought immediate relief from pain, but this is a short-term effect. More sessions may be needed to continue pain relief, and the number of sessions you need will vary based on the severity of the pain you experience. See Part Three to find a qualified acupuncturist in your area.

Pain Medications and Medical Treatments

CORTICOSTEROIDS: The traditional approach for carpal tunnel syndrome that does not respond to other approaches is to relieve the pain with corticosteroid injections.

The evidence: A 2008 review of the use of corticosteroid injections for carpal tunnel syndrome looked at 12 studies with 671 participants. Researchers found that a corticosteroid injection is useful for relieving carpal tunnel syndrome pain for up to 1 month. An additional injection did not provide any more benefit. What's more, one study found that the use of oral pain medication and splinting was as effective as corticosteroids at relieving pain.[18]

How it works: A corticosteroid injection brings a dose of anti-inflammatory medication directly to the source of the pain, so it relieves it quickly. As studies have shown, though, the medication can be relatively short lived as a treatment.

What you need to know: There are some risks involved with repeated injections to the same part of the body, so discuss these concerns seriously with your doctor when determining your carpal tunnel syndrome treatment. Although the occasional injection might be helpful for immediate pain relief, it is hardly the long-term solution to managing carpal tunnel syndrome.

SURGERY: If the pain is severe and persists for longer than 6 months, surgery might be the best option for carpal tunnel syndrome.

The evidence: A 2008 review of 317 patients in four studies showed that surgery was generally more effective than nonsurgical approaches to treating carpal tunnel syndrome. The risk of complications from surgery was also relatively low.[19]

How it works: The surgical procedure usually involves cutting the ligament in your wrist that is pressing on the nerve and causing the pain.

What you need to know: The outcome from carpal tunnel surgery is generally good, but, as with all surgeries, there are complications and a long recovery period. You may experience numbness, stiffness, weakness, or pain in your hand or wrist for several weeks to several months.

Other Strategies

SPLINTS: Options range from wearing an over-the-counter wrist splint at night to getting fitted for a custom splint system, such as a Dynasplint, by your doctor.

The evidence: The Dynasplint, which is prescribed by a doctor and worn for a specific amount of time each day, was quite effective in a 2009 study of 156 patients. (In the study, patients wore the splint for 15 to 30 minutes twice a day.)[20]

How it works: Splints seem to hold your hand and wrist in the right orientation to stretch and elongate the ligaments. This relieves the pressure they put on the nerve. Over time, it seems that they may be able to correct the misalignments that cause carpal tunnel syndrome pain.

What you need to know: For mild carpal tunnel syndrome that has lasted less than 10 months, try wearing an over-the-counter night splint to see if you gain relief. This holds your hand in the correct position as you sleep, which can help stretch the ligament and bring relief. The amount of time you'll need to wear this splint varies depending on the seriousness of your symptoms. For more serious carpal tunnel syndrome, talk to your doctor about your splinting options, such as the Dynasplint.

> ## Quick Tip
>
> For office workers, setting up your workspace ergonomically is a simple step to prevent carpal tunnel syndrome. Your computer screen should be about 2 feet from your eyes. The top of your documents should be at eye level. Your keyboard should be resting flat or slightly elevated. Most important, your wrists should be kept straight while typing. "The hand and wrist should float in the air when you type, similar to playing the piano," says Chantal Donnelly, massage therapist and professor of physical therapy.

Stress Fractures and Metatarsal Injuries

At first, it may start as subtle foot pain, usually while taking part in your favorite athletic activities. Once you stop the activity, the pain subsides, and you forget about it.

Over time, the amount of pain you feel grows, until it's present even when you're not in motion. This overuse injury is known as a stress fracture, and it's problematic precisely because of its subtlety; you may have a stress fracture for quite a while before you even know it.

Stress fractures are also known as metatarsal injuries because they are most commonly microfractures in the metatarsal (weight-bearing) bones of the foot, though they can also occur in the legs. They often occur when you start a new exercise and try to do too much too soon. Adding intensity to one of your usual exercises is another good way to cause a stress fracture.

A stress fracture requires rest, simple therapies to ease pain and swelling, and then gradual reintroduction to exercise. Read on for the simple strategies to get back in the game as quickly and safely as possible.

Is It a Stress Fracture?

Stress fractures can sometimes be difficult to identify because of how slowly they develop, but they will gradually begin to send you warning signs that something is wrong. Watch for the folllowing:

- Subtle pain develops while exercising, then ceases afterward, and might only occur at a specific time of the workout, usually early on.

- The pain increases in intensity or in duration over time.

- You feel pain even at rest.

- A specific spot on the foot is sensitive and painful to the touch.

- The pain is accompanied by swelling of the foot.

Though the doctor will start with a physical examination, an x-ray is the typical test for detecting the stress fracture. The fracture may not be apparent until 3 to 4 weeks after it occurs. Magnetic resonance imaging or bone scans might also be used to detect a subtle fracture.

Fast Relief Now

You can't heal a stress fracture alone, but you can certainly do some things to manage the pain and prevent it from getting worse.

1. **Cease the activity, and rest the foot as much as possible.** Rest prevents the injury from getting worse.

2. **Use an over-the-counter pain reliever.** This can be Tylenol, Advil, Aleve, or other brands. No one brand has been proven to be more effective than the others at treating the pain of a stress fracture.

3. Apply ice packs. Use them three to four times a day, 10 minutes at a time. Ice reduces pain and swelling.

Relief at Last

Stress fracture treatment is fairly straightforward, yet it can be frustrating for the dedicated athlete. Here are your marching orders to get back in the game as quickly as possible.

Step 1: Try over-the-counter pain relief, ice, and rest. This is the front-line treatment for reducing pain and stopping the progression of the fracture.

Step 2: Ask your doctor if more treatment is needed. In some cases, a boot or brace and crutches might be needed to help the foot heal. A cast or surgery are required in more severe cases.

Step 3: Start back into exercise slowly. Non-weight-bearing activities like swimming are a good way to get back into exercise while avoiding a recurrence.

Pain Prevention Strategies

Food and Supplements

CALCIUM AND VITAMIN D: Stress fractures aren't always related to sports. Sometimes older people with osteoporosis or reduced bone density for other reasons can get stress fractures. An adequate calcium and vitamin D intake is crucial for preserving strong bones well into your life. Now emerging research is showing that supplementation of these two crucial nutrients might help young people, too.

The evidence: In a 2009 study of 5,201 female navy recruits, the study subjects received either 2,000 milligrams of calcium and 800 IUs of vitamin D (about twice what is normally recommended for adults) or a placebo daily. The supplement group had a 20 percent lower incidence of stress fractures than the placebo group.[21]

How it works: Both nutrients are known to strengthen bones, so getting an adequate intake is critical to bone health. This is especially true among the elderly as osteoporosis becomes a greater concern.

What you need to know: You can get an adequate daily intake of calcium from dairy products as well as some leafy green vegetables, beans, and fish. The primary source of vitamin D is safe exposure to sunlight. You may also want to consider taking a daily multivitamin or a separate vitamin D supplement to ensure an adequate dose. The 2,000 milligrams of calcium cited in the study above are much more than what is typically recommended, so you may want to ask your doctor what types of calcium or vitamin D supplements, and how much, might be right for you.

Exercise and Movement Therapies

GENTLE EXERCISES: When you're ready to get back into action, the evidence is pretty clear that non-weight-bearing activities are effective for ensuring that the injury heals completely before returning to intense activity.

The evidence: Although rehabilitation often begins after the patient has been pain free for 2 weeks, the evidence indicates that the first 4 weeks are the most vulnerable time after the injury. That's why the exercise in the initial recovery process needs to be low-impact and supervised.

How it works: Intense activity is likely what caused the stress fracture in the first place, and though it's hard for many athletes to hear, it can also prevent it from healing. By taking your time and being gentle as you get back into activity, you can improve your prognosis significantly.

What you need to know: Work with a physical therapist on the proper rehabilitation program for you. One effective treatment that's sometimes used is a water workout program that begins with 2 weeks of deep-water running, 2 weeks of shallow-water running, 2 weeks of water exercises like jumps and squats while holding weights, and then a return to low-impact exercises like cycling and using stairclimbers and elliptical machines.

Pain Medications and Other Medical Therapies

SURGERY: In some instances, surgery is necessary to hold the bones of the foot in the proper position while they heal properly.

The evidence: Studies have shown that surgery can sometimes speed the rate of healing of a stress fracture, and technological advances continue to develop. A 2010 study discusses a new internal fixation technique using screws that successfully healed eight patients without complications.[23]

How it works: This surgical procedure is called internal fixation. Pins, screws, or plates are used to fuse the bones together during the healing process.

What you need to know: Surgery is typically regarded as a last resort for stress fractures that other methods won't resolve, and, as with any surgery, there are risks involved. But for severe stress fractures, the surgery can speed healing and help you return to your favorite activities. Weigh these pros and cons with your doctor when discussing surgery.

Other Strategies

NON-WEIGHT-BEARING ACTIVITIES: Most people don't like to hear it, but resting the injury by sticking to activities that put no pressure on the foot is far and away the greatest way to ensure healing and a return to activity.

The evidence: A 2009 review of previous stress fracture studies compared conservative non-weight-bearing treatment, surgery, and weight-bearing treatment for stress fractures. Non-weight-bearing activities were far and away the most successful treatment, with a 96 percent success rate, compared to surgery at 82 percent.[24]

How it works: It doesn't get much simpler than this: Stay off the foot and it has a chance to heal on its own without the risk of aggravating the injury.

What you need to know: Recovery times vary greatly depending on the extent of the fracture, so work closely with your doctor on when it's appropriate to return to activity.

SHOE INSOLES: Over-the-counter shoe insoles might help prevent stress fractures for vigorous activities, though more studies are needed in athletes.

The evidence: A review of five studies that examined the use of insoles in military personnel showed that using the insoles reduced the incidence of a stress fracture among the study participants.[25]

How it works: Shoe insoles add extra cushioning and protection to the feet during strenuous activities, preventing the kind of damage and injuries that can lead to stress fractures.

What you need to know: A number of over-the-counter insoles are available. Choose one that is comfortable, supportive, or recommended for your particular activity. You can also order insoles specifically tailored to your individual foot. You'll want to talk to your doctor about this option.

BOOTS, BRACES, OR CASTS: Simply put, immobilizing the foot in a brace or boot while it heals seems to be more effective than surgery for a successful outcome in stress fractures.

The evidence: Based on a 2009 review, conservative non-weight-bearing treatment, which often included immobilizing the foot in a brace or boot, was more successful than surgery at treating stress fractures. The study authors said that recovery was typically achieved in 6 weeks.[30]

How it works: Since it can be so hard to avoid putting weight on your foot, these tools certainly make it easier. They protect the foot and prevent you from injuring it again while it heals.

What you need to know: Ask your doctor if a boot or brace would be appropriate for healing your stress fracture properly. You'll typically have to wear it for about 6 to 8 weeks while the foot heals.

Rotator Cuff Injuries and Impingement Syndrome

You often hear of a pitcher in baseball with a torn rotator cuff from overuse of his shoulder in his throwing motion. But regular folks can get rotator cuff injuries, too. You can get them from playing sports like golf, tennis, or racquetball. Sometimes poor posture over time can cause shoulder pain. Or overexerting yourself while pushing and pulling something too heavy can do the trick. In short, you don't have to throw 90-mile-per-hour fastballs to hurt your rotator cuff.

One of the most common types of rotator cuff injury is known as shoulder impingement, which is caused by tendinitis or bursitis. It can cause limited movement and pain in the shoulder when you try to move it. If left untreated or severely strained, you can experience a rotator cuff tear just like a pitcher.

In most cases of rotator cuff injury, conservative treatments like rest, ice, massage, and over-the-counter pain relievers will do the trick. When you feel up to it, exercise is also critical for keeping the shoulder limber and restoring its usefulness. For more severe rotator cuff injuries, several viable medical options are available, including a promising new one called reverse ball-and-socket prosthesis.

Is It a Rotator Cuff Injury?

If your rotator cuff is hurt, the good news is that it's pretty easy to identify the symptoms of the injury.

- You have pain or tenderness in the shoulder area, particularly when rotating it or moving your arm over your head.

- You experience a loss in the range of motion of your shoulder.

- You don't feel like using your shoulder very often.

- Your shoulder feels weaker than usual.

Your doctor should have no trouble diagnosing a rotator cuff injury with a simple physical examination. He will probably poke and prod at the area of the pain a bit and test your range of motion. Depending on the severity of your pain, he may use x-rays, magnetic resonance imaging, or ultrasound to find the specific source of the pain around the joint.

Fast Relief Now

1. **Find a cool solution.** Wrap a bag full of ice cubes in a towel and secure it to your shoulder with another towel or an elastic band. Leave it there for 15 to 20 minutes, and do this every few hours as needed.

2. **Follow with hot.** After 2 or 3 days, replace the ice treatment with a hot pack and follow the same process to keep the shoulder limber.

3. **Treat the pain.** Take an over-the-counter pain reliever according to the manufacturer's directions.

4. **Rest the shoulder.** As much as you can, avoid any activities that will further aggravate and potentially reinjure your shoulder.

5. **As it improves, try gently stretching your arm.** More information on how to do this is provided on page 277.

Relief at Last

Rotator cuff injuries range from minor pain that you can treat yourself to more serious, debilitating shoulder injuries that require treatment or even surgery from your doctor. Here is your sequence of treatments to try.

Step 1: Use pain relievers, ice, heat, and rest for mild pain. Reduce the pain with ice, take over-the-counter pain relievers like Tylenol, Advil, and Aleve, rest, and then keep the shoulder limber with heat.

Step 2: Stretch as able. Once your shoulder starts to improve, it's critical to keep it limber and useful by starting a program of gentle stretches. We'll provide you with more specific stretching advice below.

Step 3: Ask your doctor about further treatment. Corticosteroid injections are sometimes used to address severe inflammation and pain. Sometimes surgery may be required.

Pain Prevention Strategies

Exercise and Movement Therapies

STRETCHING: Once you're able, stretching is the best way to effectively heal the shoulder and return it to its previous range of motion and function.

The evidence: A growing volume of research is showing the effectiveness of stretches known as joint and soft tissue mobilization techniques for rehabilitating the shoulder. Specifically, a 2007 study showed that 15 patients who tried the techniques as part of their rehabilitation regimen showed much greater shoulder improvement than a group who did basic range-of-motion stretches.[26]

How it works: One simple exercise you can do is to stand and clasp your hands behind your back. With your arms straight, slowly lift them upward. Hold for 15 to 20 seconds, and repeat 3 or 4 times.

Another one that helps is to hold the hurt arm out and bend the elbow at 90 degrees so that your hand is pointing up. Hold on to the end of a broomstick with the hand of your hurt arm, and with your other hand pull the bottom of the broomstick toward the front of the body. Do this stretch slowly and gently, for 15 to 20 seconds, and repeat 3 or 4 times.

What you need to know: Ask your physical therapist about joint and soft tissue mobilization techniques to heal your shoulder. Avoid any activities or aggressive stretches that overexert the muscles and joints of the shoulder.

Touch Therapies

ACUPUNCTURE AND MASSAGE: The combination of acupuncture and massage might be helpful for those with shoulder injuries.

The evidence: Forty Chinese patients with shoulder impingement received treatment with a combination of acupuncture and tuina therapy, an ancient Chinese form of massage. Twenty-seven patients had complete relief of symptoms, and all but one of the patients gained at least some relief from the treatment.[27]

When it comes to massage alone, a separate study of 29 patients with shoulder pain who received six massage sessions showed significant reduction in pain and improvement in function over a control group that received no treatments.[28]

How it works: Though they are distinct treatments, both acupuncture and massage seem to bring relief through a combination of relaxation and stress reduction, as well as specific treatment of the inflamed tissue related to the pain.

What you need to know: If you don't have a tuina therapy specialist in your area, a combination of acupuncture therapy and soft tissue massage therapy from two separate specialists might be right for your shoulder pain. Just be sure to inform them of your injury so that you can receive the appropriate treatment.

Pain Medications and Medical Treatments

STEROID INJECTIONS: For severe shoulder pain and inflammation, an injection of corticosteroids like prednisone directly to the site of the pain is a standard treatment.

The evidence: This has been shown to be an effective treatment in a number

Reverse Ball-and-Socket Prosthesis

If you have a torn rotator cuff or extremely severe shoulder pain, surgery is the appropriate medical option to repair the torn tendon or damaged shoulder. Now an effective artificial shoulder known as a reverse ball-and-socket prosthesis is available for patients whose shoulder pain is so severe that other treatments aren't helping. In a 2009 study of 48 patients who received these artificial shoulders, 89 percent of the patients rated their outcome as good or excellent after 3 years of having the artificial shoulder.[30]

of studies. Most recently, a 2010 study showed that a shot of prednisone was significantly more effective at reducing shoulder pain than an injection of a nonsteroidal anti-inflammatory drug known as tenoxicam in a study of 58 patients.[29]

How it works: Corticosteroids are powerful anti-inflammatory medications, and injecting them right at the source of the pain can bring almost immediate relief.

What you need to know: As with many injections, there are some potential side effects of corticosteroid injections, and repeated injections can cause damage to shoulder tendons. Though they provide immediate relief, you may need more injections in the future to reduce further pain.

Other Strategies

SCAPULA TAPING: Scapula taping, a taping technique performed by physical therapists that properly positions the shoulder and restricts its movement, has been effective at reducing pain and improving rehabilitation from a shoulder injury.

The evidence: In a 2009 study, 22 subjects were split into groups that either received standard physical therapy or scapula taping and physical therapy. The group that got the taping showed immediate pain reduction at a much greater level than the group that only received physical therapy.[31]

How it works: When taped properly, the shoulder's movement is restricted, preventing further injury. It also helps position the shoulder properly to assist with healing.

What you need to know: Talk to your physical therapist about taping and its use in treating your specific shoulder injury. The therapist may give you more specific details about how to tape the shoulder yourself at home. The taping technique will vary slightly based on your unique shoulder injury.

Myofascial Pain

Everybody experiences muscle pain from time to time. But when that pain continues unabated for days on end, it's known as myofascial pain. Rather than a specific strain or tear, this pain can be traced back to what are known as trigger points. These are tight bundles of fibers located within the muscles throughout the body. Though an injury or overuse may originally have injured the muscle, the trigger points will continue to radiate pain long after the injury has occurred.

At first, the pain is confined to the muscles, and the trigger points may even be sensitive to the touch. Over time, this can lead to pain in other parts of the body, including headaches, back pain, and arm and leg pain. It's more common among women than men.

Gaining relief from myofascial pain starts with rest, then doing gentle stretches to alleviate the pain. Massage and other touch therapies are also helpful. When other methods fail, a few different medical techniques can directly address the trigger points and bring relief to pain right at the source.

Is It Myofascial Pain?

A simple muscle strain is one thing, but myofascial pain can be a completely different animal. Here is what to look for.

- Deep pain in a muscle that persists for several days or gets worse over time

- Stiffness in the muscle, or joint stiffness in nearby joints

- A specific spot that's particularly sensitive and may feel like a knot

Since the trigger points are the key to myofascial pain and are what differentiate it from other types of pain, your doctor may feel your muscle to try to identify those trigger points. Then he may manipulate them to see what types of pain they produce.

Fast Relief Now

Persistent muscle pain may require a more extensive approach to healing, but there are some strategies you can use to gain relief from the flare-ups in the short term.

1. **Rest the aching muscle as much as possible.** If you find that you have to move the part of your body that hurts, keep the movements slow and gentle.

2. **Try gentle stretching exercises for the affected muscle.** Depending on where it hurts, you can slowly and carefully try to stretch it out for just a few seconds to see if that brings you any relief.

3. **Use over-the-counter pain relievers.** Tylenol, Advil, Aleve, and others are all satisfactory choices here. Use them according to the manufacturer's directions, but don't take them for more than 5 consecutive days.

4. **Practice visualization or meditation to reduce stress and relax.** Try closing your eyes and breathing deeply and slowly to forget about the pain, or picture yourself in a calming, soothing place where the pain is far away.

Stress can also play a role in causing myofascial pain, so self-relaxation techniques like deep breathing, meditation, and visualization can all be helpful. Jennifer Pells, PhD, a staff psychologist at Structure House in Durham, North Carolina, advises closing your eyes, breathing in deeply, pausing, and then saying "relax" to yourself as you slowly exhale. Repeat as needed.

Relief at Last

Self-care techniques are critical to curbing your myofascial pain. The help of other experts like massage therapists, acupuncturists, physical therapists, and doctors completes the picture. Here's your full prescription.

Step 1: Try gentle stretches and relaxation techniques. Stretches will target the muscles to relieve the pain at the source. For many people, relaxation techniques can eliminate the stress that contributes to the pain.

When to Call the Doctor

The key difference between a standard muscle strain and myofascial pain is its persistence. If it doesn't go away or you have any of the following symptoms, you need a doctor's help.

● You experience muscle pain that doesn't go away after a week.

● The pain is interfering with your daily activities.

● Self-care measures are doing nothing to relieve the pain.

Step 2: Tune in to touch therapies. Both massage and acupuncture have helped people successfully quell myofascial pain.

Step 3: Seek more extensive approaches. Doctors can use injections to target the affected trigger points or prescribe more serious pain medication than OTCs if needed.

Pain Prevention Strategies

Exercise and Movement Therapies

GENTLE STRETCHES: Gentle stretching exercises, guided by a physical therapist, are an effective treatment method for many types of myofascial pain.

The evidence: A recent review of the studies of physical therapy for myofascial pain concluded that physical therapy overall is useful for relieving pain and symptoms.[32]

How it works: Stretches lengthen and elongate the muscles, which can bring relief to the sharp and painful trigger points that are causing the pain.

What you need to know: Considering the various types and locations of myofascial pain, your best bet is to work closely with a physical therapist to determine the best exercises for you.

Touch Therapies

MASSAGE: The type of massage therapy that is commonly used to treat myofascial pain is known as myofascial release, and it is often done by a physical therapist.

The evidence: A 2010 survey of 332 physicians who treat myofascial pain showed that myofascial release therapy performed by a physical therapist had moderate but helpful results. The researchers believe more study is needed in the area.[33]

How it works: A myofascial release massage works much like acupuncture in that it focuses pressure specifically on the painful trigger points to bring relief to painful symptoms.

What you need to know: Find a physical therapist or massage therapist in your area who can perform myofascial release. You may feel some relief after the first session, though more sessions may be needed depending on the nature and extent of the pain you are experiencing.

FOAM ROLLER STRETCHES: A few programs advocate stretching exercises while placing a soft foam cylinder known as a foam roller behind your back or

Botox for Myofascial Pain

Injecting Botox at the trigger points may be an effective way to curb myofascial pain. In a 2007 study of five different methods of treatment, Botox proved the most effective, beating such approaches as gentle stretching.[35]

legs to self-relieve your myofascial pain. This is known as self-myofascial release.

The evidence: A 2009 review article concluded that myofascial release techniques using a foam roller can relieve pain and muscle spasms and improve flexibility and are an inexpensive and easy-to-learn treatment option.[34]

How it works: The large foam roller places your body in the proper position to stretch the muscles in a way that activates the trigger points. It's a form of self-massage that releases trigger points and provides relief.

What you need to know: You can ask your physical therapist about self-myofascial release. Many therapists can guide you through a program you can do at home. A relatively new pain-relieving technique called the MELT method also advocates the use of foam rollers to alleviate myofascial pain. You can learn more about it at www.meltmethod.com.

ACUPUNCTURE: Acupuncture is a great way to gain relief from myofascial pain with a safe, effective, and proven method of treatment.

The evidence: A 2007 study compared 27 patients with myofascial pain who received either a real acupuncture treatment tailored to their pain or a sham treatment. The real acupuncture treatment was significantly more effective at relieving the pain.[36]

How it works: Experts aren't exactly sure how acupuncture works, but some theorize that it increases blood flow to the afflicted part of the body to speed healing. Studies of acupuncture for myofascial pain have shown successful results.

What you need to know: Seek out a qualified acupuncturist in your area. (See Part Three for resources.) Patients typically see their acupuncturist about once a week while in active treatment. You may begin to feel relief within a session or two, but it might take more sessions to bring your pain to a resolution.

Mind-Body Therapies

RELAXATION TECHNIQUES: Deep breathing, meditation, and visualization are all useful in dealing with the stress that can lead to myofascial pain flare-ups.

The evidence: The best results may come from being part of a group class that teaches you the basics of these techniques, at least at first. In a 2007 study of 26 people with myofascial pain, 65 percent of those who took a group cognitive-behavioral therapy course that focused on stress management techniques experienced an improvement in their symptoms.

How it works: Relaxation techniques can get you through pain flare-ups by helping you focus on other things. Over time, leading a more relaxed, less stressful lifestyle can actually lead to a reduction in pain.

What you need to know: You don't need an expert to practice relaxation techniques. "Stop whatever you're doing, close your eyes and begin to picture a place, scene, or event that you associate with pleasant feelings, calm sensations, and a relaxed attitude," says Dr. Pells. "Insert yourself into the image, and really imagine that you're there, including what you see around you, what pleasant sounds you hear, and any other sensations you'd have in that situation. Allow yourself to stay with the image for a few minutes, just breathing naturally and softly." See Chapter 5 for a simple guided imagery exercise you can try, and see Part Three for CDs, DVDs, classes, and other resources to learn different relaxation techniques.

Pain Medications and Other Medical Treatments

TRIGGER POINT INJECTIONS: The standard medical treatment for relieving myofascial pain at the source is known as a trigger point injection. This involves inserting a needle in and around the trigger point to relieve the pain. The doctor may also inject a numbing medication like lidocaine during this process.

The evidence: A 2009 study compared the effects of trigger point injections using lidocaine and a placebo in 60 patients. The study showed that those who received the trigger point injections showed the most significant reduction in pain and improvement in function.[37]

How it works: If this technique sounds similar to acupuncture, that's because it is. A 2008 study from the Mayo Clinic showed that though acupuncture and the Western notion of trigger point therapy for myofascial pain evolved through different channels to become what they are today, they essentially treat myofascial pain the same way.[38]

What you need to know: Patients usually experience relief after one visit, but they may need follow-up visits if the pain returns. These injections are generally safe, but some people are allergic to the numbing agents in the injections. In these instances, a dry needling technique can be used.

Patellofemoral Pain Syndrome

The kneecap, or patella, may get all the attention, but one other critical part of your knee joint is the patellar cartilage. This bundle of cartilage that rests under the kneecap acts as a shock absorber, letting your knee move comfortably from place to place.

Whether it's from misalignment, injury, or old age, sometimes this cartilage gets worn down and loses its effectiveness over time. It happens a lot in runners and other athletes, but sometimes it happens in older people as a complication of arthritis. It's known as patellofemoral pain syndrome.

As with many injuries, rest, ice, and strengthening exercises are the proper course of treatment for most cases of patellofemoral pain. But what's interesting about knee pain is that recent research has noted that it's not necessarily the knee that is causing the pain, even though that's where you feel it. "Current research suggests that patellofemoral pain results from a weakness in the gluteal muscles," says Donnelly. "Strengthening the glutes improves pelvic stability, which improves lower limb alignment and decreases the overuse of the quadriceps muscles."

Stretching and strengthening exercises in the quadriceps and hips have also been helpful in reducing knee pain. And a cutting-edge knee taping method helps many people gain pain relief and an improvement in function. Read on for your full knee pain prescription.

Is It Patellofemoral Pain Syndrome?

Patellofemoral pain syndrome often starts as a dull, achy pain when you bend your knee or walk up stairs. Over time, the intensity of the pain can increase, as well as the instances when you feel it. Eventually you might even experience knee pain while at rest. Here are the signs and symptoms to watch for when it comes to knee pain.

- Increased knee pain while walking up and down stairs

- Knee pain while kneeling or squatting, or after sitting for a long period of time

- A sensation of bone-on-bone grinding when you move your knee

- Knee stiffness and lost mobility

Most often, patellofemoral pain can be diagnosed by a doctor with a physical examination alone. He may feel the knee as you move it to see if there is a grinding sensation. Having you move, jump, or squat can also help him determine if a muscle weakness or bone misalignment is at issue. Finally, he may recommend an x-ray or MRI to determine more specifically what the source of your pain is.

Fast Relief Now

The good news about patellofemoral pain is that in most cases these steps will not only provide relief but actually put a stop to the pain entirely. More severe knee pain might require additional steps and help from your doctor.

1. **Rest the knee and avoid painful activities.** If you can't rest, take great care to move gently and slowly to avoid reinjuring the knee.

2. **Take an over-the-counter pain reliever.** Tylenol, Advil, Aleve, and others have all been shown to be helpful when taken according to the manufacturer's directions. Avoid taking them for more than 5 consecutive days.

3. **Ice it down.** Wrap an ice pack in a towel and hold it on the knee with an elastic band for 10 to 20 minutes, as needed.

4. **Begin gentle exercises as the knee starts to heal.** We'll walk you through one simple possibility that will help on page 286.

When to Call the Doctor

While mild knee pain can be treated with self-care strategies, these are all signs that the condition might be more serious and needs treatment from a doctor.

- You experience a popping or snapping sound followed by knee pain.
- Your kneecap looks visibly misaligned.
- Your knee locks up and can't move.
- Your knee feels loose or wobbly when you put weight on it.
- Your knee hurts even at rest or when not putting weight on it.
- The pain is severe or interfering with your daily activities.
- It is accompanied by fever, chills, or redness.

Relief at Last

If you experience patellofemoral pain, you can try several self-care strategies first. If those don't work, see your doctor for additional treatment methods.

Step 1: Stop the pain before it gets worse. This is the first step toward relief and reversal of symptoms if you have mild knee pain.

Step 2: Try acupuncture or massage therapy. Both treatments have been shown to be effective at treating knee pain.

Step 3: Talk to your doctor. Over-the-counter pain relievers and some medications can bring immediate pain relief. In more severe cases of knee pain, surgery is sometimes an option.

Pain Prevention Strategies

Exercise and Movement Therapies

STRETCH AND STRENGTHEN: Once the short-term pain subsides, stretching and strengthening exercises are the best way to reduce pain and return your knee to its previous function. Exercises for the quadriceps muscles are commonly used, as well as exercises for the hip, hamstring, calf, and iliotibial band (a band of muscle that runs from your rear to just below your knee).

The evidence: In a 2009 study of 69 patients with patellofemoral pain syndrome, the patients were placed into two groups that received different types of quadriceps exercises, or a control group that did no exercise. After 8 weeks of treatments, the patients who exercised their quadriceps showed a vast improvement in pain and function over the control group.[39]

How it works: One simple exercise you can try at home is a quad strengthening contraction: Sit on the edge of a chair, extend your legs, and put your heels on the floor. Then simply tighten your thigh muscles for a count of 10, relax for 3 seconds, and repeat. Try to do two to three sets of 10 if you can.

What you need to know: Talk to a physical therapist about what quadricep and other strengthening exercises would be appropriate for you. Avoid any exercises that require you to bend your knee.

Touch Therapies

TRIGGER POINT THERAPY MASSAGE: A form of massage known as trigger point therapy that focuses on bundles of nerves known as trigger points within the muscles has shown promising results for the treatment of patello-femoral pain syndrome.

The evidence: In a 2010 study, 27 patients received 15 sessions of trigger point therapy directly at the knee region over the course of 6 months. They not only experienced a significant reduction in pain, but also a reduction in the grinding feeling typically experienced by those with patellofemoral pain.[40]

How it works: Trigger point therapy seems to work a lot like acupressure or acupuncture by directly focusing pressure and massage at the source of the pain to break up scar tissue and treat the affected joint.

What you need to know: Chiropractors and some massage therapists special-ize in trigger point therapy. Find a specialist in your area if you're interested in trying this technique. (See Part Three for more information.) You may experi-ence immediate relief, but more treatments will be needed to gain lasting relief over the long term. Because of the risk of injury from trigger point therapy, your best bet is to start with the help of a professional. She will often teach you trigger point techniques that you can use on your own at home to treat the condition.

Pain Medications and Other Medical Treatments

SURGERY: In rare, severe instances, surgery might be appropriate to repair the damaged knee. The two most common options are arthroscopy, in which an arthroscope is inserted through a small incision in the knee to remove frag-ments of damaged cartilage, and realignment, in which the components of the knee joint need to be repositioned to relieve pain and pressure.

The evidence: According to a recent study, a realignment surgical procedure called medial patellofemoral ligament overlap and lateral patellar retinaculum release might be the most effective treatment for patients with patellofemoral pain. In a study of 100 patients, those who received the medial patellofemoral ligament overlap and lateral patellar retinaculum release had better outcomes from surgery.[41]

How it works: Realignment surgery involves cutting and repositioning some of the muscles and bones in the knee to achieve better positioning. In the long term, this should alleviate pain in people with severe knee pain.

What you need to know: As with most surgeries, there are some risks involved, as well as stiffness and soreness for a few weeks to months as your knee heals. Work closely with your doctor to determine which surgical proce-dure is most appropriate for your knee pain.

Arthroscopy is a surgical procedure sometimes used to treat knee pain, but a recent study calls its effectiveness into question. Fifty-six patients received arthroscopy plus exercise for their patellofemoral pain or exercise alone. Those in the exercise program alone faired just as well as those who received surgery.[42]

Other Strategies

TAPING: "The quick fix for patellofemoral pain is taping the kneecap using a technique made popular by a physical therapist named Jenny McConnell," says H. James Phillips, PhD, a professor of physical therapy at Seton Hall School of Health and Medical Sciences in South Orange, New Jersey.

The evidence: The McConnell taping technique has indeed been shown effective at reducing pain in a number of studies. A 2010 study showed why this might be the case. In a study of 14 patients, the taping technique actually shifted the patella into its proper position in many of the study subjects.[43]

How it works: Taping the knee restricts its movement to prevent further injury. It also moves the components of the knee into their proper position to assist in healing.

What you need to know: At first, McConnell taping should be performed by a physical therapist. The therapist may show you how to perform the taping technique properly on yourself at home.

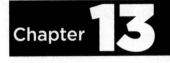

Chapter 13

Pelvic Pain

Menstrual cramps, fibroids, endometriosis, vulvodynia, pelvic inflammatory disease, interstitial cystitis/painful bladder syndrome, chronic prostatitis/chronic pelvic pain in men

C hronic pelvic pain affects a huge proportion of the population. From the monthly irritation of menstrual cramps to the often hourly pain and irritation of interstitial cystitis, it has many faces—and most of them are female. Although chronic prostatitis may affect around 15 percent of men,[1] and interstitial cystitis up to another 6 percent,[2] studies suggest that up to 80 percent of all women suffer from menstrual pain and one in five women also suffers from pelvic pain that isn't related to her cycle.[3]

Fortunately, even as doctors are finally becoming aware of how common chronic pelvic pain is, they're also discovering an entirely new range of ways to treat it. Some exciting new options for treatment take advantage of these facts:

● Physical therapy and exercise can play an important role in the treatment of many chronic pelvic pain conditions, since symptoms often seem to arise from dysfunction in the muscles of the pelvic floor. Regular exercise can also help stabilize hormone production and release the endorphins that are nature's painkillers.

- Dietary modifications can be effective pain relievers for some individuals with chronic pelvic pain, particularly those with interstitial cystitis and other forms of bladder irritation. After all, what you put into your body must come out, and when it does, you don't want it to hurt.

- Hormonal control is particularly useful for the many chronic pelvic pain conditions seen in women that are caused by dysfunctions in the menstrual cycle. Regulating menstruation can be an effective way of reducing the symptoms of not just menstrual cramps, but fibroids and endometriosis as well.

Over the past few years, there has been a growing interest in the use of nontraditional and individualized therapies for the treatment of chronic pelvic pain. From the recognition that Botox[4] can be used to release the muscle constriction that may be involved in vulvodynia and interstitial cystitis to an acknowledgment of the profound effects that traditional Chinese herbs can have on menstrual cramps,[5] it has become clear that effective treatment of chronic pelvic pain means focusing on the individual and thinking outside the box.

Menstrual Cramps

If you're a woman, you've probably had menstrual cramps, otherwise known as dysmenorrhea. Although exact numbers vary from survey to survey, estimates are that somewhere between half[6] and three-quarters[7] of the female population suffers from menstrual cramps. For most women, the pain is something they can live with, but as many as 1 in 10 has cramps that are severe enough to regularly interfere with her quality of life.

Fortunately, menstrual cramps aren't something that you just have to cross your legs and suffer through. As doctors start to gain a better understanding of why the uterus cramps, they are developing an increasing number of things you can do about it.

Is It Menstrual Cramps?

Pain associated with menstruation is nothing to laugh about. This type of pain is difficult to mistake for anything else. If you have the following symptoms while you're menstruating, then it's a pretty safe bet that you're experiencing menstrual cramps.

- Constant or intermittent lower abdominal pain
- Cramping

- Exhaustion

- Nausea

- Diarrhea

Most scientists think that menstrual cramping is caused by the overproduction of prostaglandins by the uterus. Prostaglandins cause muscle contractions, but they can also circulate throughout the body and lead to the other symptoms associated with menstruation. Women with severe menstrual symptoms are thought to have higher levels of prostaglandins in their menstrual fluid than women who don't experience as much pain.[8]

Fast Pain Relief

If it's that time of the month, and you're starting to wonder if it would really be so impractical just to rip your uterus out of your body and fling it across the room, step back and take a deep breath. There are things that you can do to control your pain.

1. **Take an NSAID.** Whether you prefer ibuprofen, naproxen, or something more esoteric, nonsteroidal anti-inflammatory drugs are great for period pain relief. That's because they don't simply numb your body. They actually interfere with production of the prostaglandins that cause your uterus to cramp.[9]

2. **Apply heat.** Although researchers aren't sure exactly why applying heat to your lower abdomen can soothe the pain in your uterus, many women do find that topical heat is an effective way to relieve menstrual pain.[10] These days, you don't even have to tether yourself to a heating pad or worry about a leaking hot water bottle. There are several options for stick-on, portable heating devices that can keep your body warm and your pain down as you move through your day.

3. **Get TENS, not tense.** Several studies have shown that women who are under stress have more painful periods,[11, 12] and finding ways to relax may help you reduce your menstrual symptoms. However, for some women the real secret may be TENS—transcutaneous electrical nerve stimulation, a technique for passing electricity across the skin that has been shown to relieve menstrual cramps effectively.[13] If you regularly suffer from severe cramps, talk to your doctor about whether this type of therapy may be right for you.

Relief at Last

The cutting edge of menstrual pain treatment is all about stopping cramps before they start. There are numerous things you can try to reduce the impact of menstrual pain on your life.

Step 1: Get your body moving. Doctors and scientists aren't certain why a regular program of exercise can help with period pain, but it certainly seems to.[14] It's not about weight loss. It's about engaging in a low- to moderate-intensity exercise program several times a week. This can reduce the severity of your menstrual cramping and, as a pleasant side effect, also improve the rest of your health.

Step 2: Explore alternative therapies. From vitamin E[15] and magnesium[16] supplementation to Chinese medicinal herbs,[17] there's good evidence that alternative therapies may be just as effective as, or even better than, traditional medical remedies for menstrual pain. These treatments may not be for everyone, but many women can get real help.

Step 3: Take control of your period. If pain relief and prevention don't work well enough to give you back control of your life, then try taking control of your period. Oral contraceptive pills and other hormonal contraception methods generally have the side effect of lighter, thus less painful, periods.[18] In addition, extended-cycle or continuous regimens can reduce the number of periods you have each year, and fewer periods means less frequent pain.[19]

Pain Prevention Strategies

Food and Supplements

CHINESE MEDICINAL HERBS: Chinese herbal medicine is designed to be tailored to the individual and adjusted as necessary throughout the period of treatment. Some well-known herbs used for the relief of menstrual pain include Chinese angelica root, Chinese motherwort, cattail pollen, salvia root, fennel fruit, licorice root, and cinnamon bark.

The evidence: A systematic review of 39 randomized controlled trials of Chinese medicinal herbs found that they were often more effective at reducing pain and overall symptoms than many NSAIDs, oral contraceptive pills, and acupuncture. However, the included studies were not of high quality.[20]

How it works: Traditional Chinese herbs may have numerous effects, including lowering prostaglandin levels, increasing endorphin production, and blocking calcium channels. These actions could result in reduced cramping and diminished pain.[21]

What you need to know: Chinese medicinal herbs have been shown to have positive effects on menstrual pain, and it would not be surprising if other herbal remedies could affect pain as well. However, since many herbs can interact with prescription drugs, make certain to talk to your doctor or pharmacist before starting to take anything new.

MAGNESIUM: Magnesium is the fourth most abundant mineral in the body and plays a role in hundreds of biochemical processes.

The evidence: A systematic review of dietary and herbal therapies found that there was good evidence for magnesium supplementation in the management of menstrual pain.[22]

How it works: Although the exact mechanism by which magnesium supplementation reduces menstrual pain remains uncertain, there is evidence to suggest that it may reduce prostaglandin production.[23]

What you need to know: Magnesium supplementation can be dangerous for individuals with kidney disease, and very large doses of magnesium can lead to adverse effects such as diarrhea and abdominal cramping. The upper limit for supplemental magnesium is currently set at 350 milligrams a day for adult women.[24]

FRENCH MARITIME PINE BARK EXTRACT: French maritime pine bark extract (Pycnogenol) has been investigated as a natural pain reliever for numerous chronic conditions, including painful menstruation.

The evidence: In one placebo-controlled trial, Pycnogenol was found to reduce the need for menstrual cramp relief in women with moderate to severe menstrual pain, but not in those with mild menstrual pain.[25]

How it works: Pycnogenol has anti-inflammatory properties and is a COX-2 inhibitor.[26] It works in a way similar to pharmaceutically produced NSAIDs.

What you need to know: The efficacy of Pycnogenol seems to grow over time when it is used as a regular dietary supplement. However, there is currently no data on the safety of long-term use.

VITAMIN E: Vitamin E, an antioxidant, is quite commonly taken as a supplement. More than 10 percent of American adults take more than 400 units of vitamin E a day.[27]

The evidence: Starting 2 days before the expected start of their periods and continuing through 3 days after they began, 278 15- to 17-year-old girls were given either 200 units of vitamin E twice daily or a placebo. Blood loss, duration of menstrual cramping, and severity of cramping were all significantly lower in the vitamin E group.[28]

How it works: Vitamin E can inhibit the production of arachidonic acid, which is a precursor of prostaglandin production.

What you need to know: Five hundred units of vitamin E is approximately 20 times the recommended daily allowance for an adult female. There is some evidence that long-term high doses of vitamin E could be dangerous; however, short-term use of up to 1,100 units a day is thought to be safe.[29]

Exercise and Movement Therapies

EXERCISE: Exercise is often recommended as a therapy for menstrual cramps, although severe cramps can make working out difficult.

The evidence: A study looking at menstrual symptoms in 250 university students before and after a 12-week exercise program found that participation in the program significantly decreased the pain of menstrual cramps as well as some premenstrual symptoms.[30]

How it works: The mechanisms by which exercise may reduce menstrual pain are not well understood, although some scientists think the effects are a result of increases in endorphin production and/or alternations in steroid hormone levels. Exercise may also reduce the levels of the cramp-inducing prostaglandins.

What you need to know: There are more than 50 years of studies examining the use of exercise for menstrual symptom relief, and the results have been largely positive.[31] Although a few studies have shown no benefit to exercise, there is no good reason not to give it a try. The evidence that it works may not be terribly strong,[32] but it certainly won't do any harm.

Touch Therapies

HEAT: Many women swear by heating pads as a method of reducing their menstrual pain. However, only recently has there been scientific evidence showing that heat works.

The evidence: When women were randomized to receive either low-level heat, ibuprofen, heat and ibuprofen, or a placebo, all three active treatments showed significantly better pain relief than placebo, and combining heat and ibuprofen relieved pain significantly faster. The average time to noticeable pain relief with the combined treatments was only 1.5 hours compared to 2.8 for ibuprofen alone.[33] Other studies have found heat to be even more effective than traditional painkillers for menstrual pain relief.[34]

How it works: How heat reduces menstrual pain is not well understood. Some hypotheses include an increase in local blood flow, relaxation of the muscles of the uterus, or changes in nerve sensitivity.

What you need to know: When using a heating pad or other heat-producing device, make certain to follow the instructions, including those about not sleeping with a heating pad, to avoid burning your skin.

TRANSCUTANEOUS ELECTRICAL NERVE STIMULATION: Transcutaneous electrical nerve stimulation (TENS) uses electrical pulses to provide pain relief. Both high-frequency and low-frequency pulses can be used.

The evidence: One recent study investigating a portable unit that is small enough to be clipped to clothing found that 86 percent of women had lower pain scores during cycles when they were using the TENS device than in cycles when they weren't. Six months after the study ended, more than half

On the Horizon

Alternative Therapies

Several alternative therapies for the relief of menstrual cramps have shown promising results in preliminary trials but lack sufficient, consistent evidence to warrant a recommendation of their use.

Aromatherapy: One randomized, placebo-controlled trial found abdominal massage with aromatherapy (lavender, clary sage, and rose in almond oil) could significantly reduce the severity of menstrual cramps.[35]

Spinal manipulation: Several studies have investigated the use of chiropractic spinal manipulation for relieving moderate to severe menstrual cramps. Although in two small studies participants experienced some relief of pain, a larger study showed no effect from manipulation.[36]

Thiamin: In 1996, a large, randomized, controlled trial found that 3 months of 100 milligrams a day of vitamin B_1 supplementation could eliminate painful periods in a sample of Indian women.[37]

Zinc: There is anecdotal evidence that 30 milligrams a day of zinc may be able to reduce menstrual cramps in some women.[38]

---

of the women were still regularly using the device at least every other menstrual cycle.[39]

How it works: It is thought that TENS units may interrupt the painful nerve signals from the uterus before they can get to the spinal cord. TENS may also cause the release of endorphins, which are natural painkillers.

What you need to know: Although several studies have shown positive effects of high-frequency TENS on menstruation pain, there is no support for low-frequency TENS.[40]

ACUPUNCTURE AND ACUPRESSURE: Acupuncture and acupressure are traditional Chinese medicine techniques that are gaining wider acceptance as methods of pain relief.

The evidence: A randomized, controlled trial of the "Relief Brief," a type of underwear with pads sewn in to put pressure on pain-relief acupressure points, found that it could significantly improve pain in women with menstrual cramps. The average number of pain pills taken by the acupressure group dropped from six pills a day to two pills a day, but did not change in the control group. In addition, more than 90 percent of women in the acupressure group reported at least a 25 percent reduction in pain severity, compared to only 8 percent of controls.[41]

How it works: According to traditional Chinese medicine, acupuncture and acupressure can realign the energy flow in the body.

What you need to know: Although there have been numerous studies of other forms of acupuncture[42] and acupressure[43] for the relief of menstrual cramps, the studies have not generally been of high quality. However, what evidence there is supports their use.

Mind-Body Therapies

RELAXATION TECHNIQUES: Several studies have demonstrated that women with high stress levels are more likely to experience menstrual cramping.[44, 45]

The evidence: Although the results are not consistent, research has shown that relaxation may be able to reduce pain and improve women's ability to go about their daily activities.[46]

How it works: Stress and anxiety can reduce an individual's ability to cope with pain and can also make pain seem more intense. Relaxation training can improve women's ability to deal with stressful aspects of life.

What you need to know: The evidence for the use of relaxation to control menstrual pain is still tentative. However, since stress has clearly been associated with discomfort during menstruation, finding ways to limit its effects on your life seems like a good idea.

Pain Medications and Other Medical Treatments

NONSTEROIDAL ANTI-INFLAMMATORY DRUGS (NSAIDS): NSAIDs, such as aspirin, ibuprofen, and naproxen, are many women's choice as a first-line therapy for menstrual pain relief.

The evidence: A systematic review of over 70 randomized controlled trials of various NSAIDs for menstrual pain relief found that they are significantly more effective than placebos. There is no real evidence for the use of one NSAID over another. Naproxen, ibuprofen, aspirin, and several other COX-1 inhibitors were all similarly effective at reducing cramps.[47]

How it works: By inhibiting COX-1, NSAIDs lower the amount of prostaglandin available to the uterus. This reduces the extent of cramping and relieves the pain of cramps.[48]

What you need to know: Long-term use of NSAIDs can damage the lining of the GI tract and cause serious side effects including nausea, headaches, and dizziness. It is a good idea to limit use of these drugs only to days when you really need them.

COMBINED ORAL CONTRACEPTIVES: Combined oral contraceptives, which include both estrogens and progesterones (as opposed to the minipill, which is progesterone only), are not only an effective way of preventing pregnancy, they also are a good way to reduce the pain of menstrual cramps.

The evidence: A number of studies have shown that combined oral contraceptives seem to be slightly more effective in reducing menstrual pain than placebo drugs. However, the strength of the evidence is mild, and these drugs may not be suitable for all women.[49]

How it works: Oral contraceptive use interferes with prostaglandin production. Women who use combined oral contraceptives also have less thickening of their endometrium over the course of the menstrual cycle and less cramping during menstruation.

What you need to know: Women who smoke should not use combined oral contraceptives because of an increased risk for blood clots. Although serious adverse events can also occur in nonsmokers using these drugs, they are less common. It is important to discuss the potential risks of long-term oral contraceptive use with your doctor so that you can decide whether this type of medication is right for you.

Choosing to Bleed Less Often: Continuous and Extended-Cycle Contraception

One way in which hormonal contraception can reduce menstrual cramping is by reducing the frequency of menstruation. Although typical combination oral contraceptive use involves 21 days on the drug followed by 7 days off to induce menstruation, there is no real biological need to follow that schedule. There are several extended-cycle and continuous contraceptive regimens that can reduce the number of periods a woman has to four a year, or stop menstruation entirely. For women who experience severe menstrual cramping and other problems associated with their periods, this type of contraceptive use may be a good option.[50]

Fibroids

Fibroids are the most common tumor seen in women, affecting at least 30 to 50 percent of the female population.[51] These noncancerous growths, also known as uterine leiomyomas, originate in the muscular wall of the uterus and can cause serious symptoms, including pain, heavy periods, and abnormal menstrual bleeding.

Fortunately, even though the pain associated with fibroids can be severe, most women with fibroids have no symptoms at all and do not need to be treated. In fact, it is thought that far more than half of women with fibroids will suffer no noticeable complications from them. Therefore, women with asymptomatic fibroids do not need medical or surgical intervention unless they are trying to get pregnant and the fibroids are large enough to have an impact on their fertility.[52]

The greatest concern of many women with fibroids is that they will need to have a hysterectomy. Although hysterectomy is the only way to be certain that fibroids will not recur, surgery that extensive is rarely necessary. Unless your symptoms are severe and do not improve with less invasive treatment, there is generally no need to consider removal of your uterus.[53] Some older women who have already finished having children may consider hysterectomy the easiest way to deal with their pain,[54] but if your doctor is pressuring you into getting a hysterectomy when you do not want one, don't hesitate to get a second opinion.

The truth is, the current thinking in fibroid treatment is that less is more. Just because a fibroid is present does not mean it's a problem. If women, particularly young women who wish to have children in the future, can get symptom relief with medical options, then there is no reason for them to undergo surgery.

When to Call the Doctor

Fibroids aren't usually an emergency condition. In fact, many women don't know they have them until they are discovered in the course of a regular pelvic exam. However, if you have heavy, painful periods that interfere with your ability to function you should make an appointment to discuss them with your doctor. You should also talk to your doctor if:

- The length of your menstrual cycle has suddenly changed
- The severity of your menstrual pain has become significantly worse
- You are experiencing abnormally heavy bleeding during your period or bleeding between periods
- You have trouble urinating or have painful urination
- You have a feeling of heaviness or bloating in your lower abdomen

Is It Fibroids?

If you have heavy, painful periods that interfere with your ability to live a normal life, it's important to discuss them with your gynecologist. These symptoms may be a result of any one of a number of gynecological conditions, including fibroids.

Most women discover they have fibroids either when their gynecologist finds one during a routine pelvic exam or when their doctor is looking for the cause of heavy periods or other gynecologic symptoms. If your doctor feels fibroids on your uterus, she might recommend that you undergo follow-up with ultrasound or MRI to get a better idea of their size, shape, and possible impact on your health, but additional testing is usually not required if you have no symptoms.

When you talk to your doctor about your painful periods, make certain to mention the length of your menstrual cycle, how long your periods last, how many pads or tampons you go through each day, if period pain affects your quality of life, and if you have bleeding between cycles. This information will help your doctor determine what type of fibroid treatment, if any, is necessary.

Fast Pain Relief

The pain from fibroids usually comes in the form of severe cramping and heavy bleeding during your menstrual period. Fortunately, many women are able to treat their menstrual cramps using drugs such as ibuprofen and acetaminophen. Other standard pain-relief strategies for menstrual pain, such as heating pads, may help as well. (See the section on menstrual cramps on page 290 for more information.)

Relief at Last

Cutting-edge fibroid treatment may involve no cutting at all. These days, whenever possible doctors often try to treat the symptoms of fibroids with the least invasive therapy they can find. However, there are several things you should consider when determining your treatment options.

Step 1: Assess the severity of your symptoms. If your symptoms are mild, then there may be no reason to treat your fibroids at all. Fibroids are benign tumors, and if they're not causing problems there is no medical reason you need to worry about them. Conversely, if the bleeding associated with your fibroids is too much to cope with, you should consider discussing the use of hormonal contraceptives with your doctor. Levonorgestrel-containing IUDs and Depo-Provera injections may be able to reduce heavy periods or even stop your menstrual bleeding entirely. Certain types of combined oral contraceptive pills could also help you control your bleeding, but there is little data on their use as a fibroid treatment.

Step 2: Determine whether your future childbearing plans affect your treatment options. Depending on where you are in your reproductive life, different types of surgical and nonsurgical fibroid treatments have different levels of risk. If you want to have children in the near future or later in life, discuss that fact with your doctor so that she can help you choose the best option for preserving your fertility. If you don't want to have children or already have all the children you want, then you will have more treatment options.

Step 3: Consider waiting for nature to take its course. Your fibroid symptoms will usually go away when you stop menstruating. If you are reaching the age at which your mother hit menopause and your symptoms are mild, waiting to see what happens may be a good choice.

Step 4: Explore hysterectomy. Although less extensive surgeries can be useful for reducing symptoms, a hysterectomy makes symptoms extremely unlikely to recur. For some women with severe symptoms and no need to preserve their uterus, it can be a good option.

Risk Factors for Uterine Fibroids

Numerous factors affect a woman's risk of developing uterine fibroids. These include:

- **Reproductive history:** A first period at an early age, short menstrual cycles, a later first pregnancy, a low number of pregnancies, and no history of breastfeeding are all associated with an increased risk of fibroids. In other words, it seems that anything that causes women to have more menstrual periods during their lives also increases their risk of developing leiomyomas.[55]

- **Race:** Several studies have found that black women are approximately three times as likely to have fibroids as white women and almost twice as likely to have a hysterectomy. Black women also tend to have larger and more numerous fibroids and their fibroids are more likely to be symptomatic.[56] The increase in risk seems to be the result of a combination of genetic, behavioral, and environmental factors.

- **Diet:** There is some evidence that diet may also affect fibroid risk, possibly through the ways in which food interacts with hormone metabolism. For example, a large prospective study found that black women who consumed large amounts of dairy products had a lower risk of developing fibroids,[57] while women who followed a high glycemic index/glycemic load diet suffered from increased risk.[58] Researchers have also linked fibroid risk to consumption of red meats,[59] ham, and alcohol,[60] while consumption of large amounts of green vegetables has tentatively been shown to be protective.

- **Lack of exercise:** One large study found that women who exercised more were less likely to have fibroids, which may be because exercise can lower circulating sex hormone levels.[61]

Outside of medical and surgical treatments, the best thing you can do to reduce the impact of fibroids on your life is to stay as healthy as possible. There is some evidence that diet and exercise can affect a woman's risk of developing fibroids. So eat well, work out, and read on to learn about the many tricks you can try to keep fibroids from taking over your life.

Pain Prevention Strategies

Medications and Other Medical Treatments

LEVONORGESTREL-RELEASING INTRAUTERINE DEVICES: The levonorgestrel-releasing intrauterine device (Mirena) is a prolonged-release hormonal IUD that was developed as a long-acting implantable contraceptive. It works well in women with fibroids, although they have a slightly increased risk of device expulsion compared to women in general.[62]

The evidence: In one study of 32 women with fibroids, women with IUDs had significantly reduced blood loss within 3 months of insertion, and by 6 months the reduced blood loss was equivalent to that seen after thermal balloon ablation—the destruction of the lining of the uterus to stop menstrual bleeding. The effects lasted through the end of the study year.[63]

How it works: Continuous release of progesterone by the IUD causes many women using the device to have lighter periods or cease menstruating entirely. Because of this, the common fibroid symptoms of painful periods and excess menstrual blood loss are reduced or eliminated. The IUD may also lower the risk of new fibroids, but there is no good evidence that levonorgestrel-releasing IUDs reduce fibroid size.[64]

What you need to know: A pilot study of medroxyprogesterone acetate (Depo-Provera), another type of synthetic progesterone, found that it was also effective at controlling excessive bleeding from fibroids. In addition, this treatment significantly reduced the average size of both uterus and fibroids.[65]

MIFEPRISTONE: Mifepristone is a synthetic steroid hormone that has antiprogesterone effects. It is best known for its use in medical abortions.

The evidence: In one randomized controlled trial, patients on 10 milligrams a day of mifepristone saw significant declines in menstrual blood loss (94.8 percent), painful periods, and uterine and fibroid volume (26 to 32 percent compared to zero percent in the placebo group). In addition, by the end of 3 months of treatment, 84 percent of treated women had ceased menstrual bleeding entirely.[67]

How it works: Mifepristone blocks the action of progesterone in the body to short-circuit the menstrual cycle. It potentially may

> ## On the Horizon
>
> ### Oral Contraceptives
>
> Long-term use of oral contraceptives has been tentatively linked to a reduced risk of uterine fibroids.[66] Since combination contraceptive pills, which contain both estrogen and progesterone, are often used to control heavy or irregular menstrual bleeding, their use could theoretically also reduce some of the most noticeable symptoms of fibroids. However, they have not been directly investigated as a fibroid treatment.

More Invasive Fibroid Treatments

If medical treatments for fibroids are unable to reduce your symptoms sufficiently, or if the physical location and size of your fibroids are impairing your fertility, there are several treatment options that actually remove or destroy the growths.

- **Focused ultrasound:** High-energy sound waves can be focused on fibroids to heat them to high enough temperatures to kill the cells of the tumors.[68]

- **Radio frequency ablation:** In this procedure, a needle is introduced into the fibroid and then the tip is heated to kill the fibroid.

- **Uterine artery embolization:** Particles, such as gelatin beads, are injected into uterine arteries to block off the blood supply to fibroid tumors, which can cause them to shrink or die.[69] The evidence is inconsistent as to whether uterine artery embolization is an effective way to preserve fertility in women who need treatment for symptomatic fibroids.[70]

- **Myolysis:** Like uterine artery embolization, myolysis cuts off the blood supply to a fibroid. However, instead of blocking arteries, the fibroids are partially or fully destroyed with heat or cold, reducing blood flow. There is less research on the long-term outcomes of this technique, however, it is probably not the best choice for women who wish to become pregnant because it can cause uterine scarring.[71]

- **Myomectomy:** Surgical removal of one or more fibroids, which leaves the uterus intact, is called myomectomy. There is some data suggesting that myomectomy may be able to help women who have experienced fibroid-related fertility problems carry an infant to term, [72] however, the science remains unclear.[73] Depending on the number and type of fibroids present, it may be difficult to remove them all while leaving the muscle of the uterus sufficiently intact to support a pregnancy.

- **Hysterectomy:** Removal of the uterus is the only guaranteed method for preventing regrowth of fibroids. When it is an option, vaginal hysterectomy is associated with shorter hospital stays and less blood loss than abdominal hysterectomy.[74] Laparoscopic hysterectomy has similar advantages.[75]

also directly reduce the growth of progesterone-sensitive fibroid tissue. Other related drugs seem to have similar effects.[76]

What you need to know: Several other studies have confirmed mifepristone's effects on menstrual bleeding, but not its ability to reduce fibroid and uterus size. However, the improvements in bleeding seem to be the most important for maintaining women's quality of life.[77]

OTHER HORMONELIKE DRUGS: Gonadotropin-releasing hormone (GnRH) agonists and aromatase inhibitors have both been shown to slow fibroid growth by interfering with ovarian estrogen production.

The evidence: Women in a small trial of anastrozole, an aromatase inhibitor, given 1 milligram a day for 12 weeks, had average reductions in uterine volume of 9 percent. They also had shorter, less painful periods.[78]

How it works: GnRH agonists reduce the activity of the ovaries directly, while aromatase inhibitors act slightly later in the process of estrogen metabolism. In either case, the resulting reduction in estrogen can slow the growth of, or even shrink, estrogen-sensitive fibroids and also affect the menstrual cycle to reduce the pain associated with bleeding.

What you need to know: GnRH agonists can have serious side effects when used long term, including loss of bone density. Right now, they are only approved for short-term use before fibroid surgery. Reducing the size of fibroids makes surgical removal easier, although there are some concerns that these drugs may sometimes shrink small fibroids too much, making them too small to visualize and treat.[79] Those fibroids might then be more likely to recur when drug treatment is stopped after surgery.

Other Strategies

WATCH AND WAIT: If your symptoms are mild and fibroids are having minimal or no impact on your life, then there may be no need to do anything at all about them.

The evidence: Fibroids are benign tumors that only very rarely become malignant, particularly in premenopausal women. If you have no symptoms or your symptoms can be controlled by occasional use of over-the-counter painkillers, then there is no reason to pursue more extensive treatment.[80]

What you need to know: If you have been diagnosed with fibroids and intend to have children, talk to your doctor about whether early treatment might have benefits for your fertility. Many women can successfully get pregnant and carry a baby to term with fibroids, but, depending on their type and location, fibroids can sometimes cause fertility problems.[83] Since it is easier and less damaging to the uterus to remove fibroids when they are small, watch-ful waiting may not be the right option for everyone.

Endometriosis

If you're one of the nearly 10 percent of women who suffers from endometriosis,[84] you know that the pain it causes can wreak havoc on your life. Endometriosis is a major public health problem that has been estimated to cost the United States more than $20 billion a year in health care costs and lost productivity.[85]

Endometriosis occurs when cells that normally make up the lining or inner membrane of the uterus—the endometrium—escape the uterus and begin to grow on other organs inside the pelvis and abdomen. Doctors aren't entirely certain why this happens in some women and not in others; however, both genetic and environmental factors seem to play a role. In general, anything that increases the number of periods you have throughout your life—such as having a short menstrual cycle or an early age of menarche—increases your risk. So do lifestyle factors such as smoking and lack of exercise.[86]

The new thinking in endometriosis treatment is that pain relief needs to be tailored to your individual life situation and goals. Which surgical and medical treatments are appropriate depends greatly on whether and when you want to have children as well as the particular ways you experience pain.

Fortunately, the number of options you have available is growing almost every day.[87]

Is It Endometriosis?

Any woman with chronic pelvic pain needs to be evaluated by a gynecologist. Although not all pelvic pain is an emergency, only a doctor can diagnose whether you are suffering from an acute infectious condition like pelvic inflammatory disease or a more chronic condition like endometriosis. The symptoms of many pelvic pain disorders are quite similar and it can be hard to distinguish between them without physical examinations and testing. The most common symptoms of endometriosis include:

- Painful menstruation (dysmenorrhea)
- Heavy periods
- Bleeding between periods
- Pain during sex (dyspareunia)
- Chronic pelvic pain
- Pain in the lower abdomen and back

In many women, the pain associated with endometriosis waxes and wanes with the menstrual cycle. This is because the extrauterine endometrial tissue

When to Call the Doctor

If the pain of endometriosis is severe enough to affect your quality of life, you should definitely make an appointment with your doctor. There is no reason you have to live with debilitating pain. Other symptoms that should lead you to call your doctor include:

- Sudden, severe pelvic pain
- Pain during intercourse
- A change in how painful your periods are
- Pain when you go to the bathroom or difficulty controlling your bladder
- Blood in your urine or stool

continues to respond to hormones just like the endometrium does—by growing and bleeding. However, some women with endometriosis have constant pain throughout the month while others have no noticeable symptoms at all. In fact, a reasonably large fraction of women with endometriosis never know they have it until they have trouble conceiving. Endometriosis is found in up to 50 percent of infertile women.[88]

Fast Pain Relief

If you suffer from severe endometriosis pain, long-term control usually requires either surgery to remove endometriosis lesions or prescription medications to regulate your hormone levels and turn off your menstrual cycle. There is some evidence that NSAIDs and other over-the-counter painkillers can provide short-term relief in some women with chronic pelvic pain,[89] but many women need stronger options for long-term pain relief.

Relief at Last

Figuring out the best way to treat your endometriosis pain has a lot to do with first determining how that pain affects your life. Effective treatment for chronic, continuous pelvic pain may be quite different than treatment for pain that varies with the hormonal changes of your menstrual cycle. Still, when you break it down, there are three basic options for endometriosis treatment.

> **Step 1: Focus on the pain**. Dealing with pain isn't simply a matter of finding the right painkillers. Although figuring out what type of pain relief works for you is important—whether that's OTC painkillers, prescription opiates, or natural pain-relief regimens—it is only the first

»More Research Needed

NSAIDs for Endometriosis

Nonsteroidal anti-inflammatory drugs are the most common front-line therapy for endometriosis; however, there is little evidence to support their use. Although NSAIDs are known to be effective painkillers, there have been very few studies of them in women with endometriosis, and those studies had only equivocal results.[90] If NSAIDs are effective at relieving your pain, there is no reason to stop using them, but insufficient evidence exists to support their current rate of use.

Depression and Endometriosis

The chronic pelvic pain and infertility problems that many women with endometriosis experience can be extremely stressful. Several studies have recently demonstrated that the prevalence of anxiety and depression in women with endometriosis is extraordinarily high.

One study of 144 women with surgically confirmed endometriosis found that 87 percent of them qualified for a diagnosis of depression and 64 percent had high levels of anxiety.[91] Another study of 100 women found that the prevalence of depression was more than twice as high in women whose endometriosis caused them chronic pain than in women who had been pain free for at least 3 months—86 percent compared to 38 percent.[92]

Chronic pelvic pain is hard to live with, and you shouldn't have to do it alone. If you're having trouble dealing with the emotional consequences of your endometriosis, seek help. Not only is emotional stress unpleasant in and of itself, depression and anxiety can also make it harder to deal with pain. Reducing your stress and anxiety levels could significantly improve your quality of life.

step. A holistic approach to pain management that also addresses the emotional side effects of chronic pelvic pain can make endometriosis a lot easier to live with.[93] Taking the time to deal with your pain can also encourage your body to heal itself. In up to a third of women with endometriosis, the condition resolves spontaneously.[94]

Step 2: Break the menstrual cycle. Endometriosis lesions are made up of hormonally sensitive tissues, similar to the ones that line the uterus. Symptoms often become worse as these tissues swell and bleed over the course of the menstrual cycle. Therefore, medications that regulate hormone levels, such as continuous-dose oral contraceptives and progesterone implants or injections, can improve a sufferer's quality of life. This type of therapy usually needs to be continued long term in order to maintain effectiveness.[95]

Step 3: Remove the excess tissue. The location of excess endometrial tissue can have profound effects on symptoms. By pressing on organs such as the bladder and otherwise distorting the internal anatomy, growths of endometrial tissue can cause sensitivity and pain. Removing these lesions can resolve pain and improve fertility, two factors that are both closely related to quality of life.[96]

These options can be used alone or in combination to come up with an individualized endometriosis treatment regimen that is right for you. Furthermore, a few years down the line you may have even more choices. There are several new therapies in development that address other factors that may be involved in causing endometriosis symptoms, such as inflammation.[97] In addition, ongoing research on alternative medicine treatments for pain and other symptoms may open new doors for endometriosis patients who would prefer to avoid pharmaceutical and surgical treatments altogether.

Pain Prevention Strategies

Food and Supplements

HEALTHY DIET: The prospective Nurses' Health Study found that women who had high trans fat intake were 48 percent more likely than other women to develop endometriosis, while high omega-3 intake was associated with reduced risk.[99] Case-control studies have also found a positive association between endometriosis and high levels of red meat consumption, while increased consumption of fruit and green vegetables may be protective.[101]

The evidence: One small randomized controlled trial comparing postsurgical dietary supplementation with vitamins, minerals, lactic acid ferments (probiotics similar to those found in yogurts), and fish oil to continuous oral contraceptives found that dietary therapy could improve nonmenstrual pelvic pain and quality of life, but not menstrual-associated pain.[103]

How it works: There is evidence that women with endometriosis are under significant oxidative stress, and it is possible that improving a woman's dietary antioxidant balance may slow development of endometrial lesions.

What you need to know: These associations are only tentative, however, eating a healthy diet that is low in trans fats, rich in green vegetables, and includes fish oil supplements is unlikely to do anything but improve your overall health.

Pain Medications and Other Medical Treatments

PROGESTERONE TREATMENTS: There are several types of progesterone analogues that are used in the treatment of endometriosis.

The evidence: A study of long-term use of a levonorgestrel-releasing IUD (Mirena) found that at 3 years, 56 percent of women were still using the device. Most women who discontinued did so between 6 and 12 months of first use, because of irregular bleeding or lack of improvement in symptoms. However, those women who chose to keep using the IUD saw consistent reductions in pain and blood loss over the study period.[104] A randomized controlled trial of the levonorgestrel-releasing IUD after surgery also found that it could reduce the number of painful periods when compared to no treatment.[105]

How it works: Continuous use of progesterone turns off the menstrual cycle by suppressing hormone production in the ovaries.

What you need to know: The levonorgestrel-releasing IUD is not the only long-acting progesterone used for the treatment of endometriosis. The once-a-month injectable contraceptive Depo-Provera has also been shown to have similar effects in reducing pain and blood loss.[106] There are also several types of daily progesterone pills used for treatment[107] that may be useful for women who are reluctant to commit to longer-acting contraceptives.

COMBINED ORAL CONTRACEPTIVES: Combination oral contraceptive pills, which contain both estrogen and progesterone analogues (as opposed to the minipill, which is progesterone only), can be used not just to prevent pregnancy but to control the menstrual cycle.

The evidence: One large 2010 study comparing continuous hormone use to intermittent hormone use to placebo found that continuous use was extremely effective at reducing the recurrence of painful periods but not pain during sex.[108] This confirmed similar results seen in two earlier studies of continuous hormone use.[109, 110]

How it works: Continuous use of combined oral contraceptives is capable of stopping menstruation in most women for the duration of their time on the drug.

What you need to know: The vast majority of studies of oral contraceptives as an endometriosis treatment have examined their usefulness in pain and recurrence after surgery. There is little data on combined oral contraceptives as a primary treatment for endometriosis.[111]

GNRH AGONISTS: Leuprolide (Lupron) is the GnRH agonist most commonly prescribed to women with endometriosis. Another GnRH agonist that has been tested for endometriosis is goserelin (Zoladex).

The evidence: The first randomized controlled trial of leuprolide found that the frequency of painful periods decreased from 97 percent to 7 percent after 6 months.[112] Pain relief from GnRH agonists has been shown to be similar to relief from both progesterone treatments and danazol (Danocrine) in several studies.[113]

How it works: GnRH agonists turn down hormone production in the ovaries. This stops menstrual bleeding and helps with endometriosis pain by reducing the growth of endometrial tissue both inside and outside the uterus.

What you need to know: GnRH agonists can have serious side effects, including loss of bone density and memory impairment. Before starting to take one, be sure to discuss the potential consequences with your doctor.

DANAZOL: Danazol (Danocrine) is a synthetic androgen, a hormone that promotes male characteristics.

The evidence: Several studies have demonstrated that danazol can effectively reduce pain caused by endometriosis both on its own and as an adjunct to surgery.[114]

How it works: Danazol decreases steroid hormone production in the ovaries, lowering estrogen levels and creating a pseudomenopause. It also interferes with FSH (follicle-stimulating hormone) and LH (luteinizing hormone) secretion. Through this combination of effects it restricts the growth of endometrial tissue and reduces the symptoms of endometriosis.

What you need to know: Side effects of danazol are similar to the ones you would experience going through menopause—including hot flashes, vaginal dryness, mood swings, and changes in libido. You might also experience weight gain, facial hair growth, and other effects from the increase in male hormones.

AROMATASE INHIBITORS: Aromatase inhibitors such as anastrazole (Arimidex) have been tested as endometriosis treatments in numerous studies. The mechanism by which these drugs reduce estrogen levels is different from that of other hormonal medications.

The evidence: A 2008 systematic review of eight studies of aromatase inhibitors found there was good evidence that these drugs can be effective in

Hysterectomy

Although removing the uterus can effectively stop the symptoms of endometriosis in many women, it is not a guaranteed cure. It is possible for endometrial tissue to remain in the pelvic cavity and continue causing symptoms after surgery.[115] If you continue to have cyclical pain after hysterectomy, this may be the cause.

reducing pain, shrinking endometrial lesions, and improving patients' quality of life. However, most of the studies of aromatase inhibitors have either been small or of low quality.[116]

How it works: Aromatase inhibitors primarily suppress estrogen production in the peripheral tissues. Estrogen production in the ovaries is reduced but not eliminated, which means that these drugs may have fewer side effects than GnRH agonists. In addition, since women with endometriosis often express aromatase abnormally in their endometrial tissue, these drugs may have additional direct effects on symptoms.[117]

What you need to know: Side effects from aromatase inhibitors are similar to those seen during menopause.

LAPAROSCOPIC SURGERY: Laparoscopic surgery is a minimally invasive surgery that involves the use of multiple small incisions to minimize surgical trauma. There are several types of laparoscopic surgery used for endometriosis including ablation, excision, and neurectomy/nerve ablation.

The evidence: A study that followed 135 women for up to 5 years after surgical excision of endometriosis found that the surgery significantly reduced menstrual pain and pain during sex for most women, although a quarter of women found that their pain got worse. The surgery also seemed to improve fertility, but 36 percent of women needed follow-up surgery.[118]

How it works: Most types of laparoscopic surgery primarily focus on removing extrauterine endometrial tissue. Excision cuts away problematic tissue while ablation burns it with heat from lasers or electrical current. Surgery can also be used to interrupt the function of the pelvic nerves, but benefits of that type of surgery may not outweigh severe complications, which can include loss of bladder and bowel control.[119]

What you need to know: Surgery to excise or ablate endometrial tissue can effectively reduce symptoms in many women, but it is rarely a permanent cure. Several studies of laparoscopic excision have found that approximately

40 percent of women experience a recurrence within 6 months,[120] and that number increases over time.[121]

Vulvodynia

Scientists estimate that more than 2.4 million women in the United States may suffer from chronic vulvar pain.[122] Vulvodynia, also sometimes known as vulvar vestibulitis syndrome, affects mostly women of reproductive age and can cause chronic pain lasting for months or years. Although vulvar pain is not only sexually related, it can have major effects on a woman's ability to enjoy her sexual life.[123, 124]

Vulvodynia can leave women feeling depressed, angry, frustrated, and unhappy with their sex lives,[125] but there are things that doctors can do to help. From physical therapy to pain relievers to retraining your body's response to pain, there are numerous ways to reduce the effects that vulvodynia has on your quality of life.

Is It Vulvodynia?

Vulvodynia is characterized by chronic discomfort, including burning, stinging or irritation of the vulva that has no obvious medical cause such as skin disease or infection. For some women the pain is widespread, but for others it is localized in very specific places, such as the entrance to the vagina.

Vulvodynia can be characterized as provoked, spontaneous, or mixed. Women who have provoked vulvodynia only have pain when their vulva is touched or manipulated, while spontaneous vulvodynia pain can occur without any contact at all. You may have vulvodynia if:

- Inserting a tampon causes pain around the opening of your vagina

- Intercourse is painful

- You are uncomfortable riding a bicycle or sitting for long periods of time

- Tight clothes and underwear make your skin hurt

If you think you might have vulvodynia, it's important to talk to your doctor about when the pain started and what makes it better and worse. To diagnose you, your doctor will touch various areas of your vulva with a cotton swab to determine the location and severity of your pain. Your doctor may also ask you questions about tampon insertion,[126] or about how the pain has affected your sex life with your current and previous partners, in order to get a better understanding of your symptoms.

Although vulvodynia is not associated with sexually transmitted disease or STD risk factors, it is important to tell your doctor if you have had an STD in the past. You should also inform him if you have been treated or have treated yourself for recurrent yeast infections, which have been found to be associated with vulvodynia in some women.[128]

Fast Pain Relief

Every woman's experience with vulvodynia is different. However, whether your pain only occurs during sex or happens every time your skin is touched in a certain location, there are several tricks you can use to reduce your pain.

1. **Try a local anesthetic cream.** Topical anesthetics containing lidocaine have been shown to reduce pain effectively in some women with vulvodynia. However, avoid anesthetics containing benzocaine or diphenhydramine since these products can further irritate your skin.[129]

2. **Lubricate your vulva.** If pressure from clothing and underwear hurts your skin and causes it to burn, try coating your vulva with a thin layer of vegetable oil or petroleum jelly. These substances can serve as a barrier to protect delicate skin from irritation.

3. **Avoid causing problems by anticipating them.** Although it's completely normal to worry about what might provoke vulvodynia pain, doing so can actually make your pain worse. Studies have shown

that the impact of vulvodynia may be greatest in women who are fearful about their pain. Try to make smart choices about clothing, soaps, and sexual activity, but don't look for things to go wrong. The more confident you are about your ability to deal with situations that may lead to pain, the less likely they are to cause problems.[130]

Relief at Last

Step 1: Be kind to your vulva. Sometimes the best thing you can do to treat your vulvodynia is keep your vulva clean and dry. Making good hygiene choices can be a very effective way to reduce the intensity of your pain and how often you experience it.

Step 2: Avoid the stimuli that cause you pain. If you've noticed that certain soaps, activities, or even types of clothing make your pain worse, it's a good idea to avoid them as long as doing so does not affect your quality of life.

Step 3: Explore direct therapy options. Pelvic floor exercises, physical therapy, and even cognitive-behavioral therapy may be able to help you either reduce your pain or find better ways of coping with it.

Pain Prevention Strategies

Exercise and Movement Therapies

PELVIC FLOOR EXERCISES WITH BIOFEEDBACK: When combined with biofeedback techniques, exercise can help some women rehabilitate the function of their pelvic floor muscles.

The evidence: A study comparing biofeedback to lidocaine treatment found that both techniques were equally effective at reducing pain and improving sexual function.[131] Other research has also shown positive effects from biofeedback training.[132]

How it works: In some women, vulvodynia may be caused by hyperirritability of the pelvic muscles. Biofeedback techniques for vulvodynia treatment use objective measurements of muscle activity to help women retrain those muscles' function. Combining exercise with biofeedback allows women to be more certain they are performing prescribed exercises correctly and to see real-time analysis of their effects.

On the Horizon

Future Treatment Options

There are a number of treatments for vulvodynia that have only been discussed in case reports or tested in limited numbers of women. Still, some of them show quite a bit of promise.

Acupuncture and acupressure: Acupuncture is becoming somewhat widely accepted as a general technique for relieving chronic pain, but specific evidence for vulvodynia is lacking. Two small studies of acupuncture[133] and acupressure[134] have shown some benefits, but the research was not of high quality.

Botox: Botulism toxin can interrupt nerve signals, causing relaxation of potentially hyperactive and painful muscles as well as direct pain relief. Several small studies have found positive results when using it as a vulvodynia treatment[135] although there was no assessment of a potential placebo effect.

Capsaicin: Capsaicin is the chemical that makes hot peppers hot, and it can also cause a warming sensation when applied to the skin. Topical capsaicin treatment has been tentatively shown to improve vulvodynia symptoms in some women, although the mechanism by which it does so is not understood. It is often used in topical muscle relaxation products, but exposure to capsaicin can also desensitize nerves.[136]

Gabapentin: Gabapentin is an anticonvulsant drug that is used for treating a number of chronic pain disorders. At least one small study has found that systemic use may be able to reduce pain symptoms in women with vulvodynia.[137] Studies of topical use are also promising.[138]

Vaginal dilators: Vaginal dilators are an accepted therapy for vaginismus, painful involuntary vaginal contractions, and preliminary research shows that they may be able to help some women with vulvodynia as well.[139] Fear of pain during sex can, paradoxically, cause the body to tense up and make penetration more painful. These devices may be able to help women recondition their expectations of pain.

Yoga: Yoga, Pilates, and similar types of exercise often focus on strengthening the pelvic floor muscles as part of practice,[140] although that fact is not usually mentioned on a day-to-day basis in the classroom setting. Pelvic floor muscle retraining has been shown to reduce vulvodynia pain in the context of biofeedback studies, and any form of exercise that effectively works these muscles may be another way to improve symptoms.

How to Be Kind to Your Vulva

According to the American College of Obstetricians and Gynecologists,[131] if you experience vulvodynia pain, you should:

1. Wear only 100 percent cotton underwear during the day and skip underwear entirely at night

2. Keep any potentially irritating substances away from your vulva, including douches, perfumes, and detergents

3. Clean your vulva only with water, and use mild soap on the rest of your body

4. Pat your skin dry after bathing instead of rubbing or using a hair dryer, and apply a thin layer of emollient such as petroleum jelly to hold moisture in

5. Use cotton pads during your period if regular ones are irritating

6. Make certain to use sufficient lubrication when you have sex

7. Rinse and pat dry your vulva after you use the bathroom

What you need to know: A long-term follow-up survey of the use of biofeedback in patients with unprovoked vulvodynia found extremely positive results. All of the patients who responded to the survey had become pain free after treatment, and 89 percent had remained completely pain free at time of follow-up 3 to 5 years later. The rest had had only one or two intermittent bouts of pain, which were associated with identifiable causes, such as yeast infections, and resolved on their own.[142]

PHYSICAL THERAPY: Physical therapy is widely recommended as a treatment for vulvodynia. Like biofeedback-based exercise training, it focuses on retraining the muscles of the pelvic floor.

The evidence: Several small studies have found that physical therapy can improve pain and sexual function associated with vulvodynia.[143, 144] The use of physical therapy is also supported by the research on biofeedback, since these techniques are often used as part of treatment.

How it works: In addition to retraining the pelvic muscles to resolve hyperactivity, physical therapy may also involve the use of heat and cold for pain relief, therapeutic ultrasound, training in the use of vaginal dilators, and other interventions to release muscle tension and improve physical and sexual health.

What you need to know: A nationwide survey of physical therapists found that 42 percent of them had experience treating patients with vulvodynia. Most women were treated in weekly sessions lasting 45 minutes to an hour for 2 to 4 months.[145]

Mind-Body Therapies

COGNITIVE-BEHAVIORAL THERAPY: If you have a chronic pain syndrome like vulvodynia, fear of experiencing pain can not only make you afraid of doing anything that might set your symptoms off but hyperaware of any sensation that might turn into pain. Unfortunately, while such reactions make perfect intellectual and emotional sense, they can actually make your symptoms worse.[146] That's why cognitive-behavioral therapy (CBT) and other types of psychotherapy can be effective ways for women with vulvodynia to deal with their symptoms.

The evidence: Several studies have found that CBT can reduce pain severity and improve sexual functioning.[147, 148] Although the extent of reduction in pain may not be as great as with some medical and surgical treatments, cognitive-behavioral therapy may be more acceptable to women who prefer less invasive approaches.

How it works: Cognitive-behavioral therapy for vulvodynia includes educational components as well as training in ways to minimize and cope with pain and improve the quality of a patient's sex life. Therapies may also include relaxation and distraction techniques and instruction in communication skills that can facilitate healthy, stress-free sexual conversations with partners.

»More Research Needed

Low-Oxalate Diets

Oxalate is a chemical naturally produced by the body, which is also present in certain food products such as black tea, chocolate, and many dark green leafy vegetables. For many years it was thought that high levels of oxalate in the urine could predispose women to vulvar pain because it is a chemical irritant. However, two studies that examined the question in detail found no association between either urinary oxalate levels[149] or dietary oxalate[150] and vulvar pain. Some guidelines still recommend a low-oxalate diet for women with vulvodynia, but there is little evidence to support that recommendation.[151]

On the Horizon

Antidepressants

There is some evidence that antidepressants may be an effective form of treatment for some individuals with vulvodynia[152]—as they are for people with many pain syndromes. This may be because in some individuals vulvodynia is a somatoform pain disorder that arises from pain-processing problems in the brain.[153] Although there is evidence that vulvodynia may be a somatoform pain disorder in certain individuals,[154] there is also data that chronic vulvar pain may be a result of measurable, local changes in inflammation,[155] nerve density, and/or muscle hyperactivity.[156] Thus, antidepressants may not be a good option for everyone.

What you need to know: Since CBT teaches skills for pain management and coping, the effects of a therapy program can last beyond the period of treatment. In fact, ongoing practice of the skills learned in these programs can continue to decrease pain and symptoms over time.

Pain Medications and Other Medical Treatments

LIDOCAINE OINTMENT: Lidocaine is an anesthetic that can be used for topical pain relief.

The evidence: In one study, 61 patients with vulvodynia applied a 5 percent lidocaine ointment nightly and slept with a lidocaine-covered cotton ball pressing against the entrance to their vagina for 7 weeks. At the end of treatment, twice as many women were able to have sexual intercourse, and levels of sexual and general pain had diminished significantly.[157]

How it works: Lidocaine interrupts nerve signaling, causing numbness in the areas to which it is applied.

What you need to know: Daytime use of lidocaine ointments and gels has also shown promise, although they may need to be applied more frequently.[158] It is also important to know that results on lidocaine's efficacy are mixed. A newer study showed no improvement when lidocaine was compared to placebo.[159]

Pelvic Inflammatory Disease

More than 800,000 women in the United States are diagnosed with pelvic inflammatory disease (PID) each year, and the annual cost of diagnosing and treating this condition is nearly $2 billion.[160]

Although women may discover they have PID because of chronic pelvic pain symptoms, PID is usually an acute problem. Most often caused by untreated sexually transmitted infections such as gonorrhea and chlamydia,[161] which have ascended up through the vagina and cervix to infect the upper genital tract, PID is a disease that requires immediate medical attention. Left untreated, it can lead to complications such as chronic pelvic pain, ectopic pregnancy, infertility, and, in rare cases, even death.

Fortunately, for most women, PID is caught relatively early and can be treated on an outpatient basis with antibiotics and follow-up. Although these women remain at increased risk of reinfection, that risk can often be managed with behavioral changes including STD testing and consistent condom use. However, for some women PID can have long-term complications.

These complications are not directly caused by the organisms responsible for the original infection. Instead, they are caused by the body's inflammatory response. Swelling and infection in the fallopian tubes, also known as salpingitis, can lead to permanent scarring, blocking off part or all of one of the tubes and increasing the risk of infertility and ectopic pregnancy.[162] Fibrous adhesions, which glue the reproductive organs to each other, can also form, leading to pain when you move.[163]

Treatment for chronic pain from pelvic inflammatory disease primarily focuses on choosing the right antimicrobial therapies to knock out all possible sources of underlying infection. In severe cases of PID, surgery may even be necessary to reach walled-off areas of infection that are not effectively treated by oral or intravenous antibiotics. Finally, laparoscopic surgery may be able to reduce pain from pelvic adhesions,[164] although the benefits must be carefully weighed since the surgery itself can cause additional adhesions to form.

Is It Pelvic Inflammatory Disease?

If you have moderate to severe lower abdominal pain with tenderness and fever, then you fit the standard profile of a patient with PID. However, not all women with PID have fevers, and many of them find their pain overshadowed by other complaints such as:

● Abnormal vaginal discharge

● Frequent urination

● Bleeding between periods

● Bleeding after sex

● Lower back pain

Diagnosis of PID usually requires a pelvic exam, and may also require laparoscopic surgery to examine the inside of the pelvic cavity for inflammation

> ## When to Call the Doctor
> If you have symptoms of PID, it is important to bring them to the attention of your doctor as quickly as possible. This is particularly true if you have pelvic pain accompanied by a fever and chills.

and damage. However, for women at the highest risk of PID, sexually active women under the age of 25, the condition will often be presumptively diagnosed and treated if you have lower abdominal pain combined with pain in your pelvic organs during a bimanual exam.[165] Bleeding from the cervix and certain types of cervical discharge can also lead to the diagnosis of PID, but laparoscopic visualization of the inside of the pelvic cavity remains the most effective way to look for signs of inflammation and other damage.[166]

Be prepared to tell your doctor about your sexual history—including whether you practice safe sex and the last time you and your partner were tested for STDs. You should also mention any changes in your vaginal odor and whether you douche or use any other feminine hygiene products. Although you may find the conversation uncomfortable, it is important to be as honest as possible. The better their understanding of your risk factors, the faster your doctors can figure out a diagnosis and get you appropriate treatment. The faster you get treatment, the less likely it is that your PID will cause long-term consequences such as infertility and chronic pain.

Fast Pain Relief

If you are experiencing lower abdominal pain and think you might have PID, then you need to get to a doctor as soon as possible. Although over-the-counter painkillers and other pain-relief techniques may improve your symptoms, acute PID requires immediate medical attention. The best way to relieve your current pain and to reduce the risk of experiencing chronic pain in the future is to treat the underlying cause of your PID as soon as possible. Treatment might be as simple as a prescription for oral antibiotics, but you might need to be admitted into the hospital for intravenous medication or surgery.

Relief at Last

The best way to avoid the painful symptoms of PID is to avoid getting an infection in the first place or to avoid a new infection that could make a second episode more likely. That's why your relief at last plan is as follows.

Step 1: Get screened regularly for chlamydia, gonorrhea, and other STDs. It doesn't matter who you are. If you have sex, you're at risk of getting an STD. Fortunately, the most common STDs can now be detected with urine tests without the need for a pelvic exam.[167]

Step 2: Always use latex or polyurethane condoms when you have sex. Unless you are in a long-term, mutually monogamous relationship and both of you have been tested for STDs and come up negative, unprotected sex can put you at risk of PID. When used properly, condoms are an effective way to prevent chlamydia and gonorrhea, the two most frequent causes of PID,[168] and they may also be able to reduce your risk of bacterial vaginosis, which has also been linked to pelvic infection.[169]

Step 3: Don't douche. If your vaginal odor changes, that means it's time to go to the doctor—not to break out the vinegar. An unpleasant vaginal odor is often the only symptom of a sexually transmitted infection. Douching could force that infection up through your cervix, which greatly increases the risk of its becoming PID.[170]

Step 4: Always finish your antibiotics. One reason that some women are prone to chronic PID is that their infections have become surrounded and blocked off by scar tissue, which makes them hard to treat without either intravenous antibiotics or surgical drainage. That's why when you're prescribed antibiotics for a sexually transmitted infection, you always want to finish the whole prescription—even if you feel better before it's done. Finishing the prescription increases the likeliness that the antibiotic will clear the whole infection, not just part of it, and will also reduce the likelihood of the infection becoming antibiotic resistant.

Step 5: Don't let embarrassment keep you from the doctor. One study found that the risk of infertility and other long-term problems was three times higher in women who put off seeking treatment for abdominal pain and other PID symptoms.[171] That's why it's a good idea to get to the doctor sooner rather than later.

Pain Prevention Strategies

Pain Medications and Other Medical Treatments

ORAL OR INTRAVENOUS ANTIBIOTICS: Broad spectrum antibiotics are used to treat the underlying causes of pelvic inflammatory disease.

Laparoscopic Surgery for PID

Laparoscopy is most often indicated for severe cases of PID or after medical management of mild to moderate PID has failed.[172] The main benefit of laparoscopic surgical techniques is that they allow doctors to directly visualize any damage to the pelvic organs and get a better idea of its cause. During surgery, doctors can also drain any abscesses that are at risk of rupture and remove adhesions that may lead to future problems with pain and fertility. However, except in severe cases, the evidence is mixed about whether surgery for the sole purpose of removing adhesions is helpful or if adhesion removal should only be attempted as a part of diagnostic or other laparoscopy.[173]

The evidence: A randomized controlled trial of outpatient versus inpatient antibiotic therapy for women with mild to moderate PID found that both types of treatment were equally effective at curing infection and preventing future symptoms. Over a 3-year follow-up period, pregnancy rates were also similar between the two groups, meaning that both types of treatment were similarly effective at preserving fertility.[174]

How it works: Antibiotics kill off the bacteria and other microorganisms that are the most frequent causes of pelvic inflammatory disease. Once the infection is gone, inflammation goes down and symptoms generally improve. However, antibiotics will not treat any existing scarring.

What you need to know: Because the specific organisms that are causing your PID may sometimes be difficult for your doctor to identify, PID is often treated with several antibiotics that together will cure the most frequent causes of the disease. Most women can be treated on an outpatient basis, but women with severe PID or signs of abscess may need to be admitted to the hospital for intravenous antibiotics and monitoring.[175] No matter what type of antibiotics you are given, it is important to follow up with your doctor for further testing, since sometimes infections can be resistant to treatment.

Interstitial Cystitis/ Painful Bladder Syndrome

It is difficult to tell how many people in the United States suffer from interstitial cystitis/painful bladder syndrome (IC/PBS). Depending on the diagnostic definition used, prevalence estimates range from 0.5 percent to 12 percent of women and up to 5 percent of men.[176, 177, 178] Part of the problem is that there's no real consensus on what IC/PBS is. Some doctors define it as chronic pelvic pain and problems with urination urgency and frequency that have lasted at least 3 months, while others only diagnose interstitial cystitis when patients have pain as the bladder fills that is relieved by urination.[179]

In any event, chronic pelvic pain and urinary problems are far more common than most people think, and there is a growing belief that the confusion about how to define interstitial cystitis is simply a reflection of the wide range of problems that can cause painful bladder symptoms. Interstitial cystitis has been linked to everything from damage to the bladder lining that leaves the nerves susceptible to irritation from urine,[180] to hyperactivity in the pelvic floor muscles that causes pain and misinterpretation of signals from the bladder,[181] to immune system dysfunction.[182]

Fortunately, increased understanding of the many factors that can play a role in the development of interstitial cystitis has also led to an explosion of new research into treatments. From medications and supplements to physical therapy, treatment for interstitial cystitis has become all about determining what works best for each individual, to reflect the fact that everyone is affected differently by the disease.

Is It Interstitial Cystitis/Painful Bladder Syndrome?

If you have chronic pain in your lower abdomen and are constantly running to the bathroom to urinate, then you may have interstitial cystitis/painful bladder syndrome. The hallmarks of IC/PBS include:[183]

Are Interstitial Cystitis and Painful Bladder Syndrome the Same Thing?

The diagnosis of painful bladder syndrome was initially developed to describe individuals who had some of the symptoms of interstitial cystitis but did not fit the full case definition. However, over time it became clear that interstitial cystitis is a very heterogeneous disorder and that the case definition might simply be too restrictive. These days, the umbrella diagnosis of interstitial cystitis/painful bladder syndrome is generally used to refer to all cases of bladder pain that cannot be linked to another cause.[184]

- Pain in the pelvic area—ranging from the lower abdomen to the upper thighs—that is usually improved by bladder emptying
- Frequent urination, including the need to get up at night to use the bathroom one or more times
- An urgent need to urinate caused by pain, pressure, or discomfort
- Pain or discomfort during urination
- Pain during sex

Not all people with interstitial cystitis have all these symptoms, and many of them overlap with those of other illnesses, including urinary tract infections, yeast infections, endometriosis, and vulvodynia.[185] That's why if you have the symptoms of interstitial cystitis it's important to bring them to the attention of your doctor. Only a doctor will be able to tell you if your pain comes from interstitial cystitis or another cause.

When you seek out a diagnosis, you should be prepared to talk to your doctor about how often you urinate, how urgently you feel you need to use the bathroom, and if you get up at night to urinate. You should also be ready to discuss any pain you have in your lower abdomen, whether your pain gets worse during sex, and if you experience urine leakage when you are under stress.

After asking you questions about your urination patterns, the first thing that your doctor will probably do is test your urine to make certain your pain isn't caused by an infection. Your doctor may then want to examine your bladder, either by inspecting it with a small camera inserted through your urethra or by filling it with various solutions to see if the lining is intact. Although neither

When to Call the Doctor

If you have pelvic pain, pain during urination, pain during sex, or frequent urination, it is important to get checked out by a doctor. These symptoms of interstitial cystitis/painful bladder syndrome can also be symptoms of other health conditions. An examination is the only way to be certain what is causing your pain. Call right away if you also have:

- A fever
- Pain in your lower abdomen
- Cloudy urine

Recurrent Urinary Tract Infection . . . Or Is It?

If you have been diagnosed with recurrent urinary tract infections (UTIs) but antibiotics aren't helping, talk to your doctor about whether you may actually have interstitial cystitis. Since UTIs are so common, many doctors will diagnose them based on symptoms alone, without first testing for the presence of an infection. However, the symptoms of interstitial cystitis are nearly identical to those of a UTI, so anyone experiencing repeated episodes of UTI symptoms should be checked to be sure an infection is present. This is true even for people who have been diagnosed—via bacterial culture—with a UTI in the past. A UTI can predispose you to future cystitis.

test is necessary for a diagnosis of interstitial cystitis, or is positive in every person who has cystitis, they can help to rule out other health conditions and identify the most likely course of treatment.[186]

Fast Pain Relief

For many people with interstitial cystitis, the worst part of the disease is feeling tied to the bathroom. However, for others it's the pain that's the real problem. Here are some methods you can try for relieving the painful symptoms of IC/PBS.

1. **For mild, intermittent flare-ups, try taking an NSAID.** Nonsteroidal anti-inflammatory medications like ibuprofen relieve pain by inhibiting the production of prostaglandins. This may reduce inflammation and lower tension in your bladder and pelvic floor.

2. **If you think your pain is caused by something you ate, drink some water.** Diluting your urine with water may reduce the concentration of whatever is irritating your bladder.

3. **Try placing a heating pad or ice pack on your perineum.** This technique, recommended by the Interstitial Cystitis Association,[187] may help relax the muscles surrounding your bladder and urethra. In addition, heat may confuse pain receptors, making them stop their signals.[188]

4. **Learn techniques for relaxing your pelvic floor muscles.** If your interstitial cystitis pain seems to be linked to pelvic floor dysfunction,

try talking to a physical therapist about exercises and other techniques that you can use to release your pelvic floor muscles when you feel a painful flare-up coming on. Research on men with chronic pelvic pain syndrome[189] has shown that regular practice may be an effective way to reduce your symptoms.

Relief at Last

The trick to treating your interstitial cystitis effectively may be figuring out its underlying cause, something that can differ from person to person. How do you go about maximizing your efforts to minimize your pain?

Step 1: Try to identify anything that makes your pain worse. If your interstitial cystitis has regular flare-ups, it may be worth keeping a diary of what you eat, drink, and do to see if you can figure out what makes the pain get worse. Some women's symptoms are set off by menstruation and stress, while other people's may be related to food allergies. Tracking your symptoms could help you find a way to reduce them. The Pain Diary in Part Three may help you do this.

Step 2: Be willing to experiment with different treatment options. Oral pentosan polysulfate may be a great fix for people whose interstitial cystitis is linked to bladder permeability issues. However, it probably won't do all that much good for people whose pain is linked to hyperactivity in the

Interstitial Cystitis in Men

Although interstitial cystitis is frequently discussed as a disease of women, it does occur in men, but at much lower rates—one-third to one-fifth of those seen in women. However, those rates may be so low in part because many men with the symptoms of interstitial cystitis/painful bladder symptoms are diagnosed as having chronic prostatitis or chronic pelvic pain syndrome instead.[190] That's why if you're a man who has been diagnosed with either chronic prostatitis or interstitial cystitis you may benefit from researching the treatments recommended for both conditions. There is a lot of overlap between the symptoms of the two syndromes, and treatments that help one may also help the other.[191] The truth is, the nature of both conditions is so poorly understood that they may even be the same disease![192]

muscles of their pelvic floor. Not all interstitial cystitis treatments will work for everyone, and multimodal therapies[193] that simultaneously address several potential causes may sometimes be the best option.

Step 3: Don't let worrying about your bladder make your symptoms worse. Stress can make feelings of pain and urgency associated with interstitial cystitis even more uncomfortable,[194] so it's important to do what you can to keep a positive outlook. Although doctors no longer think that most interstitial cystitis symptoms are related to affective disorders such as stress and depression, treating such problems may be able to improve your ability to cope with your pain.

The fact that not everyone with interstitial cystitis responds to every treatment means that finding the treatment that works for you may not be easy. However, making the effort can definitely improve your quality of life.[195] There is something out there that can help. You just have to discover it.

Pain Prevention Strategies

Food and Supplements

THE IC DIET: If you have interstitial cystitis, it may be a good idea to drink at least six to eight glasses of water each day to try to eliminate foods that could be irritating your insides.

The evidence: Although there is no solid scientific evidence that altering your diet can improve IC symptoms, dietary changes are one of the most frequently recommended treatments for IC. There is also a good deal of anecdotal evidence from individuals with IC suggesting that dietary changes can be helpful.

How it works: It is thought that some people with IC have damage to the lining of their bladder that can cause urine to irritate the nerves in the bladder wall. Removing irritating foods from the diet can make urine less stimulating. In addition, increasing fluid intake can dilute the concentration of any noxious substances, hopefully making bladder filling less painful. It may seem paradoxical that drinking more water could make you have to go to the bathroom less often, but some people have found that it actually works.

What you need to know: Potentially irritating foods include such items as citrus fruits, spicy food, coffee, tea, carbonated drinks, and alcohol. Since smoking has also been tentatively linked to interstitial cystitis,[196] eliminating cigarettes from your routine might also help.

CystoProtek

The first-line medical therapy for interstitial cystitis is the oral drug pentosan polysulfate, a complex sugar that mimics the lining of the bladder. Based on similar principles, the Cysto-Protek oral supplement contains two other components of the bladder lining—hyaluronic acid and chondroitin sulfate—as well as the plant-derived flavonoid quercetin, which may affect fluid accumulation in the bladder. In one study, 227 women and 25 men whose interstitial cystitis had not responded to other treatments took four CystoProtek capsules a day for approximately 1 year. By the end of treatment, levels of pain had decreased by approximately one-half.[197] An earlier small study of 6 months of treatment also showed a positive effect.[198] However, the evidence for its use is still quite preliminary, particularly since there is a strong placebo effect for IC/PBS treatments. Although the treatment is supported by evidence that both hyaluronic acid[199] and chondroitin sulfate[200] can be useful as intravesical treatments.

Touch Therapies

PHYSICAL THERAPY: Physical therapy for interstitial cystitis may be more useful for those patients who have tenderness or other dysfunction in the muscles of their pelvic floor than for those individuals whose disease can be explained by bladder permeability changes.

The evidence: In one study examining 26 men and women with interstitial cystitis, investigators found that myofascial physical therapy was more effective at reducing pain, urinary urgency, urinary frequency, and overall symptom scores than general massage, although the study was too small for most of the differences to reach statistical significance.[201] Another small study found that 7 out of 10 patients with interstitial cystitis experienced symptom relief from pelvic floor manual physical therapy.[202]

How it works: Lower pelvic pain and bladder urgency may be caused by spasms and hyperactivity in the muscles of the pelvic floor in some people. Trigger point release and other forms of myofascial physical therapy can help relieve excess tension in these muscles, reducing pain and restoring function. In addition, physical therapy may include instruction on exercises that patients can practice at home to retrain the muscles of the pelvic floor.

What you need to know: Myofascial physical therapy on the muscles of the pelvic floor may require internal massage of the vagina or rectum. If this sort of contact makes you uncomfortable, then these techniques may not be right for you. However, you may still find some benefit in other stress-relieving techniques, such as guided imagery.[203]

Pain Medications and Other Medical Treatments

PENTOSAN: Pentosan polysulfate (Elmiron) is a drug that strengthens the lining of the bladder and can decrease the permeability problems often seen in patients with interstitial cystitis.

The evidence: Numerous studies have shown pentosan to be effective at reducing pain and other symptoms of interstitial cystitis, and it has been approved by the FDA for treatment of IC/PBS.[204]

How it works: Pentosan binds tightly to bladder skin cells and reduces the permeability of the bladder lining. This may reduce irritation by urine by blocking access to the nerves. In addition, pentosan may also work by stabilizing mast cells and reducing inflammation.

What you need to know: There is some evidence that pentosan may be most effective for those individuals whose interstitial cystitis is caused by bladder permeability issues. Therefore, people who are nonreactive during potassium sulfate bladder testing—which shows whether the bladder lining is damaged—may be better served by other treatments.[206]

AMITRIPTYLINE: Amitriptyline (Elavil) is a tricyclic antidepressant that is also used for the treatment of neuropathic pain. There is mixed evidence for its use in treating interstitial cystitis.

The evidence: A small randomized controlled trial of up to 100 milligrams a day of amitriptyline found that it was much more effective at reducing symptoms of pain and urgency than placebo.[208] Other studies, however, have shown no improvement over placebo treatment except possibly in patients on the highest doses of the drug.[209]

How it works: It is thought that tricyclic antidepressants such as amitriptyline may alter signaling in the nerves that control the feelings of pain and

On the Horizon

Botox for Interstitial Cystitis

Although botulism toxin is best known for its use in smoothing out forehead wrinkles, it is also increasingly being used to treat a wide variety of chronic pain conditions. The toxin works by blocking neurotransmitters, which can stop the transmission of pain and also result in relaxation of the muscles the nerves control. To date there have been at least 10 trials of intravesical Botox treatment, of which 8 have shown some positive short-term effects.[205] Long-term follow-up studies, however, suggest that the benefits of Botox wear off in most people within a few months, meaning that repeat treatments would probably be necessary.[207]

urgency in the bladder. In addition, amitriptyline lowers mast cell histamine production, which may reduce inflammation and discomfort.

What you need to know: Amitriptyline treatment has mild, unpleasant side effects, including dry mouth and weight gain, which may occur in up to 80 percent of users.[210] It also seems to be effective only in a subset of patients with interstitial cystitis, possibly for reasons related to genetics.[211]

BLADDER INSTILLATION/INTRAVESICAL THERAPY: This type of therapy involves filling the bladder with either saline or medicated fluids through a urethral catheter.

The evidence: Numerous studies have shown that intravesical therapies can provide mild symptom relief for some individuals with interstitial cystitis. However, the evidence does not yet conclusively support this type of therapy.[212]

How it works: Instilling fluids into the bladder can be used both to stretch the bladder and to medicate it directly.

What you need to know: Because intravesical therapy requires repeated catheterizations, it may increase the risk of bacterial cystitis. In addition, although many drugs have been tested for intravesical therapy, the only one currently approved by the FDA for interstitial cystitis treatment is dimethyl sulfoxide (DMSO). DMSO is thought to have both anti-inflammatory and muscle relaxant properties. Other tested drugs have various proposed mechanisms including reducing bladder permeability (hyaluronic acid, heparin, chondroitin, pentosan), altering the immune response (bacillus Calmette-Guérin), and directly anesthetizing (lidocaine).

Other Strategies

INVASIVE NERVE STIMULATION: Electrical stimulation of the nerves that control the bladder may be able to help some individuals whose interstitial cystitis doesn't respond to other treatment.

The evidence: Several small studies of a permanently implanted sacral nerve modulation device have demonstrated that it can effectively reduce the number of times individuals need to urinate. It also has been shown to reduce pelvic pain and improve quality of life.[213] However, this surgery is not for everyone. Permanent implantation should only be attempted after temporary stimulation has been shown to have a positive effect, and many people still end up needing repeat surgeries.[214]

How it works: Electrical stimulation can alter the function of the nerves that control the bladder. In addition to interrupting pain and urgency signals, it may encourage retraining of the pelvic floor muscles.

What you need to know: Although most recent studies have examined the use of sacral nerve stimulation—which was approved by the FDA for use in patients with urinary urgency/frequency problems in 1999—there is some evidence that noninvasive transcutaneous electrical nerve stimulation (TENS) may also have positive effects on bladder dysfunction.[215]

BLADDER TRAINING: Bladder-training programs focus on helping individuals with interstitial cystitis expand their bladder volume so that they can go longer between episodes of urination and relieve bladder distension discomfort.

The evidence: A study in which 361 patients were treated with medical bladder distension followed by training focused on delaying urination for progressively longer intervals showed impressive results. Although at baseline 87 percent of patients felt pain when their bladder was full and 70 percent had problems with urgency, by 8 weeks after distension and training only 14 percent experienced full bladder pain and 13 percent were bothered by urgency. Patients also significantly decreased the number of times they went to the bathroom during the day and at night.[216] Another smaller pilot study, which incorporated similar training and a medication component, also showed positive results.[217]

How it works: Bladder-training programs may involve both medical distension of the bladder, using saline or other intravesical treatments, and patient-directed bladder filling involving carefully scheduled fluid intake and urination. The goal of these programs is to increase the capacity of the bladder slowly so that patients can go longer between episodes of urination. In addition, it is thought that progressively increasing the time between urinations may be able to retrain the body's perception of what level of bladder fullness is felt to be urgent.

What you need to know: Although medical distension of the bladder has been studied quite frequently, and with mixed results, there is less research on the effects of patient training to increase the time between urinations. There is a great deal of logic behind the training process, but it would benefit from additional research support.

Chronic Prostatitis/ Chronic Pelvic Pain in Men

Millions of men seek help for chronic pelvic pain every year. Although some of these men can be successfully treated with antibiotics, over 90 percent of prostatitis cases fall under the umbrella of chronic prostatitis/chronic pelvic pain syndrome (CP/CPPS), also known as Category 3 prostatitis. Chronic, nonbacterial prostatitis is the most common form of chronic pelvic pain in men, and more than 1 out of every 10 men will experience it at some point during their lives.[218]

Unlike benign prostatic hyperplasia, whose prevalence increases with age, CP/CPPS occurs just as often in younger men.[219] They are definitely two different diseases. Benign prostatic hyperplasia is characterized by prostate enlargement, but although a minority of men with CP/CPPS have noticeable inflammation of their prostate, pain in most men has no obvious cause.[220]

In fact, the newest thinking about chronic prostatitis is that it may not have anything to do with the prostate at all. Instead, it seems that what was initially identified as prostate pain may have more to do with excess tension in the muscles of the pelvic floor.[221] That's why the current focus on therapies for CP/CPPS is moving away from treating the prostate and toward drugs and techniques that can help men gain control over those muscles and relax away their pain.

Is It Chronic Prostatitis?

Chronic prostatitis/chronic pelvic pain syndrome is defined both by the pain it causes and by the fact that it cannot be clearly diagnosed as any other disease. Although chronic prostatitis is a highly individualized syndrome, the most common symptoms include:

- Pelvic pain, including rectal, scrotal, perineal, urethral, and testicular pain as well as pain deeper inside the pelvis

- Problems with urination, including frequent urination, difficulty urinating, and a feeling that you are unable to empty your bladder completely

- Ejaculatory pain

Not all men with chronic prostatitis will experience all symptoms, and not all men who have these symptoms have chronic prostatitis. Diagnosing chronic prostatitis is mostly a matter of excluding all the other diseases that could potentially cause these symptoms. This means that, after talking to you, your doctor will test you for various infections as well as make sure that you don't have bladder stones, obstructions in your urinary tract, or the early stages of cancer.[222]

When you visit your doctor, be prepared to tell him where your pain is located, how it affects your ability to urinate and ejaculate, and any history you have of urinary tract infections. He will also want to know when your pain started and how it affects your quality of life.[223] Answer honestly, even about

Types of Prostatitis

- **Category 1: Acute bacterial prostatitis:** Characterized by fever, painful urination, muscle aches, and positive bacterial culture. It can usually be treated effectively with antibiotics.

- **Category 2: Chronic bacterial prostatitis:** Similar to Category 1 prostatitis, this lasts for a longer period of time. Men with this type of prostatitis also frequently have recurrent urinary tract infections.

- **Category 3: Chronic prostatitis/chronic pelvic pain syndrome:** Patients have long-term pelvic pain and pain on urination but do not have an identifiable bacterial infection or other obvious cause for their pain. This is the most common type of prostatitis. It can be further divided into Categories 3a and 3b. Men with 3a CP/CPPS have signs of inflammation, but men with 3b do not.

- **Category 4: Asymptomatic inflammatory prostatitis:** This causes inflammation of the prostate but has no symptoms. It is usually detected during evaluation for other health problems.[224]

sexual symptoms. The more information you can provide, the more likely it is that your doctor will be able to help.

Fast Pain Relief

If you have chronic pelvic pain and difficulty urinating or ejaculating, it's understandable that you want pain relief right now. Although most available treatments for prostatitis take a little while to reach their full effect, there are a few things that you can try for short-term pain relief.

1. **If your pain is mild to moderate, try an over-the-counter NSAID.** NSAIDs, like ibuprofen or naproxen, relieve pain by inhibiting the COX-1 enzyme. This reduces prostaglandin production, which may help to release tension in the muscles of your bladder and pelvic floor. However, these drugs are not necessarily suitable for chronic pain relief. If you find yourself needing to take a higher dosage than what is recommended on the package, or taking the drugs for a longer period of time, then talk to your doctor about other treatment options. NSAIDs should primarily be used for temporary pain relief while you're getting your symptoms under control.[225]

2. **If your pain is more severe, a prescription painkiller may help.** Studies have shown that prescription painkillers such as celecoxib (Celebrex) may be a reasonable option for short-term symptom relief. Although in one study the COX-2 inhibitor did not improve urinary function, 200 milligrams a day was shown to reduce pain and help with overall quality of life in men with chronic pelvic pain syndrome.[226]

3. **Explore alternative therapies.** Acupuncture,[227] TENS,[228] and physical therapy[229] have all been shown to have positive effects on the pain of chronic prostatitis without the possible side effects of long-term NSAID use. In addition, these therapies may be able to address the underlying causes of your symptoms, providing long-term benefits rather than just a quick fix for your current pain.

Relief at Last

NSAIDs are only effective painkillers while you are taking them. Long-term therapy for chronic prostatitis focuses on relieving the reasons for your symptoms instead of just stopping you from noticing them.

Step 1: Understand the cause of your pain. Just because you have prostatitis symptoms does not necessarily mean that you have prostatitis. If you have pelvic pain, or problems with urination and ejaculation, it's a good idea to be thoroughly checked out by your doctor. There may be a clear, medical cause for your pain that is easy to treat, but there's no way for you to determine that on your own.

Step 2: Learn to relax your muscles. Prostatitis, particularly the noninflammatory Category 3b variety, often seems to have less to do with the prostate and more to do with the muscles of the pelvic floor. Physical therapy, biofeedback training, and structured exercise programs may be able to help you get control over the problematic muscles and, by doing so, relieve your symptoms.

Step 3: Try to relieve your stress. Emotional stress can make preexisting physical pain worse and can even cause you to develop new symptoms. Reducing the amount of stress in your life may both relieve your symptoms and make them easier to deal with. Pain is hard enough to cope with when you're not also worried about other things.

Step 4: Explore pharmaceutical options. For some men with prostate pain, drugs such as alpha blockers or anti-inflammatory medications may be a good option for treatment. For others, antidepressants may provide long-lasting pain relief. Medication may not be your first choice for prostate pain relief, but you shouldn't hesitate to use it if it's something that can improve your life.

Pain Prevention Strategies

Food and Supplements

POLLEN EXTRACTS: Commercial pollen extracts marketed as Cernilton, Prostat, and Poltit have been used to treat benign prostatic hyperplasia, and there is also some evidence for their use in prostatitis patients.

The evidence: One randomized controlled trial found that 12 weeks of oral treatment with the pollen extract Cernilton significantly reduced symptoms

What's in a Name?

There's a growing belief that interstitial cystitis and chronic prostatitis/chronic pelvic pain syndrome may be the same disease. The conditions show a large amount of symptom overlap and neither has a clearly definable cause.[230] However, in general, women are more likely to be diagnosed as having interstitial cystitis/painful bladder syndrome and men are more likely to be diagnosed as having chronic prostatitis/chronic pelvic pain.[231] Although there is certainly recognition that interstitial cystitis affects men, specific research studies on its treatment in men are few and far between. Fortunately, what literature there is suggests that treatments for CP/CPPS, as well as treatments for interstitial cystitis in women, may help men with interstitial cystitis as well.

and improved quality of life compared to treatment with placebo.[235] A similar trial of 6-month use of another pollen extract, Prostat/Poltit, found that it was also quite effective.[236]

How it works: Cernilton has been shown to have anti-inflammatory properties. It may also reduce muscle cramping by lowering prostaglandin production.

What you need to know: Neither study looked at how long the effects of the pollen extracts lasted after patients stopped taking them, so it is unclear whether patients may have to continue taking the pills indefinitely. They also did not examine the efficacy of the pills until patients had been taking them for at least 6 weeks. Prostat/Poltit and Cernilton are different versions of the same drug.

SAW PALMETTO: Saw palmetto is an herbal product that has traditionally been used to treat a variety of genital and urinary problems, including prostate disorders.[237]

The evidence: A randomized controlled trial comparing saw palmetto supplementation alone to a combined treatment with saw palmetto, selenium, and lycopene (Profluss) found that both treatments could significantly reduce pain and white blood cell count. However, the combined treatment was more effective and could also reduce prostate-specific antigen levels and improve urinary flow rates.[238]

How it works: Saw palmetto is thought to inhibit an enzyme that converts testosterone into the stronger hormone dihydrotestosterone. It may also have anti-inflammatory properties.[239]

What you need to know: Although it is widely used, some studies have questioned the efficacy of saw palmetto treatment alone. This is particularly true for long-term use since at least one study found it to be most effective during the first 3 months of treatment.[240] Its pharmaceutical equivalent, finasteride (Proscar/Propecia), may work better in some people.

Touch Therapies

ACUPUNCTURE: Several trials have investigated the use of acupuncture for men with chronic prostatitis with some promising results.

The evidence: A randomized controlled trial comparing acupuncture with sham acupuncture in 89 patients found that patients receiving real acupuncture were almost twice as likely to report symptom improvements as those in the sham group.[241] However, those people who responded to sham acupuncture saw the same level of pain relief.

How it works: In the randomized controlled trial, the acupuncture points chosen were ones that are supposed to improve overall energy as well as bladder voiding. The authors commented that acupuncture may work by affecting nervous system mechanisms involved in CP/CPPS. However, another small study found that acupuncture could measurably reduce the pooling of blood in the pelvis—pelvic venous congestion—seen in some men with CP/CPPS and hypothesized that it might also have additional effects on muscle hyperactivity.[242]

What you need to know: See Part Three for information on how to find a licensed acupuncturist.

MYOFASCIAL PHYSICAL THERAPY/TRIGGER POINT THERAPY: Myofascial physical therapy, or trigger point therapy, uses directed massage to release tension and spasm in the muscles of the pelvic floor and abdomen. Unlike acupressure, which is designed to alter the energy flow of the body, trigger point therapy acts directly on tense or irritated muscles.

The evidence: A small randomized controlled trial comparing trigger point therapy to general massage found that trigger point therapy was substantially more effective at relieving symptoms, including pain and frequency of urination.[243] Trigger point therapy has also been shown to have positive effects on erectile and ejaculatory function.[244]

How it works: Many men with CP/CPPS have elevated levels of tension, even spasm, in their pelvic floor and surrounding musculature. This tension can cause pain and bladder problems, and releasing it with trigger point massage may improve a number of CP/CPPS symptoms. In addition, trigger point therapy often includes a training component to help men practice relaxing their pelvic floor muscles at home.

What you need to know: Trigger point therapy for CP/CPPS involves the therapist inserting a finger inside your rectum for internal massage, as well as other contact that some men perceive as intimate. If you are uncomfortable receiving a rectal exam, then this type of therapy is not appropriate for you.

Mind-Body Therapies

BIOFEEDBACK TRAINING: Biofeedback training for chronic prostatitis uses structured feedback to help you strengthen your pelvic floor muscles and retrain your bladder.

The evidence: In one study of biofeedback-based retraining, severity of pain and other symptoms were significantly reduced and the average interval between episodes of urination increased from 0.88 hour to 3 hours.[245] Other studies have shown similar results.[246]

How it works: Biofeedback techniques help men learn how to contract and release the muscles of the pelvic floor. Over time, this can not only increase bladder control but reduce pain by addressing the muscle function abnormalities seen in many men with CP/CPPS.

What you need to know: Several studies have shown biofeedback techniques to be effective at reducing the symptoms of CP/CPPS. However, biofeedback requires significant and consistent effort on the part of the patient and may not be a good option for everyone. See Part Three for help finding a biofeedback practitioner near you.

Pain Medications and Other Medical Treatments

ALPHA BLOCKERS: Alpha blockers are drugs that block alpha-adrenergic receptors—the receptors that, when stimulated, cause the body to produce adrenaline/epinephrine and are associated with the fight-or-flight response. They include drugs such as tamsulosin (Flomax), alfuzosin (Uroxatral), and doxazosin (Cardura).

The evidence: In a small randomized controlled trial, patients who were treated with doxazosin for 3 months found that their pain, quality of life, and other symptom scores improved considerably from baseline. Placebo users also saw minor improvements, but the drug was significantly more effective.[247]

How it works: Alpha blockers promote relaxation of the smooth muscle surrounding the prostate and also reduce inflammation.

What you need to know: Alpha blockers are generally considered safe for long-term use in individuals with benign prostatic hyperplasia and are a reasonable option for CP/CPPS. However, the evidence for their use is not consistent. Although several studies have shown quite positive results, other studies have shown them to be no better than placebo.[248]

FINASTERIDE: Finasteride (Proscar/Propecia) is a drug that inhibits the action of 5-alpha reductase, an enzyme that converts testosterone to the more active dihydrotestosterone. Dihydrotestosterone is important for the development of male sexual characteristics and may also affect sexual behavior. Genetic males born without 5-alpha reductase often appear to be female or have ambiguous genitalia.

The evidence: When 64 men were randomized to treatment with either 5 milligrams a day of finasteride or 325 milligrams a day of saw palmetto and followed for 1 year, the men receiving finasteride had significantly improved pain levels and quality of life at all time points. However, the drug did not affect bladder emptying or frequency of urination.[251]

How it works: Dihydrotestosterone can cause enlargement of the prostate, but finasteride may also be able to decrease prostate pain and inflammation by other mechanisms.

What you need to know: Finasteride is widely used as a treatment for benign prostatic hyperplasia. Evidence for its use in CP/CPPS is not as strong.

PENTOSAN: Pentosan polysulfate is a complex sugar that mimics part of the lining of the bladder. It has been approved for the

On the Horizon

Nerve Stimulation for Prostate Pain

In 2009, a research study looked at the efficacy of posterior tibial nerve stimulation for reducing pain associated with CP/CPPS in men resistant to other therapies. This technique is thought to alter the function of the nerves that control the bladder.

The treatment showed impressive results. Active therapy improved pain and symptoms, at least partially, in 100 percent of patients, while sham therapy had little to no effect.[249] The extent of pain relief was also greater than that seen with most currently available therapies.[250] The research is in its early stages, but posterior tibial nerve stimulation may turn out to be an important CP/CPPS treatment in the future.

Other types of electrical stimulation, such as TENS[252] and electro-acupuncture,[253] have also been used to reduce the pain associated with prostatitis, and an implantable sacral neuromodulation device has been FDA approved for the treatment of related symptoms.[254]

Heat Therapy

Various types of heat therapy for CP/CPPS have been explored, including the following:

1. **Transrectal microwave hyperthermia:** A microwave antenna is inserted through the rectum into the prostate and used to heat the tissue.

2. **Transurethral microwave hyperthermia:** In this procedure, the microwave antenna is inserted through the urethra instead of the rectum before being heated.

3. **Dilation of the prostate with a heated balloon**

4. **Transurethral needle ablation (TUNA):** A needle is inserted through the urethra into the prostate and then heated to kill off part of the tissue.

Although many of these techniques are used to treat benign prostatic hyperplasia and several of them have shown limited success in small trials for men with CP/CPPS, a recent review of the evidence[255] suggested that right now, these therapies should not be considered except as a last resort—particularly since the prostate may not be responsible for prostatitis after all, and each of these techniques can have significant side effects.

treatment of interstitial cystitis, a disease that is thought to be closely related to CP/CPPS.

The evidence: In a randomized controlled trial, more individuals on pentosan than on placebo reported a global improvement in their symptoms (37 percent versus 18 percent), although the extent of improvement was the same in both groups. Prostatitis-specific improvements, such as improvements in urination and ejaculation, were also seen to a greater extent in treated individuals, although the difference was not statistically significant.[256]

How it works: Pentosan has anti-inflammatory properties and may reduce pain through its effects on local inflammation. It may also reduce irritation linked to bladder permeability issues.

What you need to know: Several other small studies also have reported mild positive effects for pentosan in CP/CPPS patients. However, there is little information on how long the effects of the drug last once you stop taking it.

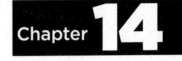

Chapter 14

Digestive and Gastrointestinal Pain

Heartburn and gastroesophageal reflux disease (GERD), gallstones, ulcers, irritable bowel syndrome, diverticulitis, kidney stones, inflammatory bowel disease, Crohn's disease, and ulcerative colitis

When all's well within the 30 feet of tubes, valves, and muscle that make up your digestive system, the only sensations you usually notice are hunger, fullness, the urge to visit a restroom, and perhaps the desire for another slice of double chocolate birthday cake. When something's amiss, however, the outcome can be severe and disabling.

You may contract the corkscrew-shaped bacterium that causes stomach ulcers. You may develop a kidney stone, and feel it scrape slo-o-owly down a narrow passageway to your bladder. You may face serious complications caused by inflammatory bowel disease, or find your job and social life interrupted by the diarrhea and constipation of irritable bowel syndrome. You may wonder what to eat to avoid another attack of heartburn or diverticulitis, or find yourself weighing the pros and cons of joining the half-million Americans a year who opt for gallbladder-removal surgery.

In all, the digestive and gastrointestinal pain conditions in this chapter affect over 100 million Americans. It's a sign of the size and complexity of your body's food-processing plant. As research reveals new causes and promising new treatments, keeping it healthy and pain free is more possible than ever before.

For example, it makes sense that food choices would affect pain in your digestive system directly. And, indeed, there's new evidence that dietary changes can help all these conditions, either by easing pain or preventing a return of symptoms. But the food tips experts recommend today are far different from what you'd have heard in the past, with more emphasis now on healthy fiber, balanced meals, and less red meat for easing many digestive pains. (Getting more good bacteria is important now, too.)

As scientists learn more about the profound connections between the digestive system, the nervous system, and the brain, it's not surprising that mind-body therapies are also emerging as powerful pain relievers for digestion problems. From relaxation and guided imagery to hypnotherapy and meditation, there's plenty of proof that while these problems aren't "all in your head," you can use the healing power of your brain to calm and improve the way your gastrointestinal system works.

In this chapter you'll also find the latest on medications and procedures with the best track record for helping these conditions, and how to combine them with drug-free strategies to ease pain today and stay pain free for years to come. (You'll also get all the news about treatments to think twice about or to avoid completely.)

Heartburn and Gastroesophageal Reflux Disease (GERD)

Is one tiny pill really all you need to squelch the pain of acid indigestion? Television commercials, highway billboards, and magazine advertisements want you to think so, as they tout the ability of newer heartburn drugs called proton pump inhibitors (PPIs) to singlehandedly douse the agonizing fires of heartburn.

These drugs are top sellers in the United States and around the world, generating billions of dollars in annual sales for drug companies. But as more and more people experience the pain of heartburn and the damaging effects of its more serious cousin, gastroesophageal reflux disease (GERD), it's becoming clear that lasting relief takes more than a little pill.

What you really need is a strategy that attacks the root causes of heartburn on all fronts.

In this chapter, you'll discover the best ways to use heartburn drugs—from simple antacid tablets to prescription-strength PPIs—safely and effectively to neutralize stomach acids. But that's just the beginning. You'll also find a wide range of proven, drug-free strategies that attack the real causes of the growing epidemic of heartburn and GERD: pressure in your stomach and a faulty stomach "valve" that lets acids escape into your esophagus.

Heartburn drugs can't do that; in fact, the biggest sellers don't work well for 30 percent of the people who try them[1,2] and leave about 40 percent with breakthrough pain several times a week. What really works? Sensible steps like losing weight, getting more exercise, eating stomach-friendly foods, and trying out complementary medicine techniques like relaxation and acupuncture. (By the way, we're not going to hand you a boilerplate list of forbidden foods. The conventional wisdom about what sets off heartburn has been proven all wrong!)

If you rely on medications to control heartburn and GERD, now is the perfect time to broaden your relief strategy. Research shows that using nondrug techniques can bring more relief without increasing your drug dosage. And plenty of former heartburn sufferers say that healthy changes can even reduce or eliminate your need for medication—important because emerging research is discovering that some heartburn drugs are dramatically overused and can cause serious side effects.

Is It Heartburn or GERD?

As many as 44 percent of adults get heartburn once a month; 14 percent have it weekly, and for 7 percent it's a daily problem. The trouble? A less-than-stalwart lower esophageal sphincter (LES). This muscular valve at the top of your stomach is supposed to keep stomach acids from escaping upward into your esophagus. But if it relaxes at the wrong times or is pushed by too much pressure in

When to Call the Doctor

Antacids may provide temporary relief, but it's worth seeing the doctor if heartburn happens more than two to three times a week or has been an on-and-off problem for months or years; if you've been taking antacids regularly for more than 2 weeks; if you've been upping the amount of other heartburn drugs you take; or if nothing is helping.

your stomach (thanks to a heavy meal or to lying down too soon after eating), or if you have another medical problem such as a hiatal hernia or a stomach that empties slowly, your LES can't hold back the acid. It backwashes into your throat and you feel that familiar burning sensation. Smoking, alcohol, some foods, and some medications can also help acid escape.

The pain may be in your throat or chest. It may be worse after a meal, when you bend over, or at night (research shows that stomach acids grow more acidic during the night; when you're horizontal, gravity can't help keep these juices where they belong). A chronic cough and/or chronic laryngitis can also be signs of heartburn or GERD.

So which is it, and which should you worry about? Occasional heartburn is no cause for alarm. But heartburn becomes more severe—and is considered GERD—when chronic acid backwash damages the delicate tissue lining of your esophagus. This can lead to a sore throat, coughing, wheezing, nausea, laryngitis, and in some cases even increase your risk for cancer.

It's likely that your doctor will be able to diagnose heartburn or tell if it's becoming GERD based on your symptoms (such as a chronic cough or laryngitis). He may check your esophagus with an endoscope—a long, thin tube—or with x-rays to look for damage caused by GERD. Sometimes, medical tests such as an esophageal pH probe study—which measures acidity in your esophagus for 24 hours—or a wireless version that doesn't require the probe are done to see if acid backwash is the cause of your symptoms.

Your doctor will also rule out other medical conditions that could be causing your pain, including heart disease.

Fast Pain Relief

The drugstore—or even the pack of chewing gum in your purse or desk drawer—offers lots of relief from heartburn pain. That's great news, but we've got a caveat. Now that several effective remedies once available only by prescription are sold over the counter, it's easy to treat heartburn at home for too long. The problem: You're risking damage to your esophagus. That's why it's important to take steps to prevent future heartburn and to see your doctor if pain persists.

1. **Chew gum after a meal.** Working your jaws with a stick of chewing gum doubles the amount of heartburn-soothing saliva you produce and swallow. Chewing gum can neutralize nasty stomach acids for up to 3 hours after a meal. If you have occasional heartburn or find pain coming on when you're out of antacids, try it.

2. **For mild heartburn, start with an antacid that contains an alginate.** Regular antacids (like Maalox, Mylanta, Gelusil, Rolaids, and Tums) work by absorbing and neutralizing stomach acids. But in a Baylor College of Medicine review of 10 studies, these eased heartburn pain by just 11 percent, while those containing alginic acid (such as Gaviscon-2 and Genaton) eased the pain of mild heartburn by 60 percent. Alginates form a protective layer on top of the acids in your stomach, helping to prevent backwash into your esophagus. Take after a meal for best results.

3. **For more severe heartburn, try an acid-reducing H2 blocker.** If your heartburn doesn't respond to antacids, you owe it to yourself to see your doctor. In the meantime, it's okay to use an over-the-counter version of an H2 blocker (such as Axid, Pepcid, Tagamet, and Zantac) for 2 weeks for temporary relief.

   H2 blockers ease mild heartburn about 40 percent of the time. By reducing the acidity of your stomach "juices," they give the delicate tissue in your esophagus a break from heartburn's corrosive backwash and help it heal about 80 percent of the time. H2 blockers work best when taken before you eat that pepperoni pizza or ask the boss for a raise. In other words, take an H2 blocker before you expose yourself to anything you know triggers your heartburn.

4. **If you've been diagnosed with GERD, take a proton pump inhibitor.** Stronger than H2 blockers, these drugs are available over the counter (brands include Aciphex, Nexium, Prevacid, Prilosec, and Protonix) and by prescription. They work by stopping production of 90 percent of stomach acid, which provides plenty of relief. If you've been diagnosed with GERD and your esophagus has been irritated or damaged by acid backwash, a PPI can also help repair it in 4 to 7 weeks.

> ## Quick Tip
> Stomach juices become more acidic between 10 p.m. and 6 a.m., which is one reason why 75 percent of people who take the strongest heartburn drugs get "acid breakthrough" in the middle of the night. You can stop nighttime heartburn by skipping cola drinks (in one study, having one a day increased risk for nighttime heartburn 24 percent); avoiding food 2 to 3 hours before going to bed; and elevating the head of your bed by 6 to 10 inches by putting it up on blocks or using wedge pillows to raise your head and upper chest up.

PPIs are serious medicine and should be used under a doctor's care. Some experts think PPIs are used too often and that regular antacids or H2 blockers will work just as well, with fewer risks, for many people. Overuse raises your risk for pneumonia and infection with the bacteria *Clostridium difficile*.

5. **Eliminate your trigger foods.** Wondering what to have at your next meal? Be smart. If coffee, five-alarm chili, and pizza with the works fire up your heartburn, it's time to trade 'em in for milder fare. Doctors used to warn patients with reflux away from many edible culprits, but the new thinking is that triggers are a personal matter. Figure out what yours are and steer clear.

6. **To ease nighttime heartburn, think "up."** We mean stay up for at least 3 hours after your last meal or big snack. Heartburn is worse if you lie down with a full stomach. And when you do turn in, try elevating your bed on blocks or raising your head up with several pillows or a foam wedge so that gravity can help keep your stomach acids where they belong.

Relief at Last

There's plenty you can do to protect yourself from future heartburn pain, so start today. These steps are essential whether you're bothered by mild heartburn or must take medications to help stop severe GERD.

Step 1: Start with lifestyle changes. Skip big meals, don't lie down for at least 3 hours after eating, cut out your personal heartburn trigger foods (we'll show you how to spot them), lose weight, bump up your fiber intake, cut back on salt, start a regular exercise routine, and stop smoking. Each of these strategies is proven to reduce heartburn and GERD. Combining them could eliminate your acid backwash pain, or at least make it less frequent and less severe, without medication. But even if you need drugs to help control heartburn or GERD, following these lifestyle strategies will help you keep things under control with the smallest possible dose. In addition, controlling diabetes and/or asthma can also help you get heartburn and GERD under control.

Step 2: Learn a progressive muscle relaxation exercise. Stress boosts heartburn pain two ways—by increasing stomach acid and by boosting your sensitivity to pain signals. Dial both back by practicing relaxation; in one study it eased symptoms significantly.

Step 3: Work with your doctor to set up a heartburn medication plan. Yes, there are plenty of strong, over-the-counter drugs—such as H2 blockers and PPIs—to ease the pain. But there's growing evidence that PPIs are overused, raising risk for serious side effects such as bone fractures. By reducing the acidity of your digestive juices, these medications can buy time for delicate tissue in your esophagus to heal. They can also give lifestyle changes a chance to start working. But taking them long term raises risks for side effects.

Step 4: Add acupuncture. If you need more relief than you're getting from the strongest heartburn drugs (PPIs), adding acupuncture may help, research suggests.

Pain Prevention Strategies

Food and Supplements

HIGH-FIBER FOODS: Eating more fruit, vegetables, and whole grains can douse the flames of acid reflux—and not just because this healthy eating strategy can help you lose weight. The fiber they contain seems to have a direct effect on muscles that control acid backwash.

The evidence: In a Swedish study of 3,153 people, those who ate high-fiber breads had half the risk of GERD compared to people who ate low-fiber breads.[3] When researchers at the Houston Veterans Affairs Medical Center scanned the esophaguses of 164 people, they found that those who ate more fruits, veggies, whole grains, and beans were 20 percent less likely to have signs of erosion of delicate tissues there caused by reflux. At higher risk: people who took in more fat, protein, and calories.

How it works: Fiber may help by soaking up excess amounts of nitric oxide, a compound that relaxes muscles in the digestive system.

On the Horizon

No-Cut Valve Repair for Severe Heartburn

Doctors sometimes recommend that people with severe heartburn consider a surgical procedure to keep stomach acids from backwashing into the esophagus. Called fundoplication, it involves tightening the lower esophageal sphincter, the valve between the top of the stomach and the esophagus. Some hospitals are beginning to offer an incisionless version of this surgery, in which doctors work through the mouth and use a camera and light on a long tube to see what they're doing. There are fewer complications, shorter hospital stays, and little or no need for antacids and other heartburn drugs afterward.

What you should know: Why not turn trouble foods into high-fiber helpers? Instead of two slices of pizza, have one slice piled high with vegetables along with a side salad, for example. Or enjoy a piece of fresh, sweet seasonal fruit instead of a bottle of soda.

STAY AWAY FROM YOUR PERSONAL TROUBLE FOODS: Trigger foods aren't the same for everyone, which means that a one-size-fits-all list of no-no's from your doctor is an outdated concept. However, it's likely that some foods and drinks do fan your heartburn flames. Figuring out what they are and avoiding them or eating them in smaller quantities (and never close to bedtime) is still an important comfort strategy.

The evidence: When researchers from Stanford University reviewed over 100 studies of lifestyle remedies for heartburn they concluded that avoiding chocolate, mint, spices, grease, and late-night noshing weren't proven to help.[4] But plenty of other research, and the experience of digestive disease specialists, suggests that for some people these are exactly the foods they should avoid.

How it works: No one's sure why skipping some foods clears up heartburn pain for some people yet has no benefits for others. Experts say some foods, such as mint, may relax the muscle that keeps food in your stomach. Others, like acidic drinks and spicy stuff, may simply be irritating.

What you need to know: Identify your personal problem foods, then skip 'em or cut way back. Possible culprits include citrus fruits, chocolate, fizzy drinks, coffee and tea, drinks with caffeine or alcohol, fatty and fried foods, garlic and onions, mint flavorings, spicy foods, and tomato-based foods like spaghetti sauce, salsa, chili, and pizza.

HOLD THE SALT: Extra-salty foods—such as processed foods, restaurant and fast-food items, and foods preserved with salt—don't just raise your blood pressure, they also contribute to heartburn pain.

The evidence: Swedish researchers found that people who ate extremely salty foods just three times a week were 50 percent more likely to have acid reflux than those who avoided them. Salting your food raised risk 70 percent.

How it works: Researchers don't yet know why salt increases heartburn pain. One possibility: People who use more salt may simply be eating more foods that ignite heartburn.

What you need to know: Cutting back on salt at the table and in cooking is important, but the best way to trim your intake is to eat fewer processed foods and restaurant meals, the source of nearly 80 percent of the sodium in the American diet.

Exercise and Movement Therapies

MOVE: Even a little bit of exercise can have a big, positive effect on heartburn, perhaps by speeding digestion or by keeping you upright so acid is discouraged from backwashing.

The evidence: People who exercised for as little as 30 minutes a week were 50 percent less likely to have heartburn than people who rarely exercised, Swedish researchers report.[5]

How it works: Exercise may work by helping to move food more quickly through your digestive system. Or it might just be that staying upright—whether you're walking, playing tennis, or working out to your favorite aerobics DVD—lets gravity keep stomach acid down where it belongs.

What you need to know: A stroll after a big or late meal can prevent heartburn, too. In one study, people who walked for an hour after munching a big breakfast reduced their heartburn 17 percent compared to people who sat still after eating.

Touch Therapies

ACUPUNCTURE: For plenty of people, even strong, acid-reducing proton pump inhibitors don't fully control heartburn pain. Now there's evidence that adding the ancient healing art of acupuncture can fill the gap.

The evidence: When 30 people with persistent heartburn received a double dose of PPIs or took their regular dose and had two acupuncture sessions a week for 8 weeks, the acupuncture group saw a larger decrease in reflux during the day and at night. In this University of Arizona study, taking more PPIs did little to ease breakthrough pain.[6]

How it works: Acupuncture may help by preventing the lower esophageal sphincter from opening up when it shouldn't, say researchers from the Royal Adelaide Hospital in Australia. In one experiment, electrical stimulation acupuncture at the Neiguan point (also called P6 by acupuncture practitioners) prevented the LES from opening when it shouldn't 40 percent of the time.[7] The Neiguan point is located between the tendons on the inside of the wrist, about 2 inches up from your hand.

What you need to know: The Neiguan point is used extensively in acupuncture and acupressure to prevent and relieve nausea. You can try pressing this spot firmly for a minute, or sign up for more extensive acupuncture treatment with a licensed practitioner. See Part Three to find an acupuncturist in your area.

Mind-Body Therapies

PROGRESSIVE MUSCLE RELAXATION: It's no secret that stress dials up heartburn pain. But the conventional wisdom that says tension boosts production of stomach acids is only part of the story. Stress can increase levels of stomach acids,[8] but it turns out that it also increases pain sensitivity significantly, which makes your heartburn feels worse.[9]

The evidence: In one University of Alabama at Birmingham study, 20 people with heartburn saw symptoms improve after they tried a muscle relaxation exercise.

How it works: Relaxation seems to help in two ways. It reduces stress, which can make you less sensitive to acid backwash pain. It can also cut the amount of acid splashing up against your esophagus, researchers found.[10]

What you need to know: The breathing and muscle relaxation exercises in Part One could help you cut stress and reduce heartburn symptoms.

Pain Medications and Medical Treatments

ANTACIDS: Over-the-counter antacids (Tums, Maalox) and antacids containing alginates may be all you need to stop the pain of infrequent heartburn. They're great for stopping symptoms quickly.

The evidence: Even digestion experts reach for antacids. In one nationwide study of gastroenterologists, 78 percent said they'd choose an antacid if heartburn woke them up at night. Other research suggests they ease moderate heartburn pain in about an hour.[11]

How it works: Antacids make your stomach acid less acidic so that it's not as irritating. Types that also contain alginates help prevent acid from backwashing into your esophagus.

What you need to know: Take antacids about an hour after you eat or when heartburn begins; they work fast and could be less helpful if taken on an empty stomach. Liquids offer quicker relief, but chewables may be more convenient to carry around. Different types can cause different kinds of side effects: Magnesium-based antacids can cause diarrhea and aluminum-containing varieties may cause constipation. So if one type causes discomfort, try another.

H2 BLOCKERS: These acid-reducing drugs aren't as strong as proton pump inhibitors and shouldn't be taken for long periods of time. Heartburn that's not responding to home treatment merits a closer look by your doctor. But if you're taking a PPI and are experiencing breakthrough pain, H2 blockers (such as Tagamet HB, Pepcid AC, Axid AR, and Zantac) can help. These drugs work by blocking histamine, a chemical that triggers acid secretion in the stomach.

The evidence: H2 blockers ease symptoms in just a few weeks for 70 percent of people who take them, say researchers who reviewed dozens of heartburn relief studies.[12]

How it works: H2 blockers reduce the production of stomach acids and can be taken just before a big meal or stressful event to help prevent breakthrough pain.

What you need to know: It takes 30 to 90 minutes for H2 blockers to work so they're best taken before a big meal or a stressful event that you think will set off heartburn. Although some doctors prescribe H2 blockers along with PPIs to reduce nighttime heartburn, research shows that this strategy isn't very effective.

ANTACIDS AND H2 BLOCKERS: This can be a winning combination if you tend to get heartburn after a meal or have breakthrough heartburn pain at night.

The evidence: In one study from the Oklahoma Foundation for Digestive Research, 26 people who got heartburn four times a week took an antacid, an H2 blocker, or both. Researchers measured their heartburn symptoms and stomach acid levels and found that the combination therapy worked best. In another study, people who took an antacid and an H2 blocker for 2 weeks saw symptoms ease 52 percent, while those who just took an antacid rated their relief at 44 percent.[13, 14]

How it works: This mix of medications gives heartburn a one-two punch. Antacids get to work quickly but also wear off fast. H2 blockers take a little longer to kick in but can keep heartburn at bay for 6 to 24 hours.

What you need to know: Some OTC heartburn remedies already combine these two medications, such as Pepcid Complete.

PROTON PUMP INHIBITORS: You may need an acid-stopping PPI if your doctor says you have GERD, as acid reflux threatens to damage delicate tissue in your esophagus. These drugs are extremely effective because they lower acid levels in the stomach by as much as 90 percent. That's brought much-needed relief for many people whose severe heartburn isn't helped by other strategies.

But too many people are using these strong medications when they don't really need them. Digestive disease experts say 25 to 70 percent of heartburn sufferers on PPIs would do just as well with antacids, H2 blockers, and lifestyle changes. Thanks to heavy marketing by drug makers, the popularity of the drugs among doctors because of their effectiveness, and the easy availability of low-dose OTC versions, people continue to flock to PPIs. That's a problem, because more serious side effects are coming to light, including extra risk for bone fractures, pneumonia, and tough-to-treat digestive system infections with the bacteria *Campylobacter enteritis* and *Clostridium difficile*.[15]

The evidence: In a Swedish study, 73 percent of heartburn sufferers got significant relief within 7 days of starting a PPI. And 86 percent said symptoms were completely gone, or reduced to mild, after 16 days.[16] In a West Virginia University study of 268 people with GERD, those who took a PPI were almost twice as likely to be symptom free as those who took an H2 blocker.[17] Other research shows that for people whose GERD has damaged the esophagus, a PPI can be as effective as surgery for healing eroded areas.[18]

How it works: PPIs work by interfering with tiny molecular pumps on cells in the lining of the stomach that secrete stomach acid.

What you need to know: PPIs are best prescribed for 4 to 8 weeks to heal damaged areas of the esophagus. They can also ease chronic laryngitis and chest pain caused by acid reflux and are good at easing heartburn brought on by exercising. For best results, take your PPI a half-hour before eating; food is needed to turn on proton pumps so that PPIs can do their job.

For most people who use PPIs, it's safe to use an antacid and an H2 blocker also, as needed for breakthrough pain. Talk to your doctor first, though. PPIs can interact with drugs such as warfarin (Coumadin) and diazepam (Valium).

Other Strategies

LOSE WEIGHT: If you're overweight, losing a few pounds is a surefire way to reduce the intensity and frequency of heartburn episodes. In contrast, gaining weight can make the pain far worse.

The evidence: Being overweight increased risk for heartburn 80 percent in a German study of 7,124 people[19] and tripled odds for heartburn in a Harvard School of Public Health study of over 10,000 women. The good news? Shedding 27 pounds cut reflux episodes 40 percent in the same study.[20]

How it works: Extra weight and extra body fat around your midsection put extra pressure on the lower esophageal sphincter (LES), the muscular valve that's supposed to prevent stomach acids from washing up into your esophagus.

What you need to know: Some experts say losing as little as 5 pounds can soothe heartburn symptoms. Eating smaller meals can have an immediate benefit, too, because less food means less pressure on your LES.

QUIT SMOKING: There are so many good reasons to quit smoking, from better heart health and lower risk for cancer to protection against serious lung problems like emphysema. Now there's evidence that kicking the habit cools heartburn, too.

The evidence: Longtime smokers in a Swedish study of over 3,153 people were 70 percent more likely to have heartburn and GERD than nonsmokers.[21] In one study from the Hayden Veterans Administration Medical Center in Arizona, people who quit smoking for just one day had a significant drop in heartburn episodes.[22]

How it works: Tobacco makes heartburn worse for several reasons. Chemicals in tobacco smoke weaken the valve between your stomach and esophagus. Smoking also provokes coughing, which puts pressure on the valve and contributes to acid backwash. It also increases your body's production of stomach acid and reduces levels of saliva, which neutralizes stomach acids that splash upward.

What you need to know: The most effective quitting strategy uses a smoking cessation drug like bupropion, nicotine replacement products (patches, sprays, gum), and counseling. Be aware that nicotine replacement products could temporarily increase heartburn for some people.

CONTROL ASTHMA: Three out of four people with asthma also have acid reflux. The connection? Coughing and difficulty exhaling may trigger the backwash of stomach acid into the esophagus. Controlling asthma may ease heartburn symptoms.

The evidence: Studies show that treating GERD can improve asthma symptoms significantly. According to the American Academy of Allergy, Asthma & Immunology, controlling asthma may improve heartburn, too.

How it works: Airway obstructions that reduce pressure in your lungs may also encourage stomach acids to travel upward into your esophagus. Asthma drugs that widen airways may relax the valve that's supposed to keep stomach acids where they belong. That means you're not only dealing with asthma, but heartburn problems, too.

What you need to know: If you have asthma and heartburn that won't go away, be sure to tell your doctor. Uncontrolled reflux can make asthma worse.

TAKE CHARGE OF DIABETES: High blood sugar with type 1 and type 2 diabetes can damage nerves throughout your body, including those that control how quickly or slowly your stomach empties after a meal. Slow stomach emptying, called gastroparesis, can cause heartburn or make it worse.

The evidence: Some research suggests that better blood sugar control can help keep your stomach up to speed, which in turn could cool off heartburn pain.

How it works: Food that stays in your stomach can flow upward into your esophagus more easily. Keeping it moving lowers the risk.

What you need to know: Eating small meals, taking medications to improve stomach emptying, and controlling your blood sugar can all help.

Gallstones

Every year, about a million Americans experience the telltale belly pain of a gallbladder attack. A deep ache or a long, sharp jab, it begins somewhere in the upper right-hand section of your abdomen and may spread to your upper back. It starts out small, then builds to a painful crescendo that can sustain itself for hours before it fades away.

What's happening? Most gallbladder problems start in a digestive fluid called bile. Produced in your liver, this yellow-brown liquid is stored in your gallbladder until needed for the digestion of fat in the foods you eat. But if your liver blends too much cholesterol into your bile or if your gallbladder can't squirt its contents into your small intestine effectively, the cholesterol begins to form crystals that grow into stones. About 80 percent of gallstones are made of cholesterol; the rest are pigment stones made up of other components of bile including calcium salts and bilirubin—broken-down red blood cells.

Within hours, days, or weeks of a gallbladder attack, a half-million people a year wind up in an operating room having their gallbladder removed. Saying good-bye to this little organ causes no hardships; your liver produces the bile and surgeons hook up a duct so it gets to your intestines as needed. The upside? No repeat gallstone attacks and no chance of complications such as perforated gallbladder, an inflamed pancreas, and even gangrene if infection sets in.

But if you're among the half-million who don't (or can't) have surgery, or if you have "silent" gallstones (with no symptoms) that could act up in the future,

ThinkTwice:
The Gallstone Flush

Two-thirds of a cup of olive oil and one-third of a cup of lemon juice sound like ingredients for a tasty salad dressing, but it's also the recipe for a "gallstone flush" widely touted online and in some natural health books as an alternative to gallbladder surgery.

Proponents claim that drinking this concoction at night triggers gallbladder contractions that force out stones. They also claim you'll see proof the next morning: clumps of greenish "stones" in your bowel movement. Trouble is, these stones are actually olive oil soap, formed when the olive oil and lemon juice interact with digestive juices, say researchers from New Zealand who analyzed such stones brought in by a woman who'd tried this home remedy.[23]

A gallstone flush may not be dangerous, but it could be painful. Your gallbladder contracts in response to fat in a meal. Downing a huge quantity (like all that olive oil) could lead to strong, prolonged contractions—a problem if a stone blocks the duct leading from your gallbladder to your intestines. A better plan: If you're experiencing gallbladder attacks, talk with your doctor about surgery, or, if the stones must come out but you're not a good candidate for surgery, about a medication, such as ursodeoxycholic acid (Actigall) or chenodiol (Chenix), that can dissolve the stones over time.

it's important to do all you can now to reduce your risk for a repeat attack in the future.

You're up against big odds. The chances of new gallstones in the next few years are 50-50 if you've had nonsurgical treatments such as taking a gallstone-dissolving medication or undergoing a stone-shattering shockwave procedure called extracorporeal shockwave lithotripsy. Doing nothing is a gamble: Your odds for a repeat attack are about 70 percent if you decide simply to wait and see what happens after a first attack. (Thirty percent of people who've had one gallstone attack never have another.) If you have silent stones (often discovered during a medical scan for another purpose), your odds for a gallbladder attack within the next 10 years are one in four.

The best way to stay pain free? Don't rely on questionable home remedies like drinking vinegar or the olive oil and lemon juice "flush" widely touted on the Internet as an overnight cure. The results you'll see when you visit the bathroom in the morning aren't gallstones at all. They're actually a crude type of olive oil soap, New Zealand researchers reported recently!

Luckily, new research has uncovered plenty of surprising strategies that can really help—from avoiding crash weight loss programs and yo-yo dieting to eating the right type of fat, and from exercise to making an easy medication swap if you're a woman using hormone therapy for menopausal symptoms.

Is It Gallstone Pain?

Gallstones may be smaller than a grain of salt or grow to the size of a golf ball. Most never cause trouble. But if a stone blocks or becomes trapped in the duct between the gallbladder and the intestines, the resulting pain is a gallbladder attack. Gallstone pain can appear in different areas.

- **Abdominal pain caused by gallstones:** This is usually located in the upper right-hand section of your belly and may radiate to your upper back. It quickly grows in intensity and lasts 4 to 6 hours. You may also have nausea and vomiting. A gallstone attack often happens after eating a high-fat meal, which triggers contractions of the gallbladder that can send stones or even cholesterol-laden sludge into the bile duct.

- **Cholecystitis:** Inflammation of the gallbladder itself can be a onetime event, or, if your gallstones aren't treated, become a chronic condition that can damage your gallbladder. About 1 in 10 people with active gallstones develop this problem, which happens when a stone completely blocks the bile duct. If it lasts 6 hours or longer, it's probably acute cholecystitis. You may also have nausea and vomiting, fever and chills, and the muscles on the right side of your abdomen may grow tight and hard after a few hours.

- **Biliary pancreatitis:** This occurs when a gallstone lodged in the bile duct also blocks the duct leading to the pancreas. This can lead to infection and even damage your pancreas. Once you have one bout, your odds for repeat pancreatitis are about 60 percent—a major reason doctors recommend gallbladder surgery early for many people.[24] Symptoms are the same as for other gallstone problems: tummy pain, nausea, and vomiting. But you may also feel pain in the upper left-hand side of your abdomen or in your back, and the pain may be sudden, sharp, and severe. You may even feel a squeezing sensation.

To diagnose gallbladder problems, your doctor may use abdominal ultrasound or a computed tomography (CT) scan to look for stones. Other tests can find gallbladder inflammation and blockages in the duct between your gallbladder and small intestine. These include magnetic resonance imaging (MRI);

hepatobiliary iminodiacetic acid (HIDA) scan, also called cholescintigraphy or a hepatobiliary scan, which uses a radioactive tracer dye to follow the passage of bile from your liver through your gallbladder to your small intestine; and endoscopic retrograde cholangiopancreatography (ERCP), which uses a long, flexible, lighted tube called an endoscope, along with special dyes and x-ray equipment so your doctor can see your bile ducts. Sometimes small gallstones can be removed during an ERCP check.

Your doctor may also order blood tests to help check for complications such as infection, jaundice (yellowing of the skin caused by a buildup of bile in the bloodstream), or inflammation of the pancreas.

Fast Pain Relief

Don't treat gallstones or other gallbladder problems by yourself at home. Call your doctor or to go to the emergency room if your abdominal pain is severe. As described above, it's important to be checked for infection, inflammation, and other complications and to get prompt treatment. Since all gallbladder pain can be severe, it's impossible to tell on your own whether it's "just" gallstones or something more complex that will require surgery or other help.

If you are not hospitalized and/or don't have infection or signs of inflammation, your doctor may recommend these steps for at-home pain relief.

1. **Take a pain reliever.** An over-the-counter pain medication like ibuprofen, acetaminophen, or aspirin may be all you need, or your doctor may prescribe a stronger, prescription pain drug.

2. **Take antibiotics as directed to prevent infection.** If your doctor prescribes an antibiotic, be sure you take all of it even if you start feeling better sooner.

3. **Don't eat for a few hours, then have a low-fat meal or stick with liquids.** After a meal, your gallbladder contracts to send bile into your intestines for the digestion of fats. Avoiding food, especially fats, could prevent painful contractions.

Relief at Last

You and your doctor have three options for dealing with gallbladder problems. Here's the best strategy for each.

Step 1: If you don't want surgery now, do all you can to prevent gallstones from growing larger and to stop new ones from forming. Avoid crash diets and yo-yo dieting, get more good fats and a special type of fiber, and make time for exercise. Women using hormone therapy to control menopausal symptoms should consider switching from pills to a skin patch. *Note:* These steps won't shrink existing gallstones or encourage them to pass, but they might help you sidestep or delay future attacks.

Step 2: If you've had several attacks, or your gallbladder is inflamed, or you'd like to simply avoid future problems, choose surgery. Gallbladder surgery is generally low risk and minimally invasive; it is usually performed through a few small incisions. It stops or significantly eases pain 92 percent of the time.

Step 3: If you cannot have surgery because you are frail or have weakened immunity, consider a stone-dissolving drug or stone-blasting treatment called lithotripsy. These drugs are better than nothing, but less effective than surgery. The drugs can take up to 2 years to work and stones return in up to half of the people who try them. Lithotripsy is even less successful; stones return 70 percent of the time and many people end up having surgery anyway.

Pain Prevention Strategies

Food and Supplements

AVOID CRASH DIETS: Being overweight increases your risk for developing gallstones, but losing pounds too quickly is an even bigger risk.

The evidence: Researchers say losing more than 1½ pounds per week increases risk. So does weight cycling—losing pounds then regaining them. In one Harvard School of Public Health study of 47,000 women, those whose yo-yo dieting took off and put back on 5 to 9 pounds increased their risk for gallstone problems that required surgery by 20 percent; those who cycled through a 20-pound loss and gain increased their odds by 69 percent.[25]

Shedding pounds via weight loss surgery raises risk, too. In one Cleveland Clinic study of nearly 800 people who had weight loss procedures such as gastric bypass and gastric banding, those who lost more than 25 percent of their excess weight raised risk for gallstones fourfold.[26] Some surgeons remove the gallbladder during weight loss surgery for this reason.

How it works: Losing weight slowly seems to keep your gallbladder more active in a good way, because you're eating enough to trigger contractions after every meal. Extremely low-calorie diets seem to allow bile to pool in the gallbladder, setting the stage for cholesterol to begin to clump together.

What you need to know: Instead of slashing calories drastically, add more exercise. Other research suggests that getting at least 30 minutes of exercise 5 days a week lowers your odds for gallbladder pain by 34 percent.[27]

EAT MORE GOOD FAT, LESS SATURATED FAT: Plant-based fats—the good-for-you monounsaturated fats found in nuts, olive and canola oil, and avocados, for example—and omega-3 fatty acids found in fish, flaxseed, and walnuts all seem to lower risk for active gallbladder problems.

The evidence: In one University of Kentucky study that followed more than 45,000 men for 14 years, those who ate the most of these good fats were 18 percent less likely to have gallbladder problems.[28] Harvard School of Public Health researchers have found that men and women who snacked on an ounce of nuts—packed with healthy monounsaturated fats—five times a week were 30 percent less likely to have active gallbladder disease than those who rarely ate those tasty little nuggets.[29, 30]

In contrast, several studies show that diets packed with saturated fat—the kind found in fatty meats; full-fat dairy products like whole milk, cheese, and ice cream; and palm and coconut oils—can raise gallstone risk.

How it works: Good fats—such as nuts, olive oil, and fish oil—seem to make bile less likely to form stones by keeping cholesterol dissolved and discouraging clumping, research shows.[31, 32]

What you need to know: This dietary strategy might help you cut your risk for developing new gallstones, but it won't affect stones you already have.

EAT MORE INSOLUBLE FIBER: You may be able to sidestep a rocky future by choosing whole grain breakfast cereals (such as oatmeal), whole grain bread, and whole grain pastas instead of types made from refined flour.

The evidence: In another Harvard study, of 69,778 women, those who ate the most insoluble fiber—the type found in whole grains—were 17 percent less likely to develop problematic gallstones or need gallbladder surgery than those who took in the least. Every 5-gram increase (about the amount in two slices of whole grain bread a day) lowered risk 10 percent.

How it works: Fiber may help by reducing the amount of bile acid produced by the liver.

What you need to know: Nuts, vegetables like tomatoes, cucumbers, and squash, and fruits such as apples and berries are also good sources of insoluble fiber. Most of this fiber is in the skins, so eat nuts and produce with the skins on (wash fruits and veggies first) when possible.[33] Or look for a fiber supplement that contains insoluble fiber, such as one made from wheat bran—and be sure to take it with plenty of water to avoid discomfort!

Exercise and Movement Therapies

REGULAR EXERCISE: Don't just sit there, move! Regular physical activity discourages the formation of gallstones.

The evidence: In a Harvard School of Public Health study of over 45,000 men, those who exercised regularly lowered their risk for gallstone attacks by at least 20 percent.[34] Getting up and moving around during the day helps, too, especially if you tend to spend most of your time sitting down—whether you're at work, at home surfing the Internet, watching TV, or reading a book. Harvard researchers report that sitting for more than 40 hours a week increases your odds for a gallstone attack by 42 percent and sitting for over 60 hours each week more than doubles them.[35]

How it works: Brisk exercise switches on genes in your body that change the chemistry of your bile so that it has more bile acids and less cholesterol. This is good because a high ratio of cholesterol sets the stage for gallstones, report researchers from the University of Illinois.[36]

What you need to know: Aim for 30 to 45 minutes of brisk activity most days of the week, the level shown in studies to reduce risk for new gallstones.

Pain Medications and Medical Treatments

GALLBLADDER SURGERY: Fortunately for people with gallbladder problems, removing this organ usually has no downside beyond softer stools and more frequent bowel movements. (Surgeons connect the bile duct directly from the liver to the small intestine during the procedure so that you still have a supply of bile on hand for digesting fats.) The upside? No more gallbladder problems or complications.

Today, 90 percent of gallbladder surgeries, called cholecystectomies, are performed laparoscopically—usually through four tiny incisions in the abdomen—rather than in major surgery with big abdominal incisions and long recovery times.

The evidence: Researchers and surgeons report that the procedure is safe, has the lowest rate of gallstone recurrence (although sometimes stones already lodged in the bile ducts can act up after surgery), and stops or reduces pain significantly 92 percent of the time.

How it works: Removing the gallbladder not only gets rid of most gallstones and gallbladder inflammation, it also removes risk for even more serious complications such as inflammation of the pancreas and of the interior of the abdomen.

What you need to know: Up to 15 percent of people who undergo this procedure still have pain, nausea, vomiting, or bloating afterward—in part a result

> ## Quick Tip
> If you're using hormone replacement therapy to cool off menopause-related hot flashes, your pills could be aggravating your gallstones. In one new study, risk quadrupled for women who used HRT for over a year.[37] Luckily, a simple swap can help. When British researchers checked the health records of over one million women, they found that HRT pills increased the odds for a serious gallstone attack—the kind that lands you in the hospital—by 79 percent, while a hormone skin patch raised risk by just 17 percent.[38] So while both raise risk, the patch may be a better option if you need relief from menopausal symptoms. Switching helps because the patch sends lower doses of estrogen into your bloodstream.

of bile leaking into the abdomen, gallstones forced into the bile duct by surgery, or stones that had already moved into the duct. Some people need additional surgery or other procedures to correct problems.

ORAL DISSOLUTION THERAPY: Dissolving stones with the drugs ursodeoxycholic acid (Actigall) or chenodiol (Chenix) may be your best bet if you need gallstone treatment but can't undergo surgery because of other serious health conditions or frailty.

The evidence: In one study, people who took Actigall saw pain ease by 56 percent within 3 months. Stones were reduced in size by 59 percent in a year.[39]

How it works: These drugs slowly dissolve gallstones but can't prevent recurrences. Gallstones return within 5 years for one-quarter to one-half of all people who use these medications.[40]

What you need to know: These drugs must be taken for up to 2 years and only work on small, cholesterol-based gallstones. They may cause diarrhea, and chenodiol may also raise your blood cholesterol levels temporarily.

Ulcers

Stop blaming stress, pepperoni-and-chile-pepper pizza, or even stomach acid (even though it's strong enough to dissolve metal!). These old-time "causes" of ulcer pain miss the mark and can leave you hurting instead of healing.

For decades, wrong thinking about the real culprits responsible for ulcers led to plenty of antacid-chomping and milk-chugging but little lasting relief. Today, thanks to plenty of new research—including a dramatic experiment in which a pioneering Australian scientist infected himself with a controversial "ulcer bug"—we know that stress, food, and digestive juices sure can make things worse. But the bad actors that actually wear away the tough-as-kryptonite lining of your stomach are surprisingly commonplace, yet totally devious.

The first is a "bug" called *Helicobacter pylori*. This spiral-shaped bacterium exists in many human stomachs; by age 60 half of us have been infected with it. About 10 percent of the time, an *H. pylori* infection causes an ulcer. Most ulcers are the work of *H. pylori*. But it wasn't until the late 1990s that this understanding became widely accepted. Research shows that even today people with ulcers may not receive the most effective treatment for eradicating it unless they know to ask. That's crucial, because if you don't completely knock out this bug, you're at risk for a painful encore.

The second cause? Over-the-counter and prescription nonsteroidal anti-inflammatory pain relievers (NSAIDs). Americans pop 30 billion NSAID tablets and capsules each year, and we've all heard the warnings about upset stomachs and even bleeding that can result. NSAIDs cause a lot of ulcers, but not everyone who takes these pain pills is at risk. (We'll talk more about who should worry in a minute.)

NSAIDs lead to ulcers by the same mechanism that allows them to stop headaches, mute joint pain, and ease backaches. These drugs block enzymes called COX-1 and COX-2 that normally help produce prostaglandins, which cause pain and inflammation. Trouble is, COX-1 enzymes also ensure that your stomach is coated with a thick layer of mucus to protect it from harsh, acidic digestive juices. Without it, the acids can literally eat holes in your stomach lining, sometimes creating ulcers on their own and sometimes allowing *H. pylori* to cause trouble.

You're at high risk for an NSAID-related ulcer if you take these pain pills and are over age 65, if you also take a corticosteroid or a blood-thinning medication (such as Coumadin), if you take higher than recommended NSAID doses, or if you take more than one type on a regular basis (such as a low-dose aspirin for heart attack prevention plus ibuprofen for joint pain). One in four high-risk NSAID users will develop an ulcer and as many as 1 in 25 will develop serious ulcer complications such as bleeding and perforations of the stomach wall—unless they know what to do. Once an ulcer heals, risk for a repeat attack is high if you keep on taking NSAIDs.

The fix goes back to the premise of *Relief at Last*: doing all you can to ease pain without relying solely on drugs, and using the medication you do need safely and wisely. In this case, it might mean looking into new ways to prevent or ease a headache or a migraine, to reduce knee pain with weight loss and exercise so you don't need as much medication, or to learn the mind-body techniques that can reduce backaches. If you're taking NSAIDs for any of those reasons and are experiencing tummy troubles, we urge you to give these and the other research-proven strategies in this book a try.

If you can't cut out or cut way back on NSAIDs, we've got a Plan B: Take a stomach-protecting drug along with your pain reliever. New research shows that this strategy can allow you to keep on taking your pain reliever (good news if you have arthritis or another chronic pain condition) without risking an ulcer.

The third major ulcer-maker worth worrying about is cigarette smoking. Toxic chemicals in tobacco smoke boost levels of stomach acid, hamper the natural turnover of cells in the stomach lining, and hamstring your body's efforts to heal damaged tissue—a triple whammy that could land you with a slow-healing ulcer in no time. In one Centers for Disease Control and Prevention study of 2,851 women, 10 percent of smokers developed ulcers—double the rate of nonsmokers. Continuing to smoke after your first ulcer heals raises your odds for another significantly.

Is It an Ulcer?

The pain profiles for stomach ulcers and duodenal ulcers (ulcers at the top of the small intestine) are slightly different. You may have a stomach ulcer if you get a gnawing pain soon after eating and if antacids provide some, but not much, relief. The pain may be at your midsection, high on the right side of your abdomen, or anywhere in your tummy. You may have a duodenal ulcer if pain occurs hours after eating and/or at night and if eating or taking antacids relieves it. The pain may radiate to your back.

You may also feel full soon after starting a meal, have a heavy, bloated feeling in your abdomen, vomit, or have unexpected weight loss. One signature sign of an ulcer: pain that wakes you up between midnight and 3 a.m., when the body normally ratchets up acid levels in digestive fluids. Two-thirds of duodenal ulcers and one-third of stomach ulcers send this nighttime signal. You may also have signs of a bleeding ulcer such as black, tarry stools—an "alarm symptom" that merits a call to the doctor immediately. Your doctor will ask you about NSAID use and likely also test your breath, your blood, or your stool for signs of an *H. pylori* infection. Often, the results along with

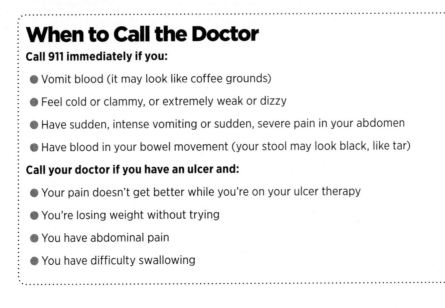

When to Call the Doctor

Call 911 immediately if you:

- Vomit blood (it may look like coffee grounds)
- Feel cold or clammy, or extremely weak or dizzy
- Have sudden, intense vomiting or sudden, severe pain in your abdomen
- Have blood in your bowel movement (your stool may look black, like tar)

Call your doctor if you have an ulcer and:

- Your pain doesn't get better while you're on your ulcer therapy
- You're losing weight without trying
- You have abdominal pain
- You have difficulty swallowing

information about your NSAID use give your doctor enough information to prescribe treatment.

If you have any signs of bleeding, of a stomach perforation, or of an obstruction, your doctor may recommend a more invasive test to assess the damage. You may have an endoscopy, in which she will thread a long, slim tube equipped with a light through your mouth and into your stomach and small intestine to take a look and to get tissue samples. Or you may be asked to swallow a chalky liquid containing barium, which shows the presence of trouble on an x-ray (called an upper GI series).

Fast Pain Relief

These steps may help while you're waiting to see the doctor.

1. **Take an antacid.** Drugstore antacids can soothe ulcer pain fast by neutralizing stomach acids so they can't burn exposed nerves in an ulcer. Types containing sodium bicarbonate or calcium carbonate (such as Caltrate or Tums) may be most effective. Use antacids only for temporary relief until you start medical treatment. Antacids can't kill *H. pylori*, and using them long term to dull the pain could allow the infection to flourish and cause more damage. Once you've started antibiotic therapy, stop taking antacids, which can interfere with the action of your drugs and lead to an incomplete cure.

2. **Switch from NSAIDs to acetaminophen.** Acetaminophen (such as Tylenol) won't irritate your stomach (but stick with recommended doses to avoid liver problems). Other options to discuss with your doctor if you must continue taking low-dose aspirin or another NSAID are to add an acid-suppressing proton pump inhibitor or a stomach-protecting drug called misoprostol (Cytotec), described below.

3. **Steer clear of alcohol, caffeine, and other irritating foods.** Edibles and beverages can't cause an ulcer. But while your ulcer is healing it makes sense to avoid foods that could irritate sensitive spots in your stomach or duodenum.

Relief at Last

We want you to be free of ulcer pain now and for years to come. To get there, follow this antiulcer strategy:

Step 1: Use "triple therapy" to wipe out *H. pylori*. Two antibiotics plus an acid-suppressing proton pump inhibitor can cure an ulcer in 14 days when *H. pylori* is present. (If you don't have an *H. pylori* infection, skip the antibiotics.)

Step 2: Add a probiotic supplement to help ease the side effects of ulcer-clearing antibiotics. Beneficial bacteria can't eliminate ulcer-causing bad bacteria on their own, but they can help keep you comfortable and minimize problems like diarrhea while you're wiping the bad guys out.

Step 3: Protect your stomach from NSAID damage. Switch to acetaminophen or reduce your dose to the lowest level possible. Adding a stomach-protecting drug is crucial if NSAIDs played a role in the rise of your ulcer. Sticking with this plan is key to keeping future ulcers at bay.

Step 4: Quit smoking. Continuing to smoke raises your risk for a relapse because chemicals in smoke seem to help *H. pylori* gain a foothold in the lining of your stomach and duodenum.

Food and Supplements

PROBIOTICS: Unfortunately, taking a supplement containing "good bacteria" isn't enough to eradicate the *H. pylori* or stop it from drilling holes in your stomach. But research shows that taking a specific probiotic while you're taking antibiotics to wipe out bad bugs can keep you comfortable.

The evidence: In one Italian study of 41 children taking antibiotics for stomach ulcers, those who also took a probiotic supplement containing *Lactobacillus reuteri ATCC 55730* had significantly less gastrointestinal distress than those who got a placebo.[41] Some experts suspect taking a probiotic along with antibiotic therapy could also help eradicate *H. pylori* more quickly and effectively, but more research is needed.

How it works: Probiotic supplements help sustain colonies of beneficial bacteria in your digestive tract that could otherwise be wiped out by antibiotics. Good bugs promote healthy digestion and can help prevent diarrhea.

What you should know: The probiotic *L. reuteri* is widely available online and in health food stores.

Pain Medication and Medical Treatments

TRIPLE THERAPY: Before the 1990s, peptic ulcers were almost never cured. That all changed when, in one of the most dramatic stories in 20th-century medical research, an Australian doctor swallowed a large "helping" of *H. pylori* bacterium in order to document what would happen next. The researcher, Barry Marshall, MD, had already shocked the scientific world by publishing a research paper with a pathologist named Robin Warren, MD, revealing the presence of the bacterium in people with stomach ulcers. At the time, scientists believed no living thing could survive in the high-acid environment of the human stomach.

Marshall developed a preulcerous condition called gastritis—inflammation of the stomach lining. Later research proved that antibiotics could treat ulcers, and the two men shared the Nobel Prize in medicine for their discovery. Since 1994, the National Institutes of Health has been recommending antibiotic therapy for ulcers, a move that can eradicate this annoying and sometimes life-threatening digestive problem.

If tests reveal an *H. pylori* infection—present in 80 to 90 percent of ulcers, including those caused by NSAIDs—the gold standard of treatment is a 14-day course of three drugs: two antibiotics and an acid-reducing proton pump inhibitor.

The evidence: Triple therapy has a cure rate of 85 to 90 percent. If you're careful afterward with NSAIDs, triple therapy also has a great track record for preventing reinfection and formation of new ulcers.[42, 43] Two antibiotics are better than one at wiping out nasty, stomach-burrowing *H. pylori*: In one Japanese study of 34 people with peptic ulcers, 89 percent who got triple therapy were cured versus 59 percent of those who took one antibiotic plus a PPI. Among those with duodenal ulcers, triple therapy fixed 91 percent while using two drugs helped just 70 percent.[44]

How it works: While the antibiotics take care of *H. pylori*, the proton pump inhibitor inhibits the release of acid from cells in the lining of your stomach. This reduces stomach acidity by 90 percent, giving painful, eroded areas of your stomach lining a chance to heal.

What you need to know: The usual triple therapy combination consists of the antibiotics amoxicillin and clarithromycin plus a PPI such as omeprazole (Prilosec), lansoprazole (Prevacid), rabeprazole (Aciphex), or esomeprazole (Nexium). If you're allergic to penicillin and cannot take amoxicillin (a related antibiotic), your doctor may prescribe metronidazole (Flagyl).

A few weeks after you finish up, a breath test or stool check can determine whether *H. pylori* has been completely knocked out. Your doctor may recommend continuing triple therapy longer if breath tests show your ulcers haven't completely healed. If this doesn't work, it may be time for quadruple therapy: That's triple therapy plus the addition of a stomach-coating bismuth product such as Pepto-Bismol or a third antibiotic.[45]

If your doctor prescribes just one or two medications—instead of three or four—to heal your ulcers, find out why. There's growing evidence that using fewer than three medications is far less effective.

STOP NSAIDS OR ADD A STOMACH-PROTECTING DRUG: Stomach and intestinal checks show that one in five NSAID users has stomach or duodenal ulcers; every year, up to 1 in 25 people who use NSAIDs on a daily basis develop serious ulcer complications like bleeding or a hole in the stomach wall.[46, 47]

The evidence: In a study of over 3,000 people, British researchers found that those who had taken NSAIDs recently were 2 to 30 times more likely to have bleeding ulcers than those who avoided these pain relievers. Over-the-counter and prescription drugs that can raise risk include buffered aspirin, ibuprofen, naproxen, and oxaprozin, as well as combination remedies such as Alka-Seltzer and Goody's Powder.[48]

How it works: NSAIDs create the perfect conditions for a stomach or duodenal ulcer; they weaken the layer of protective mucus on the inner wall of the stomach so that stomach acids can invade more easily. What should you do? Switch to acetaminophen for chronic pain relief; if that doesn't work for you, take the lowest possible NSAID dose as infrequently as possible.

What you need to know: If you must continue taking an NSAID to reduce the pain of another health condition such as arthritis, add a proton pump inhibitor (PPI) such as Prilosec, Prevacid, Aciphex, Protonix, or Nexium, which all reduce acid levels in the stomach. Taking one with your pain reliever could cut your odds for a bleeding ulcer by 54 percent, research shows. Another stomach-protecting option is the drug misoprostol (Cytotec), which you can take long term along with an NSAID.[49] In one review of the research, this drug reduced the risk for stomach ulcers by 74 percent and for duodenal ulcers by 53 percent among people taking an NSAID.[50] But there are drawbacks: Up to 40 percent of the time, it causes diarrhea and abdominal pain, and it must be taken four times a day.

A PROTON PUMP INHIBITOR, AN H2 BLOCKER, OR BOTH: If your ulcer was caused by NSAIDs and you have no signs of an *H. pylori* infection, your doctor may skip the antibiotics and prescribe a proton pump inhibitor or an acid-suppressing H2 blocker such as cimetidine (Tagamet), ranitidine (Zantac), famotidine (Pepcid), or nizatidine (Axid). Some recommend taking both.

The evidence: Experts say that 4 or more weeks of this double treatment provides better pain relief and healing of the stomach lining than either drug can deliver on its own. Studies show that H2 blockers can heal 70 percent of ulcers caused by NSAIDs; PPIs can heal 80 to 100 percent in 4 to 8 weeks.[51, 52]

How it works: PPIs shut down the mechanism inside cells that dumps acid into your stomach. H2 blockers shut down histamine, a compound that stimulates the secretion of stomach acid. The combination reduces stomach acid significantly around the clock, allowing healing to begin.

What you need to know: If you have to keep on taking an NSAID during your ulcer treatment, your doctor may ask you to keep taking a PPI for 8 weeks or longer.[53]

Other Strategies

STOP SMOKING: Chemicals in tobacco smoke raise your risk for developing an ulcer and get in the way of ulcer healing in several ways. Continuing to smoke increases your risk for a repeat and of serious ulcer complications like bleeding and perforations of the stomach.

The evidence: Smoking doubled the risk for developing ulcers in one study that followed the health and lifestyle habits of 2,851 women for 12 years. Men are at similar risk.[54]

How it works: Smoking increases the production of stomach acid, raising ulcer risk.[55] Researchers have found that compounds in tobacco smoke also help NSAIDs and *H. pylori* bugs do more damage by blocking the ability of your stomach lining to heal itself. In one study, compounds in tobacco smoke stopped cells from dividing and moving into damaged areas.[56]

What you need to know: We know quitting's tough. The best strategy for many people is a combination of a smoking cessation drug, nicotine replacement therapy, and counseling or a support group.

Irritable Bowel Syndrome

What's behind the cramps, pain, bloating, diarrhea, and constipation of irritable bowel syndrome (IBS)? If you're among the one in five adults with this uncomfortable and sometimes life-limiting condition, finding real answers could bring lasting relief.

Avoiding foods that trigger symptoms and taking a wide variety of medications—from laxatives and antidiarrheals to antidepressants and spasm-calming drugs—can keep you comfortable. But these conventional approaches don't work for everyone. Why? There's growing evidence that they don't influence some of the factors working behind the scenes to cause IBS. The good news is that simple therapies including mind-body relaxation techniques, supplements, foods containing beneficial bacteria called probiotics, and a nonabsorbable antibiotic, can help. Combining several of these strategies with IBS medications recommended by your doctor can do more to relieve IBS than drugs alone.[57] These techniques may even allow some people to stop taking some medications entirely.

Is It IBS?

Symptoms of IBS include:

- Abdominal pain

- Bloating

- Gas

For some people, constipation is a prominent symptom—with small, hard stools that are difficult to pass without lots of straining and cramping. For some, diarrhea is a bigger problem—sometimes with frequent, nearly uncontrollable urges to get to the bathroom pronto. For others, IBS fluctuates between bouts of diarrhea and constipation.

There's no lab test for IBS, but your doctor may order stool checks, blood tests, or even x-rays to rule out other abdominal problems such as inflammatory bowel disease, diabetes (which can slow down the movement of food in your digestive system), lactose intolerance, infections, the use of medicines that cause constipation or diarrhea, or an over- or underactive thyroid.

Signs that it really is IBS include:

- Abdominal pain for 12 weeks out of the past year

- More than three bowel movements a day or fewer than three a week

- Pain that improves when you have a bowel movement

- Changes in the look or frequency of your bowel movements when you have a flare-up

---

IBD or IBS?

Inflammatory bowel disease (IBD) and irritable bowel syndrome (IBS) sound so similar they could be the same problem. Both cause diarrhea, constipation, and pain. And some of the same drug-free strategies, such as dietary changes, encouraging "good" bacteria, relaxation, and antibiotics, can help both.

But, in fact, they're very different conditions. In IBD, inflammation, infection, and ulcers damage the digestive system. Sometimes the damage is so severe that surgery is necessary. In IBS, the basic machinery of your digestive system isn't harmed, but the parts don't work properly.

- Hard, lumpy stools you have to strain to pass, or loose, mushy stools

- Passing whitish mucus with your stool.

Pain Relief

Keep your medicine cabinet stocked with the natural and over-the-counter remedies recommended here, so you're ready when the discomfort of IBS strikes.

1. **For diarrhea, take loperamide (Imodium).** You can take this up to four times a day for relief. If you know that stress brings on diarrhea, you can start taking loperamide before a stressful event (like a big meeting at work or a major exam at school).

2. **For constipation, take an osmotic laxative (one that contains the active ingredients magnesium citrate, lactulose, or polyethylene glycol, such as Miralax or the prescription drug Lactulose) as directed on the package.** If these don't work, contact your doctor. Avoid stimulant laxatives (types containing senna or cascara, such as Dulcolax or Ex-Lax); they can cause severe cramping and pain.

3. **For abdominal pain and cramping, try enteric-coated peppermint oil capsules.** These have been proven to reduce muscle spasms. (For details, see the next section.)

4. **For more severe tummy pain, ask your doctor about the drugs dicyclomine (Bentyl) or hyoscyamine (Levsin), which ease muscle spasms in your gastrointestinal tract.** They work by relaxing the walls

When to Call the Doctor

Contact your doctor if you have any of these signs that IBS may be getting worse or that you may have another digestive problem as well.

- Your symptoms aren't responding to lifestyle changes or are getting worse.
- You're unintentionally losing weight or don't have an appetite.
- You're tired all the time.
- Abdominal pain doesn't feel better after a bowel movement or passing gas.
- The pain is in one area.
- There's blood in your stool.

of your intestines. You may have to try several to find the one that's best for you.

5. **For gas and bloating, try simethicone (Mylanta, Gas-X).** There are no studies to prove it, but this drugstore remedy, available as a liquid or in tablet form, may help ease gas and is worth a try at least once.

Relief at Last

These steps can help you avoid flare-ups and ensure that your digestive system functions smoothly and painlessly on a daily basis.

Step 1. Use a food diary to find, then eliminate, your personal trigger foods. Some Web sites and books recommend that you simply cut out lots of potential trouble foods. But that could leave you with a limited and less-than-nutritious diet, and could even mean denying yourself foods you like that aren't making trouble. A better plan: Personalize your trigger food list by first keeping a food and symptom diary for 2 weeks. When you spot potential problem foods, eliminate them one at a time and see if symptoms improve. Our Pain Diary in Part Three may help you pinpoint triggers.

Step 2: Encourage good bacteria. Probiotic supplements (and/or yogurt with live active cultures) can bolster colonies of "good bugs" in your digestive system proven to reduce inflammation and quiet your symptoms. Slowly increasing the amount of soluble fiber in your diet—from foods like beans, barley, pears, and oatmeal (and a fiber supplement if you can't get enough soluble fiber from food)—helps by creating probiotic-friendly conditions.

Step 3: Relax your mind and your digestive system with a mind-body therapy. Gut-focused hypnotherapy, cognitive-behavior therapy, progressive muscle relaxation, and yoga are all proven to reduce pain and ease IBS symptoms dramatically. It's worth adding at least one of these serious relaxation techniques to your tool kit of IBS-control strategies.

Step 4: Ask about the nonabsorbable antibiotic rifaximin (Xifaxan). There's growing evidence that an overgrowth of bacteria in the small intestine can trigger IBS flare-ups for up to 84 percent of people with IBS.[58] In studies, rifaximin eased symptoms significantly, and the benefits continued for at least 10 weeks.

Step 5: Still having pain and other symptoms? Ask your doctor about an antidepressant. Antidepressants don't just ease depression. They're widely prescribed for IBS because they can relieve pain and improve most other symptoms including diarrhea, constipation, bloating, nausea, and that sense of urgency that makes you want to stay close to a bathroom. Antidepressants are usually given to people with moderate to severe IBS that doesn't respond completely to healthy lifestyle changes and other treatments. They can take 4 to 6 weeks to work, but often you need only a low dose to get relief.

Food and Supplements

KEEP A FOOD DIARY TO SPOT TROUBLE FOODS: Up to two-thirds of people with IBS say some foods and drinks trigger their symptoms.[59] Instead of eliminating a laundry list of foods, find out what bothers your digestive system and cut out the worst offenders one at a time.

The evidence: In one study, 150 people who stopped eating their personal trigger foods experienced a 26 percent reduction in pain and other symptoms.[60]

How it works: Research suggests that some foods seem to trigger an immune reaction—a food sensitivity that could be related to IBS symptoms. When British researchers ran blood tests on 132 people with IBS and 42 people without IBS after they ate 16 common foods, they found higher levels of the antibody IgG after the IBS group ate beef, lamb, pork, soybeans, and wheat.[61]

What you should know: Common problem foods that might set off pain and diarrhea include alcohol, chocolate, caffeinated beverages such as coffee and sodas, medications that contain caffeine, dairy products, and sugar-free sweeteners such as sorbitol or mannitol. For some people, high-fat foods also cause pain. Gas and bloating may get worse after eating beans, broccoli, cabbage, and cauliflower, too. Some people with IBS cannot digest gluten, a protein found in grains like wheat, rye, and barley; eating these grains can set off an immune reaction that can damage the small intestine.

Before you eliminate any food, make sure it's a troublemaker by keeping a food diary. For 2 weeks, track your symptoms as well as what you eat at meals and for snacks. Note the time of day and how long symptoms lasted. When you've got 14 days' worth of information, start looking for patterns. If you find some foods that always seem to lead to discomfort, eliminate the one that seems like the biggest troublemaker. If symptoms improve, try eliminating a second problem food. But be sure not to restrict your diet too much; you need a healthy mix of produce, whole grains, low-fat dairy, lean protein, and good fats for optimal health.

SOLUBLE FIBER: Found in oatmeal, pears, dried beans, barley, and fiber supplements such as psyllium (Metamucil), soluble fiber forms a soothing gel in your intestinal tract that can help with diarrhea, constipation, and pain. Adding more fiber isn't the right IBS relief strategy for everyone; for some it can increase pain,[62] but for others slowly boosting fiber intake can bring relief.

The evidence: In a Dutch study of 275 people with IBS, those who added 2 teaspoons of psyllium powder a day to their diets saw symptoms including pain, diarrhea, and constipation improve by 59 percent compared to those who got a fake (placebo) powder made from rice. Those who got a supplement of insoluble fiber (the kind found in whole grains as well as corn and other vegetables) saw some improvement as well, but soluble fiber seems especially helpful for IBS.[63]

How it works: Soluble fiber multitasks in your digestive system. It can ease diarrhea by holding stool together and improve constipation by making bowel movements softer and larger so that they move more easily when muscles in the walls of your intestines contract.

What you need to know: Go slowly when adding fiber to your diet. Add one new high-fiber food per week or start with a small dose of a soluble fiber supplement that you mix with water. Water is key to comfort; without it, extra fiber in your digestive system can cause gas, constipation, and cramping.

PEPPERMINT OIL CAPSULES: Peppermint is an age-old herbal remedy for soothing tummy troubles. Now there's proof that it can help with IBS pain. If needed, you can take it for several weeks to keep pain and spasms at bay during and after a flare-up.

The evidence: In one Turkish study of 90 people with IBS who took a peppermint oil capsule or placebo three times a day for 8 weeks, one-third of the peppermint group saw abdominal pain ease significantly.[64] In another study, 57 people with IBS who took two peppermint oil capsules twice a day for 4 weeks got at least a 50 percent drop in pain and other symptoms.[65]

How it works: Compounds in peppermint oil can ease muscle spasms, including fast, painful contractions of the muscles in the walls of your intestinal tract.

What you need to know: Studies of this remedy use enteric-coated peppermint oil capsules rather than peppermint tea or peppermint leaves. The capsules are designed to withstand digestion in your stomach. That way, the oil is delivered to your intestines. If you're having active diarrhea, the oil could cause anal burning.

PROBIOTICS: Your gastrointestinal system normally plays host to a healthy balance of trillions of bacteria. IBS symptoms may rear up when bad bacteria begin to colonize the upper reaches of your small intestine, an area that's usually a low-bug zone. The beneficial types in probiotic capsules and in yogurt could help right the balance.

The evidence: In one North Carolina study of 44 people with IBS, those who took a probiotic supplement containing *Bifidobacteria lactis* and *Bifidobacteria bifidum* (also found in yogurts containing live active cultures) for 1 week got a 50 percent reduction in pain, intestinal spasms, constipation, and diarrhea. In a Korean study of 70 people with IBS, probiotics eased tummy pain and pain during bowel movements by an average of 31 percent.[66]

How it works: Good bacteria—which may be in short supply in the intestinal tracts of people with IBS—have been shown in lab studies to reduce pain sensations in the intestinal wall. There's also evidence that probiotics quiet

Where the Good Bugs Are

From yogurt and dairy drinks to pills, powders, and capsules, probiotics come in many forms and contain a dizzying variety of good bacteria with strange-sounding names. It can be a challenge choosing one. These buying tips can help.

- **Look for a science-based product.** Good-quality products give you the exact names of the strains of bacteria they contain, the amounts, and often, if you check manufacturer Web sites, published studies that back up their products.

- **Get the right probiotic organisms for your condition.** Specific strains of probiotic bacteria at specific doses have shown promise for relieving painful digestive disease conditions. It's smart to look for those. You'll find examples throughout this chapter, but here are some probiotics to seek out for specific conditions.

   Diverticulitis: *Lactobacillus acidophilus, Lactobacillus casei, Lactobacillus plantarum, Saccharomyces boulardii* and *bifidobacteria*
   Irritable bowel syndrome: *B. infantis 35624*
   Inflammatory bowel disease: *Lactobacillus GG, E. coli* strain Nissle 1917, VSL#3, *Saccharomyces boulardii*
   Ulcers: *Lactobacillus reuteri* (to help ease side effects of antibiotic therapy)

immune system activity in the intestines, which can cause pain and other symptoms when in high gear.[67]

What you need to know: There are many probiotic supplements containing different mixes of bacteria on the market. Types that have improved IBS in research studies include *Bifidobacteria* strains (as mentioned above) as well as *Lactobacillus* strains, both found in many yogurts with live active cultures and many common probiotic capsules and powders.

Exercise and Movement Therapies

YOGA: With a few simple poses—there's no need to bend yourself into a pretzel—yoga can relax you and your nervous system enough to ease IBS symptoms.

The evidence: Daily at-home yoga was as effective as the diarrhea-stopping drug loperamide for IBS with diarrhea in a group of 25 men, researchers from India report.[69]

How it works: Yoga may ease diarrhea by calming down your nervous system and easing overactive bowel activity, say researchers from the All India Institute of Medical Sciences, New Delhi.

What you need to know: Yoga participants practiced a set of 12 basic, relaxing poses (including Camel Pose, Zen Pose, Cat Cow Pose, and Triangle Pose) as well as a calming breath exercise twice a day. For a simple stress-relieving yoga routine, turn to Part Three.

Mind-Body Therapies

GUT-FOCUSED HYPNOTHERAPY: Not a party trick, medical hypnotherapy has serious

On the Horizon

Anorectal Biofeedback Therapy

If painful constipation is part of your constellation of IBS symptoms, retraining the muscles of your pelvic floor with a biofeedback technique called anorectal biofeedback therapy could help. This approach helps you learn to contract and relax muscles that may not be working in a coordinated way.

It really works. When 25 Australian women with IBS tried this technique, 75 percent said their IBS pain and constipation improved.[68] The reason? Chronic constipation in IBS may be the result of pelvic floor dyssynergia, in which the muscles used in a bowel movement don't operate in a synchronized way.[70] Training with small water balloons (not real stool) plus a biofeedback probe to help you tell what's happening can get your muscles working as a team again.

Anorectal biofeedback therapy is available at some large medical centers.

benefits and such a great track record for easing IBS symptoms that the American Gastroenterological Association has approved its use for this painful condition and England's National Institute of Clinical Excellence recommends it for IBS when medications fail.

The evidence: Five sessions of gut-focused hypnotherapy helped reduce pain and diarrhea in one British study and the benefits lasted at least 3 months, British researchers report. While improvements did fade over time, the hypnosis group needed less medication to control its IBS than another group of study volunteers who didn't undergo hypnosis.

How it works: Hypnotherapy may help simply because it relaxes your digestive system. Plenty of research shows that this can improve pain, diarrhea, bloating, gas, and constipation.

What you need to know: Medical hypnotherapy won't put you into a trance or make you do crazy things. You'll feel extremely relaxed yet alert, and open to suggestions and images from a trained hypnotherapist about helping your gastrointestinal system work better. For more information about finding a qualified medical hypnotherapist, turn to Part Three. You can also find hypnotherapy programs for IBS on CDs for home use from Healthy Audio Limited (www.healthyaudio.com).

COGNITIVE-BEHAVIORAL THERAPY: Aimed at helping you identify and cope with the everyday stresses that can make IBS flare up, cognitive-behavioral therapy (CBT) can help you learn relaxation techniques, change thinking patterns that dial up stress, and problem-solve solutions to your personal tension triggers.

The evidence: CBT that's focused on easing IBS symptoms really works. In one University of Buffalo study of 75 people with IBS, those who took a CBT self-study course or met with a counselor saw pain ease by as much as 90 percent and bowel symptoms ease by up to 80 percent.[71]

How it works: Learning to overcome stress helps relax your digestive system and turns down the volume on pain signals that are amplified when you're tense and anxious. CBT can also help you feel more in control of your IBS, instead of overwhelmed.

What you need to know: In some studies, CBT worked best in conjunction with a variety of IBS medications.

PROGRESSIVE MUSCLE RELAXATION: Letting go of bodywide muscle tension doesn't just feel good or help you fall asleep faster, it may also put a damper on IBS pain.

An Antibiotic for IBS

There's growing evidence that an overgrowth of bacteria in the small intestine may be the hidden source of IBS pain, bloating, and gas. Now, researchers say a nonabsorbable antibiotic (it stays in your intestines rather than entering your bloodstream) already widely used to treat inflammatory bowel disease might help with IBS, too.

In two new studies of 1,200 people with IBS, researchers found that those who took the antibiotic rifaximin (Xifaxan) for 2 weeks had significantly less pain, bloating, and gas. Thirty-seven percent saw symptoms improve by at least 50 percent. Benefits continued for at least 10 weeks after treatment stopped—a first for IBS drug therapies.

Rifaximin seems to help by killing off excess bacteria in your small intestine that may be churning out gas after you eat a meal.[72] It's still being studied but is FDA approved for traveler's diarrhea and widely prescribed for other bowel conditions.

The evidence: Researchers from the Center for Stress and Anxiety Disorders at the State University of New York at Albany found that people with IBS who performed progressive muscle relaxation exercises regularly were five times more likely to get a break from pain and abdominal cramping than those who didn't.[73] It was a very small study, but relaxation can't hurt and could help.

How it works: Stress and tension can make pain feel stronger; relaxation seems to turn down the volume on pain signals transmitted to your brain, research suggests.

What you need to know: For more information and a full-body muscle relaxation exercise, turn to Chapter 5.

Pain Medication and Medical Treatments

ANTIDEPRESSANTS: Several types of antidepressants seem to help reduce pain and ease the diarrhea and constipation of IBS. These medications are often prescribed even if you're not depressed, though research suggests that some types work better than others.

The evidence: Tricyclic antidepressants such as amitriptyline (Elavil), imipramine (Tofranil), desipramine (Norpramin), and nortriptyline (Pamelor) have been used to help ease IBS pain and diarrhea for more than a decade. Newer selective serotonin reuptake inhibitors (SSRIs), once believed to help IBS, are proving to be less effective, though they may help somewhat in people who are taking them for depression.

How it works: Antidepressants block pain messages sent from nerves in the walls of your intestines to your brain. Tricyclic antidepressants can also help firm up loose bowel movements.[74]

What you need to know: If your doctor recommends an antidepressant, you may need to take it for 6 months to a year or longer. Side effects vary with the drug you take, but can include anxiety, decreased sex drive, fatigue, weight gain, dry mouth, and headaches.

Diverticulitis

If you avoid vegetables, wrinkle up your nose at whole grains, and tend to load your plate instead with low-fiber fare like white bread, white rice, French fries, cheese, and meat, beware: You're following the recipe for diverticulitis to a T.

Fiber keeps bowel movements soft, big, and regular. Skip it and you're likely to end up with small, hard stools and constipation as well as an unseen danger: high pressure in your large intestine as you and your body work hard to push a bowel movement along. Over time this extra pressure creates tiny, bulging pouches in your intestines called diverticula—the lining of your intestines bulges out in areas where the walls are weak. An estimated 30 percent of people in their fifties and sixties have diverticula—as do half of all those in their seventies and eighties.

These little sacs usually don't cause any trouble. But if they become infected and inflamed, you will wind up with intense pain, fever, nausea, and constipation or diarrhea.[75] This is diverticulitis, and it can lead to complications such as bleeding, dangerous internal blockages, and even holes in the walls of your intestines.

In the past, people with diverticulitis were told to avoid high-fiber foods (like popcorn, nuts, and seeds). They were also told that one in five people with diverticulitis ultimately needs surgery to remove the damaged section of bowel. Today, digestive disease experts have a better handle on how to prevent problems and, for many people, how to avoid surgery.

The new thinking? High intestinal pressure can lead to repeat attacks, so getting plenty of fiber is essential. Research shows that most people can eat corn, seeds, and nuts, too. Adding beneficial bacteria as a supplement or in yogurt protects against damage and can help damp down inflammation. Eliminating an overgrowth of bacteria in your small intestine with a special antibiotic, it turns out, may help, too. And for diverticulitis that keeps coming back, experts now recommend taking an inflammation-fighting drug that could lower your odds for needing surgery.

Is It Diverticulitis?

Your abdominal pain may be diverticulitis if:

- It's located in the lower left-hand side of your abdomen

- It hurts more after you eat

- It comes on quickly and intensely (though some diverticulitis begins as a mild ache that grows more severe over 2, 3, or 4 days)

- It eases up when you have a bowel movement or pass gas

Since the pain comes and goes, it's tempting to try to tough out an attack of diverticulitis at home. Don't do it! It's important to see your doctor so that she can rule out other digestive system conditions such as appendicitis, food poisoning, hemorrhoids, inflammatory bowel disease, even uterine fibroids or colon cancer. Your doctor can evaluate your diverticulitis in order to decide on the best treatment so that you won't have complications or to control things if you already do.

In order to diagnose diverticulitis, your doctor will probably ask you about your bathroom habits, your diet, and medications you're taking that could be causing symptoms or could make you constipated for long periods of time. Your doctor may also run tests to confirm her diagnosis. Options include a barium enema, in which you're given an enema containing tracer dyes that let your doctor see your colon on an x-ray; flexible sigmoidoscopy, in which your doctor uses a long, thin tube with an attached light and video camera to examine your rectum and the lower part of your colon; colonoscopy, like a sigmoidoscopy but more extensive, allowing your doctor to view your entire colon; or a computed tomography (CT) scan, a more detailed x-ray that reveals more information about the presence of inflamed or infected pouches in your intestinal wall.

Fast Pain Relief

Some people need prompt hospitalization so that serious or even life-threatening complications of diverticulitis can be treated. But more often these steps can help you feel comfortable again.

1. **Take a pain reliever.** An over-the-counter type like ibuprofen (Motrin) or acetaminophen (Tylenol) may be all you need. If your pain is more

severe, your doctor may prescribe a short course of a stronger pain reliever. Take these exactly as directed; prescription pain relievers like codeine can cause constipation, which will make your diverticulitis worse.

2. **Give your bowels a rest with a clear liquid diet.** Sticking with water, tea, broth, and clear fruit juices can help your colon heal. After 2 to 3 days, it's usually okay to reintroduce bland, low-fiber foods such as applesauce, rice, saltine crackers, plain noodles, white bread, baked chicken or fish, gelatin, soups, and cooked vegetables.

3. **Take antibiotics as directed.** Your doctor may prescribe any of a number of antibiotics to heal the infection in your colon, such as ampicillin, gentamicin, metronidazole, piperacillin, clindamycin, or ceftazidime. Be sure to finish the entire prescription even if you start feeling better before all your pills are gone. Stopping early could allow the infection to return and lead to a new attack.

Relief at Last

After a first bout of diverticulitis, three out of four people never have another.[76] You can increase the odds that you'll end up in this lucky, pain-free club by taking these important steps.

Step 1: **Increase the fiber in your diet.** Boost it slowly so you stay comfortable, but be sure to add more fiber-rich produce and whole grains each week and consider adding a fiber supplement if you can't get to 30 grams every day. Fiber is the best way to keep pressure in your intestines low and to reduce your risk for more diverticula and more inflammation of the ones you have already.

Step 2: Eat danger foods less often and in smaller quantities. Processed foods high in fat, sugar, and refined carbohydrates can raise your risk for another attack. So can diets packed with red meat and processed meat products (like hot dogs, lunch meat, and sausage). These foods cause problems when they dominate your plate and leave little room for high-fiber good stuff. But that's not the only reason to avoid them. It turns out these foods also encourage the bacteria in your digestive system to release compounds that may weaken your intestinal walls just enough to boost the risk for pouches to form.

Step 3: Snack on yogurt or pop a probiotic supplement. Beneficial bacteria—the probiotics found in yogurt and in supplements—help damp down inflammation in your intestines. The good bugs may also help keep your intestinal walls strong and pouch-proof.

Step 4: Ask your doctor about the antibiotic rifaximin (Xifaxan). There's growing evidence that an overgrowth of bacteria in your small intestine may fuel frequent attacks of diverticulitis by sending bacteria along that infect the diverticula, the tiny pouches bulging from the intestinal wall. Rifaximin fights this overgrowth. Since little is absorbed into your bloodstream, levels stay higher in your intestines, a plus that means fewer antibiotic side effects and more bacteria-controlling power.

Step 5: If diverticulitis keeps coming back, ask about an inflammation-fighting medicine, too. Prescription drugs called 5-amino salicylic acids (5-ASAs) can help keep a lid on inflammation and prevent repeat attacks of diverticulitis. Taking one long term along with an antibiotic could help you avoid flare-ups and complications for years on end and reduce the need for bowel surgery.

Pain Prevention Strategies

Food and Supplements

FIBER: Surprised to see fiber at the top of our list? While this indigestible component of fruit, vegetables, and whole grains can increase pain and discomfort during a flare-up, it's proven to keep symptoms at bay once an attack ends. Here's why: Getting 30 grams a day—double the amount most of us manage to take in—could cut your odds for repeat attacks in half.[77]

The evidence: In a British study of 100 people who had been hospitalized with diverticulitis, 90 percent who switched to a high-fiber diet were still symptom free 7 years later.[78] In another study, people who got more fiber had less pain during bowel movements, and abdominal pain became less severe and less frequent as well.[79]

How it works: Fiber makes bowel movements softer and fluffier so they slide along easily in your intestines rather than pressing and grinding the way hard, dry stool can. Muscles in the walls of your intestines have to work harder when your stool is small and compact; this creates extra pressure in your intestines that can create new diverticula or inflame existing pouches.[80] In contrast, intestinal pressure is lower when you eat plenty of fiber.

But that's not all. Dietary fiber also acts as a prebiotic, creating the perfect environment in your intestines for beneficial bacteria that help regulate your immune system, thereby soothing inflammation. Fiber also helps preserve the protective layer of mucus on your intestines' inner walls.

What you need to know: It's usually okay to start increasing your fiber intake a month after a flare-up. Check with your doctor first to see what's right for you. If you weren't in the habit of eating a lot of high-fiber foods before your flare-up, build up slowly, as adding lots of fiber at once to your diet can be uncomfortable. See how your body responds to new, fiber-rich edibles. If a particular food causes pain or discomfort, stop eating it and try something else. Drinking at least eight 8-ounce glasses of water a day can help, too.

FIBER SUPPLEMENTS: If you find you're not getting 30 grams of fiber every day from food, add a powdered fiber supplement that you mix with water.

The evidence: In one study, 60 percent of people who got 18 grams of fiber a day from a bran supplement were symptom free. Other studies show that getting more fiber can help with constipation and lower colonic pressure, which protects the lining of the intestines from further damage and inflammation.[81, 82]

How it works: Like the fiber in food, the fiber from a supplement softens and bulks up your stools and speeds up transit time—the time it takes for stool to make its way through your intestinal tract.

What you need to know: Many types of fiber may help. Since cellulose-rich foods are beneficial, consider a supplement containing cellulose such as Benefiber or Unifiber. See how your body responds, though. A supplement containing soluble fiber, such as psyllium (Metamucil), which forms a gel in your digestive system, may be more soothing.

HEALTHIER SNACKS: Processed foods high in fat, sugar, and other refined carbohydrates could increase your odds for an attack. The healthy stuff lowers them.

The evidence: In one study, people who ate fruits such as peaches, blueberries, apricots, apples, and oranges reduced their risk for a diverticulitis attack by as much as 80 percent. In contrast, those who munched French fries, cookies, or a small bag of chips five or six times a week boosted their chances for a flare-up by as much as 69 percent.[83]

How it works: Fresh fruit delivers all the soothing, protective powers of fiber. Junk foods contain little or no fiber but are packed with fats that research suggests may weaken intestinal walls and promote the formation of diverticula.

What you need to know: Always pay attention to your own body's responses to foods. If a particular fruit (or any food) irritates your digestive system, try another.

Foods That Fight Diverticulitis

Produce and whole grains containing a form of fiber called cellulose protect the inner lining of your intestines from damage that boosts odds for diverticulitis flare-ups, say Harvard School of Public Health researchers.[84] These include:

FOOD	SERVING	TOTAL FIBER	CELLULOSE
Beans (legumes)	½ cup	6.7 grams	2.79 grams
Peas	½ cup	4.4 grams	2.14 grams
Tomato sauce	½ cup	4.2 grams	1.97 grams
Potatoes with skin	1 cup	4.2 grams	1.60 grams
Apple	1 medium	3.7 grams	1.03 grams
Carrots	½ cup	2.6 grams	0.97 gram
Whole grain cereal	1 cup	6 grams	0.68 gram
Banana	1 medium	2.7 grams	0.50 gram
Whole grain bread	1 slice	1.1 grams	0.33 gram
Orange	1 medium	3 grams	0.30 gram

CHICKEN OR FISH INSTEAD OF RED MEAT: Opting for fish, chicken, or vegetarian sources of protein like beans or tofu instead of a burger, steak, or hot dog is a smart move.

The evidence: According to Greek researchers, a diet focused on red meat doubles risk.[85] Other research suggests that a meat-heavy diet might increase odds 25 times higher than normal![86] And having a 4- to 6-ounce serving of beef, pork, or lamb 5 to 7 nights a week tripled risk in one Harvard study. Processed meats are bad news, too. The same study found that a weekly hot dog raised odds 86 percent; a serving of lunch meat five to six times a week nearly doubled risk.[87]

How it works: Red meats increase oxidative stress and seem to trigger bacteria in your colon to release damaging substances that weaken the walls of your intestines, allowing pouches to form.

What you need to know: Research suggests that having some chicken or fish may not raise risk as much, but regardless of your protein choice, be sure you're also getting plenty of fiber. One of the big problems with any meat-heavy diet is skimping on fiber-rich whole grains, fruit, and veggies.

PROBIOTICS: Beneficial bacteria—the probiotics found in yogurt and in supplements—are emerging as important players in cutting-edge strategies to stop flare-ups.

The evidence: In one study, most people who took a supplement containing the gut-friendly bacterium *Lactobacillus casei* regularly were still symptom

---

Popcorn and Seeds Are Okay!

For many years doctors have warned people with diverticula to avoid nuts, seeds, and popcorn over worries that small, hard foods could lodge in the pouches and kick-start the inflammation, infection, and pain of a diverticulitis attack. But that's all changed. When University of Washington researchers checked up on 47,288 men, they found that those who munched these treats at least twice a week were 20 percent less likely to develop diverticulitis than those who ate them less than once a month. The reason? All are packed with digestion-friendly fiber, and nuts and seeds contain good fats that may even help soothe inflammation.

Of course, if you're just recovering from a flare-up, go easy. It may be a while before you're ready to munch a big bowl of popcorn while watching a movie!

free when researchers checked on them a year later.[88] In contrast, those who stopped taking this probiotic supplement saw symptoms return. *L. casei* is found in many types of yogurts containing live active cultures and is also available as a supplement.

How it works: Your intestinal tract is home to trillions of bacteria. They help with digestion, absorption, and even help control your immune system and protect the fragile inner lining of your intestines. By encouraging the growth of friendly types, you get benefits that can help prevent diverticulitis flare-ups—such as faster passage of stool, protection against damage to intestinal walls, and prevention of inflammation.

What you need to know: Other probiotics that soothe and protect your intestines include *Lactobacillus acidophilus, Lactobacillus plantarum, Saccharomyces boulardii* and *bifidobacteria*. If you take a supplement, follow package directions. In studies, probiotics work best when used along with medications that control inflammation, such as mesalamine.[89]

Exercise and Movement Therapies

REGULAR VIGOROUS EXERCISE: There's no doubt: Regular exercise cuts the risk for diverticulitis.

The evidence: In one study, physical activity lowered odds for diverticular disease by 48 percent. In another, from the University of Washington, people who got serious exercise several times a week—such as running—were 46 percent less likely to experience bleeding from diverticulitis.[90]

How it works: A good workout may cut risk by helping to prevent constipation.

What you need to know: Activity that works up a sweat and raises your heart rate, such as a brisk walk, a fast ride on an exercise bike, or a challenging exercise class or DVD, may be the most protective. Getting exercise and adding fiber to your diet is even better: When Harvard School of Public Health researchers tracked 47,678 men, they found that those who got the least activity and ate the least fiber were $2\frac{1}{2}$ times more likely to develop diverticulitis as those who got the most of both.[91]

Pain Medications and Medical Treatments

RIFAXIMIN: The antibiotic rifaximin (Xifaxan) stays in your gastrointestinal tract—it's not absorbed into your bloodstream—and battles overgrowths of bacteria that experts suspect can trigger flare-ups.

The evidence: In an Italian study of 307 people with diverticulitis, those who took rifaximin plus a fiber supplement regularly for 2 years had less pain, bleeding, bloating, and fewer other symptoms than those who only got the fiber.[92]

How it works: There's emerging evidence that an overload of bacteria in the small intestine can trigger flare-ups of diverticulitis. Signs of small intestine bacterial overgrowth (also known as SIBO) include bloating, gaseousness, and diarrhea or constipation. Wiping out these bad bugs with an antibiotic that stays in your intestinal tract is proven to help.[93]

What you need to know: Rifaximin is often prescribed along with a fiber supplement and/or the anti-inflammatory medicine mesalamine to better prevent repeat bouts of diverticulitis and to control discomfort. You may have to take it off and on for a year to get the benefits.[94]

5-AMINO SALICYLIC ACIDS (5-ASAS): Digestive disease experts are discovering that medications called 5-aminosalicylic acids (5-ASAs), long used to control Crohn's disease and ulcerative colitis, can be extremely effective at preventing recurrences of diverticulitis.[95]

The evidence: In a yearlong Italian study of 268 people with diverticulitis, those who took 800 milligrams of the 5-ASA drug mesalamine (Asacol) for 10 days a month were less likely to have signs of a flare-up such as upper or lower abdominal pain or tenderness, bleeding, bloating, nausea, diarrhea, or fever than those who took an antibiotic.[96] Other research suggests that combining mesalamine and the antibiotic rifaximin works better than either drug alone.[97]

How it works: Mesalamine short-circuits diverticulitis flare-ups by soothing the intestinal lining and preventing inflammation.

What you need to know: Some people take mesalamine long term, either every day or several times each month for several months or even years, to prevent flare-ups. It is often prescribed along with the antibiotic rifaximin to prevent the two causes of repeat attacks: inflammation and infection.

SURGERY: One in five people with diverticulitis may ultimately need surgery, though new medications mean those numbers are dropping. Emergency surgery to remove infected sections of your large intestine—called a partial colectomy—can be life-saving if you're experiencing serious complications such as ruptures, heavy bleeding, widespread infection, inflammation of other organs such as your bladder or uterus, intestinal blockages, and breakthrough perforations in the intestinal wall (holes called fistulas) that allow infection and stool to escape into your abdomen.

But digestive disease experts are beginning to question elective surgery for people whose diverticulitis might be controlled with medication instead. In the past, a partial colectomy was recommended if you'd had two serious flare-ups (or one serious attack before age 50). The goal was to prevent complications. Now there's evidence that these nonemergency procedures often don't help.

The evidence: In one Irish review of the results of elective surgery for diverticulitis, the researchers concluded that the procedure doesn't save lives or lower risk for complications. They estimate surgeons would have to operate on 18 people to prevent one diverticulitis-related medical emergency.[98] Risk for a flare-up

Is Your Pain Reliever Triggering Diverticulitis?

Many over-the-counter and prescription drugs can set the stage for a flare-up of diverticulitis. If you're taking one and are experiencing symptoms, talk to your doctor about alternatives.

Drugstore pain relievers: Ibuprofen, aspirin, naproxen, and prescription-strength NSAIDs can cause GI bleeding. Using aspirin several times a week doubled risk for diverticulitis symptoms in one Harvard Medical School study. Ibuprofen and other nonsteroidal anti-inflammatories (like naproxen) quadrupled it and acetaminophen raised risk 13 times higher than normal.[99]

Opioids: Narcotics like morphine, codeine, oxycodone, and others are notorious for causing constipation, which raises risk for a flare-up, too.

Other constipating drugs: Antacids that contain aluminum or calcium, antidepressants, antihistamines, calcium channel blockers, diuretics, and iron supplements also raise risks.

in the 15 years after elective surgery is about 16 percent, Dutch researchers say.[100] Instead of operating after two flare-ups, the scientists say doctors should look for signs of trouble like recurring bleeding, narrowing of the lower part of the large intestine, or existing fistulas—breaks in the intestinal wall.[101]

How it works: Surgery removes damaged areas of the intestines. It can save your life if you have the serious complications mentioned above, such as heavy bleeding and widespread infection, but may not be useful if you don't.

What you need to know: If your doctor recommends elective surgery, ask whether the inflammation-fighting 5-ASA drug mesalamine (Asafol) plus the antibiotic rifaximin (Xifaxan) is a good alternative for you. There's growing evidence that it can keep flare-ups and serious complications at bay for years or perhaps permanently, eliminating the need for surgery for some people.[102]

Other Strategies

LOSE WEIGHT: Once rare in people under the age of 50, diverticulitis is on the rise thanks to the growing obesity epidemic. Maintaining a healthy weight could help you avoid developing diverticulitis in the first place and might help you sidestep a recurrence.

The evidence: When University of Maryland researchers checked scans of people who came to an emergency room with abdominal pain, they found that carrying extra weight and having a large waist increased diverticulitis risk.[103] In another study, overweight men were 78 percent more likely to have diverticulitis than lean men.[104]

How it works: Overweight may be a risk factor simply because it's a sign of a low-fiber, high-fat diet and a sedentary lifestyle.

What you need to know: Weight loss has not yet been studied as a way to avoid flare-ups. But slimming down by following a high-fiber diet filled with fruit, vegetables, and whole grains could help.

Kidney Stones

Imagine a sharp rock stuck inside a garden hose. Turn on the tap and water pushes the rock along slowly, scratching and scraping the hose as it moves through.

That's what happens when a kidney stone lodges in one of the long, thin tubes that carry urine from your kidneys to your bladder. It's a pain like no other, and can go on for days or even weeks as the stone makes its way out of your body. The journey is agonizing. Ultimately, 90 percent of kidney stones exit your body on their own. The rest need medical intervention. But once you've passed a kidney stone (and heaved a big sigh of relief), the story's not over, because it's time to prevent the next one.

If you're among the 15 percent of adults who develop these miserable miniboulders, your odds for a repeat attack in the next 5 years are as high as 50 percent, so the pain could easily return. But it doesn't have to. If you're trying to avoid an encore attack or want to hasten the passage of a stone that's causing problems right now, new research shows that there's plenty you can and should be doing. The right moves go far beyond conventional advice like chugging lots of water!

New research shows that what you eat and drink can play a big role in whether you develop one of these stones, but the best antistone diet may surprise you. (Some clues: Milk and cheese are back on the menu, along with lemonade and even diet soft drinks, but meat, salt, and sugar could cause trouble.) Other research shows that the usual exit strategy when you have a stone—rest, water, and lots of painkillers—isn't always effective. Adding a drug usually prescribed for high blood pressure, it turns out, helps more stones find their way out of your body, reducing the odds that you'll need a medical procedure to remove one.

Is It a Kidney Stone?

The telltale sign that a kidney stone has lodged in one of your ureters—the tubes that carry urine from your kidneys to your bladder—is pain in your side. It may start small, then build to waves of excruciating agony. Your symptoms are a clue to where the stone is: A stone at the top of your ureter may cause pain in your upper abdomen; a stone that's reached the middle may cause pain in your side and at the front of your abdomen; a pain that's nearing the bottom of your ureter may also make you feel like you have to urinate very frequently, or make it very difficult to do so.

Kidney stones can be as small as a grain of sand (in which case they'll pass unnoticed) or as rotund as a marble. They form when your urine becomes supersaturated with stone-forming salts and when levels of stone-inhibiting compounds are in short supply. Seventy to eighty percent are made of calcium and a material called oxalate. The rest include struvite stones, made from magnesium and ammonia, usually in people with kidney infections; uric acid stones; and, rarely, stones made from cystine, an amino acid present in the urine of people with a rare, inherited condition called cystinuria.

Your doctor will rule out other causes of abdominal pain such as gallstones, appendicitis, diverticulitis, a hernia, constipation, or an aneurysm in an artery. She will also make sure that there aren't other obstructions in your ureters. To confirm that your pain is caused by a kidney stone, your doctor may test your urine for the presence of tiny crystals. She'll also do an imaging test to look for stones. While ultrasound and x-rays are more commonly used because equipment is more widely available, they can miss up to 80 percent of stones. A computed tomography (CT) scan is best, spotting stones 95 to 100 percent of the time. Imaging tests help your doctor determine the size and location of the stone and make decisions about the best treatment for you.

Fast Pain Relief

One telltale sign that a kidney stone is behind your pain is that over-the-counter pain relievers do little to relieve it. That's another important reason to contact your doctor if you suspect a stone's on board. She will most likely recommend that you:

1. **Take a prescription narcotic such as codeine or morphine so you stay comfortable while the stone is passing.**

2. **Drink 2 to 3 quarts of water per day.** Lots of fluids means lots of urine, which will help wash the stone out of your body. (Your doctor may want you to use a strainer when you urinate so the stone can be caught and analyzed. Knowing the type you have can help determine what you should do to avoid another one.)

When to Call the Doctor

Call your doctor right away if you have any warning signs of a kidney stone or of a stone with an infection, such as:

- Extreme pain in your back or side that will not go away
- Blood in your urine
- Fever and chills
- Vomiting
- A burning sensation during urination
- Urine that looks cloudy or has an unusual odor

Although some stones can be managed at home with pain relievers, seeing a doctor for help can ensure that you avoid complications such as a serious infection or damage to a ureter.

3. **Try medical expulsive therapy.** Ask your doctor whether you can also take a calcium channel blocker such as nifedipine (Adalat, Procardia, Afeditab, Nifediac) or an alpha blocker such as tamsulosin (Flomax), terazosin (Hytrin), or doxazosin (Cardura) to boost the odds that your stone will pass. You'll usually get a 4-week prescription. If the stone hasn't passed by then (your doctor will check your kidneys, ureters, and bladder regularly to be sure the stone isn't causing damage), you'll be referred to a urologist.

4. **Try extracorporeal shockwave lithotripsy.** If your stone measures more than about one-fifth of an inch (5 millimeters) and is located at the top or middle of your ureter, there's little chance it will pass on its own; your chances rise to just 25 percent if it's located lower down. Under these circumstances—or if a stone doesn't pass in 2 to 4 weeks, blocks urine flow, is getting bigger, or is damaging your kidneys or causing bleeding—your doctor may schedule you for extracorporeal shockwave lithotripsy, a procedure that uses shock waves to break the stone into tiny pieces that can pass easily from your body. Extremely large stones may require surgical removal.

Relief at Last

These steps can help you avoid future kidney stones.

Step 1: Drink plenty of fluids every day. You need enough to pass 2 to 3 quarts of urine a day (your urine should be pale). Start with water but don't stop there. If you've had a calcium oxalate stone, sipping sugar-free lemonade or even diet citrus-flavored soda as part of your daily fluid quotient could help even more by increasing stone-discouraging citrate levels in your urine.

Step 2: Prone to calcium oxalate stones? Get plenty of calcium-rich foods but steer clear of calcium supplements. It turns out that dairy foods and other calcium-containing edibles actually help control levels of oxalates, lowering stone risk. But calcium supplements don't help in the same way and may increase your odds for new stones.

Step 3: Follow an eating plan full of fiber and low in sodium, sugar, red meat, and processed meats. This eating strategy can cut your risk for kidney stones by at least 50 percent, studies show. It helps on several levels—by reducing compounds in urine that promote stone formation such as uric acid and excess calcium, while increasing levels of stone-discouraging compounds like citrate.

Step 4: Avoid the right oxalate-rich foods. In books and online you'll find long lists of high-oxalate foods to avoid in order to lower your chances for calcium oxalate stones. But it turns out that only eight—beets, chocolate, nuts, rhubarb, spinach, strawberries, wheat bran, and tea—actually raise oxalate levels in your urine. If you're prone to calcium oxalate stones, these are the ones to avoid.

Step 5: Ask about a potassium citrate supplement. Taken daily, potassium citrate—available over-the-counter and as a time-release prescription drug[105]—can lower stone risk by blocking the formation of calcium crystals. Don't take it if you don't need it. This supplement makes your urine less acidic; your doctor may have to test the acidity of your urine periodically to be sure it stays between 6 and 7. Lower and higher pH levels can encourage stone formation.

Food and Supplements

WATER: It's not the only step you should take, but sipping plenty of water—enough so that you produce 2 quarts of urine every day—can cut your risk for future stones significantly.

The evidence: In one study, men who drank the most water were 30 percent less likely to develop kidney stones compared to those who drank the least.[106] In another, women who drank the most water cut stone risk 32 percent.[107]

How it works: Drinking more water will make your urine more dilute, which can prevent minerals from aggregating to form new stones or add on to existing ones hiding in your kidneys. More water also means more urine, which could wash tiny stones out of your kidneys before they have a chance to get big and cause trouble.

What you need to know: Tired of plain water? Regular and decaf coffee are okay, but steer clear of sugary sodas, fruit punches, and sweetened iced teas, as sugar raises stone risk. Go easy with black tea as well as cranberry, grapefruit, and orange juice. There's some evidence they also up your odds for stones by raising oxalate levels in your urine. Drinking just one glass of grapefruit juice a day raised stone risk 37 percent in one large study. Risk fell 8 to 10 percent for every daily cup of coffee people in the study drank.[108]

If your doctor determines that you're producing cystine stones, you'll need about a gallon of water per day and may be asked to drink a third of it through-out the night so that your urine is dilute at all times.

CALCIUM-RICH FOODS, BUT NOT CALCIUM SUPPLEMENTS: As we mentioned earlier, high-calcium foods like low-fat or fat-free milk, yogurt, and cheese actually help protect against the formation of new calcium oxalate stones. This reverses old medical advice to avoid calcium-rich foods, but it doesn't apply to calcium supplements, which raise risk for stones.

The evidence: In two large Harvard School of Public Health studies of 45,000 men and 92,731 women, those who got the most high-calcium foods were about 30 percent less likely to develop kidney stones than those who got the least. In these and other studies, taking calcium supplements raised risk by 20 percent for women but not for men.[109]

How it works: Calcium-rich dairy foods seem to control levels of oxalates in the bloodstream, an effect that may be a result of the potassium and phosphate they contain. In contrast, getting calcium by itself, as in a supplement, seems to raise risk.

What you need to know: Be sure your bones are protected: If you're prone to calcium oxalate stones and can't take calcium supplements, go for three servings of low-fat or fat-free dairy products a day to meet your calcium needs—generally, 1,000 milligrams a day for men, 1,200 to 1,500 milligrams a day for women.

LEMONADE: No citrus fruit contains more stone-preventing citrates than lemons, an observation that's led urologists to test "lemonade therapy" for stone prevention. Doctors already prescribe potassium citrate to stone-prone patients to reduce their risk, and new research suggests that if you can't or don't want to take this supplement (side effects can include nausea, bloating, gas, and some-times even vomiting and diarrhea), lemonade might be a good alternative.

The evidence: In a study from Duke University's Comprehensive Kidney Stone Center, 22 people with recurrent kidney stones tried daily lemonade or potassium citrate for a year. At the end of the study, the lemonade group saw a sevenfold reduction in new kidney stone formation.[110] Other studies show that drinking lemonade increases levels of potassium citrate in urine, but not quite as high as supplements do.[111]

How it works: Potassium citrate binds with calcium in your urine, prevent-ing the development of tiny crystals that become the foundation for calcium oxalate kidney stones. It also keeps your urine from becoming overly acidic, discouraging the formation of uric acid and cystine stones. Lemonade works

Diet Soda Fights Stones

Could sipping citrus-flavored diet soda cut your risk for future kidney stones? A recent University of California, San Francisco, study says that these thirst quenchers show promise because they contain large amounts of citrate, a compound that inhibits the formation of the most common type of kidney stones: calcium oxalate stones.

This study simply analyzed the ingredients of commercially made beverages; it didn't test whether they'll actually work. But supplements of potassium citrate are used to lower stone risk in people with low citrate levels. And reaching for a citrusy diet drink may be a better choice than sweetened soda, tea, or fruit punch, all of which have been shown to increase kidney stone risk. High-citrate drinks in the study included Diet Sunkist Orange, Diet 7Up, Sprite Zero, Diet Canada Dry Ginger Ale, Sierra Mist Free, Diet Orange Crush, Fresca Grapefruit, and Diet Mountain Dew.[112]

the same way, and also helps simply because drinking more fluids helps flush out tiny crystals before they can become big stones.

What you need to know: Urologists at the University of Wisconsin-Madison recommend that many of their kidney stone patients make their own sugar-free or low-sugar lemonade by mixing 1 cup of lemon juice with 7 cups of water, then sweetening it with a low- or no-calorie sweetener. (Don't use regular lemonade. Excess sugar in your diet raises stone risk, too.) In one study, the urologists found that lemonade therapy increases citrate levels in urine enough to discourage stone formation, but that adding potassium citrate supplements seemed even better.[113] There's new evidence that the citrates in orange and grapefruit juice also help, so feel free to swap in a glass of one of these citrus fruits as part of your daily fluids.

FIBER: In addition to lots of water and calcium-rich foods, pile on the fruit, vegetables, and whole grains every day. High-fiber foods lower kidney stone risk—just skip those that are high in oxalates.

The evidence: When researchers combined information from three long-term studies of diet and stone risk involving more than 200,000 people, they found that this eating strategy cut the odds for problem stones in half.

How it works: The experts admit that their findings were a bit puzzling, because some fruits, vegetables, and nuts contain oxalate, which is found in the most common type of kidney stone. But these foods also raise urinary levels of citrate, which may discourage the growth of calcium oxalate stones.[114]

What you need to know: Some experts recommend steering clear of high-oxalate foods known to raise oxalate levels in the body, such as nuts, rhubarb, spinach, and wheat bran.

CUT BACK ON RED MEAT AND PROCESSED MEATS: Eating beef and processed meats like sausage, bacon, ham, lunch meat, and hot dogs increases kidney stone risk, so it makes sense to swap in more poultry, fish, and vegetable-based proteins like dried beans.

The evidence: A diet packed with red and processed meats raised stone risk 34 percent in one Harvard School of Public Health study.[115]

How it works: Red meat is rich in purines, which break down to form uric acid in your bloodstream and urine. High uric acid levels encourage the formation of uric acid stones, a less common type of stone that can develop if you're dehydrated too often, eat lots of red meat, have gout, or have a genetic predisposition. Meanwhile, processed meats are usually high in sodium, also recently proven to increase kidney stone risk by raising calcium levels in urine.

What you need to know: Try not to eat more than 6 ounces of meat a day—about the size of two decks of cards.

CUT BACK ON SALT: Americans consume more sodium than ever before, most of it from processed foods, restaurant meals, and fast-food edibles. Cutting back could help you stay stone free, new research shows.

The evidence: Low-salt eating plans reduced the amount of calcium in the urine of people prone to developing kidney stones in one recent Italian study of 210 people.[116] In another Italian study that compared a low-salt, low-meat diet to a traditional low-calcium diet for people who tend to develop calcium oxalate stones, researchers found that reducing sodium and meat cut kidney stone risk in half.[117]

How it works: As we mentioned above, sodium triggers the release of calcium into urine. That's bad news, because at high levels calcium in your urine can combine with oxalate to form kidney stones.

What you need to know: Stick to no more than 2,400 milligrams of sodium a day if you're at risk for kidney stones. Eating fewer processed foods and restaurant and fast-food meals—all of which are high in sodium—can help.

POTASSIUM CITRATE SUPPLEMENTS: Available as tablets or as a liquid, potassium citrate can help cut your risk for calcium oxalate stones significantly.

The evidence: Research shows this supplement can cut stone formation by 90 percent.[118]

How it works: As we mentioned earlier, potassium citrate increases citrate in your urine. This can stop the formation of calcium crystals that become calcium oxalate stones and balance the acidity of your urine, discouraging the formation of uric acid stones.

What you need to know: Your doctor may ask you to test your urine to be sure the pH—the measure of acidity and alkalinity—stays between 6 and 7. At lower and higher pH levels, stones are more likely to form.

Inflammatory Bowel Disease, Crohn's Disease, and Ulcerative Colitis

For reasons scientists have yet to understand, the two types of inflammatory bowel disease—Crohn's disease and ulcerative colitis—cause out-of-control inflammation of the lining of the intestines. This leads to chronic pain, diarrhea, constipation, bleeding, damage, loads of stress, fatigue, and often surgery.

IBD can easily take over your life: In one survey of 1,000 people with Crohn's disease, respondents said they had diarrhea for an average of 225 days per year and spent 38 days a year in the hospital.[119] In another national survey of 1,000 people with ulcerative colitis, 40 percent reported incapacitating symptoms like bloody diarrhea and severe pain 180 days of the year. Twenty percent had had surgery in the previous 5 years, with many undergoing two or more procedures and a third opting for removal of their entire colon.[120]

Even if your IBD is mild, these unpredictable conditions can throw your life into complete disarray. Crohn's disease and ulcerative colitis can go into remission for months or even years, only to flare up again without warning. The pain and bowel changes make just leaving your house difficult and can get in the way of your love life, your social life, your job, and your ability to feel whole and healthy. In the same surveys, one in four said IBD imposed way too many limits on their lives.

Meanwhile, new understandings about the way your intestinal tract works are leading to better ways to diagnose, treat, and control IBD pain so that you can reclaim your life.

It starts with getting a faster, more accurate diagnosis. Early diagnosis means better treatment, fewer relapses, and less pain. But many people with IBD visit five or more doctors before[121] the real cause of their abdominal distress is discovered. Now, IBD advocacy groups say that if you have cramping abdominal pain, diarrhea, and other signs of trouble such as constipation or weight loss, it makes sense to go directly to a gastroenterologist, a doctor who specializes in diseases of the gastrointestinal system. These specialists are tuned in to telltale signs of

IBD and will more readily deploy a full range of tests that can pinpoint the real problem. These tests can also tell your doctor whether you have Crohn's disease or ulcerative colitis so he can tailor your treatment.

You've also got more treatment choices than ever before. Back in the 1950s, IBD treatment meant taking a steroid. Today, seven different classes of drugs—from diarrhea-stopping remedies to high-tech "biologics" that target specific inflammation-triggering proteins and enzymes with precision—mean your chances for stopping a flare-up and staying in remission are better than ever before. New drugs help people whose IBD hasn't responded to older medications.

These days, healing doesn't end with drugs. Foods help, too. There's more and more evidence that encouraging the growth of beneficial bacteria in your intestinal tract helps control inflammation. Taking probiotics, friendly bacteria in yogurt and supplements, and prebiotics, types of fiber (such as inulin and pectin) that these good bugs like to eat, can help keep IBD in remission, research shows. (Of course, you won't want to add fiber to your diet during a relapse, in the early days of remission, or if you have a narrowing of your intestines.)

There's also strong evidence that you can enjoy extra pain relief without taking more medication simply by learning how to reduce stress. We're not saying stress causes IBD. It doesn't! But there's plenty of evidence that chronic daily stress (from a tough commute to a difficult boss to money worries) and big, sudden, high-tension jolts (a loss, a divorce, even a new home, job, or addition to your family) raise odds for a relapse. And there's growing proof that reducing stress and using your mind to send soothing signals to your digestive system can help ease pain.

Is It IBD?

Early signs of IBD include:

- Cramps and abdominal pain
- Diarrhea
- Weight loss
- Abdomen that may feel swollen and tender
- Rectal bleeding
- Urgent need to use the bathroom over and over again, yet production of little stool

In Crohn's disease, virtually any part of your digestive tract from your mouth to your anus may become inflamed, but it most often affects the lower portion of the small intestine, called the ileum. Several areas may be inflamed at once. Swelling leads to diarrhea and pain and can also narrow your intestines (which could cause dangerous blockages), poke microscopic holes in the walls, or lead to the formation of fistulas, ulcers that burrow into neighboring organs like the bladder or vagina and can cause infections.

In ulcerative colitis, ulcers develop where inflammation has killed off cells in the lining; these can bleed and become infected. Inflammation also leads to diarrhea, which can be bloody and frequent.

Doctors use a variety of tests to confirm a diagnosis of IBD. Blood tests such as a complete blood count (CBD) look for signs of infection as well as anemia and mineral deficiencies (resulting from absorption problems and chronic diarrhea) that can point the way to an IBD diagnosis. Stool studies can detect bacterial infections that might be associated with IBD or with other look-alike conditions. And your doctor may also want to take a look by performing a colonoscopy and taking tissue samples for biopsy to confirm IBD. Examining the intestines with a long, flexible lighted tube linked to a TV camera and taking tissue samples for testing is the gold standard check for IBD, according to the American Society for Gastrointestinal Endoscopy. It can also help your doctor distinguish ulcerative colitis from Crohn's disease about 85 percent of the time.

If your intestinal tract is too inflamed and irritated for a colonoscopy, your doctor may use capsule endoscopy, a test in which you swallow a capsule containing a tiny camera and wireless transmitter that look for signs of trouble, or a sigmoidoscopy.[122] You may be asked to follow a bowel-cleansing liquid diet, use enemas, or drink special bowel prep liquids beforehand to clear out the colon before the test.

Other checks used to diagnose IBD include computed tomography (CT) or a magnetic resonance imaging (MRI) scan, which can help your doctor find complications outside the walls of your intestinal tract, like abscesses or openings called fistulas. Your doctor may give you a barium enema or have you swallow a barium preparation, then look for signs of trouble using x-rays. This technique can help find problems higher up in your small intestine.

Fast Pain Relief

These steps can help you begin to bring the pain and diarrhea of IBD under control, but be sure to consult your doctor. Several prescription medicines (listed below) can help control flare-ups and bring you back into remission.

1. **Loperamide (Imodium):** Over-the-counter diarrhea remedies containing loperamide can help your intestines absorb more fluids

and help your sphincter better control the release of bowel movements. Don't use loperamide if you have bloody diarrhea, if your entire colon is inflamed (a condition called active pancolitis), or if you or your doctor suspect you have an intestinal infection.

2. **Prescription antidiarrhea and antispasmodic drugs:** Your doctor may prescribe the antidiarrheals cholestyramine (Questran) or diphenoxylate and atropine (Lomotil) and/or an antispasmodic drug such as dicyclomine (Bentyl). These prescription drugs can help control some types of diarrhea by helping your intestines absorb more fluids and damp down muscle spasms that cause pain.

3. **A low-fiber, low-residue diet:** Cutting fiber and foods that leave behind a residue such as many fruit juices and even milk gives your intestinal tract a rest during a flare-up. Cut out whole grain breads and cereals, dried beans, potatoes with the skin, nuts and seeds, raw fruits and vegetables, as well as all berries, broccoli, brussels sprouts, cabbage, cauliflower, corn, peas, raisins, winter squash, and any vegetable with seeds. You should also avoid tough, fibrous cuts of meat, limit or eliminate fat, and cut back on or cut out milk.

   The foods you can eat include white bread and cereal, crackers and noodles made with refined (white) flour, white rice, fruit and

When to Call the Doctor

Call right away or go to the emergency room if you experience any of these.

- Loss of a large amount of blood via rectal bleeding (enough that it worries you) in a short period of time
- Diarrhea that leaves you dehydrated (you'll be extra-thirsty, tired, have a dry mouth, and dark, scant urine)
- Dizziness
- Fainting
- Intense abdominal pain so that you can't move
- Waves of tummy pain after eating
- Nausea and vomiting that doesn't seem to stop
- A sudden fever over 102°

vegetable juices that are pulp free, milk, yogurt, pudding, ice cream, and strained creamy or broth-based soups, tender meat, chicken, turkey, fish, or egg dishes, oils, margarine, butter, jelly, honey, or syrup. (Have no more than 2 cups of dairy products per day.)

It's best to follow this eating plan until inflammation heals and then add the healthy foods on this list back into your diet very slowly.

4. **Prescription anti-inflammatory drugs:** Reducing swelling and tenderness decreases diarrhea, bleeding, and pain. Depending on the severity of your Crohn's disease or ulcerative colitis, your doctor may prescribe an aminosalicylate drug such as mesalamine (Asacol, Pentasa, Rowasa) or sulfasalazine (Azulfidine), a corticosteroid such as prednisone, and/or an immunosuppressant such as azathioprine (Imuran), mercaptopurine (Purinethol), or methotrexate (Rheumatrex) if you aren't helped by steroids and even broad-spectrum antibiotics to calm down the immune response in your intestines.

Relief at Last

Help your digestive system heal and avoid relapses with these proven steps.

Step 1: Ask your doctor about newer IBD drugs. Steroids may help end a flare-up fast but newer medications are a better choice for keeping you in remission with fewer side effects. What you take will depend on the severity of your symptoms, so discuss them all with your doctor. Choices range from aminosalicylates to control inflammation in mild IBD to strong immune-suppressing drugs called immunomodulators and high-tech medications called biologics that target specific immune system compounds. Be sure to ask about antibiotics as well. Even if you don't have an active infection, controlling bacteria in your small intestine could help ease inflammation by quieting an overactive immune system. Some studies show that taking two antibiotics works as well as a steroid for easing Crohn's disease symptoms.

Step 2: Take a probiotic supplement containing strains of *Lactobacillus* and/or *E. coli* Nissle 1917. These beneficial bacteria have been proven to soothe inflammation in your digestive system. In one study, they worked as well as an aminosalicylate drug for keeping ulcerative colitis in remission.

Step 3: Follow the right diet. Once your IBD is in remission, you may be able to add high-fiber foods back into your diet—a good move because they can help keep you regular and provide fuel for beneficial bacteria in your intestinal tract that put a damper on inflammation. (It's wise to avoid cola drinks, chocolate, and big helpings of red meat and even fish, as there's some evidence that eating lots of animal protein could triple your risk for developing IBD.[123] It might play a role in flare-ups, too). Other foods may be on or off your menu depending on the severity of your disease at any given time. We've got advice on how to include the healthy stuff so that your diet provides the nutrition you need.

> ## Quick Tip
>
> **If you want to encourage more IBS-soothing good bugs to take up residence in your digestive tract, it makes sense to feed them well. Their favorite foods: carbohydrates that we humans can't really digest but that bacteria love to munch on. There are prebiotic fibers in bananas, berries, asparagus, garlic, wheat, oatmeal, barley, flaxseeds, tomatoes, onions, chicory, greens, and dried beans.**

Step 4: Take stress reduction seriously. One of the most exciting developments in IBD research is growing evidence that reducing stress—especially in ways aimed at relaxing your digestive system as well as your mind—translates into tangible pain relief. Progressive muscle relaxation and a type of medical hypnosis called gut-directed hypnotherapy are proven to ease pain and help keep people in remission, sometimes with lower doses of medication.

Step 5: Take a stroll. By reducing stress and possibly improving digestion, gentle exercise is a proven pain reliever for people with Crohn's disease and ulcerative colitis. The key? Take it easy. Vigorous workouts can set off symptoms for some people with IBD, but several studies show that low-intensity activity has real benefits.

Food and Supplements

YOGURT AND PROBIOTIC SUPPLEMENTS: Encouraging healthy colonies of beneficial bacteria in your digestive system is a smart, inflammation-fighting move.

The evidence: When 34 people with mild to moderate ulcerative colitis took a probiotic supplement for 8 weeks, 53 percent said they felt completely better and another 24 percent felt somewhat better, report University of Alberta researchers. In another Canadian study, people with ulcerative colitis and Crohn's disease who ate yogurt every day for a month had less inflammation in their intestinal tract, blood tests showed.

How it works: Probiotics influence your immune system in ways that dial

Good Foods/Bad Foods for IBD

There's no single, perfect diet for everybody with Crohn's disease and ulcerative colitis, or even one diet that a person with inflammatory bowel disease should follow at all times.

Take fiber, for example. During a flare-up, it's smart to soothe your bowels with a low-fiber diet. Many, but not all, people with IBD add fiber back in once they're in remission, to help regulate bowel movements, to get all of the nutrients found in high-fiber produce and whole grains, and to encourage the growth of beneficial bacteria in their intestines. But for people with strictures in the lower small intestine, a high-fiber diet could ramp up pain. A low-fiber or liquid diet may be the way to go.

Absorption problems and a limited diet can lead to nutritional gaps for people with IBD. Your best move? Ask your doctor about a vitamin/mineral supplement and about a referral to a certified dietitian who can devise a nutrient-packed eating plan that's right for you.

In the meantime, pay attention to these foods.

Dairy products: A third of people with Crohn's disease and 20 percent with ulcerative colitis have trouble digesting lactose, a type of sugar found in milk and many other dairy products. The good news is that the bloating and cramping you feel may seem like the start of a relapse, but usually they're not.

What to do: Ask your doctor about a test to find out if you're lactose intolerant. If you are, using lactase enzyme tablets or drops can predigest the lactose in milk. Yogurt and hard cheese are usually okay because they're lower in lactose. If you skip dairy products, take a calcium supplement to be sure you have plenty of this important, bone-building mineral on board.

High-fiber foods: Fruits, vegetables, whole grains, and nuts come packed with plenty of fiber, along with other vitamins, minerals, antioxidants, and other nutrients your body needs. But for some people too much fiber could trigger a flare-up.

What to do: Before you give up on high-fiber foods, try softening them up first by back inflammation. Fostering the good guys helps reduce the ranks of less-beneficial types that encourage inflammation, too.

What you need to know: The supplement used in the University of Alberta studied contained eight types of *Lactobacillus* bacteria, the same kinds found in many yogurts with live active cultures. It is also available from several

---

steaming, baking, or stewing them. And, of course, skip those you know you can't tolerate.

High-fat foods: From butter and ice cream to French fries and peanut butter, high-fat foods (even healthy fats) accelerate the movement of stools through your intestines, which could make diarrhea and pain worse. If you're having trouble digesting fat, an issue with some types of Crohn's disease, these foods could trigger a type of diarrhea called steatorrhea.

What to do: First, go easy on foods high in saturated fats such as fatty meats, whole milk, cheese, and ice cream. If you can, eat small amounts of good fats like peanut butter, avocados, fatty fish like salmon, and olive and canola oil. The fats in these foods are healthy for your heart and help prevent diabetes so are worth keeping in your diet if possible.

Caffeine: It doesn't just wake up your brain! The caffeine in coffee, tea, and cola drinks (and hidden in other foods like some noncola sodas, chocolate, and even some medicines) speeds the transit time of food in your intestines. This can irritate the lining and make diarrhea worse.

What to do: Switch to herbal teas that don't contain caffeine. Some, such as chamomile, may even help soothe your intestines.

Alcohol: Beer, wine, cocktails, and shots can all irritate the delicate lining of your digestive system and interact with IBD medications.

What to do: Some people can tolerate one drink with a meal; others cannot even have a small amount of alcohol without feeling discomfort. It's important to discover your own comfort zone, then stay in it.

Artificial fats and sweeteners: Fake fats such as Olestra and low- or no-calorie sweeteners such as sorbitol, mannitol, and maltitol can trigger diarrhea.

What to do: Gotta satisfy a snack food craving? Choose baked chips (or make your own baked French fries) instead. Choose naturally sweet foods like fruit instead of sugar-free stuff with artificial sweeteners, or sweeten drinks with a teaspoon of the real thing.

supplement makers as a supplement called VSL#3. Meanwhile, another probiotic called *E. coli* Nissle 1917 (ECN for short) was as effective as mesalamine, a 5-ASA drug used to control IBD, at keeping ulcerative colitis in remission in one German study.[124] (One brand name you can try is Mutaflor, www.mutaflor.us.)

VITAMIN D SUPPLEMENTS: People who take steroids to help control Crohn's disease and ulcerative colitis often have low blood levels of vitamin D. New research suggests that this could aggravate IBD.

The evidence: A new McGill University study finds that low levels of vitamin D might leave your body, and particularly your intestinal tract, vulnerable to attacking microbes, which raises risk for Crohn's disease. Your skin produces vitamin D when exposed to sunlight, but most people don't get enough time in the sun to make as much as experts now think we need. Meanwhile, researchers from the Medical College of Wisconsin have found that people with low levels of vitamin D often had more active disease.[125]

How it works: Vitamin D helps fortify your innate immune system, the body's first line of defense against invading bacteria and other organisms. It helps activate genes that alert this system to the presence of invaders and that direct production of microbe-fighting compounds called beta-defensin and NOD2. Problems with both have been linked with Crohn's disease.

What you need to know: So far, studies suggest that getting enough vitamin D might help prevent Crohn's disease. But since getting 1,000 to 2,000 IU a day of this vitamin is suggested for overall health, it can't hurt and might help.

AVOID SULFUR- AND SULFITE-RICH FOODS: Foods naturally rich in sulfur such as red meat, and those with added sulfites such as many wines and some fruit juice, can raise risk for a relapse of ulcerative colitis.

The evidence: In a study of 191 people with ulcerative colitis, researchers

»More Research Needed

Fish Oil Capsules

There are plenty of good reasons to include omega-3 fatty acids in your diet regularly by eating fish, munching on walnuts and flaxseed, or taking fish oil capsules. They're proven to protect your heart, for example. But despite early signs of promise, and despite the fact that one in five people with IBD take them, a large international study that followed 738 people with IBD for about a year found that fish oil didn't keep people in remission.[126]

from England's Newcastle University found that those who ate the most red meat were five times more likely to have a painful relapse than those who ate the least. Alcoholic beverages tripled relapse risk and eggs raised it by 30 percent.[127]

How it works: Foods that contain sulfur compounds may irritate or even erode the lining of the small intestine. This happens when bacteria interact with the sulfur to produce hydrogen sulfide, which damages the intestinal lining.

What you need to know: Sulfites occur naturally when beer and wine are made; more is sometimes added to wine to speed aging. Sulfites can also be found in some baked goods, soup mixes, jams, pickled foods, many condiments, vegetable juices, apple and sparkling grape juice, dried fruit, and potato chips. To find sulfites on an ingredients list, look for the words *sulfur dioxide, potassium bisulfite, potassium metabisulfite, sodium bisulfite, sodium metabisulfite,* or *sodium sulfite.*

SKIP COLA BEVERAGES AND CHOCOLATE: When Dutch researchers looked at dietary triggers for inflammatory bowel disease, these modern snack foods emerged as troublemakers. But citrus fruits were soothing—so snack on an orange instead!

The evidence: Digestive disease experts from Holland's University Hospital in Maastricht looked at the eating habits and relapse rates of 688 people with IBD and 616 people without this disease. They found that sipping cola drinks and nibbling on chocolate doubled risk for ulcerative colitis and for Crohn's disease.[128]

How it works: Experts aren't sure why these foods lead to relapses but suspect the real issue may be that they've replaced protective foods like fruit and vegetables in modern diets.

What you need to know: Chewing gum also increased Crohn's disease risk by 50 percent in the study.

Exercise and Movement Therapies

EASY WALKING: Afraid exercise could lead to a flare-up? While many people with IBD—and their doctors—have shied away from physical activity for fear it could make symptoms worse, a growing stack of research shows that gentle exercise has real benefits for people who are in remission or who have mild symptoms.

The evidence: A half-hour walk three times a week helped improve pain and other symptoms for 12 people with Crohn's disease in a study from the

University of Manitoba in Canada.[129] During the 12-week walking program, study volunteers had no flare-ups, either. In another Canadian study of 32 people with IBD, this time from the University of Western Ontario, those who followed the same easy walking routine said their symptoms improved, and those who didn't walk reported that theirs grew worse.[130] A British study of 32 people with Crohn's disease got similar results.

How it works: Gentle exercise reduces stress, the researchers say. It may also help normalize digestion.

What you need to know: A low-intensity routine, such as taking a short walk every day, seems to be better than a vigorous routine, especially if you're not used to exercise. Of course, if you're able to exercise at a higher intensity without discomfort, keep it up. The benefits of exercise are too important to miss out on.

Mind-Body Therapies

RELAXATION: It's not all in your head. Although tension and anxiety do not cause IBD, they sure can make it worse. People with IBD have long known this, and recent research confirms the connection. In one new Canadian survey of 552 people with Crohn's disease or ulcerative colitis, researchers found that stressful times doubled the risk for a flare-up.[131] Taking time to learn a deep relaxation exercise, such as a breathing exercise or progressive muscle relaxation, could help you keep things under control.

The evidence: In one Spanish study of 45 people with Crohn's disease, those who took a stress management class enjoyed a significant drop in abdominal pain, constipation, and bloating and were still feeling better a year later.[132]

How it works: Stress activates your sympathetic nervous system, which can make inflammation of the lining of your intestinal tract worse. Stress hormones may even allow harmful bacteria to thrive in your intestines.

What you need to know: Finding time to relax can help you feel more in control of IBD, something that translated into better bowel health for 30 people with Crohn's disease or ulcerative colitis in one recent Northwestern University study.[133] Try the progressive muscle relaxation in Part One to get started.

HYPNOTHERAPY: In gut-focused hypnotherapy, you learn to relax your mind and your body—including your digestive system. You also send your body suggestions designed to encourage better bowel functioning. In one study, participants imagined that their intestines were like an orderly English garden with wide, easy-to-navigate paths.

The evidence: In several small studies, hypnotherapy improved inflammatory bowel disease significantly.[134] In one British study of 15 people with severe IBD who tried 12 sessions of hypnotherapy, symptoms went into remission for four volunteers and were reduced to mild for another eight. Sixty percent no longer needed steroids to control their symptoms.[135]

How it works: Hypnotherapy reduces stress and can also improve the healthy functioning of your gastrointestinal system, boost immunity, and reduce inflammation.

What you need to know: You won't be asked to cluck like a chicken or meow like a cat! During sessions with a trained, certified medical hypnotherapist you'll feel deeply relaxed and focused, as you would during prayer or meditation, leaving your mind receptive to suggestions that could improve bowel health. If you'd like to try hypnotherapy, be sure to work with a medical hypnotherapist with experience working with people with inflammatory bowel disease. It may take several sessions to get relief. For more information, turn to Part Three.

Pain Medications and Medical Treatments

CORTICOSTEROIDS: Used to ease IBD since the 1950s, steroids such as prednisone and budesonide (Entocort) shut down inflammation fast, making them the usual first-choice drugs for reining in moderate to severe relapses of Crohn's disease and ulcerative colitis. The downside? They don't work for everyone, and they can be a double-edged sword when they do. Long-term use of steroids raises your risk for serious side effects—a concern for many people with IBD who are dependent on these drugs to avoid a relapse.

The evidence: In one study of 176 people with active Crohn's disease, prednisone and budesonide brought over half into remission in 10 weeks.[136]

How it works: Steroids work by inhibiting the activity of cytokines and T cells, two components of your immune system that normally boost levels of inflammation.

What you need to know: Steroids are far from perfect. They don't work 20 to 30 percent of the time. They should only be used for 8 to 12 weeks, then tapered off to avoid serious side effects like high blood pressure, infections, a swollen face, weight gain, mood swings, and even weakened bones, insomnia, and cataracts. Don't try to go cold turkey. Stopping steroids abruptly can cause abdominal pain, diarrhea, muscle and joint pain, and could even trigger a new flare-up. If you have ulcerative colitis, a steroid enema could bring relief with lower risk for side effects because less of the drug is absorbed into your body.

If you're among the 20 to 30 percent of people whose IBD flares up even if they taper off steroids slowly,[137] one strategy that might help is to start taking an immune-modulating drug (described below) before trying to quit your steroid, experts say. If you have Crohn's disease, you may be able to avoid taking steroids by using one or a combination of two antibiotics to control flare-ups (also described below).

AMINOSALICYLATES: If you have mild to moderate Crohn's disease or ulcerative colitis, drugs such as mesalamine (Rowasa) and sulfasalazine (Azulfidine) could help control a flare-up and prevent relapses, too. Aminosalicylates are more effective for preventing relapses in ulcerative colitis than in Crohn's disease.

The evidence: One type, sulfasalazine, helps up to 80 percent of people with ulcerative colitis get better and stay symptom free.[138] If you're allergic to sulfa drugs, other types such as mesalamine, balsalazide, and olsalazine are also extremely effective. For example, mesalamine helps up to 55 percent of people with Crohn's disease go into remission.[139]

How it works: Aminosalicylates contain the active ingredient 5-aminosalicylic acid (5-ASA), which helps control inflammation.

What you need to know: Your doctor may prescribe an aminosalicylate along with a steroid to control a flare-up. For mild flare-ups, an aminosalicylate plus an antibiotic (or two) may be all you need to control symptoms and get back into remission. For ulcerative colitis, an enema or suppository can help, and your doctor may suggest you use one along with aminosalicylate pills.

ANTIBIOTICS: Even if you don't have an active infection, antibiotics such as metronidazole (Flagyl, Protostat) and ciprofloxacin (Cipro) can help bring Crohn's disease into remission and keep it there.

The evidence: Research shows that these antibiotics can help about half the people who use them go into remission.[140] In one study, the combination of both antibiotics worked as well as the steroid prednisone for easing symptoms of Crohn's disease.[141]

How it works: They help by knocking back intestinal bacterial infections that happen frequently in Crohn's disease. This quiets down immune system reactions that fire up inflammation in your intestines.

What you need to know: Antibiotics are often recommended for mild to moderate Crohn's disease, especially if aminosalicylates don't work. After a course of antibiotics, which may last about 8 to 16 weeks, your doctor may recommend an aminosalicylate to prevent relapses. Antibiotic side effects include a metallic taste in your mouth and diarrhea. Antibiotics are also used to help heal fistulas, openings between internal organs caused by inflammation and infection in Crohn's disease. But when they are stopped, about half of all fistulas return. Antibiotics may not work on resistant strains of bacteria. Antibiotics are usually not used to treat ulcerative colitis.

IMMUNOMODULATORS: Strong, immune-suppressing drugs such as azathioprine (Imuran), mercaptopurine (Purinethol), and methotrexate (Rheumatrex) can put severe Crohn's disease and ulcerative colitis into remission when aminosalicylates fail. If you've been dependent on steroids, these drugs can help you finally get off them, or reduce your dose, without risking a flare-up.

The evidence: In one Scottish study of 32 people whose Crohn's disease didn't respond to other drugs, weekly methotrexate injections brought 71 percent into remission in 16 weeks. Among those who had been dependent on steroids, 26 percent stopped completely and 41 percent reduced their doses.[143] In other research, azathioprine and mercaptopurine have helped 50 to 70 percent of people with tough-to-treat forms of Crohn's disease go into remission, too.

How it works: These drugs block immune system reactions that cause inflammation.

What you need to know: By damping down your immune system, immunomodulators leave your body more vulnerable to infection, but they're still considered safer than steroids for long-term use.[144] It may take 4 months for immunomodulators to put IBD into remission; sometimes doctors prescribe them for long-term use to keep IBD in remission. However, they're not always effective at preventing future flare-ups. Other side effects include nausea, vomiting, diarrhea, stomach ulcers, skin rashes, and even liver inflammation.

BIOLOGICS: The newest drugs for IBD, these include adalimumab (Humira), certolizumab pegol (Cimzia), infliximab (Remicade), and natalizumab (Tysabri). Because they selectively knock down specific compounds, they're considered safer than corticosteroids, which suppress your whole immune system.

The evidence: In one study of 108 people whose Crohn's disease didn't respond to other drugs, 81 percent improved significantly with 4 weeks of infliximab.[146] These drugs are the first also to help people with Crohn's disease who have fistulas, holes in the intestinal wall that tunnel into a nearby organ.[147] They can also help relieve symptoms and prevent relapses of moderate to severe ulcerative colitis.

How they work: Given by injection or intravenous infusion, these genetically engineered medicines target proteins and enzymes that increase levels of inflammation in the body.

What you need to know: There's evidence that combining a biologic with an IBD-friendly eating plan gets better results than the drug alone: In one Japanese study of 110 people, 68 percent who took Remicade and avoided trigger foods saw significant improvements in 4 months compared to 32 percent who took the drug but didn't change their eating habits.[148] People with weakened immune systems, heart failure, or high risk for infections aren't good candidates for these drugs because they weaken the immune system. Other side effects include headaches, flulike symptoms, nausea, and skin rashes.

SURGERY: About three out of four people with Crohn's disease and one in three with ulcerative colitis will eventually need surgery. It's a big decision, but surgery is recommended if your IBD doesn't respond to medication or if you have complications such as blockages, major bleeding, or perforations (literally holes) or abscesses in your intestines. In the past, surgery was a last resort for out-of-control IBD because it was a major procedure that involved big incisions, long healing times, and could mean you would need an ostomy bag, worn outside the body to collect waste from your bowels. Today, minimally invasive procedures and techniques mean faster recovery, fewer complications such as adhesions (painful scar tissue in your abdomen), more precise removal of damaged sections of the intestines (leaving more healthy tissue in place), and fewer postsurgery problems.

The evidence: Is surgery worth it? In one Spanish study, people who had surgery for Crohn's disease reported that their quality of life was equal to that of people whose disease was in remission; pain and bowel problems were low and everyday activities were easier to do.[149] Some experts suggest choosing surgery sooner, rather than enduring years of worsening disease. In one Swedish study of 139 people with Crohn's disease, having surgery earlier meant fewer complications and relapses.[150]

How it works: If you have ulcerative colitis, removal of your colon and anus (a procedure called a proctocolectomy) cures the disease. But Crohn's disease surgery, which removes damaged portions of the intestines, is not a cure; symptoms return within 5 years for half of all people who have surgery. Half of these will need surgery again.

What you need to know: Procedures range from simply draining an abscess or widening areas of the small intestine that have grown narrow to taking out the entire colon. Some people need an ostomy bag afterward, which collects waste from the small intestine through an opening in the abdomen. But a newer procedure called restorative proctocolectomy has done away with that. After your procedure, your doctor will probably recommend that you take medications to keep you in remission as long as possible.

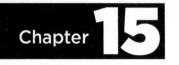
Nerve Pain

Diabetic neuropathy, shingles, Lyme disease, trigeminal neuralgia and complex regional pain syndrome (CRPS), Raynaud's phenomenon

S tinging and burning. Jolting like an electric shock. Tingling, as if your foot or fingers have fallen asleep. The agonizing aches of nerve pain are unique. An estimated 20 million Americans live with this searing pain, the result of nerve damage caused by an accident, an injury, a medical condition such as diabetes, an infection such as shingles, or even medications such as che-motherapy drugs, HIV/AIDS medications, and some antibiotics.[1]

Nerve pain can make sleeping under a light blanket or wearing your favorite sweater excruciating. If you have trigeminal neuralgia—facial pain—you may have trouble eating, smiling, talking, or drinking hot or cold beverages. Nerve damage after a bout of shingles—a rash caused by the chickenpox virus—can make even the whisper of a breeze across your neck feel like needles. Complex regional pain syndrome—nerve damage usually caused by an injury or stroke—leaves you with extreme pain and joints or limbs that become immobilized (unless you sign up for physical therapy).

Its causes are usually well known and researchers are discovering new ways to relieve it all the time. Yet nerve pain is often more severe and more difficult to treat than joint, muscle, digestive, or headache pain, and may be even trickier to diagnose. That's a big problem, because getting a good diagnosis is crucial to finding relief. But even the most common and well understood type of nerve pain—diabetic neuropathy, which affects about half of all people with type 1 and type 2 diabetes[2]—went undiagnosed up to 69 percent of the time in a study of nearly 7,400 people with diabetes.[3] Even when doctors do spot it, less than half of the people with diabetic neuropathy get real relief.[4]

Often, a person experiencing nerve pain stands in her own way of feeling better, too. You may not realize your pain is the result of nerve damage and may spend years trying to ease it with drugstore remedies that often are not effective on their own. In one survey of 147 people with neuropathic pain, just 6 percent were taking the most effective pain-blocking medications—nonopioid drugs that are gaining wide recognition as important weapons in the nerve pain–relief arsenal. (You'll read more about these throughout this chapter.) Nearly half were using drugstore pain relievers. These might help with mild nerve pain, but even in this survey most people said their medications weren't helping enough.[5]

Three Top Causes of Nerve Pain

Most nerve pain is caused by one of these factors.

- **Trauma:** Physical injury—from a car accident, a sports injury, or a household accident like cutting your hand on a broken glass or falling off a ladder—can slice through nerves. It can also damage their ability to send accurate pain signals by compressing, crushing, or stretching them.

- **Bodywide diseases, infections, and metabolic problems:** Diabetes, kidney problems, cancer, and other systemic diseases can also damage nerves. High blood sugar and other metabolic changes that come with diabetes are responsible for about a third of all nerve pain in the United States. Several viruses, including herpes zoster—the shingles virus that can appear decades after you've had a chickenpox infection—as well as the AIDS virus, Epstein-Barr virus, cytomegalovirus, and herpes simplex can damage nerves, triggering searing pain. Lyme disease, transmitted by ticks, can also cause nerve damage within just a few weeks of infection. A vitamin B_{12} deficiency can also damage nerves.

- **Drugs and toxins:** Some chemotherapy drugs, HIV/AIDS medications, and antibiotics can cause nerve damage. So can exposure to heavy metals like lead and mercury, environmental pollutants, and other toxins.

One reason nerve pain is tough to diagnose or to spot on your own is that it produces so many different pain symptoms. People with neuropathy say the pain is on par with burning yourself and leaves them never feeling like a "real person."[6] It's severe. It may burn, tingle, jolt, or stab. It can also be accompanied by numbness, or by pain produced by sensations as slight as a breeze across your skin or the brush of a light cotton shirt across your arm. You may even have spontaneous and unpredictable pain sensations, provoked by nothing at all.

The reason for this wide variety of symptoms is that peripheral neuropathy damages several different types of nerve fibers in your peripheral nervous system, the vast net that sends signals about pain and sensation to your brain and spinal cord from everywhere else in your body. If high blood sugar, a virus, a medication, or an injury frays larger sensory nerves, you may feel numb, have trouble detecting vibrations, and even have difficulty with balance. If smaller fibers are affected, pain receptors near the surface of your skin may become overly sensitive to normally painless inputs—so the feeling of a flannel sheet across your legs in bed on a winter's night is excruciating. The nerves may even fire without any provocation, causing pain when you least expect it. They may eventually go numb, leaving you without pain's early warning signal that you've got a bad blister on your toe or a cut on your leg.

You may also have pain in your face, a condition called trigeminal neuralgia, or debilitating pain at and near the site of an injury, which makes using the affected limb difficult or even impossible, a condition called complex regional pain syndrome (CRPS). CRPS is responsible for ongoing pain after many accidents, injuries, strokes, and even sometimes surgical procedures.

Is It Nerve Pain?

There's no single test for nerve pain. Sometimes the cause is obvious—such as pain in the weeks after a shingles infection or severe ankle pain in the months after that fall while putting up the Christmas lights. Other times your doctor may have to order a variety of tests and carefully check your history to uncover the cause.

Depending on what he suspects, your doctor may ask for blood tests to check for diabetes, vitamin deficiencies, or metabolic problems such as a liver or kidney dysfunction. He may check your muscle strength or perform tests to determine whether your nerves can detect touch, temperature, pain, or vibration. A computed tomography (CT) or magnetic resonance imaging (MRI) scan may be used

Hidden Cause of Nerve Pain: Lyme Disease

Burning and tingling in your fingers and toes. Attacks of joint pain that can last for days or weeks and that may travel from joint to joint. Muscle aches. If you've had mystery pain like this for at least 2 weeks—and live in an area of the United States where there's a moderate to high risk for Lyme disease infection—it's worth asking your doctor if this tick-borne infection is the cause.

While 40 percent to 90 percent of people bitten by an infected deer tick develop a telltale bull's-eye rash or other symptoms (such as fever, chills, and body aches) that lead to a quick diagnosis, many cases are missed. The reason: Symptoms may be vague or wrongly diagnosed as everything from fibromyalgia to chronic fatigue syndrome to arthritis and even inflammatory bowel syndrome.

That's a problem, because an untreated Lyme disease infection can ultimately damage your nerves, muscles, joints, and even your digestive, respiratory, and cardiovascular systems. This can lead to pain, numbness, facial paralysis, seizures, meningitis, and brain problems like memory loss, fuzzy thinking, and mood swings.

If you've had unexplained nerve pain or numbness for at least 2 weeks, or symptoms like long-term fatigue, paralyzed muscles in your face, or signs of meningitis (stiff neck, fever, severe headaches), ask your doctor about a pair of blood tests for Lyme disease infection called the ELISA and the Western blot test, which are usually given together. High-risk regions for Lyme disease include the mid-Atlantic and New England states, parts of Wisconsin and Minnesota, and sections of northern coastal California. But infections crop up in all 50 states.

The fix? Antibiotics such as doxycycline or amoxicillin, intravenous ceftriaxone, cefotaxime, or high-dose penicillin for later-stage infections. Experts say these drugs can be extremely effective even when Lyme disease is caught late. And the sooner treatment begins, the better the results.

to look for cysts, tumors, spinal changes, or other signs of changes that could affect nearby nerves. Your doctor may also use electromyography or nerve conduction velocity tests to see how well your nerves transmit signals. A nerve or skin biopsy can also help your doctor check the health of individual nerve fibers.

The most important thing about a diagnosis? Getting one as soon as possible. The longer you and your doctor wait, the harder nerve damage is to treat and the further it may progress.

Raynaud's Phenomenon: Come In from the Cold

At the merest whisper of cold, your fingers or toes turn white or blue. They go numb or develop an itchy pins-and-needles sensation. It can happen if you touch cold water while running a bath, grip your car's steering wheel on a brisk fall morning, or pick up a cold glass of iced tea on a hot summer day.

This medical condition is called Raynaud's phenomenon.[7] It may be inconvenient and uncomfortable, but more rarely it is an early warning sign of an autoimmune disease such as lupus, rheumatoid arthritis, scleroderma, or Sjögren's syndrome. It's usually benign if it cropped up before you turned 30, but may be a symptom of another medical problem if it came along later. For that reason, it's wise to consult your doctor if you develop signs of Raynaud's.

Many people can relieve or prevent the pain of Raynaud's without medication. Experts recommend starting with these steps.

- **Keep blood vessels open wide.** Avoid smoking, caffeine, and vessel-narrowing medications. In Raynaud's, constricted blood vessels are responsible for skin color changes and discomfort. Drugs to avoid if possible include migraine

Fast Pain Relief

These steps can help you get control of nerve-related pain quickly.

1. **Start with over-the-counter pain relievers.** If nerve damage is mild, taking aspirin, ibuprofen, or acetaminophen may be all you need to get relief. However, even these drugstore remedies can have serious side effects if you take them long term. Be sure to follow package directions or directions from your doctor. Turn to Chapter 6 for advice on using these pain stoppers safely and effectively. If you have diabetes and signs of kidney damage, don't use these pain relievers without first talking with your doctor: Nonsteroidal anti-inflammatories like aspirin, ibuprofen, and naproxen can harm your kidneys if they've already been weakened by high blood sugar.

   These pain relievers block pain signals in the brain; NSAIDs also relieve inflammation. Drugstore pain relievers haven't been well studied for neuropathy, but experts say they're worth trying if your pain isn't severe.

medicines containing ergotamine, OTC cold remedies and diet pills, prescription blood pressure drugs called beta blockers, birth control pills, and some cancer treatments such as cisplatin and vinblastine.

- **Keep warm from head to toe.** Yes, it's wise to wear mittens or gloves to protect your hands. Put them on when getting frozen stuff out of the freezer, when the weather's turning nippy in the fall, or when getting into the car on a cold morning. But it's just as important to keep the rest of your body warm in order to prevent a Raynaud's episode. A warm hat, a scarf for your face and neck, warm layers, and heavy socks can help in cold weather, too.

- **Keep away from cold stuff.** Run the shower or tub until the water's warm before touching it. Use oven mitts or keep gloves in the kitchen for handling cold drinks and foods, carry a sweater or jacket so you don't find yourself shivering in an air-conditioned building in summer, and warm up your bed with an electric blanket before slipping between the sheets.

- **Keep stress low.** Moments of anxiety and tension can trigger Raynaud's, probably because stress tightens blood vessels. Experts say practicing a stress reduction technique can help. (Try the progressive muscle relaxation and meditation exercises in Chapter 5. Skip biofeedback; one well-designed study found that it really doesn't help people with Raynaud's.)[8]

It's important to expect real relief. If these drugs don't ease your pain in a day or two, call your doctor. You need—and deserve—a prescription for a stronger, more effective prescription pain drug.

2. **Try an over-the-counter pain cream.** In one Louisiana State University study of 60 people with moderately intense neuropathic foot pain (they ranked it as less than 8 on a 10-point pain scale with 10 being the most intense), a homeopathic pain remedy called Neuragen eased pain by 50 percent or more within a half-hour for 52 percent of the people who used it.[9] People with diabetic neuropathy seemed to get the most benefit; 78 percent saw pain fall by at least 30 percent. Pain stayed low for about 7 hours. This cream contains tiny amounts of six homeopathic remedies traditionally used to soothe nerve pain, including Saint-John's-wort (*Hypericum perforatum*), wolfsbane (*Aconitum napellus*), club moss (*Lycopodium clavatum*), phosphorus, poison ivy (*Rhus toxicodendron*), and rye ergot (*Secale cornutum*), as well as six essential oils including lavender, geranium, tea tree, and

bergamot. (Of course, if any over-the-counter or prescription remedy doesn't work for you, move on to something else.)

3. **If you think you have the shingles rash, see your doctor immediately and ask about starting the antiviral drug valacyclovir (Valtrex) or famciclovir (Famvir) pronto.** Shingles rash causes itchy blisters that often appear on the torso. Your odds for developing painful postherpetic neuralgia after a shingles infection are 40 percent if you're over age 50 and 75 percent if you're over age 75, so it's important to do all you can to minimize nerve damage from this virus.[10, 11, 12, 13] Starting one of these antivirals within 3 days after your rash first appears can minimize nerve damage from this herpes virus; studies show valacyclovir reduced the average time people had postherpetic neuralgia to 40 days (it worked twice as fast as a placebo) and left 81 percent pain free 6 months after their shingles infection. Famciclovir got similar results.[14] But another antiviral, acyclovir, only cut postherpetic neuralgia to 60 days and reduced pain for 74 percent.[15]

4. **Stick on a lidocaine patch, especially if you have postherpetic nerve pain.**[16] Applied to sore areas for up to 12 hours a day, skin patches that contain a gel infused with the painkilling drug lidocaine (Lidoderm) can reduce shingles nerve pain in just a few hours.[17] Doctors are also beginning to use them as "off-label" soothers for other types of nerve pain, too.

5. **Move up to a fast-acting opioid-based pain reliever if other drugs aren't helping.** There's plenty of controversy about whether opioids like morphine and oxycodone help ease nerve pain related to shingles, diabetes, trigeminal neuralgia, CRPS, and other conditions. But newer research shows that these drugs can reduce pain by 20 to 30 percent and help one out of three people who try them.[18]

Relief at Last

Taking control of nerve pain for the long haul requires patience. You may have to try several therapies or several different combinations of therapies to get relief. Don't give up and don't settle for unacceptable levels of pain. Your best bet may include drug-free strategies along with medication, so keep on working with your doctor. Here's what works.

Step 1: Talk with your doctor about which fast-relief strategies can be used long term. Some approaches that work as fast rescue relief therapies—such as OTC pain relievers, lidocaine patches, and opioid-based painkillers—may need to be adjusted or monitored if you plan to use them long term. You may have to switch to a lower dose, use a patch for a period of time and then stop for a while, or switch to an opioid that controls pain for a longer period of time.

Step 2: If you have complex regional pain syndrome, talk with your doctor about finding a physical therapy program. Pain can stiffen joints, making it more and more difficult to walk, move your arms, or even use your hands. Physical therapy can reverse this side effect so that you can keep on doing the things you want and need to do every day. You may need stronger pain relievers in order to participate in PT sessions, but the benefits are worth it.

Step 3: If you're not using an antiseizure drug or an antidepressant, ask your doctor if one is right for you. These medications help block nerve pain and are widely prescribed these days for many types of nerve damage. (You don't have to be depressed or have a seizure disorder to get the benefits.) While some experts say that the antiseizure drug pregabalin (Lyrica) may be a good first choice for diabetic neuropathy and the tricyclic antidepressant amitriptyline (Elavil) may be a good choice for postshingles nerve pain,[19] the truth is that different medications work best for different people. The side effects of these drugs may mean some aren't good options if you have other health conditions and take other medications. You may have to try several before finding the best one for you.

Step 4: If pain is severe, add an opioid pain reliever. One effective strategy is to combine a low-dose opioid with a low-dose pain-blocking drug; there's evidence that this mix works better than higher doses of just one. One option is the drug tramadol (Ultracet), which acts as both an opioid painkiller and a pain-blocking antidepressant.[20] Studies show it can reduce pain by more than 50 percent for one in five people.[21]

Step 5: Investigate dietary therapies. L-carnitine and/or alpha-lipoic acid may help ease nerve pain, especially if you have diabetic neuropathy. These probably cannot replace prescription drugs, but they can provide additional relief. Keeping your blood sugar under tight control is also important if you have diabetes-related nerve damage; it can help prevent its progression, and there's even some evidence that it can reduce pain somewhat. It may even be worth getting your blood levels of vitamin B_{12} checked. Sometimes low levels can lead to nerve damage.

Step 6: Add acupuncture. Used along with antidepressants, this ancient healing art could ease your pain by as much as two-thirds.

Pain Prevention Strategies

Food and Supplements

VITAMIN B_{12}: Low levels of vitamin B_{12} in your bloodstream can raise your risk for nerve damage and nerve pain. But don't take megadoses of this vitamin on your own. It makes more sense to take a multivitamin, eat a vitamin B–rich diet, and ask your doctor about a blood test to check your B_{12} levels first.

The evidence: Your body absorbs less and less B_{12} from food with age, thanks to a slowdown in the production of digestive acids in the stomach. An estimated 10 to 15 percent of people over age 60 are low in B_{12}.[22] Absorption may also be reduced if you take acid-blocking drugs used to ease ulcer pain and heartburn or to protect your stomach or if you take NSAIDs on a regular basis.

How it works: Not having enough vitamin B_{12} may damage the myelin sheath that covers most of the nerves in your body. Early symptoms include numbness and tingling in your feet, legs, fingers, hands, and arms. You need 2.4 micrograms of B_{12} per day; getting at least some of it from your multivitamin or from enriched foods (such as breakfast cereals with added vitamins) can help because supplemental B_{12} is in a form more readily absorbed than the B_{12} in food. Liver, clams, mussels, crab, and beef are also rich in B_{12}.

What you should know: Experts recommend that people over age 50 take a multivitamin or eat an enriched breakfast cereal containing 6 to 30 micrograms of B_{12} daily. Some nutritionists recommend getting 100 to 400 micrograms a day, especially if you're over age 50, are vegetarian, or take acid-blocking medications. Vitamin B_{12} is considered safe at these levels.

TIGHT BLOOD SUGAR CONTROL IF YOU HAVE DIABETES: Diabetes can damage the coverings on delicate nerve endings if your blood sugar stays high for long periods of time. But blood sugar is only part of the story. Experts suspect that higher than normal levels of blood fats and low levels of insulin also contribute to nerve damage. Diabetes-related weakening of tiny blood vessels that carry oxygen and nutrients to nerves also seems to play a role. For all these reasons, diabetes specialists recommend bringing blood sugar into tight control to help lower your risk of new nerve damage.

The evidence: In one small study of 50 people with diabetes, having an A1c (a measure of long-term blood sugar control) over 7 percent increased risk for early nerve damage tenfold.[23] Controlling blood sugar is the answer. In a landmark study of 1,441 people with type 1 diabetes called the Diabetes Control and Complications Trial, tight blood sugar control reduced the risk for neuropathy and slowed the progression of existing nerve damage by 57 percent.[24]

How it works: Healthy eating, regular exercise, stress reduction, and medications to lower your blood sugar (and to control the high blood pressure and high cholesterol that often come with diabetes) help control the factors that harm nerves.

What you need to know: Work with your doctor to determine the best blood sugar control goal for you.

ALPHA-LIPOIC ACID: Found in small amounts in spinach, tomatoes, broccoli, and carrots, alpha-lipoic acid (ALA) is an antioxidant long used in Europe as a supplement and even as an intravenous therapy to ease nerve pain.

The evidence: In one German study of 24 people with diabetes-related nerve pain, those who took 600 milligrams of ALA three times a day for 3 weeks got twice as much relief from burning pain as those who got a placebo.[25] In a review of four ALA studies involving 1,278 people with diabetic neuropathy, 53 percent who received intravenous ALA got relief from pain.

How it works: ALA may protect nerves by mopping up free radicals—harmful oxygen molecules that occur naturally in the body—before they can damage nerve cells. Research suggests it may also help damaged nerves repair themselves to some degree.

What you need to know: ALA also helps your cells absorb blood sugar more easily; as a result, your blood sugar levels may decrease. If you take medications to control diabetes, talk with your doctor about testing your blood sugar and making adjustments in your drug doses before trying ALA.

L-CARNITINE: An amino acid found naturally in your body, L-carnitine helps carry fatty acids from the foods you eat into your mitochondria, the tiny power stations inside cells that generate energy. Normally, your diet provides plenty of L-carnitine. But there's evidence that levels are low in some people with diabetes.[26] Some studies suggest that replacing it may help alleviate diabetes-related

Mirror Therapy for Complex Regional Pain Syndrome

Tricking your brain into believing that a hand or arm affected by CRPS is actually healthy, flexible, and pain free can boost healing, some intriguing research suggests. The switch works when you do hand or arm exercises with both your "good" limb and your affected limb. But in mirror therapy, a specially positioned mirror hides your affected limb and reverses the image of your good side. The result? You watch an image that looks healed.

In several small studies of people who developed CRPS on one side of their body after a stroke or an accident that severed nerves, several weeks of mirror therapy reduced pain by as much as 90 percent and improved mobility significantly.[30, 31] (Other research suggests a 30 to 50 percent improvement is more likely.) Mirror therapy, also known as mirror box therapy, is also used for phantom limb pain and stroke rehabilitation.

nerve pain and even fix some nerve damage. Early research suggests it may also help with nerve damage caused by AIDS drugs,[27] but it doesn't seem effective for shingles nerve pain.

The evidence: When researchers from Wayne State University in Michigan reviewed results of studies of 1,335 people with diabetic neuropathy, they found that those who took L-carnitine for a year saw significant improvements in pain. Those who took 1,000 milligrams three times a day said their pain was cut nearly in half. They also showed encouraging signs that nerve fibers were regenerating and repairing themselves somewhat.[28]

How it works: L-carnitine seems to help damaged nerves repair themselves by improving the function of energy-producing mitochondria in cells and by helping cells make use of a compound called nerve growth factor.[29]

What you need to know: People who had diabetes for 5 years or less were twice as likely to get improvements with L-carnitine as those who had diabetes for more than 10 years in the Wayne State study described above. The reason? L-carnitine may work best when nerves haven't sustained as much damage. So far, L-carnitine has not been able to reverse nerve damage or completely soothe pain. It's a promising therapy worth adding to your pain-relief arsenal, but not a good option as a stand-alone therapy.

Exercise and Movement Therapies

PHYSICAL THERAPY: If you have complex regional pain syndrome, you may find that along with the nerve pain, your limbs are becoming stiff and difficult to move. That's why physical therapy is considered a cornerstone treatment for this type of pain.

The evidence: In one study of children and teens with complex regional pain syndrome, those who got 6 weeks of physical therapy had an easier time climbing stairs and walking, and saw a 90 percent drop in pain.[32] Physical therapy seems to work best when combined with other strategies, such as cognitive therapy to help you cope with pain and the ways it has changed your life as well as pain-relieving medications and even nerve blocks. In a Case Western Reserve University study of people with complex regional pain syndrome, people who had 20 sessions of physical therapy along with counseling and pain relief saw pain tolerance improve by 50 percent and said they had better mobility and stronger muscles. Two years later, 75 percent were back to work.[33]

How it works: Physical therapy keeps joints and muscles flexible.

What you need to know: You may need stronger pain relievers just to take part in a physical therapy program, but the results are worth it. Work with your doctor to find one that's right for you. Many use specially designed exercises that help you become used to the sensation of moving and using an affected limb and also help you build strength in muscles and connective tissue so that you can put pressure on limbs and use them to bear weight once again. The goal is to regain a normal range of motion so that you can go about your daily life and get back to work, too.

Touch Therapies

ACUPUNCTURE: Using hair-thin needles to change the flow of energy in the body and relieve pain is a mainstay of traditional Chinese medicine. There's evidence that it may help with nerve pain from diabetes, cancer drugs, HIV/AIDS treatments, complex regional pain syndrome, and possibly even shingles.

The evidence: In a British study of 44 people with diabetic neuropathy who received six acupuncture treatments in 10 weeks, 34 got significant pain relief and 7 said their pain was gone. Two-thirds who had been using pain drugs were able to decrease their doses or stop taking them altogether. Benefits lasted for up to a year.[34] Combining acupuncture with other pain-relief therapies may work better than acupuncture or drugs alone. Some doctors have also found that acupuncture along with antidepressants eases pain more than either therapy alone—a promising area we hope is explored by more researchers in the future.[35]

Acupuncture might also help with nerve pain from shingles, but studies so far have had mixed results. A large acupuncture study under way in Germany of 336 people with postherpetic neuralgia should help experts know for sure how much this therapy really helps.[36] In a small study from Belgium, people who got real or fake acupuncture saw pain fall 90 percent, leading experts to speculate that even mild pressure near trigger points could improve pain.[37]

How it works: Researchers suspect acupuncture may increase levels of neurotransmitters such as serotonin, which can block pain signals coming to the brain from damaged nerves in your arms and legs.

What you need to know: Be sure to talk with your doctor before undergoing acupuncture for nerve pain relief. Turn to Part Three for information on finding a qualified acupuncture practitioner.

Pain Medications and Medical Treatments

CAPSAICIN CREAM: The ingredient that gives hot red peppers their zing can diminish nerve pain resulting from diabetes and possibly shingles, too. But be careful. This therapy can cause pain before it eases it, and you'll want to be extremely careful to wash your hands after using it to avoid getting irritating cream in your eyes, mouth, or elsewhere.

The evidence: Capsaicin cream diminished pain by 59 percent in one study of people with diabetic neuropathy, published in the journal *Archives of Internal Medicine*.[38] In one study of 99 cancer patients with nerve pain resulting from surgery, those who applied capsaicin cream four times a day for 8 weeks felt pain ease by 53 percent.[39] There's evidence that it can ease postherpetic neuralgia, but you may need to use extra pain relievers at first because capsaicin increases pain before it decreases it.

How it works: Capsaicin prompts pain-sensing nerve fibers to release a neurotransmitter called substance P, which is involved in sending pain signals to your brain. The extra substance P at first increases pain, but then pain decreases, and stays low, when levels drop.[40] To become effective, capsaicin cream must be applied four or five times a day for up to 4 weeks.[41]

What you need to know: You'll have to put up with some discomfort before pain relief kicks in, because the extra substance P that capsaicin frees temporarily sends even stronger pain messages to your brain. Be sure to wash your hands thoroughly after each use, to avoid getting the stinging cream in your eyes or on mucus membranes in your mouth or nose.

If you'd rather not slather on cream so often, a prescription-strength patch containing about 11 times more capsaicin than OTC creams may be a good alternative. Recently approved by the FDA to control shingles nerve pain,

Qutenza is applied in the doctor's office and left in place for an hour. You can repeat it every 3 months. In a study of 402 people with shingles pain, researchers from the University of Wisconsin found that 42 percent of those who used the high-dose patch got a 30 percent reduction in pain within 8 weeks compared to 32 percent who used a lower-dose formula. The downside: You may need pain-relief medication during or after your treatment to keep you comfortable until the capsaicin depletes the pain-transmitting substances in the nerves in your skin. The capsaicin in this patch is so strong that your doctor has to wear protective gloves to apply it![42]

LIDOCAINE PATCHES: Infused with the painkilling drug lidocaine (Lidoderm), these patches are recommended for nerve pain after a bout of shingles and are also beginning to be used for diabetes-related nerve pain.[43] These prescription patches can be a good option if you can't tolerate the side effects of antidepressants, anticonvulsants, or opioid drugs, or would rather not use them.[44]

The evidence: In two studies of people with shingles nerve pain, those who used a lidocaine patch said they began feeling better after 30 minutes. After 2 weeks, 84 percent got moderate to complete relief.[45] And in one study of 210 people with diabetic neuropathy, lidocaine patches seemed to ease pain as successfully as the antiseizure drug pregabalin (Lyrica). Both improved pain for 68 percent of those who tried one of these therapies.[46]

How it works: Lidocaine seems to help by preventing the transmission of nerve signals from your skin to your spinal cord and brain. It does that by stopping the exchange of ions between cells that allows signals to travel along nerve fibers.

What you need to know: Each lidocaine patch measures 4 inches by 5$\frac{1}{2}$ inches, and you can wear up to three at the same time. They're left on the area where you're experiencing nerve pain for about 12 hours, then have to be removed for 12 hours. They can then be applied again.

ANTIDEPRESSANT DRUGS: Antidepressants are effective for many types of neuropathy, but not because they lift depression. These drugs ease pain by changing levels of neurotransmitters in your brain, which can turn down pain intensity. One type that increases levels of pain-blocking serotonin and norepinephrine is duloxetine (Cymbalta), the first medication approved by the FDA to treat diabetic neuropathy. Other experts say that an older tricyclic antidepressant called amitriptyline (Elavil, Tryptizol, Laroxyl, Sarotex) should be your doctor's first-line choice for easing the pain of postherpetic neuralgia. Antidepressants are less effective for nerve damage related to HIV/AIDS medications.[47] Other antidepressants sometimes prescribed for neuropathic pain include imipramine (Tofranil), desipramine (Norpramin, Pertofrane), venlafaxine (Effexor), bupropion (Wellbutrin), paroxetine (Paxil), and citalopram (Celexa).

The evidence: In one review of 21 studies of antidepressants for neuropathic pain, researchers from England's University of Oxford found that they lift pain by at least 50 percent for 30 percent of people who use them.[48] In one study, amitriptyline, one of the most effective antidepressants for nerve pain, relieved pain for 74 percent of the people who used it.[49] In a British review of six studies of duloxetine for diabetes-related nerve pain, researchers found that one in six people who took the drug saw pain improve by at least 50 percent in 12 to 13 weeks.[50]

How it works: The neurotransmitters serotonin and norepinephrine turn down the volume on pain signals traveling from your spinal cord to your brain. Antidepressants make more of these neurotransmitters available in your brain, which means stronger protection against pain signals.

What you need to know: Older tricyclic antidepressants (they got their name from their chemical structure) such as amitriptyline, imipramine, and desipramine may be more effective for easing nerve pain than newer selective serotonin reuptake inhibitors (SSRIs) like fluoxetine (Prozac). Side effects—including nausea, drowsiness, constipation, and lack of appetite—may make some antidepressants impossible to continue taking. It's worth trying a different type in that case; different drug formulations affect people differently. Many people with nerve pain take their antidepressant dose in the evening to soothe overnight pain and improve sleep.

ANTICONVULSANT DRUGS: Drugs that prevent seizures have also been proven to ease the pain of diabetic neuropathy, trigeminal neuralgia, and shingles nerve pain. Antiseizure drugs have been used for nerve pain for at least 50 years, but risk for serious side effects like liver damage, double vision, and headache kept many people away. Now, newer versions of these pharmaceuticals work for nerve pain with a lower risk of reactions.

The evidence: Two out of three people who try antiseizure drugs for nerve pain can expect to get relief, say researchers who reviewed 12 studies involving 404 people for the evidence-based medicine review organization called the Cochrane Collaboration.[51]

How it works: Experts don't completely understand why antiseizure drugs block nerve pain but suspect they work by muting overly excited nerve fibers so they can't send pain signals to your brain.

What you need to know: Over time, anticonvulsants may become less effective; your doctor might switch you to a different one or increase your dose. The anti-seizure drug doctors often prescribe first for nerve pain, carbamazepine (Tegretol, Carbatrol) can trigger side effects including fatigue, nausea, vision problems, and dizziness. In people of Asian and South Asian ancestry, carbamazepine can also cause potentially fatal skin reactions. As a result, your doctor may order a genetic test to see if you're at risk before prescribing it.[52]

Newer drugs such as gabapentin (Neurontin) and pregabalin (Lyrica) (approved by the FDA for diabetic neuropathy) are often more widely prescribed because they have fewer side effects. Other antiseizure drugs your doctor might prescribe include oxcarbazepine (Trileptal), tiagabine (Gabitril), and topiramate (Topamax).

OPIOID DRUGS: If antidepressants and antiseizure medications don't work for you or don't provide complete relief, your doctor may recommend that you add on or switch to an opioid pain reliever such as oxycodone, morphine, or methadone. Following your doctor's directions is important to get the best results and to cut your odds for side effects like drowsiness and nausea.

The evidence: In one review of 23 studies of opioids for nerve damage pain, researchers found that the drugs reduced pain by at least 13 percent.[53] And when researchers from the University of California, San Francisco, tested high- and low-dose opioids for people whose nerve pain wasn't soothed by other medications, they found that the stronger versions reduced pain by 36 percent, the weaker by 21 percent.[54] Study volunteers also felt calmer and slept better.

How it works: Opioids bind to pain receptors in your brain so that pain signals, in effect, bounce off and can't be felt.

What you need to know: Combining a low-dose opioid with a low-dose antiseizure drug eases pain better than a higher dose of either drug, according to a study published in the *New England Journal of Medicine*.[55]

Opioid side effects such as constipation, nausea, vomiting, drowsiness, and dizziness prompted 11 percent of people in drug trials to drop out.[56] It's important to take opioids around the clock to prevent breakthrough pain. If you wait and take your next dose when pain has started again, it could be more difficult to control.

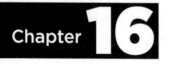

Chapter 16

Cancer Pain

Bone, nerve, organ, or muscle pain

I t may be a dull ache, waves of punishing, knifelike jolts, or a tingling, pins-
and-needles sensation that just won't quit. It may come on slowly, arrive only
at night, or hit you so hard there's no time to head it off. Pain is cancer's common denominator; it affects at least 60 percent of people with newly diagnosed
or intermediate-stage cancers and up to 95 percent with late-stage cancers.

Triggered both by the disease itself and by cancer-related medical tests and
treatments, pain makes the challenge of living with cancer infinitely more difficult. Pain can cost you your job, strain your marriage, lead to depression, and
even lower your chances of beating cancer if it prompts you to call an early halt
to a medical test or delay your next round of treatment.

No one has to live with cancer pain in the 21st century. Experts now say that
90 percent can be eased with simple strategies, the rest with more advanced
treatments. Yet less than half of the people coping with cancer pain get real
relief. When the American Cancer Society reviewed comments from 360 call-
ers to a pain hotline in 2008 and 2009, it saw a disturbing trend: Seventy-six
percent said they'd told their doctors about their cancer pain, yet most were still
living with moderate to severe levels.

The pain relief gap is huge. In one study of 421 Minneapolis-area women
with late-stage ovarian cancer, half weren't receiving the right pain relievers.[1]

When doctors at the University of Texas M. D. Anderson Cancer Center in Houston interviewed 93 people receiving radiation, 66 percent said they'd had pain since starting their treatment but just half got relief.[2] The answer? Closing the gap begins with new attitudes, experts say.

Start by promising yourself you won't grin and bear it. Pain specialists now urge patients to talk openly and in detail about their pain instead of suffering in silence. If you track your pain, rate its intensity, and discuss your experiences, your doctor will know whether your relief plan is working or needs a tweak.

Next, keep an open mind about pain-relieving drugs. Fears of addiction have kept many people with cancer—and their doctors—away from painkillers. But when used safely and effectively, these medications can help you get back to living your life, without leaving you hooked.

Finally, stop thinking that pain relief is all about drugs. Nondrug strategies are just as important. We'll be honest. They probably will not take the place of your pain medications. But a growing stack of research proves that they can bring relief when drugs alone can't and may allow some people with milder pain to reduce doses. They help control flare-ups. And they address pain-related problems that drugs can't even begin to fix, such as soothing emotional reactions that intensify pain, easing depression triggered by chronic aches, giving you a sense of control, and letting you find ways to feel good about your body and your life again. In this chapter you'll find out about the most powerful, research-proven strategies for solving the cancer pain puzzle.

What Type of Cancer Pain Is It?

Understanding why, where, and when you have cancer pain can help you and your doctor find the best solutions. Here's what you need to know.

Why does it hurt?

Cancer pain has three main causes:

- **The type and stage of your cancer:** Many early-stage cancers, such as those of the breast, prostate, and colon, are virtually painless. In contrast, others become painful early on, such as pancreatic and lung cancer. And most late-stage cancers cause pain if tumors have infiltrated bone or are pressing on nerves, organs, or muscle. This can also trigger inflammation, which causes swelling and makes nerves more sensitive. The pain may be different depending on where a tumor is located. A small tumor near a nerve or near your spinal cord may be extremely painful, but a large tumor somewhere else may cause very little discomfort.

- **Cancer-related medical tests:** These include biopsies, spinal taps, and bone marrow tests. Some can be infamously agonizing. For example, prostate cancer biopsies—which use a long, hollow needle to extract tissue samples from a man's prostate gland—cause mild to severe pain for 65 percent to 90 percent of men, prompting some to leap off exam tables before the procedure is finished. Often, anesthesia isn't even offered.

- **Treatment:** Surgery, chemotherapy, radiation, and other therapies can harm healthy tissues while waging their all-out war against your cancer. For example, if you have lymph nodes removed during breast cancer surgery, nerve damage may cause a cold or hot sensation of pins and needles that persists for weeks, months, or even years. At the same time, fluid buildup can make your arm on the side of the lymph node removal

Rate Your Pain

If you're experiencing daily cancer pain, talk with your doctor about a personalized pain-relief plan. Designing one should be a collaboration between you and your doctor or cancer care team. It's up to you to tell your doctor about your pain—when it happens, how it feels, where it is in your body, and how severe it is, as well as about how well any medications you now take are or aren't controlling it. Don't be shy or try to tough it out. It's important to be honest about how your pain feels, about whether it interferes with everyday living, and about how you're coping mentally and emotionally. Don't try to be a model patient who never complains. Your doctor or pain control team need to know how you're doing.

Keeping track of your pain is crucial for helping you and your doctor assess whether your plan is working. The only way to know is to keep track of your pain on a daily basis. Record when you felt pain, where the pain was, how it felt, and how long it lasted. You can use a notebook, add the info to your daily calendar, or copy the sample Pain Diary in Part Three.

Use a pain rating scale to assess the intensity of your pain, too. Some scales use a 1 to 10 rating system, with 1 being blissfully pain free and 10 being the worst pain you can imagine. Some scales are a series of faces, ranging from happy to extremely upset. (See Chapter 1 for more information about pain scales, with examples.) Choose one and make sure your doctor has a copy of the scale in your medical records, so you can refer to it at your appointments. A scale gives the two of you a common language for discussing your pain levels and will help your doctor understand your needs.

swollen and achy. Prostate surgery can lead to pain on urination as well as rectal pain, as the prostate is located next to the rectum.

Radiation therapy and chemotherapy can ease—or cause—pain. Both are sometimes used to target tumors pressing on nerves, and radiation may ease symptoms caused by cancers of the bones, brain, nerves, blood vessels, and spine. But radiation can irritate your skin and the lining of your mouth, even cause adhesions—internal scarring caused when tissues stick to surrounding organs, bones, muscle, or other tissue. Chemotherapy can also damage nerves, especially in the feet and hands.

Where will it hurt?

Cancer pain can affect many body systems. Research shows that 80 percent of the time cancer pain occurs in at least two places in the body; 30 percent of people have pain in three or more spots. These include:

- **Bone pain:** The most common type of cancer pain, this affects 60 to 80 percent of people whose cancer has spread. If cancer cells invade bone, they cause tissue damage that triggers a dull throb.

- **Nerve pain:** Also known as neuropathic pain, this is the result of damage to nerves or of pressure on nerves or the spinal cord. It may feel like a burning, tingling, or crawling sensation. If a tumor spreads to the spine, it can compress the spinal cord, causing back and neck pain, too. Surgery, radiation, and chemotherapy can all cause nerve pain as well.

- **Organ or muscle pain:** This may feel sharp, aching, or throbbing. Soft tissue pains can be tough to locate, too. A pain in your back may be the result of kidney damage, for example, or a swollen liver may make your shoulder hurt.

When will it hurt?

Many people with cancer experience chronic "background pain" along with flare-ups of intense, short-lived breakthrough pain.

Background pain may feel like a dull ache or a constant sharp pain. It may be mild or agonizing, but is usually present for at least 12 hours most days. It can get in the way of your interest in everyday life, keeping you away from friends, events, and places you enjoy. For some people, background pain also leads to an avoidance of further cancer treatments. Traditionally, doctors have relieved it with long-acting prescription drugs called opioids. Today, adding a second (and sometimes a third) drug targeted at specific types of pain has proven even more effective than opioids alone.

Breakthrough pain feels sharp, shooting, and/or radiating. It's sudden and usually unpredictable, but is sometimes triggered by simple activities like getting dressed. The usual duration is 30 to 60 minutes, though it may linger for several hours. Any type of cancer can cause breakthrough pain, but the risk is higher if your cancer affects bones or nerves. New fast-acting pain medications promise better relief from breakthrough pain.

Fast Pain Relief

Even if you take medications and use other strategies to help calm and control background pain, you may still experience flare-ups of breakthrough cancer pain. If they're frequent, talk to your doctor about whether your daily pain-relief strategies need an upgrade. During a flare-up, these strategies can help.

1. **As soon as you realize a flare-up is beginning (or you know it's coming), use the rescue pain medication prescribed by your doctor.** Don't wait. Taking your medication as soon as possible will get you the most relief the fastest and at the lowest dose. Your best option for quick relief is a fast-acting opioid-based painkiller such as a fentanyl-based lozenge, dissolvable oral patch, or sucker (yes, it's like a medicated lollypop). Although 98 percent of people with breakthrough cancer pain rely on pills for fast relief, these drugs take 20 to 30 minutes to begin

working, and that's too long during a flare-up. You'll get faster relief with fentanyl, which is about 100 times more potent than morphine,[3] the other widely used drug for breakthrough pain. It reaches your nervous system in 3 to 5 minutes[4, 5] when absorbed through the thin skin inside your mouth and starts easing pain in 10 minutes, research shows.[6] These lozenges, patches, and suckers are also metabolized quickly, with effects wearing off in a few hours—making them ideal for pain spikes, which usually last 30 to 60 minutes. They're also good if you have trouble swallowing, nausea, or gastrointestinal problems as a result of your cancer or your cancer therapy.

Options available in the United States include: a lozenge you suck on, called a fentanyl buccal tablet (Fentora), a fentanyl "sucker" called oral transmucosal fentanyl citrate (Actiq), and a tiny fentanyl patch called a buccal soluble film (Onsolis) that dissolves in your mouth. Immediate-release morphine, oxycodone, and hydromorphone may cost less but work more slowly.[7]

2. **Make yourself comfortable.** Many people find that certain movements or body positions tend to bring on pain. When a flare-up begins, don't try to push through the pain. Take a break and get comfortable by sitting down, lying down, or changing your position. Research shows that this simple act can bring significant relief. In an Italian study of 302 people with cancer pain, published in the *Journal of Pain and Symptom Management*, 44 percent reported that movement was a trigger. The researchers report that when volunteers stopped the movement, pain decreased or stopped completely for 66 percent.[8]

3. **Distract yourself with guided imagery.** Breathing deeply as you imagine yourself transported to your own personal "happy place"— beside a blue ocean, in a summer meadow, or atop a towering mountain—can also prevent a buildup of stress that can make your pain worse. Like muscle relaxation, guided imagery can also help during a flare-up by distracting you. You may even be able to use imagery exercises to imagine the pain itself diminishing. Have someone read you one of the guided imagery exercises in Chapter 5 or listen to your favorite imagery CD. (Also see Part Three for suggestions.) In one small University of Wisconsin study, 62 percent of people with severe cancer pain reported improvements with guided imagery. Benefits lasted up to an hour.[9]

4. **Relax your mind and body.** Progressive muscle relaxation (try the exercise in Chapter 5) eases physical and emotional tensions that can make pain worse. It can also help distract you while you're waiting for your rescue medicine to take effect. In one University of Wisconsin study of 26 people hospitalized with cancer pain, a 14-minute progressive muscle relaxation exercise reduced pain by at least 30 percent for 42 percent of study participants. Benefits lasted for 30 to 60 minutes. If you use this technique, don't tense muscles that are sore or that provoke pain, of course.[10] Getting comfortable is important when you're in pain.

5. **Warm up tense, aching muscles.** Breakthrough bone and nerve pain can make muscles tighten up, intensifying the ache. A heating pad with a moist setting, a hot bath or shower, adhesive-backed heat patches, or even a warm, moist towel can relax muscles and increase circulation, both of which can help ease pain. (*Cautions:* Don't use a heating pad on bare skin, and don't fall asleep with a heating pad turned on, so be careful if you're taking medications that make you sleepy. Skip areas that are receiving radiation or have in the past 6 months or where circulation is limited.) A menthol cream, lotion, or gel can also warm up and soothe tense muscles (again, skip areas exposed to radiation therapy).

6. **Cool down a sore spot.** For some people, cold therapy works better, numbing pain in sore muscles. Keep gel packs (available at the drugstore) in the freezer so they're ready to use. Or use a bag of frozen peas or corn, or ice cubes in a Ziploc plastic bag. Wrap in a towel or pillow case and apply to sore areas for 5 to 10 minutes. Of course, stop sooner if the cold causes pain or if you start shivering. (Don't use on areas of the body that are receiving radiation treatment or have gotten radiation in the past 6 months, and get your doctor's okay before using cold therapy if you're undergoing chemotherapy.)

7. **Give yourself a gentle self-massage.** When pain flares up, lightly massaging your own head, face, and neck can help you feel more relaxed, say experts from the M. D. Anderson Cancer Center. With light pressure, move your fingertips in small circles over your temples and forehead, behind your ears, and over your jaw. Cup your hands around your neck, with fingertips meeting over your spine. Gently draw your fingertips to the front. Then knead your neck muscles. (Talk with your

doctor first if you're receiving radiation therapy to areas of the body you'd like to massage, or if you have arthritis or any active cancer.)

8. **Switch on your TENS unit.** Transcutaneous electrical nerve stimulation (TENS) sends low-level electrical currents through electrodes to your skin to interrupt pain signals. You may feel a buzzing or tingling sensation instead. According to the American Cancer Society, TENS may work best if your pain is from mild nerve damage resulting from your cancer or cancer therapy.

Relief at Last

How would you like a 20, 30, or 40 percent drop in pain—without increasing your pain reliever doses? What if you could, at the same time, feel your spirits rise and your stress ebb away, so that it felt good to be alive? Complementary therapies such as guided imagery, mindfulness meditation, relaxation, and yoga can give you all these benefits and more. We've compiled the evidence for the best-studied therapies being used today to augment pain drugs.

The more you try, the better. Like drugs, not all will work well for everyone, so it's smart to test-drive several. Be patient. It may take several attempts to come up with the right combination. Go slowly. Learn one technique at a time.

Experts say that the winning combination of pain medications and nondrug therapies is the best way to conquer cancer pain. One reason? These approaches can soothe anxiety, fear, and depression—emotional states that can make your pain feel worse.[11] Because you do most of them yourself, you'll have a feeling of control over pain. This is important, because a cancer diagnosis can leave you feeling as if you have very little control over your own life.

Step 1: Find the best pain medication for you. From drugstore painkillers to strong, prescription pain pills to an unusual collection of drugs that target specific types of cancer pain in unconventional ways, medications are an important part of cancer pain relief for most people. Experts recommend a ladderlike or stepwise approach to cancer pain: starting with over-the-counter remedies for mild to moderate pain, moving up to stronger painkillers for moderate to severe pain, then adding additional drugs if you need more relief.

● For mild to moderate pain, use an over-the-counter NSAID.

● For moderate to severe pain, try an opioid.

● For nerve pain, consider adding an antidepressant.

- If antidepressants don't work, add an antiseizure drug.

- Try including a steroid for inflammation caused by nerve pain.

- For bone pain, add a bone-building bisphosphonate.

Step 2: Start trying out add-on pain control strategies. Keep using the ones that help and add new ones to replace those that don't. We can't tell you which will work best for you; your response is unique. So choose one from the many you'll read about below, see what happens, then add more. The more pain control strategies you have at your fingertips, the better. In a University of Wisconsin–Madison study of 30 people with cancer pain, those who got an MP3 player loaded with 12 different pain control strategies reported that they felt significantly less pain after using them. Among the techniques: guided imagery, relaxation, and nature sound recordings they could use to distract themselves.

Learning several strategies lets you find the ones that work best for you. It also gives you alternatives for a variety of circumstances: Active strategies like yoga may work best if you're at home and feeling energetic, for example, while listening to a distracting piece of music may work best if you're tired or at work (and can slip on headphones!).

Exercise and Movement Therapies

YOGA: Gentle yoga poses that stretch muscles and loosen stiff joints can not only leave you feeling elated after even a short session, but there's growing evidence that they act as pain relievers, too. Yoga can help you become more aware of how your body is feeling. It helps you feel connected to your body, less stressed-out, and able to spot growing tension that can sometimes lead to pain flare-ups.

The evidence: In a Duke University study of 13 women with advanced breast cancer, yoga eased pain significantly—and quickly. The women reported that pain decreased immediately after yoga sessions and stayed lower the following day, too. They also felt more invigorated and relaxed.[12] Other research shows that yoga helps lift depression and anxiety (both of which can make pain feel worse), improves sleep, boosts feelings of peace and tranquility, and works for many types of cancer pain.[13, 14]

How it works: Yoga may help with cancer pain because it relaxes muscles, gives your mind and emotions a break from worry as you pay attention to your body position in various postures, and relieves stress.

What you need to know: Look for a yoga class taught by an experienced instructor who's been trained to work with people with cancer. Check local hospitals and cancer centers for classes and ask your oncologist for a recommendation. There are many styles of yoga; those used in most studies are considered gentle, mild, or restorative and focus on easy poses as well as relaxation. Never push yourself to do more than feels right or safe in a yoga class. The most important thing is working within your body's capabilities. See Part Three for a sample routine and resources for finding a class near you.

Touch Therapies

ACUPUNCTURE: When it comes to cancer care, this ancient healing art—so old that archeologists have uncovered 5,000-year-old stone acupuncture needles in Inner Mongolia—is practically mainstream in 21st century medicine. Acupuncture cannot cure cancer, but research shows it has a good track record for helping to relieve pain as well as nausea, hot flashes, and other side effects of cancer and cancer treatments, especially when drugs fall short. Many cutting-edge cancer centers now have licensed acupuncturists on staff, specially trained to work with people who have cancer. And the American Cancer Society and the National Institutes of Health recognize it as a safe integrative medical treatment.

The evidence: Research shows that acupuncture can help relieve the nerve, bone, muscle, or organ pain related to many types of cancer—including those types in which pain is difficult to soothe, such as lung cancer.[15] In a French study of 90 people with advanced cancer whose pain wasn't fully controlled by medication, acupuncture at specific points along their ears decreased pain 36 percent, and the relief lasted for at least 2 months. The researchers used tiny, thumbtacklike needles that stay in place for weeks at a time, a practice called auricular acupuncture.[16] People in this study had pain caused by nerve damage, a type that often resists relief with drugs alone.

After surgery for colon cancer, 93 people who got pain medications plus acupuncture and massage reported their pain decreased twofold compared to people who received standard medical care in one University of California, San Francisco, study. The acupuncture and massage group also felt less depressed—good news because depression can magnify pain.[17]

Acupuncture holds promise for easing the excruciating and tough-to-treat pain flare-ups that can happen when cancer spreads to bone, British researchers say. In several small studies, people with cancer-related bone pain report that acupuncture brought significant relief.[18]

How it works: Brain scans and other research suggest that acupuncture relieves pain by stimulating the release of endorphins, the body's natural pain relievers.[19] It also interrupts the flow of pain signals to the brain, improves blood flow, and helps dial back your brain's emotional responses to pain signals, an effect that reduces the intensity of unpleasant or agonizing sensations.[20]

What you should know: Always confer with your oncologist before scheduling acupuncture and be sure to work only with a certified acupuncturist who is also trained in cancer care. At press time, just one cancer center in the United States—Memorial Sloan-Kettering Cancer Center (MSKCC)—had a training program to teach licensed acupuncturists to work with people with cancer. For a referral, contact MSKCC's integrative medicine service by phone at 646-888-0800. More and more cancer centers have acupuncturists on staff who are trained to work with cancer patients. If you don't have access to one, ask your oncologist if she can recommend a certified acupuncturist with oncology training. (Turn to Part Three for more on finding a licensed acupuncturist.) Bring treatment notes from your doctor to your first session and ask the practitioner to contact your doctor before planning your acupuncture treatment.

There's a slight risk for infection and bleeding, so some cancer experts advise against acupuncture if you're having heavy doses of chemotherapy, a bone marrow transplant, or flap reconstruction (such as after mastectomy), if you have a low white blood cell count (neutropenia) or low blood platelets (thrombocytopenia), or if you already have a fever, infection, or a tendency to bleed heavily. If you have lymphedema (a swelling of the arms or legs) after cancer treatment, make sure acupuncture is not performed on that limb.

MASSAGE THERAPY: From invigorating full-body rubdowns to gentle strokes on your feet, massage has uncommon power to soothe mind and body. Once, people with cancer were warned to avoid massage for fear it would disturb tumors, speed circulation, and provoke the spread of cancer. Today, massage therapists trained to work with cancer patients are opening the doors to the deep-down benefits of this powerful pain-relieving touch therapy.

A massage therapist's soothing hands can help you feel less alone on your cancer journey. And massage has important pain-stopping benefits; studies show it can help many types and stages of cancer and may help you get more pain relief without increasing the amount of pain relievers you take. It may even help you reduce your dose. Massage also relieves cancer-related symptoms such as anxiety, fatigue, and depression, all of which can make pain feel worse.

The evidence: Plenty of research shows that massage works for many stages and types of cancer and many types of cancer pain. In one large study of 1,290 people with various cancers, researchers from Memorial Sloan-Kettering Cancer Center in New York found that pain dropped by 40 percent after massage. The study looked at three types of massage—classic, muscle-kneading

Swedish rubdowns, light-touch massages, and simple foot rubs—and found that all helped. People felt better right away, and the effects lingered for up to 2 days. The researchers concluded that "massage therapy . . . is non-invasive, inexpensive, comforting, free of side effects and greatly appreciated by recipients."[21]

Massage helps with pain from many types of cancer. In a University of Colorado study of 380 people with advanced cancers, those who got six half-hour massages during a 2-week period reported big reductions in pain: a 1.9-point drop on a 10-point pain scale. Participants had cancers of the lung, breast, pancreas, colon, and prostate, all of which had spread to other organs or to their bones.[22]

Massage may also help you use smaller doses of pain medicine and still feel comfortable. That's what happened in a University of Minnesota study of 230 people with cancer who received massage.[23] And it can just help you feel great. People with cancer who've gotten a massage say things like "It's like a vacation from cancer," "It's my place to be in control and do something for myself," and "I'm overcome by the most amazing feelings of acceptance and peace."

Related touch therapies like Reiki, reflexology, and a type of medical massage called manual lymph drainage have also been proven to ease discomfort.

How it works: Massage seems to ease pain directly and indirectly. It triggers

Bodywork for People with Cancer

These comforting and restorative touch and bodywork therapies can soothe body and soul.

● **Reflexology:** A really terrific foot massage, reflexology is based on the belief that the foot is a map of the whole body. Applying pressure at specific spots on your sole is said to change the flow of energy in a corresponding body part. Other advocates say it feels good for a simpler reason: It improves blood flow and works the tension out of muscles. If you're in too much pain or too ill for body massage, reflexology is a good alternative.

● **Reiki and therapeutic touch:** In these touch-free bodywork techniques, a practitioner makes sweeping movements and uses special hand positions over the body to smooth and improve the flow of energy inside. There's no physical contact, and you don't have to take your clothes off. Advocates call these modalities "energy healing."

● **Body awareness techniques:** These classes, available at many cancer centers, help you become more flexible and promote a sense of wholeness and wellness. One popular form, called Feldenkrais, employs slow, gentle movements to improve body awareness. Another, the Alexander Technique, uses postures and exercises to bring the head, neck, torso, and spine into alignment.

It doesn't take a professional to give a great massage. Safe, gentle, at-home massage, given by a spouse or a caregiver, eased pain 34 percent in a recent National Cancer Institute–funded study of 97 people with cancer. It also lifted stress and anxiety by 44 percent, fatigue by 32 percent, depression by 31 percent, and nausea by 29 percent. The researchers say home massage was good for givers and receivers.

the release of dopamine, one of the body's natural pain-relieving brain chemicals, eases inflammation, relaxes muscle spasms, and increases circulation to bring more oxygen to muscles that may be tense.[24] At the same time, it invokes the relaxation response, reducing mind-body stress that can make pain feel worse.[25]

What you need to know: Check in with your oncologist before scheduling a massage, especially if you're undergoing cancer treatment or have recently finished.

Work only with a certified massage therapist (and one who is also licensed if your state requires it; see Part Three for details) who has received advanced training in cancer care. Your doctor may be able to recommend someone, or check the online locator service of the Society for Oncology Massage (www.s4om.org), which lists massage therapists who've been trained in cancer care programs recognized by the society. You can also learn some of the techniques with a DVD called *Touch, Caring, and Cancer: Simple Instruction for Family and Friends*, which was developed as part of a research study sponsored by the National Cancer Institute (www.partnersinhealing.net).

Massage therapists should avoid these areas on cancer patients: tumor sites, incisions from surgery, areas that have received radiation, skin thinned or damaged by radiation treatment, and the skin near medical devices such as an IV catheter. A therapist should use only light strokes if your blood platelet count (which can be reduced by chemotherapy) is lower than normal, if cancer is in your bones or you have brittle-bone disease (osteoporosis), if you have nerve damage in your hands or feet, if you take anticlotting drugs, or if your spine is unstable or you have fractures. Skip massage if you have neutropenia (a white blood cell count of 1,000 or less).

Mind-Body Therapies

EMOTIONAL SUPPORT: Talking about your experiences, exploring and expressing your feelings, and problem-solving can make you feel better emotionally. But a growing stack of research shows that emotional support can reduce pain and ease depression, stress, and anxiety.

The evidence: In one study of women with advanced breast cancer, those who participated in weekly group therapy sessions for 1 year reported half as much pain as those who only got conventional medical care. They also felt less tense, depressed, tired, and confused and were less likely to smoke, drink alcohol, or overeat to cope with their feelings. In their support group, they talked honestly about living with cancer—their fears, their frustrations with their doctors, and the ways their families had to adjust.[26, 27]

How it works: Emotional support may help by reducing stress and depression, proven to intensify physical pain. It can also help you feel less tired and more motivated to eat well, exercise, and get enough sleep, all of which help you feel your best and may help you cope better with pain.

What you need to know: If you're having a difficult time coping with cancer, one-on-one counseling may be your best bet. Otherwise, a support group—in person or online—may be all you need. See Part Three for resources to find a support group near you. You can find support groups in your area by using the American Cancer Society's online locator service at http://www.cancer.org/. The Web site www.cancercare.org offers free, professionally moderated support groups online. The R. A. Bloch Cancer Foundation (800-433-0464) and the Cancer Hope Network (www.cancerhopenetwork.org or 800-552-4366) match you with cancer survivors. National groups that support research and treatment for specific types of cancer also offer support services. You'll find a comprehensive list on the Web site of the National Cancer Institute (www.cancer.gov) or by phone at 800-4-CANCER.

GUIDED IMAGERY: Imagine the sights, sounds, and scents of a tropical island. The burst of tart juice when you bite into a grapefruit. Or the deep calm you feel holding hands with someone you love. These imaginary experiences can leave you feeling like you've been on a long, relaxing vacation—and they have serious pain-relief benefits for people with cancer, too.

Guided imagery involves using all your senses to put yourself into a richly imagined scene that's pleasant, relaxing, and distracting. It might be a place from your past or a beautiful scene you build for yourself, such as a sunny beach, a beautiful meadow, or a scenic mountaintop. In your imagination, you move around in this place and experience it with all your senses—its sounds, sights, smells, feel, even tastes. You find it easier to relax your mind and your body. Feelings of fear and panic ebb away. Practiced on your own with a CD of recorded exercises or with the help of a therapist, guided imagery is proven to help ease pain and to make stress, fear, and anxiety evaporate. Cancer experts say guided imagery may help you control pain with lower doses of pain medications and can help you stay calm and relaxed during pain-provoking procedures such as a bone marrow biopsy or bronchoscopy, an examination of the throat, larynx, and airways.

The evidence: Guided imagery is usually combined with relaxation techniques for best results. In a study from the Fred Hutchinson Cancer Research Center in Seattle of people undergoing bone marrow transplants, those who used guided imagery plus relaxation techniques got the most relief for a common and painful side effect called oral mucositis.[28] In a University of Wisconsin study of 40 people undergoing chemotherapy, radiation therapy, or both for cancer, researchers found that half of those who practiced guided imagery saw pain intensity drop 31 percent.[29] And according to the American Cancer Society, other research shows that guided imagery may be helpful in managing stress, anxiety, and depression, and in lowering blood pressure, reducing pain, and reducing some side effects of chemotherapy. It can also help quell anticipatory nausea and vomiting before a chemotherapy session.

How it works: A vivid image can reduce stress and even relax muscles by lowering your heart rate, slowing your breathing, and reducing levels of the stress hormone cortisol. Researchers say guided imagery can help control pain by interrupting the delivery of pain signals to your brain, by helping you stop paying attention to pain, and by reducing thoughts that magnify pain.[30]

What you need to know: For best results, practice guided imagery exercises for a few minutes every day. The more you do it, the more effective it will be—and the more it will help you if you experience a flare-up of breakthrough pain. Turn to Chapter 5 for a guided imagery exercise you can try. Part Three also has more information on finding guided imagery CDs, books, and qualified instructors. You can listen to free guided imagery exercises for cancer pain relief on the Web site of the University of Michigan Comprehensive Cancer Center at http://www.cancer.med.umich.edu/support/guided_imagery_podcasts_descriptions.shtml. Classes or one-on-one instruction with a qualified teacher can help you learn the most effective techniques for you.

HYPNOSIS: Hypnotherapy is nothing like the hypnosis you see in the movies. You won't fall into a trance or do something you'll regret later on. Instead, this form of healing hypnosis sends you into a state of deep relaxation and awareness. Performed by a medical hypnotherapist, it can help you change your attitude about cancer pain so that you feel less fear and tension. Learn it yourself and self-hypnosis can help you handle pain episodes so that they feel less intense and overwhelming.

The evidence: In a Stanford University study of 124 women with advanced breast cancer, those who learned self-hypnosis and participated in group therapy sessions for 1 year saw a much smaller increase in pain over the year than those who didn't get either therapy. Study volunteers who were the most "hypnotizable" got the biggest benefits and were most likely to use hypnosis at home when pain cropped up.[31] When researchers at Mount Sinai School of Medicine in New York hypnotized women before breast cancer surgery, the women needed less anesthesia because they felt less pain during surgery. They also had less pain, nausea, and emotional distress afterward.[32]

How it works: Self-hypnosis involves putting yourself into a deeply relaxed yet fully aware state in which you can focus on changing your experience of your pain. Medical hypnosis by a licensed practitioner works in a similar way. It's not mind control; you're aware of what's going on around you, but you feel very calm. According to the National Institutes of Health, hypnosis can help with chronic pain, fear, and anxiety.

What you need to know: Check in with your doctor before trying hypnosis and work with only with a licensed, certified hypnotherapist, such as those licensed by the National Board for Certified Clinical Hypnotherapists. For more information, turn to Chapter 5 and Part Three.

MINDFULNESS MEDITATION: Also called mindfulness-based stress reduction, this simple technique involves getting comfortable, closing your eyes, and simply following your breath as you inhale and exhale. The "mindfulness" part? Gently drawing your focus back to your breath each time your mind wanders so that you stay in the present. It may also involve scanning your body to become more aware of how each area and part is feeling. No judgments, just noticing is one of the keys of mindfulness.

The challenge? When you're in pain, it can be difficult to stay in the moment—or to want to be in the moment. But research proves that being present can be the way out, by directly easing discomfort and muting factors such as stress, worry, lack of exercise, and a bad night's sleep, which all make pain worse for people with cancer. Other types of meditation, such as transcendental meditation, prayerful meditation (such as a long, contemplative prayer that includes repeated words or sounds), and guided meditations may help, too, according to British cancer experts.

The evidence: Stress levels dropped for 1,000 women with breast cancer and men with prostate cancer who took an 8-week mindfulness meditation class, report researchers at the University of Calgary. They got more and better sleep, exercised more frequently, and drank less caffeine—suggesting they felt more energetic (and probably helping them sleep better at night!). They also showed healthy changes in levels of stress hormones.[33] In a pilot study at the Dana-Farber Cancer Institute, a meditation technique called mindfulness-based stress reduction helped 18 people undergoing stem cell/bone marrow transplantation to feel happier and calmer.[34] Pain diminished and their heart rates and breathing slowed to more relaxed levels.[35, 36] In a Canadian study of 63 people with cancer-related sleep problems, mindfulness meditation helped them fall asleep and stay asleep more easily.[37]

How it works: Mindfulness meditation reduces levels of stress hormones, relaxes the body, and teaches your mind to observe what's going on without jumping to conclusions that can make pain worse by making you feel fearful or anxious or upset. You feel calmer and more in control.

What you need to know: Using mindfulness regularly gets best results. The good news is that it doesn't have to take very long and can be practiced when you have just a few minutes while waiting for a doctor's appointment, during a work break, or between activities at home. Just remember the acronym STOP:

S: Slow down and stop.

T: Take slow, deep breaths, paying attention to how it feels when you inhale, your chest and belly expanding, and when you exhale.

O: Observe your thoughts, emotions, and body sensations.

P: Proceed with your day with awareness and curiosity.

For more on mindfulness exercises, classes, books, tapes, and CDs, see Part Three.

PROGRESSIVE MUSCLE RELAXATION: Tense and relax your muscles as you imagine stress slipping away. Breathe quietly as you calm your mind. Tension-melting techniques like these can help you better cope with cancer pain mentally and physically. Relaxation exercises are often combined with other strategies, like guided imagery, for even better results.

The evidence: Pain became 31 percent less intense and 26 percent less distressing for half of the cancer patients who practiced progressive muscle relaxation for just 2 days in a University of Wisconsin study.[38] They also felt more in control of their pain. That's good news, as most of the 16 study volunteers were undergoing cancer treatment and all were taking strong pain relievers that hadn't completely blotted out chronic cancer pain. Afterward, three out of four told the researchers they enjoyed the exercise, which involved tensing and releasing 12 muscle groups (they avoided sore spots). In a study of 60 women undergoing chemotherapy for breast cancer, South Korean researchers found that those who practiced muscle relaxation exercises and guided imagery before each treatment session were less anxious and depressed and had a better outlook on life 6 months later.[39] Relaxation has been shown to improve sleep for women undergoing chemotherapy for breast cancer, too.[40]

How it works: Progressive muscle relaxation may help reduce levels of stress hormones and inflammation in the body, both of which can play a role in chronic cancer pain.

What you need to know: Give yourself time to learn progressive muscle relaxation. One researcher says it may take up to 40 minutes in early sessions to really feel muscle tension easing, but over time you can get results faster if you've trained your mind and body to relax. Skip muscles that are sore or that make pain elsewhere in your body feel worse. To get started, try out the relaxation exercise in Chapter 5, or turn to Part Three for information on ordering books and CDs about this useful technique.

Pain Medications and Other Medical Treatments

OVER-THE-COUNTER NONSTEROIDAL ANTI-INFLAMMATORIES: Acetaminophen, aspirin, or ibuprofen may be all you need for relief if you have mild to moderate pain.

The evidence: A review of 42 studies involving 3,084 people concluded that NSAIDs were effective for cancer pain; for mild, short-term pain, they were as effective as opioids.[41]

How it works: NSAIDs like aspirin and ibuprofen help by reducing swelling and inflammation.

What you need to know: Overuse of aspirin and ibuprofen can cause gastrointestinal bleeding; overuse of acetaminophen can cause liver problems. See Chapter 6 for details.

OPIOIDS: If NSAIDs don't blunt your pain sufficiently, it's time to climb to the next rung on the pain-relief ladder: opioid drugs such as morphine, codeine, hydrocodone (available with acetaminophen as Lortab or Vicodin), hydromorphone (Dilaudid), fentanyl (Duragesic), meperidine (Demerol), oxycodone, and methadone.[42] These opioids all relieve pain in ways similar to opium—the active ingredient in morphine—and are the gold standard for cancer pain relief.

The evidence: Morphine, the most widely used cancer pain drug, is the cornerstone of the World Health Organization's guidelines for treating this kind of pain.[43] In one 2007 review of 54 studies involving 3,749 cancer patients, British researchers concluded that opioids all worked well to control pain and that some newer forms, such as skin patches, may bring relief faster than others.

How it works: Opioids boost pain tolerance and at the same time reduce the brain's perception of pain intensity and its reaction to pain signals.

What you should know: Are they safe? Opioids have a reputation for addiction, something experts say doesn't happen all that often with cancer pain. Thanks to new combination pain-relief strategies—opioids plus other medications and/or complementary therapies—your risk for problems may be lower simply because you may not have to increase the dosage to get relief. You may develop some physical dependence, which means you would need to taper off if you decided to stop taking the drug rather than simply stopping cold. Your body may build up a tolerance, though, which could mean needing larger doses to get relief. But avoiding opioids for fear of addiction, experts say, leaves many people stuck with unnecessary cancer pain.

If one opioid doesn't work, try another. Different people get relief with different types; the only way to find the one best for you is through trial and error.[44] Don't worry that using an opioid now will leave you without options if pain gets worse later on; you may develop some tolerance, but there's no ceiling dose with these drugs. If at some point you need more for pain, it will still work.

Constipation is a nearly universal side effect; plan on using stool softeners

Treatments for Stubborn, Severe Pain

If pain medications plus drug-free strategies don't relieve your pain, more invasive treatments may. These options, usually reserved for advanced cancers, include:

Chemotherapy: Anticancer drugs can shrink pain-provoking tumors.

Neurosurgery: Nerves that transmit pain signals to the brain are cut.

Nerve blocks: Pain medication is injected into or around a nerve or into the spine to block pain signals.

Radiopharmaceutical drugs: These medications, such as strontium-89 (Metastron) and samarium-153 (Quadramet), contain radioactive elements. They collect in bone and kill off invading cancer cells, easing pain. They are more effective than radiation in many places if cancer has spread to bone.

Radiation therapy: Relieves pain if cancer has spread to bone. Most effective if the pain is in one or just a few areas, can also be used to shrink tumors pressing on the spine.

Surgery: Part or all of a tumor may be removed if it is pressing on nerves, organs, or causing pain in other ways.

and a laxative daily. You may also have nausea for a short time; your doctor can prescribe medication to control it. Many people are also sleepy when starting an opioid, but this effect usually wears off in a few days.

ANTIDEPRESSANTS: If your doctor suggests one, he's not saying you're depressed or have a mental illness. A class of drugs called tricyclic antidepressants (named for their chemical structure), including amitriptyline (Elavil), nortriptyline (Aventyl, Pamelor), and desipramine (Norpramin), can help with the tingling and burning of nerve pain, research shows. They work best, pain researchers say, when taken along with an opioid.

The evidence: When researchers reviewed 50 studies of 19 antidepressants for the treatment of pain caused by nerve tissue damage, also known as neuropathic pain, they found that tricyclics brought relief for two-thirds of the people who took them.[45] These include medications such as imipramine (Tofranil), clomipramine (Anafranil, Clomicalm), desipramine, and nortriptyline.

How it works: Researchers suspect these drugs turn down the volume of pain signals sent from damaged nerves to the brain, boost the pain-relieving powers of opioids, and help you get a better night's sleep, which can help you better cope with pain.[47, 48]

What you need to know: These drugs may take several weeks to work; side effects include digestion problems and dizziness.

ANTISEIZURE MEDICATIONS: Antiseizure drugs like gabapentin (Neurontin) and clonazepam (Klonopin) could help if antidepressants aren't effective or if you can't take them because of side effects.

The evidence: In one study published in the *Journal of Pain and Symptom Management*, of 63 people with cancer-related nerve pain, those who took an

On the Horizon

Pain-Relief Nasal Spray

Vastly more potent than morphine, the drug fentanyl reaches your nervous system and begins easing pain in a matter of minutes—two to three times faster than pills—making it a top choice for the relief of breakthrough cancer pain. It's now available in the United States as a lozenge on a stick (like a lollypop) and a thin film that dissolves in your mouth, and researchers are also looking into a nasal spray version. In one recent study from the Georgia Center for Cancer Pain Management & Palliative Medicine, a fentanyl nose spritz eased pain in 5 minutes for one-third of study volunteers and in 10 minutes for another third.[46] It could be a good option for people who can't use lozenges or dissolvable films because of dry mouth, mouth sores, nausea, or vomiting.

Strong Medicine: Using Opioid Drugs Wisely, Safely, and Effectively

Worried that taking morphine or another opioid pain reliever will lead to addiction? This misconception keeps many people, and their doctors, from taking advantage of the pain relief these medications offer. If your doctor prescribes an opioid, these steps can help you get the best results.

- **Choose the right form.** Pain drugs are usually prescribed as a pill or liquid, but a skin patch, rectal suppositories, injections, or infusion pump may work better for you. Pain drugs have to reach your bloodstream in order to go to work. If you take pills but are experiencing nausea and vomiting, the medicine can't reach your digestive system in order to be absorbed into your bloodstream. If you opt for a skin patch but are sweating profusely, it won't stick to your skin, so the drug can't be transferred into your skin. If pain is severe, an infusion pump delivers the drug directly to your spinal cord for faster, longer relief. Talk to your doctor about the form that's best for you.

- **Take the full dose at the right time.** Don't let fears about pain drugs lead you to skimp by taking a partial dose or waiting longer between doses. Both can lead to more severe pain that requires a larger dose of medication. By taking the right dose at the right time, you can keep pain at bay. If pain is getting stronger before you're due to take your next dose, talk to your doctor about whether you need a larger dose or a different prescription.

antiseizure drug with an opioid had less burning, shooting pain and fewer side effects than those who took an opioid alone at a higher dose.[49]

How it works: These drugs may help by reducing oversensitivity in nerve cells that transmit pain signals to the brain.[50]

What you need to know: Side effects can include lowered white blood cell counts, dizziness, blurred vision, and nausea.

ANTI-INFLAMMATORY STEROIDS: Corticosteroids like prednisone and dexamethasone not only ease pain, they can help with appetite, which sometimes flags after cancer therapy.

The evidence: Researchers have found that steroids helped reduce the pain of advanced prostate cancer in one Columbia University study of 770 men[51] and with cancers that have spread to bone in a Case Western Reserve University study of 139 men.[52]

How it works: Steroids reduce swelling, which would ease pain by releasing pressure on nerves.

- **Stick with your plan.** Increasing your drug dose without talking to your doctor could increase your risk for side effects. Taking less could lead to withdrawal symptoms. Remember to renew your prescription before it runs out, too. And don't split, chew, or crush pain pills unless your doctor says it's okay.

- **Start taking a laxative pronto.** Opioids almost always cause constipation because they slow the pace of food through your intestinal tract. This makes stools hard. Be sure your doctor recommends a bowel regimen (usually a stool softener such as docusate (Colace) and a stimulative laxative such as bisacodyl (Dulcolax) or senna. Drink lots of water, but don't add a fiber supplement; these tend to make constipation from these drugs even more painful.

- **For better sleep, ask about a long-acting opioid.** If you have to wake up in the middle of the night to take your next dose on time, you're interrupting needed sleep. A long-acting formula might be a better bet.

- **Add other pain-relieving strategies and medications.** Plenty of research shows that adding a second drug for specific types of cancer pain (such as bone or nerve pain) and practicing a nondrug pain-relief technique works better than just taking an opioid alone.

- **Don't combine opioids with sleeping pills, tranquilizers, or alcohol.** This could make you feel confused, anxious, dizzy, or even cause breathing problems. Tell your doctor if you use any of these—and about all other medications you take—so she can advise you about avoiding problems.

What you need to know: Side effects of using steroids long term include weight gain, fluid retention, and thinning bones.

BISPHOSPHONATES: The same type of medication used to bolster fracture-prone bones in people with osteoporosis can relieve the pain of cancer that's spread to the bones. Bisphosphonates used for cancer bone pain include pamidronate (Aredia), ibandronate (Boniva), and clodronate (Bonefos).

The evidence: In one review of studies involving 1,955 men with prostate cancer that had spread to bone, 27 percent of those who took a bisphosphonate along with their other medications got pain relief.[53] In a study of advanced breast cancer, clodronate decreased pain significantly.[54]

How it works: Bisphosphonates prevent bone loss and also seem to protect bone against new invasions from cancer cells.

What you should know: Bisphosphonates may work best for advanced breast cancer and multiple myeloma and help in cancers of the lungs, prostate, and digestive system.

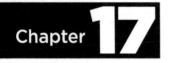

Chapter **17**

Mystery and Bodywide Pain

Chronic fatigue syndrome, fibromyalgia, mystery pain, and functional somatic syndromes

Chronic widespread pain is thought to affect up to 10 percent of the population[1, 2] and often it has no obvious cause. While some individuals with chronic, bodywide pain will eventually be diagnosed as having chronic fatigue syndrome or fibromyalgia, others will simply be told that they have a functional somatic syndrome—in other words, that their experience of pain has no obvious medical cause.

In some ways those aren't actually different diagnoses. Chronic fatigue syndrome, fibromyalgia, and medically unexplained pain are all functional somatic syndromes, as are irritable bowel syndrome and several other diseases characterized by mystery pain. In addition, some doctors question whether these are different diseases at all or simply varying manifestations of the same illness. It's a reasonable question. Even though the individual diseases have specific symptoms, many patients diagnosed with one functional somatic syndrome fit the diagnostic criteria for several others.[3] There are huge overlaps even between such seemingly disparate diseases as fibromyalgia and irritable bowel syndrome,[4] and all of the functional somatic syndromes are closely intertwined with anxiety and depression. These conditions are sometimes referred to as somatoform pain disorders.

Because of the nonspecific nature of their symptoms and the lack of an obvious underlying cause, fibromyalgia, chronic fatigue syndrome, and other functional somatic syndromes remain difficult to diagnose. Fortunately, many doctors and scientists have focused on developing new types of treatments that help people cope with their pain no matter what the cause.

If you think you may have a functional somatic disorder, the good news is that you don't need a formal diagnosis to start taking steps to improve your health. Although a formal diagnosis may help you feel more confident managing your symptoms, coping with full-body pain isn't just about identifying your condition and using that label to choose the right drug. Although medication can certainly be a big help, simple behavioral changes may be your best opportunity to get back on the road to a strong, happy, and functional life.

Chronic Fatigue Syndrome

Chronic fatigue syndrome was first defined as a condition by the Centers for Disease Control in 1988,[5] but there were no internationally standardized diagnostic criteria published until 1994. It remains difficult to diagnose, and thus estimates of how many people are affected by chronic fatigue syndrome vary. Current studies suggest that the syndrome, which is two to three times more common among women than men, may affect about 1 out of every 100 people,[6] and cases are found worldwide. It is most often seen in people between the ages of 20 and 40.

Individuals with chronic fatigue syndrome have so little energy that they can no longer live their lives in the same way they did before the disease's onset. Sleep doesn't help, exercise makes it worse, and because there is no obvious cause of chronic fatigue it can be very hard to diagnose and treat. By the time people are diagnosed with chronic fatigue syndrome, they have suffered from profound, life-altering fatigue for at least 6 months in addition to potentially experiencing a wide variety of other full-body symptoms.

Although it may take several years to get a chronic fatigue syndrome diagnosis, the good news is that most doctors no longer think that your exhaustion is all in your head. In fact, although mood disorders are beginning to seem like an important component of chronic fatigue syndrome, they are only that—a

When to Call the Doctor

Getting a diagnosis of chronic fatigue syndrome takes so long that by the time people have been able to put a name on their symptoms, they are often frustrated with the whole medical profession. However, even if you have been diagnosed with chronic fatigue, you should call your doctor if:

- You have swollen glands
- The type of symptoms you have changes
- You are unable to get sufficient sleep
- Your fatigue is accompanied by blurry vision, weight loss, or frequent urination, which could be signs of diabetes

If you have not yet been diagnosed with chronic fatigue syndrome but have long-lasting fatigue and/or the other symptoms listed below, you should visit a doctor. Early diagnosis may make it easier for you to get effective treatment.

component. Doctors have become more aware of the other aspects of chronic fatigue syndrome—including inflammation, muscle aches, sleep disorders, and cognitive problems,[7] and they are focusing their treatment on improving those specific symptoms as well as overall quality of life.

Is It Chronic Fatigue Syndrome?

Chronic fatigue is characterized by long-lasting fatigue so severe that it affects your ability to go about the tasks of everyday life. This physical and mental exhaustion is made worse by stress and does not get better when you sleep. When you have chronic fatigue syndrome:

- **You are so tired that you cannot go about the activities of your daily life.** This exhaustion occurs whether you exert yourself physically or not, and it may either continue for long periods of time or come in waves.

- **You experience other physical symptoms, including body aches, fever, and sore throat, whenever you experience fatigue.** These symptoms may vary from episode to episode and last for weeks or months.

- **You have difficulty concentrating or have problems with your memory.** You may also be depressed, have trouble sleeping, or want to sleep too much.

● **Any physical exertion leaves you feeling sick for a day or more, even if the activity used to be simple for you.**

There is currently no laboratory test for chronic fatigue syndrome, and so doctors diagnose it primarily by listening to your symptoms. If you think you may have chronic fatigue syndrome, make certain to tell your doctor about how your fatigue has impacted your ability to live your life and describe any associated pain or other physical symptoms. At that point, your doctor will probably put you through an extensive series of tests to rule out the long list of other medical and psychiatric causes that could be causing your symptoms before giving you a diagnosis.

Although there are several different sets of diagnostic criteria used in various settings, the international standard for diagnosis[8] of chronic fatigue syndrome is that:

1. A person has chronic fatigue that has persisted for at least 6 months, or intermittent, relapsing fatigue that is unrelated to exertion. This fatigue does not improve with rest and causes a significant reduction in the patient's previous levels of activity.

2. Other diseases that could cause chronic fatigue have been excluded.

3. At least four of the following symptoms have been observed, concurrently, for at least 6 months after the onset of fatigue.

> Impaired memory or concentration
>
> Sore throat
>
> Painful lymph nodes in the neck or under the arms
>
> Muscle or joint pain without swelling or redness
>
> Headaches of a new type, pattern, or severity
>
> Sleep that does not leave the person refreshed
>
> Exhaustion after exertion that lasts more than a day

Depending on the country you live in and where your doctor was trained, your chronic fatigue syndrome may have been diagnosed as myalgic encephalomyelitis. This term refers to exactly the same condition, but some people may find that a diagnosis of the more technical-sounding myalgic encephalomyelitis is taken more seriously than one of chronic fatigue.[9]

Fast Pain Relief

There is no fast relief for the exhaustion that is the primary symptom of chronic fatigue syndrome. However, there are ways to treat the associated aches and pains. The important thing is to focus on making yourself as comfortable as possible.

1. **If your fatigue comes with headaches and muscle pain, take an over-the-counter NSAID such as aspirin or ibuprofen.** The physical pain associated with chronic fatigue can be treated with painkillers. Just be careful not to overdo it. Excess use of painkillers can cause additional damage to your body, so if you find yourself wanting to take more than the recommended dose, talk to your doctor about prescription alternatives.

2. **Prescription-strength analgesics can be used to control other pain symptoms.** Pain management can significantly improve quality of life for patients with chronic fatigue syndrome.[10] Don't hesitate to talk to your doctors about treating the secondary symptoms of your illness just because fatigue is your major concern.

3. **Slow down if it gets too hard.** When you have chronic fatigue syndrome it can be frustrating not to be able to do everything you want or need to do. However, it's important to be realistic. If you feel like you are too exhausted to complete a task, take a break. It's normal to try to push through and finish things, but for patients with chronic fatigue, it's actually counterproductive. Exceeding your energy limits[11] can leave you unable to function for a day or more, so it's much better to stop and take a break and then pick up whatever you were doing again later.

Relief at Last

When you have chronic fatigue syndrome, it can be difficult even to get out of bed in the morning. Still, there are some simple coping strategies that can help you live a more full life with your exhaustion and pain.

Step 1: Pace yourself. When figuring out what you need to get done on any given day, first think about how you're feeling and how much energy you have.[12] That will allow you to choose appropriate activities and plan for any necessary breaks. You'll get more done if you're realistic about how much you can do than if you do too much and set off a flare-up.

Step 2: Move, but not too fast or too far. Chronic fatigue syndrome makes exercise exhausting, but small amounts of exercise and activity can increase your resilience and give you the ability to do more over time. Don't push yourself so hard that you make your symptoms worse, but don't let fear keep you from the things you can still enjoy in life.

Step 3: Look for ways to relax. Meditation,[13] massage, and similar relaxation techniques have been shown to have benefits for some people with chronic fatigue syndrome. Finding ways to incorporate these techniques into your life can give you more energy for the rest of the day.

Step 4: Seek psychiatric help. When your chronic fatigue is associated with specific psychological symptoms such as depression or anxiety, treating those symptoms with drugs or therapy can make your life easier by making it easier for you to cope with your physical limitations.

Food and Supplements

MAGNESIUM: Some research has suggested that chronic fatigue syndrome may be associated with low to moderate levels of magnesium deficiency. Supplementation could boost your body's magnesium stores to the normal range and improve functioning,

The evidence: In a randomized controlled trial of six weekly injections of either intramuscular magnesium sulfate or placebo, 12 out of 15 magnesium patients had improved energy levels, emotional state, and pain, but only 3 out of 17 placebo patients felt better.[14]

How it works: Magnesium deficiency is associated with weight loss, nausea, concentration problems, weakness, tiredness, and muscle pain, as well as increases in inflammatory cytokines—all of which are also seen in chronic fatigue syndrome. Recent research has also suggested that magnesium supplementation may improve the antioxidant balance of the body.[15]

What you need to know: There remains debate about whether oral magnesium supplementation is useful for people with chronic fatigue syndrome because the treatment studies used injectable and IV forms of the mineral rather than dietary supplements. In fact, at least one study has found little relationship between dietary magnesium and the level of magnesium in the body's stores. Still, eating a more magnesium-rich diet can't hurt. You can't get too much magnesium from food sources, although it is possible to get sick from excessive use of supplements.[16] Magnesium is found in foods such as green vegetables as well as many nuts and beans.

ESSENTIAL FATTY ACIDS: Essential fatty acids, also known as omega fatty acids, are dietary fats that the body needs to be healthy but can't manufacture itself. Instead, we need to get them from foods, such as various types of fish, nuts, and seeds, or from supplements.

The evidence: There have been two small placebo-controlled trials of a treatment containing a mixture of four omega-3 and omega-6 fatty acids and 10 IU of vitamin E. In one of the studies, patients saw statistically significant symptom improvements over the placebo,[17] while in the other they did not.[18]

How it works: Essential fatty acids help fight the infections that could be responsible for some cases of chronic fatigue syndrome. Viral infections can also deplete stores of these acids, which can cause problems with metabolism and clear thinking.

What you need to know: Fish oil and other omega fatty acid supplements are some of the most popular on the North American market. Among other reasons, this is because omega-3 and omega-6 fatty acid supplementation is widely accepted as being beneficial for numerous health conditions.[19] Even though the evidence of its specific effects on chronic fatigue syndrome is somewhat mixed, there is growing evidence that supplementation may be able to alleviate depression,[20] which could be useful for many chronic fatigue sufferers. To date there is no clear evidence about which specific essential fatty acids are most beneficial for many health conditions, but eating a healthy, varied diet can provide the amounts of fatty acids that most people need. The omega-3 acids found in fish are different than those found in plants; this variety may be harder to find in supplements. Taking too high a dosage of supplements may negatively impact your health, so you should talk to your doctor about what levels are appropriate for you before adding these or any other supplements to your diet.

ACETYLCARNITINE AND PROPIONYLCARNITINE: Acetylcarnitine (ALC) and propionylcarnitine (PLC) are two forms of carnitine used as energy sources for some of the most basic processes in the human body. Produced by the body, and found in many foods, carnitine also plays an important role in fatty acid synthesis.

The evidence: A small, exploratory study looked at the effects of taking 2 grams per day of these supplements in 30 patients with chronic fatigue syndrome. The scientists found that 59 percent of ALC patients, 63 percent of PLC patients, and 37 percent of patients taking both drugs felt better after 24 weeks, while 10 percent, 3 percent, and 16 percent, respectively, felt worse.

The specific type of symptom improvement was different between groups, with ALC patients having significantly improved mental fatigue and PLC patients experiencing significantly improved general fatigue. Improvement stopped when patients quit taking the drugs, and individual treatments appeared to work better than combination therapy.[21]

How it works: These drugs affect cellular energy stores. ALC is thought to primarily affect cellular metabolism in the brain, whereas PLC affects cellular metabolism in the rest of the body. This could explain the differential effects seen in the study.

What you need to know: These supplements are not currently approved for the treatment of chronic fatigue syndrome, and the study that found the positive effects was small. As with all supplements, use caution and make certain to inform your doctor of what you are taking since these products may interact with prescription drugs, such as those used to control blood clotting.

Pain Prevention Strategies

Exercise and Movement Therapies

EXERCISE THERAPY: It may seem paradoxical that exercise, which is known to make chronic fatigue syndrome symptoms worse, can actually improve overall functioning of chronic fatigue patients. However, studies suggest that a controlled exercise program can really improve your health.

The evidence: At least five controlled trials of aerobic exercise therapy[22] have shown promising results. Three studies that compared exercise therapy to either relaxation or treatment as usual found significant improvements for the exercise group in fatigue and quality of life after 12 weeks. Similar results were also seen in a study that looked at the effects of adding exercise therapy to drug treatment with fluoxetine (Prozac), although those results were not significant.

How it works: In healthy populations, exercise therapy has been shown to improve cardiovascular health, mood, and energy levels. In chronic fatigue patients it is also thought to prevent or delay further loss of muscle function that could be caused by inactivity.

What you need to know: Because exercise can make chronic fatigue symptoms worse for some patients, exercise therapy may not be the right choice for everyone. It may also be a difficult therapy to sustain. Talk to your doctor about finding a physical therapist or trainer who has experience working with chronic fatigue patients and knows how to construct an appropriate exercise program that starts slowly and builds gradually over time. Taking small, manageable steps is important because dropouts have been found to be a significant problem in several exercise therapy trials.

Touch Therapies

MASSAGE THERAPY: Many people use massage therapy for simple relaxation, but it can also have more profound physical effects.

The evidence: A small study of 20 patients[23] found that chronic fatigue patients treated with massage had less anxiety, depression, and pain than individuals treated with sham stimuli. A much larger study comparing two different types of massage in 182 patients found that both types led to substantial symptom improvements.[24]

How it works: Massage improves blood flow to tissue, encourages relaxation, and can relieve pain. It has also been shown to decrease levels of the stress hormone cortisol while increasing levels of the neurotransmitters dopamine and serotonin.[25]

What you need to know: The evidence for massage therapy as a treatment for chronic fatigue syndrome is still quite preliminary. However, given how good a massage usually feels, a few small studies may be more than enough reason to give it a try.

ACUPUNCTURE: Although the traditional Chinese medicine diagnostic system does not specifically recognize chronic fatigue syndrome as a disease, many providers will use acupuncture to try to address a patient's specific symptoms.

The evidence: Numerous studies have suggested that acupuncture may be an effective way of relieving chronic fatigue symptoms for some people.[26, 27, 28] However, most of the research that has been done is of low to moderate quality.

How it works: Chinese medicine practitioners say that acupuncture works by reestablishing proper energy flow within the human body.

What you need to know: Acupuncture practitioners in the United States are licensed and/or certified on the state level. Different states have different requirements for acupuncture practice, which may affect both your quality of care and whether your provider is covered by your medical insurance. To protect your health, you should only visit acupuncturists who can legally practice in your state. See Part Three for help in finding a licensed practitioner near you.

Other Drug Therapies

In some individuals, chronic fatigue syndrome is associated with viral infections and changes in the immune system. In these subsets of patients, research has focused on whether treating the underlying problems by attempting to cure viral infections or alter the immune response can also improve symptoms associated with chronic fatigue.

The Evidence[29, 30]

Antivirals: There is little evidence that antiviral drugs improve the health of individuals with chronic fatigue.

Immunomodulators: Four randomized controlled trials of immunoglobulins for chronic fatigue syndrome have shown varied results. Two of the studies led to improvements in symptoms and functional outcomes, a third improved immune function but not symptoms, and the fourth had no effect. Two trials of interferon-alpha had similarly mixed effects—one showing an increase in physical activity and the other an improvement in immune function but not symptoms. A single randomized controlled trial of ampligen showed some improvements in functional ability and cognitive function but not in depression.

Central nervous system stimulants: Two small randomized controlled trials of modafinil (Provigil), a nonamphetamine stimulant, were not encouraging. One found a slight improvement in fatigue with significant appetite side effects and the other showed no positive results at all. A 60-person trial of the amphetamine methylphenidate (Ritalin) did show improvement in fatigue and concentration for some patients, but the drug had no effect on pain or other aspects of mental health.

All these treatments have the potential for serious side effects and are not currently recommended for general treatment of chronic fatigue patients. Certain drugs may be indicated for patients with specific complications of chronic fatigue, but you and your doctor should discuss the potential side effects carefully before use.

Mind-Body Therapies

COGNITIVE-BEHAVIORAL THERAPY: Cognitive-behavioral therapies have shown some very promising results for the treatment of chronic fatigue syndrome. These therapies are designed to give patients practical techniques for pacing themselves and using energy wisely.

The evidence: Numerous randomized trials of cognitive-behavioral therapies

Is Chronic Fatigue Syndrome an Infectious Disease?

The causes of chronic fatigue syndrome remain poorly understood. No single risk factor, infectious or otherwise, has been consistently linked to the condition. The following is an alphabetical list of the many infectious agents that have been hypothesized as playing a role in the development of some cases of chronic fatigue syndrome, but there is a great deal of conflicting evidence. Some scientists are beginning to think that it may be the way a person's body responds to an infection[31] that is important for the development of chronic fatigue syndrome rather than the infection itself.[32, 33, 34, 35]

- Brucella
- *Chlamydia pneumoniae*
- *Coxiella burnetii*
- Cytomegalovirus
- Enteroviruses
- Epstein-Barr virus (Human herpesvirus 4)
- Group B coxsackieviruses (CVB)
- Hepatitis C virus
- Human herpesvirus 6
- Human herpesvirus 7
- Human lentiviruses
- Human T cell leukemia virus (HTLV)
- Parvovirus B19
- Spumavirus
- Toxoplasmosis
- Xenotropic murine leukemia virus-related virus (XMRV)

have found that it can effectively reduce fatigue both immediately after treatment and after short- to medium-term follow-up. Several studies have also shown benefits for depression, physical functioning, and quality of life, although the evidence there is more mixed. Cognitive-behavioral therapy may also improve the work situation of individuals with chronic fatigue syndrome. One study of 60 patients found an improvement in work status 1 year after therapy, although another showed no changes in absenteeism.[36]

How it works: Cognitive-behavioral therapies use systematic methods, including keeping a diary and building skills to help patients cope with the highly stressful symptoms of chronic fatigue syndrome. Cognitive-behavioral therapy for chronic fatigue also sometimes includes gradual increases in physical activity along with the cognitive training.

What you need to know: The most effective forms of cognitive-behavioral therapy seem to involve individual therapy that includes increases in activity, but it is not a quick fix. Cognitive-behavioral therapy is an ongoing process that requires a great deal of work on your own to have any chance of success, and it is important to seek out a therapist with a strong history of working with chronic fatigue patients.

Medications and Other Medical Treatments

ANTIDEPRESSANTS: People with chronic fatigue syndrome are at increased risk of major depressive disorders,[37] and vice versa, but the symptoms of the two diagnoses also have a lot of overlap. That's why these drugs, which have a positive effect on both depression and pain, can also help improve the health of people with chronic fatigue.

The evidence: A meta-analysis of 94 studies of tricyclic antidepressants and selective serotonin reuptake inhibitors (SSRIs) found that these drugs significantly improved the physical symptoms of chronic fatigue—including both pain and fatigue. Several small studies on the dopamine-norepinephrine reuptake inhibitor bupropion (Wellbutrin) have also shown positive effects. However, individual randomized controlled trials of specific antidepressants for chronic fatigue syndrome have had mixed results, and there is no accepted dosing strategy for these drugs in chronic fatigue patients.

How it works: Antidepressants alter the availability of neurotransmitters in the brain and the peripheral nervous system, which may change the way that pain signals are processed.

What you need to know: To date, no specific antidepressant has been approved for the treatment of chronic fatigue syndrome; however, numerous drugs are used off-label to treat people with and without separately diagnosed depression. If other therapies have been unsuccessful for you, antidepressants may be an option worth exploring.

Fibromyalgia

Chronic widespread pain, aching joints, and tender skin are the hallmarks of the condition known as fibromyalgia. Worldwide estimates are that somewhere between 0.5 and 5 percent of the population suffers from fibromyalgia,[38] which can greatly impact a person's ability to work and perform the other activities of a healthy life.

Although fibromyalgia is the most common chronic widespread pain condition, that does not mean it is easily identified. One large international study found that it took people an average of 2.3 years and 3.7 doctors until they were diagnosed.[39]

Part of the problem is that doctors still don't really understand what causes the symptoms of fibromyalgia. The new thinking is that fibromyalgia and other similar pain disorders may be caused by the brain misinterpreting other signals as pain. However, other theories are still being debated.

Fortunately, no matter what causes fibromyalgia or how hard it is to diagnose, there is an ever-expanding range of options for treatment. Thanks to pharmaceutical therapies and lifestyle remedies like exercise and massage, more and more people are finding that they can make fibromyalgia a disease to live with, rather than one that takes over their life.

Testing the Tender Points

Until recently, a person was considered to have fibromyalgia when the three following conditions were met.[40]

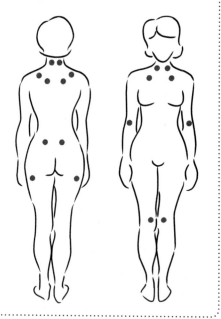

1. They had been experiencing widespread muscular pain for at least 3 months.

2. Pain was present in both sides of the body, above and below the waist, and in the axial skeleton.

3. Pain was present on digital palpation for at least 11 of the 18 tender points diagrammed at right.

Is It Fibromyalgia?

The core symptom of fibromyalgia is chronic widespread pain—pain in every quadrant of your body. In fact, according to long-standing guidelines, in order to be diagnosed with fibromyalgia you need to have pain on both sides of your body and above and below your waist. Other symptoms include fatigue, unsatisfying sleep, forgetfulness and other cognitive problems, stiffness, and difficulty managing the activities of daily life.

However, that definition may be changing. Preliminary new American College of Rheumatology diagnostic criteria published in May 2010 propose to eliminate the use of tender points in fibromyalgia diagnosis because they do not effectively identify a large enough percentage of fibromyalgia patients. Instead, people would be diagnosed by looking at two factors: the number of body areas in which they experience pain and how strongly they are affected by fatigue, waking unrefreshed, cognitive symptoms, and other somatic symptoms.[41]

For most people, fibromyalgia pain isn't constant. Symptoms wax and wane over periods of hours, days, or weeks. Some things that can cause a flare-up include:

- Abnormal levels of exercise or exertion
- Lack of sleep
- Prolonged periods of inactivity
- Exposure to cold
- Physical or psychological stress[42]

But everyone's triggers are different. If you've been experiencing chronic widespread pain and do not know why, it's important to bring it to the attention of your doctor. The symptoms of fibromyalgia are so non-specific that they could be a result of any number of other problems, potentially even one that could be easy to treat.

Fast Pain Relief

If you've been hit with a sudden surge of fibromyalgia pain and need relief right now, there are several things you can try:

1. **For quick relief of allover muscle ache, consider a hot bath.** The heat of the water can help relax your muscles and relieve some of your pain. If you have access to a spa tub, that may work even better.[43]

2. **If your pain is mild to moderate, try taking an over-the-counter painkiller.** Many people prefer NSAIDs such as aspirin or ibuprofen to acetaminophen[44] for treating their fibromyalgia pain, but it's good to experiment with several options to see what works best for you. It's also a good idea to talk to your doctor about what drugs are safest to use with any other medications you take.

3. **If you are prone to occasional severe pain, talk to your doctor.** A prescription painkiller such as tramadol might be of use. Although tramadol and other opiate painkillers can have serious side effects, particularly with regular use, they can be a useful adjunct to your normal pain control routine.[45]

Relief at Last

Sometimes the best way to get control over your pain is to make some changes to the way you live your life. Little differences can mean a lot if they give you the pain relief you need to make it through the day.

Step 1: Get regular exercise. Whether your preference is aqua aerobics or Pilates, regular exercise has been shown to have enormous benefits for people with fibromyalgia. Try to exercise at least two or three times a week, and incorporate aerobic exercise and strength work in your routine.[46]

Step 2: Find ways to relax. Fibromyalgia flares can be set off by excess stress. In addition, anxiety and depression can not only make it harder to cope with your fibromyalgia pain but make the pain itself seem worse.[47]

Step 3: Explore alternative forms of pain relief. Regular massage[48] can provide pain relief for some people with fibromyalgia. So can acupuncture,[49] hypnosis,[50] and hydrotherapy.[51] If you're reluctant to use medication, there are plenty of alternative remedies that may be able to improve your symptoms. It's simply a matter of finding the one that works for you.

When to Call the Doctor

If you have long-lasting, widespread muscular pain that isn't linked to exercise or any other clear cause, it is important to make an appointment to talk to your doctor. She can examine you to see if you have fibromyalgia or if your pain is caused by another problem that may need a different form of treatment.

Step 4: Don't be afraid to ask for medication if you need it. There are currently three FDA-approved treatments for relieving the pain and other symptoms of fibromyalgia.[52] If lifestyle therapies don't give you the relief you need, then talk to your doctor about pharmaceutical options. The most important thing is regaining the ability to live your life—not how you do it.

Pain Prevention Strategies

Food and Supplements

S-ADENOSYLMETHIONINE (SAMe): S-adenosylmethionine, or SAMe, was initially investigated as a treatment for depression. It can be produced by the body, but people with folate, methionine, or vitamin B_{12} deficiencies may also have reduced levels of SAMe.

The evidence: Oral supplementation with 800 milligrams of SAMe a day was found to significantly reduce pain, fatigue, and morning stiffness compared to use of a placebo. Placebo patients also used more pain relievers over the course of the study, but that difference did not reach statistical significance.[53]

How it works: How SAMe, reduces pain associated with fibromyalgia is not understood, although it is thought to have antidepressive, anti-inflammatory, and analgesic effects.

What you need to know: Three out of four published double-blind studies on S-adenosylmethionine showed positive results. However, two of those studies involved intravenous or injection treatment rather than oral supplementation. No new research on SAMe treatment for fibromyalgia has been published since 1998. Before taking SAMe, talk to your doctor, because this supplement may have problematic interactions with other medications including certain antidepressants.

On the Horizon

Melatonin

One of the main functions of melatonin in the human body is to control the sleep/wake cycle. Secreted at night, melatonin helps to schedule the function of bodily systems according to the rise and fall of circadian rhythms—that is, the biological clock. Since one of the hallmarks of fibromyalgia is unsatisfying sleep, two small studies have recently investigated whether supplementation with melatonin, which can regulate sleep, might also be able to improve fibromyalgia symptoms. Early results look promising. Although the two studies combined only included 25 fibromyalgia patients, every single one of them showed improvement in both sleep quality and other symptoms.[54]

Exercise and Movement Therapies

EXERCISE: Exercise is probably the single most widely researched therapy for fibromyalgia treatment. Although it can be difficult for some fibromyalgia patients to remain on an exercise program long term, it's worth the effort. These programs can have profound effects on pain, depression, and overall function.

The evidence: There have been numerous studies of strength training[55] and aerobic exercise[56] for the relief of fibromyalgia symptoms. Although many of the studies are not of high quality, the combined weight of the evidence shows quite clearly that exercise can have positive effects on pain reduction and overall health. A 2010 review of the evidence for aerobic exercise found that programs should ideally consist of low to moderate intensity land-based or water-based exercise two to three times a week for at least 4 weeks.[57]

How it works: Researchers don't entirely understand how exercise relieves pain but suspect it may have to do with the release of endorphins, which are nature's painkillers. In addition, regular exercise builds strength and increases the energy available for the pursuit of other activities. It can provide both physical and psychological benefits for fibromyalgia patients.

What you need to know: Research on exercise for fibromyalgia can be divided into two categories: aerobic exercise and strength training. A Cochrane Collaboration review of 34 studies of exercise as a treatment for fibromyalgia found that strength-training programs were most effective for reducing pain and depression, while moderate aerobic exercise was best for improving overall physical function. Both improved people's feeling of overall well-being.[58]

There has also been a great deal of research on the use of pool-based exercise in fibromyalgia treatment. These exercises have been shown to reduce pain and improve quality of life,[59] and exercising in warm water may also provide additional benefits. Water has the benefit of providing a combination of physical support and moderate resistance, which makes pool-based exercises particularly well suited to individuals with balance and movement difficulties.

Other specific forms of exercise that have shown at least mild positive effects for fibromyalgia patients include yoga,[60] Pilates,[61] and tai chi.[62] Although not all the research studies have been of equal quality, the wide range of exercises that have shown a treatment benefit suggest that individuals with fibromyalgia should primarily focus on finding types of aerobic and strengthening exercise that they like enough to stick with. Being able to keep up with a program is probably the most important factor for improving your long-term health.

See Part Three for some gentle exercise routines that may help.

Touch Therapies

ACUPUNCTURE: In recent years, acupuncture has become somewhat widely used as a method of pain relief; however, its usefulness for relieving the symptoms of fibromyalgia is still in question.

The evidence: In one well-designed, randomized controlled trial comparing acupuncture with electrical stimulation to sham acupuncture and stimulation, the 25 treated patients had significant improvements in their levels of pain, fatigue, and anxiety compared to the 25 controls. However, there was no difference between the groups in how much pain interfered with their quality of life, and the effects of treatment diminished over time.[63]

How it works: The mechanism by which acupuncture relieves pain is not well understood. Theories include improvement in the circulation, up-regulation of certain neurotransmitters, alterations in the immune response, and the release of painkilling endorphins.

What you need to know: Although several individual trials have shown small decreases in fibromyalgia pain following acupuncture therapy, there are still questions about its efficacy. Many acupuncture trials are small and/or poorly designed, and at least three separate meta-analyses that examined the combined data from multiple studies have come to the conclusion that acupuncture cannot be recommended as a scientifically validated therapy for fibromyalgia.[64, 65, 66] However, two of those meta-analyses did acknowledge that it may have a short-term effect on pain. If you do want to try acupuncture, be sure to visit a licensed practitioner. See Part Three for help finding one in your area.

MASSAGE: Many people with fibromyalgia use massage therapy for symptom relief. It can not only reduce pain, but alleviate stress and improve the quality of sleep.[67]

The evidence: There have been at least six randomized controlled trials of massage therapy as a treatment for fibromyalgia, most of which showed that massage had at least mildly positive effects on fibromyalgia symptoms.[68]

How it works: Different types of massage work in different ways, including improving lymphatic drainage, increasing blood flow, and promoting relaxation. In addition, by decreasing stress levels, massage can reduce the impact of pain on quality of life.

What you need to know: Although the studies of massage therapy as a fibromyalgia treatment have been of mixed quality, existing evidence suggests that for it to have a chance of being effective, massage needs to be performed at least once or twice a week.

THERAPEUTIC BATHING: Therapeutic bathing, sometimes called hydrotherapy, involves soaking in warm water, medicinal water, mineral water, or mud. It is most often performed at a health spa.

The evidence: A recent meta-analysis identified 10 randomized controlled trials of various types of hydrotherapy for fibromyalgia symptom relief. When the data from these studies were combined, there was moderate evidence for reduced pain and improved quality of life both immediately after therapy and during follow-up. The median follow-up time was 14 weeks.[69]

How it works: Spa therapies involving hot water and mineral baths relax the muscles and promote a general feeling of well-being. Exposure to heat from spa treatments and mud packs may also lead to the release of endorphins.[70] These factors may combine to relieve some of the anxiety and pain associated with fibromyalgia and may also improve the quality of sleep.[71]

What you need to know: In general, the studies of hydrotherapy as a fibromyalgia treatment have been small and not of high quality. However, if you have access to spa therapy and can afford it, it is generally considered to be safe and may reduce both your stress and symptoms.

Mind-Body Therapies

COGNITIVE-BEHAVIORAL THERAPY: Cognitive-behavioral therapy not only trains people to live more fulfilling lives in the presence of chronic pain, it can also help reduce that pain's intensity.

The evidence: One study of tailored cognitive-behavioral therapy found that it could provide significant reductions in pain, fatigue, and functional disability compared to people who did not receive this therapy.[72]

How it works: The ways in which the human body is conditioned to respond to pain—including avoidance, catastrophizing (perceiving pain as worse than it actually is), and an increase in physical tension—may be useful for dealing with acute pain, but they can actually cause problems when the pain in question is chronic. Cognitive-behavioral therapies focus on retraining fibromyalgia patients' responses to their chronic pain and may also provide instruction in various relaxation techniques.

What you need to know: Both group[73] and individual cognitive-behavioral therapies are widely accepted as effective for the treatment of chronic pain in individuals with fibromyalgia, but the actual data on their efficacy are mixed.

Do Breast Implants Cause Fibromyalgia?

There have been rumors linking silicone breast implants to a variety of health conditions—including connective tissue diseases and fibromyalgia—for years. Most evidence to date,[74] including several nationwide follow-up studies of implant recipients,[75] does not support those rumors. The exception is one study published in 2001, which found that ruptured implants where silicone was released into the body almost tripled the odds of self-reported fibromyalgia diagnosis.[76] However, even in that study, symptoms were not related to rupture status and there was no assessment of whether fibromyalgia diagnoses occurred before or after implantation. A follow-up study designed to confirm the results found no association between self-reported fibromyalgia and rupture status.[77]

The best evidence seems to be in support of multimodal therapies that address several types of retraining, although single-method therapies that only focus on physical relaxation training have also shown some ability to reduce pain.[78]

HYPNOTHERAPY: When used as a treatment for chronic pain, hypnotherapy usually involves a hypnotic induction followed by a suggestion encouraging either relaxation or pain relief. Hypnosis is currently being investigated as a potential therapy for a wide variety of chronic pain conditions.[79]

The evidence: In a study comparing the effects of hypnosis in which the suggestion used was directed at reducing pain to hypnosis in which the suggestion used was directed at increasing relaxation to a simple relaxation training program that did not involve hypnosis, researchers found that while all three methods significantly reduced pain, the pain-relief suggestion was by far the most effective. Hypnosis aimed at increasing relaxation was not found to be more effective than nonhypnotic relaxation training.[80]

How it works: Researchers don't entirely understand how it works, but it is clear that hypnosis can lead to real, measurable changes in the brain. The changes in blood flow to the brain observed by PET scan during one study of hypnotic analgesia suggested that the reduction in fibromyalgia pain might be owing to its effects on how pain is processed by the limbic system.[81] In addition, an fMRI study found that analgesic suggestions after hypnosis caused substantially greater changes in brain activity than the same suggestions performed without hypnosis.[82]

How Hypnosis Research May Help Explain Fibromyalgia Pain

Some people believe that the pain experienced by individuals with fibromyalgia and somatoform pain disorders is related to changes in brain activity that lead to the brain independently generating sensations of pain rather than processing external stimuli as painful. In other words, if you have fibromyalgia, your brain might produce signals saying that your leg aches without any communication of damage from that area.

A group of scientists recently investigated this theory by using fMRI to scan the brains of patients experiencing real pain, imagined pain, or pain induced by hypnotic suggestion. Imagined pain and hypnotically induced pain are measurably different phenomena. Susceptible people experience hypnotically induced pain as real, and they have the changes in galvanic skin response, heart rate, and respiration to prove it. People who simply imagine pain have no equivalent reactions.

When scientists compared the brain activation in people experiencing the three different types of pain, they discovered something fascinating. Both real pain and hypnotic pain caused activation of the thalamus, anterior cingulate, insula, prefrontal, and parietal cortices, but imagined pain did not. This suggests that activation of the brain can generate sensations of pain similar to those sensations that are a response to "real" physical stimuli, and that this pain has nothing to do with imagination.[83]

What you need to know: If you do decide to visit a hypnotherapist, plan to discuss in detail what you're looking for in terms of results—whether that's relaxation or symptom relief. It may be helpful to bring along a copy of some of the posthypnotic suggestions shown to be useful for fibromyalgia patients, such as the ones from the analgesia/relaxation study cited above. You can request a copy of the study from your local library, or see Part Three for a few samples.

RELAXATION TECHNIQUES: There are many techniques that can be used to promote physical and emotional relaxation, including meditation, guided imagery, and biofeedback.

The evidence: In one randomized controlled trial of a mindfulness-based stress reduction program, 91 patients either received eight weekly $2\frac{1}{2}$-hour mindfulness training sessions or care as usual. Individuals in the training program were also encouraged to meditate daily for at least 30 to 45 minutes and attend a 1-day meditation retreat after 6 weeks of training. At the end of the training program, meditation significantly improved the symptoms of depression in the study group. Those individuals who continued to meditate after the training program was over also saw additional reductions in their pain levels over the next 2 months.[84] Another randomized controlled trial of biofeedback in 30 patients found that after 6 consecutive days of treatment, individuals who received real biofeedback with their relaxation training had significantly greater decreases in pain and the number of tender points than those who received sham biofeedback.[85]

How it works: Physical and emotional stress can increase the perception of pain and make it more difficult to cope with. Meditation, guided imagery, and relaxation techniques are designed to reduce the mental and physical manifestations of stress and lower the impact of pain on the body. In addition, physical relaxation may directly reduce some of the tenderness and muscle pain associated with fibromyalgia. Incorporating biofeedback into relaxation training programs can give patients objective measurement of the success of their techniques and improve the efficiency of training.

What you need to know: Biofeedback can be combined with various types of relaxation training and exercise therapy programs.[86] It uses computers and other electronic devices to provide an objective measurement of different types of tension in the body. Patients can then use that feedback to learn how to relax more effectively. In particular, biofeedback for fibromyalgia often focuses on reducing muscular tension in the forearm. However, there have also been studies examining its use in reducing heart rate variability,[87] a biological marker that has been associated with stress, depression, and pain. See Part Three for resources to get you started with biofeedback, meditation, guided imagery, and other relaxation techniques.

Pain Medications and Other Medical Treatments

DUAL SEROTONIN NOREPINEHRINE REUPTAKE INHIBITORS (SNRIS): Duloxetine (Cymbalta) and milnacipran (Savella) are two of the three FDA-approved medical therapies for fibromyalgia. They are both SNRIs.

The evidence: Numerous randomized controlled trials have demonstrated the efficacy of both duloxetine and milnacipran in reducing pain and other symptoms associated with fibromyalgia. Evidence was sufficient to earn both drugs official recognition as fibromyalgia treatments by the FDA. For example, a pooled analysis of 1,300 patients in four studies of duloxetine found that average pain, maximum pain, the extent to which pain interfered with activities, illness severity, and depression all significantly improved in duloxetine-treated individuals when compared to those treated with placebo.[88]

How it works: Both drugs alter the brain's use of serotonin and norepinephrine, two neurotransmitters that are involved in the pain response. While duloxetine inhibits both neurotransmitters equally, milnacipran is somewhat more selective for norepinephrine.[89] Although they are both effective, some individuals may find that one medication works better than the other.

What you need to know: These drugs are quite effective but they can cause serious side effects, including gastrointestinal distress and headache, when used long term. In one study of 120 milligrams a day of duloxetine, adverse events caused 20 percent of the treated patients to drop out over 3 months of treatment compared to 10 percent of patients in the placebo group.[90] In a 6-month trial of milnacipran, 23 percent of patients on 100 milligrams a day and 28 percent of patients on 200 milligrams a day of the drug dropped out because of adverse events compared to 12 percent of patients in the placebo group.[91]

PREGABALIN: Pregabalin (Lyrica) is the last of the three FDA-approved medical therapies for fibromyalgia and the only one that is not a serotonin norepinephrine reuptake inhibitor. Pregabalin is classed as an anticonvulsant, but it is also used to treat a wide variety of neuropathic pain.

The evidence: An 8-week 2005 dosage study of pregabalin found that the highest amount tested—450 milligrams a day—was the most effective at reducing pain and fatigue and improving the quality of sleep.[92] A 14-week dosage study performed in 2008 increased the range studied and found that both 450 milligrams a day and 600 milligrams a day were highly effective.[93]

How it works: Pregabalin affects neurotransmitter production in ways that are not yet well understood.

What you need to know: Pregabalin can have some serious side effects including dizziness, sleepiness, headache, and weight gain. In one trial, almost 20 percent of patients withdrew from long-term (32-week) therapy because they found the side effects unacceptable. Unfortunately, the same study demonstrated that for long-term effects pregabalin therapy probably needs to be continuous.[94]

OTHER ANTIDEPRESSANTS: Although only duloxetine and milnacipran are currently approved for the treatment of fibromyalgia, other antidepressants are often used for it off-label.

The evidence: One randomized controlled trial comparing the use of

4.5 milligrams a day of the dopamine receptor agonist pramipexole (Mirapex) to placebo found that over 14 weeks, 42 percent of the treatment group reduced their pain by at least half compared to only 14 percent of the placebo group. Overall function, fatigue, and quality of life scores also improved in a much higher percentage of treated patients than controls.[96]

How it works: Antidepressants alter the function of neurotransmitters in the brain. By doing so, they may change some of the problematic ways in which individuals with fibromyalgia experience pain.

What you need to know: There have been numerous encouraging studies investigating the use of various antidepressants for fibromyalgia. One 2008 systematic review of the results of 26 randomized controlled trials of antidepressant use found that, of 13 studies of amitriptyline (Elavil), the vast majority supported its use for moderate reductions in pain and improvements in quality of life. Nine of 12 studies for various SSRIs also showed positive results.[97]

TRAMADOL OR TRAMADOL AND ACETAMINOPHEN: Many patients with fibromyalgia have episodes of acute pain that require management with painkillers.

The evidence: A randomized controlled trial investigating the use of one to two combination tramadol (37.5 milligrams) and acetaminophen (325 milligrams) tablets four times a day found that, by the end of treatment, people taking tramadol/acetaminophen had pain scores approximately 18 percent lower than those taking the placebo. In addition, almost twice as many people in the treatment group had at least a 50 percent reduction in pain (35 percent versus 18 percent). However, by day 91, twice as many people in the treatment group as in the placebo had quit because of adverse events.[98]

How it works: Tramadol (Ultram), which is often used as an adjunct therapy for acute pain in fibromyalgia, is an opiate pain reliever that also has some selective serotonin norepinephrine reuptake activity. Acetaminophen is more commonly known as Tylenol. They are sold in a combined pill under the name Ultracet.

What you need to know: Tramadol can be addictive and overdose can be highly damaging or even fatal. Furthermore, in May of 2010, the labeling for Ultram and Ultracet was changed to reflect a growing concern that these drugs may increase the risk of suicide in patients who are prone to addiction or have a history of emotional disturbance.[99]

ELECTROTHERAPY: Electroconvulsive therapy (otherwise known as electric shock therapy) is the most extreme form of electromagnetic therapy that has been investigated for use in the treatment of fibromyalgia pain. Self-administered[100] and less extensive clinic-based therapies[101] have also shown some positive effects.

The evidence: In one study of pulsed electromagnetic therapy, 56 women with fibromyalgia were instructed to spend 30 minutes a day, twice a day, lying on a mat that randomly provided either real or sham treatment. Although women in both groups experienced some improvement in pain, quality of life, and physical functioning after 3 weeks of treatment, the improvements were greater and longer lasting in the pulsed electromagnetic field group. Their symptoms continued to improve throughout the 12-week follow-up period, even after treatment had ended.[102]

How it works: There is no clear understanding of how electroconvulsive therapy and other electromagnetic therapies work. It is thought that they might alter neurotransmitter release or electrical activity in the nervous system, increase production of endorphins, or alter blood flow in the brain.

What you need to know: The two studies of actual electroconvulsive therapy in fibromyalgia patients have been quite small and neither contained a control group. One showed reductions in severe pain,[103] but the other study—in individuals with both fibromyalgia and a major depressive disorder—only showed significant effects on depression.

Mystery Pain and Functional Somatic Syndromes

It may seem hard to believe, but according to research more than 10 percent of the population experiences chronic widespread pain.[104, 105] Although for many people this pain will eventually be explained by a diagnosis of fibromyalgia, chronic fatigue syndrome, irritable bowel disease, or any of a number of conditions that cause the body to ache, for others the symptoms will remain a mystery. That can be incredibly frustrating for both patients and doctors, because when you don't know what's causing the pain, figuring out how to treat it can feel like an impossible task.

The truth is that even diagnosis doesn't always lead to answers. Chronic fatigue syndrome and similar diseases are often described as medically unexplained symptoms, because while it's clear the symptoms are real to the people who suffer from them, there is no clear explanation for why they occur. What doctors do know is that mystery pain and other unexplained symptoms are more common in women than in men. These conditions are also more common in people who are generally worried about their health, although that may be a question of putting the cart before the horse. The long-term experience of unexplained pain is draining enough to make anyone nervous.

Unexplained pain needs to be taken just as seriously as pain resulting from a clear, medical cause. The patient's experience of pain is just as real whether that pain originates from damage to the tissue or communication problems in the nerves. As doctors and scientists learn more about how pain and other physical symptoms can be hallmarks of traditionally psychiatric diagnoses, the lines between body and mind are becoming blurred.

What Is My Mystery Pain?

Pain that is severe enough to impact your quality of life calls for a trip to the doctor, particularly if that pain has no obvious cause. In the best-case scenario, your unexplained pain will only be unexplained temporarily—until your doctor tries the right test that leads him to a diagnosis. There are a number of diseases that can cause widespread physical pain but are not often seen by a primary care physician.

Even if your doctor cannot figure out what is causing your pain, he may be able to recommend appropriate treatments for pain in general. Be prepared to tell him about when your pain started, how long it has lasted, whether it has been constant or intermittent, and how it impacts the way you live your life. The better your doctor's understanding of the nature of your pain, the more likely it is that he'll be able to help.

If your doctor can't figure out a clear cause for your pain, he may diagnose you as having a somatoform pain disorder. That's medical language for "the pain doesn't have a clear physical cause, and so it's probably coming from someplace in your brain"—which is not to say that the pain is a product of your imagination.

It has become increasingly clear that depression, anxiety, and other affective disorders are associated with physical and chemical changes in the brain that may cause it to perceive pain where there is no damage.[106, 107] In fact, in some countries unexplained physical pain is the major complaint for people with depression, not

Somatoform Pain Disorder or Functional Somatic Syndrome?

People with unexplained pain are often shuttled from medical doctor to psychiatrist and back again, looking for a diagnosis. Medical doctors call conditions whose symptoms have no obvious cause functional somatic syndromes—an umbrella term that includes, among other diseases, chronic fatigue syndrome, fibromyalgia, and irritable bowel syndrome. Psychiatrists sometimes call the same group of conditions somatoform or dissociative disorders, and the two types of doctor will often have very different ideas on how to go about treating the same disease.[108]

Chronic mystery pain can be a major source of depression and anxiety and have profound effects on a patient's quality of life. Although doctors will often focus their attention on finding the cause of the pain so that it can be treated most effectively, sometimes there are no easy answers and the pain remains unexplained for years. Fortunately for people who suffer from this condition, there is a growing recognition that sometimes medically unexplained pain is a diagnosis of its own.

mental distress. One international study found that 45 to 95 percent of patients with major depressive disorder only complained of physical pain.[109]

Fast Pain Relief

When you don't know what's causing your pain, sometimes the best thing you can do is look for ways to address its symptoms.

1. **For mild, unexplained, intermittent aches and pains, over-the-counter painkillers can be your best friend.** Although chronic headaches and muscle aches are a sign that you should seek out medical attention, you can sometimes temporarily short-circuit the pain with standard painkillers.[110] However, if you find yourself taking more pills than the bottle recommends or taking them for longer than a few weeks, talk to your doctor about alternatives. Excessive use of over-the-counter painkillers can cause serious health problems.

2. **For moderate to more severe pain, talk to your doctor about prescription painkillers that you can use during a flare-up.** There are numerous drugs used to treat chronic or severe pain that can help you stomp down a bad attack and are safer to use for extended periods of time than OTC painkillers. Some of these drugs may leave you exhausted or otherwise impair your mental function, but the trade-offs may be worth it if pain relief is what it takes to get you through your day. Don't be afraid to ask your doctor to refer you to a pain management specialist if she doesn't know how to treat you safely and effectively. It's a specialty for a reason.

3. **Talk to your doctor about antidepressants and psychotherapy.** Pain is stressful, and people with mystery pain are at high risk for

depression and anxiety. Furthermore, mystery pain can be a physical symptom of some of the same biological processes that lead to those psychological symptoms. A personalized combination of antidepressants and counseling may be able to reduce your pain and improve your ability to live with it.[111]

4. Ask for help. If your pain is making it difficult or impossible to go about the activities of your daily life, don't be afraid to ask for help. Take breaks when you need them and don't push your body farther than it can safely go. Overstressing your system to make it through today is not only likely to make your pain worse, it can make it more difficult to get through tomorrow.

Relief at Last

The cutting edge of mystery pain treatment is all about accepting that pain is real and needs to be treated even when doctors don't know the cause. Of course, since mystery pain is a mystery, it means there are no surefire ways to avoid or cure it. Still, there are some things you can do to reduce the impact of any kind of pain on your life.

Step 1: Use painkillers when you need them. Although it's good to avoid unnecessary use of painkillers, sometimes you really do need them to function. Chronic pain is exhausting and can have a serious impact on your quality of life. If there's a way to safely reduce your pain levels, you should take it. You can't focus on improving your health if all you can do is think about your pain.

Step 2: Make sleep a top priority. Individuals with somatoform pain disorders have been shown to have reduced sleep quality compared to healthy controls.[112] Since lack of sleep is associated with increases in pain and a decreased ability to function while in pain, improving your sleep can do wonders for your quality of life.

Step 3: Focus on improving your mental health. Other than gender, which you have no control over, the single biggest factor associated with medically unexplained pain is your mental health. That's because the same mechanisms that control your mood also affect how you experience pain. There's a pretty good chance that the more time you spend working on your mood and practicing your coping skills, the less time you'll spend disabled by pain.

Pain Prevention Strategies

Food and Supplements

SAINT JOHN'S WORT: Saint John's wort is an herbal supplement that is often used for the treatment of anxiety and depression, although the evidence for its use is mixed. Since somatoform pain disorders and other unexplained pain are often linked to depression and anxiety, there is some suggestion that Saint John's wort may also be useful as a pain treatment, although the research is still in its early days.

The evidence: In a randomized double-blind, placebo-controlled trial, 184 patients with multiple unexplained symptoms were given either 300-milligram tablets of Saint John's wort or a placebo twice a day. After 6 weeks, 44 percent of the treatment group claimed that they were completely improved compared to 25 percent of the patients in the placebo group. In addition, 45 percent of placebo patients felt unchanged or worse, while only 17 percent of treatment patients did.[113]

How it works: The leading hypotheses for how Saint John's wort works are that it acts as an immune modulator or that it alters the uptake of serotonin in the brain, or both. The second explanation is more likely to explain any effects the herb has on depression or chronic pain, since in some studies the class of drugs known as selective serotonin reuptake inhibitors (SSRIs) seems to have similar effects.[114]

What you need to know: Saint John's wort can interact with several types of prescription medication. It's important to talk to your doctor before you start using this supplement.

Exercise and Movement Therapies

EXERCISE THERAPY: Exercise is known to have positive effects on your emotional state, possibly because production of the neurotransmitters norepinephrine and serotonin is altered during physical activity.[115] Since levels of these neurotransmitters may also be affected in people with somatoform disorders, scientists have investigated whether exercise can also improve medically unexplained pain.

The evidence: Although there is a substantial amount of evidence supporting the use of exercise for specific functional somatic syndromes such as chronic fatigue syndrome, very little research has examined its effects on medically unexplained pain. However, one study looking at how aerobic exercise and stretching affected 228 people with medically unexplained symptoms found that those patients who attended at least one training session significantly reduced their number of doctors visits and filled prescriptions over the next 6 months, although their pain was only slightly improved.[116]

How it works: The exact mechanism by which exercise improves medically unexplained pain is not well understood. However, a small study of exercise withdrawal in healthy adults discovered something interesting. When adults who were used to exercising at least 4 hours a week were told to stop for 7 days, approximately half of them developed fatigue, an increased sensitivity to pain, or problems with their mood. Those individuals who developed symptoms after stopping exercise had differences in hypothalamic-pituitary-axis hormones and immune markers similar to those reported in some patients with chronic multi-symptom illnesses. It is therefore possible that exercise moderates unexplained pain by affecting the endocrine and immune systems.[117]

What you need to know: You should always talk to your doctor before beginning a new exercise program, particularly if you have health problems in addition to your unexplained pain. It's also important to monitor your heart rate so that it stays within the range recommended for adults of your sex and age.

Mind-Body Therapies

COGNITIVE-BEHAVIORAL THERAPY: There is a great deal of support for the use of cognitive-behavioral therapies to improve the lives of individuals with unexplained pain. These types of treatment focus on helping patients examine factors that make them susceptible to pain, set off a painful episode, or make their pain worse so that they can alter the ones they have control over and accept the ones they do not.

> ### *Quick Tip*
> A 2008 study of over 37,000 Canadians found that people who identified themselves as religious had better psychological well-being scores than the general public and were significantly less likely to have a history of chronic pain. There are several theories for how being religious could lower a person's risk of chronic pain. Members of a religious community have a source of social support when they need help. Religious practices also offer some people a source of relaxation and an outlet for their stress. Finally, religion might help people develop better skills for handling the anxiety and depression that can predispose a person to chronic pain.[118]

The evidence: Numerous studies have demonstrated the efficacy of various CBT programs for the treatment of medically unexplained pain. One randomized controlled trial looking at a 10-session therapy intervention found that at the end of 3 months, 60 percent of treated patients had an improvement in their physical symptoms compared to 25 percent of patients in the placebo group. Unfortunately, the effects diminished over time. After an additional 3 months had passed, only 50 percent of treated patients were still improved compared to 31 percent of controls.[119]

How it works: In the study just mentioned, the therapy program tried to help people stop focusing on their pain through training that addressed using relaxation techniques, regulating activity levels, paying attention to emotional state, and improving communication skills. The intervention encouraged people to alter their behaviors in ways that both reduced the likelihood of pain and improved their ability to deal with it productively.

What you need to know: One small study has suggested that cognitive-behavioral therapy might also be able reduce physical symptoms and anxiety in children with medically unexplained pain.[120]

Pain Medications and Other Medical Treatments

ANTIDEPRESSANTS: Medically unexplained pain is often closely linked to affective disorders such as depression and anxiety. In addition, somatoform pain disorders have been tentatively linked to alterations in a gene

On the Horizon

Music Therapy

If you love music, you're not likely to be surprised by the suggestion that music can have profound effects on a person's emotional state, but you may be surprised that it is sometimes used as a component of medical care. Music therapy involves either listening to music or creating it as part of the therapeutic process. Several studies have indicated that music can be effective in treating a number of illnesses, including migraines, tinnitus, and chronic pain.

In one study, a group of 40 patients with chronic pain were randomized to treatment with music therapy and drug treatment or drug treatment alone. While only 35 percent of the drug therapy group reported an improvement in their symptoms, 70 percent of individuals who also received music therapy felt better. Detailed analysis suggested that the addition of music therapy not only reduced pain symptoms but also helped with psychological distress.[121]

What Is Sleep Hygiene?

Sleep hygiene is the term that scientists use to describe a series of habits that you can practice to improve your sleep. These habits include:

1. **Changes in behavior:** Pick a consistent time to go to bed and get up, avoid napping, stop all intake of alcohol and caffeine at least 4 hours before bed, and exercise regularly, preferably during the afternoon.

2. **Changes in your bedroom:** Use the most comfortable bedding that you can afford, make the room as dark and quiet as possible, and keep the thermostat set low enough to let you sleep comfortably.

3. **Changes in your mind set:** Use your bed only for sleeping and sex and find ways to leave your worries outside the bedroom.

There are other things you can do to help you fall asleep, such as drinking a little warm milk or taking a soothing bath, but this list should give you a good start. It's worth noting that although some people find it relaxing to read before bed, it may be a better idea to read someplace else until you get sleepy and head to the bedroom only when you're actually ready to sleep.

controlling serotonin transport.[122] Although other factors may be involved in this type of pain as well, the genetic link suggests that they might be amenable to treatment with antidepressants that affect serotonin uptake.

The evidence: One large study of almost 300 patients with major depressive disorder found that 60 milligrams of duloxetine (Cymbalta) used once a day significantly reduced not only the patients' average level of pain but how much pain interfered with their lives, compared to placebo.[123] Numerous other studies have also shown that antidepressants can provide relief for chronic pain.[124]

How it works: Antidepressants primarily work by altering the way in which nerves communicate. For example, selective serotonin reuptake inhibitors prevent the transmitting nerve cell from taking back the neurotransmitter serotonin once it has been released. This can increase the strength of the communication signal between nerves.

Improving neurotransmitter levels has the potential to improve a person's mood and level of pain because, in many people, medically unexplained pain seems to be linked to problems with nerve signaling—similar to what is seen in individuals with depression.

What you need to know: Antidepressants can have seriously unpleasant side effects that may outweigh their benefits. However, the side effects vary both by drug and dosage. If the first type of medication your doctor prescribes doesn't work for you, there may be other options.

Other Strategies

GET MORE AND BETTER SLEEP: When you're in pain it's hard to sleep, which makes it particularly ironic that lack of sleep can increase pain levels and reduce your ability to cope with pain's impact on your life. Fortunately, if you can find ways to improve your sleep—either through behavior modification or the use of medication—your mornings may start to look a lot brighter.

The evidence: In one population study of people with chronic widespread pain, researchers found that pain improvement over a 15-month follow-up period was tightly linked to a good night's sleep, although the scientists could not determine which change came first.[125] Another study looking at the effects of fatigue on children with chronic pain found that fatigue significantly mediated the effect of pain on the children's health-related quality of life.[126] In other words, pain didn't cause as many problems for children who slept well as it did for children who were tired.

How it works: Scientists don't completely understand why fatigue makes people more susceptible to pain, but it's clear that it does. Some of the effects may be the result of the effects of sleep loss on the immune system, but it's also clear that it's a lot harder for people to deal with their pain when they're tired.

What you need to know: There are plenty of techniques you can try to improve your sleep habits before you have to resort to medication. Still, the important thing is getting a good, restorative night's sleep—not how you manage that.

PART THREE

Tools for Pain-Free Living

There is a world of pain-relief options out there ready for you. From support groups to supplements, guided imagery to exercise, yoga to hypnotherapy, the possibilities are vast. Where can you find the best services, products, organizations, and practitioners you need? Right here in this resource guide.

After you've read about powerful pain-easing modalities in Part One and learned more about your specific pain condition in Part Two, turn to this section to put your chosen therapies into action. It's where you'll find exercise plans designed to soothe chronic pain and a reproducible Pain Diary you can use to track your pain so you can find triggers and know for certain whether a new therapy is helping, hurting, or not doing much at all.

You'll also find locator services to help you reach top practitioners, advice on how to buy the safest and most effective supplements, and recommended books, CDs, and products for pain-free living. We've included listings for specific modalities—such as yoga, acupuncture, and massage—as well as resources to help you make informed decisions about each type of pain treatment. We wish you health, happiness, and pain-free ease on your journey.

Pain Diary and Pain Scales

s we discussed in Part One, it's important to track your pain, no matter where you are in your pain journey. If you are still struggling to get a diagnosis and an explanation for your pain, taking note of when it occurs and exactly what it feels like can be an invaluable tool for you and your doctor. If you are working on identifying your pain triggers, keeping a pain diary can help you become more aware of what foods, activities, stressors, or even medications might be contributing to painful flare-ups. If you are trying out a new treatment, listening to your pain can tell you if it's working or if you need to make further adjustments to your pain management plan.

You'll want to make this diary work for you, so track only the information you find helpful. In order to keep it flexible, we've designed the questions and prompts to be open-ended. Here are some ideas how you can use each section of the page.

Weather: There are many environmental factors that can trigger pain. Use this section to note an impending storm, the temperature, or even just a change in the weather, which is something that could trigger a migraine in people who are prone to them.

My Mood: The type of mood you're in can indicate your overall sense of well-being. Included below is a word bank of moods you can draw from to help you answer this prompt—but you are not limited to just these.

aggravated	depressed	hopeful	restless
amused	discontented	hyper	sad
angry	distressed	lethargic	satisfied
annoyed	drained	mellow	scared
anxious	energetic	moody	sleepy
apathetic	exhausted	nervous	sore
blah	frustrated	numb	stressed
bored	groggy	peaceful	thankful
calm	grumpy	pessimistic	uncomfortable
cheerful	guilty	relaxed	worried
confused	happy	relieved	

Pain Scale: Rating your pain is an important part of tracking it. It's a measurement you can compare day to day and share with your doctor to assess your treatment. Fortunately, you don't have to make up your own rating system. The pain scale here is widely used and relies on numbers (0, a smiley face, is no pain, to 10, a distressed and crying face, the worst possible pain). Because your level of pain may change throughout the day, we've provided a place under each rating number to write down the time at which you noticed a change in the intensity of your pain.

Beneath the pain scale, you can answer questions to help you pinpoint what may be causing or exacerbating your pain as well as what relieves it. Be sure to note any symptoms you have in addition to pain, as they can help your doctor narrow down the cause and the best treatments.

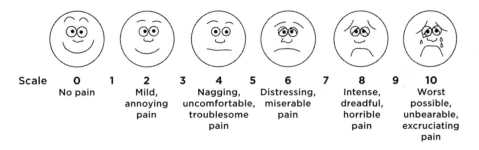

Scale	0	1	2	3	4	5	6	7	8	9	10
	No pain		Mild, annoying pain		Nagging, uncomfortable, troublesome pain		Distressing, miserable pain		Intense, dreadful, horrible pain		Worst possible, unbearable, excruciating pain

On the right-hand side of the pain diary, you can track everyday types of things, like the medications you take daily, the foods you eat, the sorts of exercise and physical activity you do, how much sleep you got the night before, and your daily stress and energy levels.

My Medications: Use this area to write down the medications you take on a daily basis, including those prescribed by a doctor, daily vitamins and supplements, and additional routine therapies such as insulin injections or weekly allergy shots. This is not the place to write down painkillers or other meds that you take as needed for pain flare-ups. Those should be noted on the left-hand side of the spread under "What did you try to relieve the pain?"

My Food Log: Use this tool to discover and eliminate trigger foods. For example, a low-fiber diet can help you ease pain during a flare-up of diverticulitis. Avoiding sulfite-rich foods like red meats and many types of wine could cut your odds of a flare-up of inflammatory bowel disease. If you have a food sensitivity or intolerance, such as to dairy products or gluten, avoiding offenders can keep you more comfortable. Take note that eliminating trouble foods works if you customize your strategy. You don't want to cut out huge categories of healthy foods that may not really be bothering your body! In one study of 150 people with IBS published in the journal *Gut*, those who stopped eating their personal trigger foods experienced a 26 percent reduction in pain and other symptoms. But the list of potential trouble foods is huge; alcohol, chocolate, caffeinated beverages, sugar-free sweeteners, and high-fat foods may set off diarrhea and pain. IBS gas and bloating may even get worse after eating otherwise healthy foods like beans, broccoli, cabbage, and cauliflower. Because triggers vary from person to person and among different disorders, it makes sense to spend time tracking down your personal pain culprits rather than cutting too much out of your diet.

My Activity Log: As with the food log, looking for patterns in your activity types and intensities can help you identify potential triggers. Use this log to write down your exercise routine and even the basic tasks you do in the course of the day that can impact your pain. In particular, overuse injuries, back and joint pain, and fibromyalgia can all be affected by tasks such as weeding a garden, biking to work, or grocery shopping. Even spending the day typing at a computer will be significant to note for someone suffering from carpal tunnel syndrome, a pain in the hands or wrists that's usually associated with office work.

My Stress Rating, My Energy Rating, and My Sleep: The benefits of rating your stress and energy levels on a daily basis are twofold. First, it requires you to be mindful of how you are actually feeling each day. Because stress is a known trigger for many chronic conditions, correlations you notice between your stress and pain levels over time can indicate that you need to introduce some effective stress-relief techniques into your self-care arsenal. If your stress level ranks above a 5, try some of the de-stressors on page 58 or incorporate your favorite go-to stress reliever.

Rating your energy is also useful. Since three out of four chronic pain sufferers contend with low energy levels, noting your daily energy can offer cues about how your pain is affecting your ability to perform basic functions like working and interacting with other people. Low energy ratings can also be clues that you are not eating well enough or are experiencing fatigue or illness. For those with

> ### *Quick Tip*
> You can also use the Activity Log to record any non-drug therapies, such as tai chi, massage, or a physical therapy session. If you want to reflect on those therapies, use the "Additional Notes" section mentioned on the opposite page.

somatic diseases like fibromyalgia or chronic fatigue syndrome, tracking energy can be a leading indicator of whether your relief at last plan is working.

Noting how many hours you sleep each night, as well as the quality of that sleep, can also help you figure out if you are getting the rest you need to confront the challenges of the day ahead. This is an ideal place to note insomnia or unrefreshing sleep, and to spark a sense of accountability for getting to bed in time to hit your sweet spot for sleep. The amount of sleep each person needs to thrive can vary widely, and journaling about your sleep can help you figure out how many slumbering hours you typically need to start the day right.

Additional Notes: Note whatever doesn't fit in the previous areas. Appointment reminders, to-do lists, test results, and reflections on your well-being throughout the day are all valuable ways to use this space, but what you want to use it for is completely up to you!

Photocopy the following pages 494 to 495 to use as often as you'd like. To keep your notes organized, try sorting your pain diary pages in a 3-ring binder or typing your logs up to file on your computer. The most important thing is to find a system that works for you and that will provide useful insight to you and your doctors so that you can get relief at last!

Pain Diary and Pain Scales

Date: _____

Weather: _____

My Mood: _____

How much pain am I in today?

Scale	0	1	2	3	4	5	6	7	8	9	10
	No pain		Mild, annoying pain		Nagging, uncomfortable, troublesome pain		Distressing, miserable pain		Intense, dreadful, horrible pain		Worst possible, unbearable, excruciating pain

Morning:

      0   1   2   3   4   5   6   7   8   9   10

Afternoon:

      0   1   2   3   4   5   6   7   8   9   10

Evening:

      0   1   2   3   4   5   6   7   8   9   10

What my pain feels like:

_____

What I was doing when the pain started or increased:

_____

What I tried to relieve the pain:

_____

Did that make a difference?

_____

Any other symptoms?

_____

Food and Activity Logs

My Medications	Dose	Time
☐		
☐		
☐		

MY FOOD LOG: What have I eaten today?

Time	List your meals, snacks, or other foods here

MY ACTIVITY LOG

Type of Activity	Duration

My Stress Rating: 0 1 2 3 4 5 6 7 8 9 10

0 = No stress   10 = Completely overwhelmed

What is making me feel stressed today?

My Energy Rating: 0 1 2 3 4 5 6 7 8 9 10

0 = Can hardly get out of bed, no energy   10 = Bouncing off the walls, too much energy

How did I sleep last night?

Additional Notes:

Exercise Routines

As you've discovered throughout this book, exercise is a cornerstone of pain management, whether it's a gentle yoga stretch, a walk around the block, a water routine in the pool, or something more vigorous. Physical activity is a healthy option for most types of chronic pain, but it's always a good idea to talk with your doctor first about any types of movement you should avoid.

A Walking Routine for People with Chronic Pain

Walking. It's the perfect exercise. You can do it virtually anywhere with no special equipment (other than comfortable, well-fitting walking shoes or sneakers). Proven to reduce stress and ease many types of chronic pain, walking is infinitely flexible. You can do your daily stroll in one continuous session or break it into several shorter walks if you're short on time or can only manage a few minutes of movement at a time.

It's always wise to check with your doctor and/or physical therapist before beginning to exercise. Walking may not be for you if you have a foot or leg injury, such as severe nerve damage, circulation problems related to diabetes, ankle sprain, Achilles tendinitis, plantar fasciitis, a stress fracture, or other conditions. People with peripheral artery disease (PAD) should be on a regimented walking program as prescribed by a physical therapist.

You'll need: Sneakers or walking shoes.

How to do it: Walk 5 or 6 days a week, adding a few minutes each week. Your goal is to build up to 30 minutes of walking on 5 to 6 days a week.

Week 1: Walk 5 to 10 minutes a day at a comfortable pace.

Week 2: Add 5 minutes, so that you're now walking for 10 to 15 minutes a day. If that's too much, try breaking it into two 5- to 7-minute walks at different times of day.

Week 3: Add another 5 minutes to each walk. You could walk for 15 to 20 minutes straight or break your walk into two to three shorter segments done at different times of day.

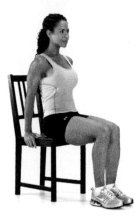

Leg Lift

1. Sit in the chair with your feet flat on the floor. Slowly lift your right leg until it's straight, counting to 5 as you lift.

2. Hold this position as you count to 5 again, then lower your leg.

3. Do this move 10 times with your right leg, then 10 times with your left leg.

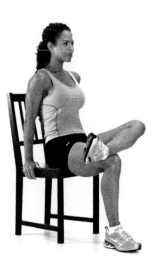

Foot Circles

1. Sit in the chair and cross your left leg over your right knee. Slowly circle your left foot in a clockwise direction 10 times, then reverse and circle slowly 10 times in a counterclockwise direction.

2. Repeat with your right leg crossed over your left knee.

Easy Squat

1. Stand behind the chair. Put your hands on the top of the chair back to help you stay balanced.

2. Slowly squat, bending your knees and lowering your hips about 4 inches. To safeguard your knees, avoid overextending them. Watch your knees as you squat. Don't let them stick out past your toes. Count to 2 as you lower and to 2 as you stand back up. (If your knees hurt, don't squat as far down. Even lowering yourself an inch or two strengthens thigh muscles and improves joint flexibility.)

3. Do this move 8 times.

Knee Raise

1. Stand beside the chair with your right hand on the chair back.

2. Raise your left knee as high as it will go, then slowly lower it again. Remember to stand tall; don't hunch over.

3. With your right hand still on the back of the chair, do this move with your right leg.

4. Repeat this move 5 times with each leg.

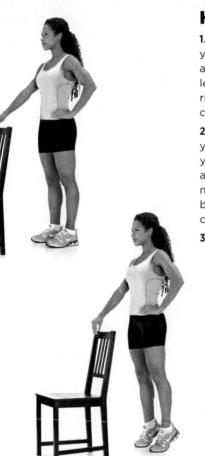

Heel Lift

1. Stand behind the chair with your feet flat on the floor and about 5 inches apart. Put your left hand on your hip and your right hand on the back of the chair.

2. Raise up onto your toes as you count to 2. Then lower until your feet are flat on the floor again as you count to 2. (If you need help with balance, put both hands on the back of the chair.)

3. Do this move 10 times.

Gentle Yoga for Pain Relief

Yoga's benefits can be long-lasting. People reported 70 percent less lower back pain 3 months after a study in which they attended a weekly yoga class and practiced at home, say researchers at West Virginia University School of Medicine. *Bonus:* It may also make you happier. This gentle routine of simple yoga stretches is great for beginners. With regular practice, you'll tone your muscles, improve flexibility, and feel younger than ever.

As with any other exercise program, you should talk with your doctor before starting to practice yoga. Certain poses may cause problems for individuals with various health conditions. A qualified yoga instructor should be able to help you find adjustments that will address your needs.

You'll need: A yoga mat and a sturdy chair.

How to do it: Perform poses in order, flowing from one to the next. It will take about 15 minutes. For a greater challenge and more benefits, do the routine twice or hold the poses longer. Repeat as often as you'd like each week.

Spinal Twist

1. Lie on your back with arms extended on the floor at shoulder height, palms down. Bring knees toward chest.

2. Keeping your knees together, exhale and lower your legs to the right side. Turn your head to look over your left arm. Take several deep breaths.

3. Inhale, bringing your legs back to center, then exhale and repeat on the opposite side.

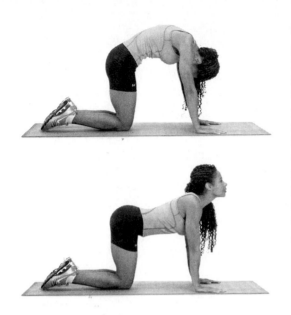

Cat Cow

1. Get on all fours, with your knees directly below hips and your hands directly below shoulders. Exhale.

2. Tucking your tailbone under, arch your spine upward like a Halloween cat, bringing your chin toward your chest.

3. Inhale, tipping your tailbone up and curving your spine downward. Look toward ceiling, expanding your chest.

4. Repeat 5 times.

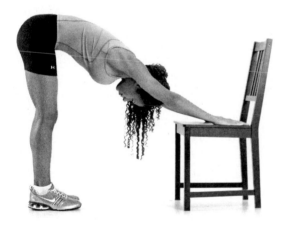

Supported Downward-Facing Dog

1. Stand in front of a sturdy chair with the seat facing you. (If it slides, place it against a wall.)

2. Bending forward from your hips, put your hands on the back of the seat and step back until your arms are extended.

3. Exhale and release your chest toward the floor, keeping your back flat and your shoulder blades pressed down.

4. Reach gently forward, head level between your arms. Inhale and gently press your heels down.

5. Exhale and move deeper into the pose, stretching through your arms while keeping your shoulder blades down.

6. Hold for 3 to 5 breaths, then walk forward and gently roll up to standing.

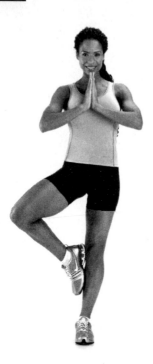

Tree Pose

1. Stand with your feet together, palms in front of your chest in prayer position. Fix gaze on a spot to help balance.

2. Inhale, placing the bottom of your right foot on the inside of your left calf, right knee pointing out to the side.

3. Hold and exhale, pressing your left foot into the floor.

4. Inhale, reaching the top of your head toward the ceiling. Hold for 3 to 5 breaths.

5. Repeat on opposite side.

Note: *To make it easier, perform with hands on hips or arms out to sides. You can also bring your right foot only to your ankle, touching the floor as needed to maintain balance.*

Water Workout

Working out in water provides the same benefits as other aerobic exercises like jogging or stair stepping, but with less stress on joints thanks to water's buoyancy. Experts recommend starting slowly, walking forward and backward in the shallow end of the pool. For variety, add these movements from the Arthritis Foundation Aquatic Program, a warm-water exercise class proven to decrease arthritis symptoms and increase mobility.

Always have the joints you are moving submerged. Waist-high water is fine for hip and knee exercises, but when working the upper body water should cover your shoulders. To up your workout's intensity, increase speed or add resistance by wearing water gloves.

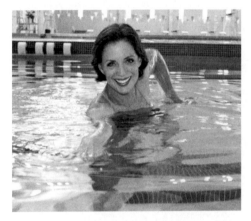

Crawl Stroke

1. In a lunge position for stability, simulate front crawl stroke. Alternate pulling slightly bent arms down and back underwater.

2. Continue for 30 seconds to a minute.

3. For added challenge, walk forward while simulating crawl stroke.

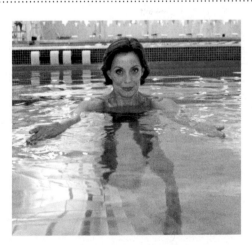

Breaststroke

1. With cupped hands, thumbs beside index fingers, sweep arms to the front of your body with palms below water.

2. Simulate breaststroke, moving your arms to your sides then downward at 45 degrees, and return to starting position as if you were drawing a heart. (Keep thumbs down to protect back and neck muscles.)

3. Continue for 30 seconds to a minute.

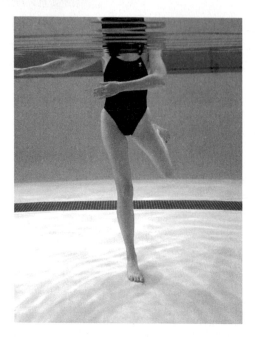

Speed Skate

1. Shift your body weight to right foot, bend your left knee, and move your left heel toward left buttock.

2. Alternate legs in a speed-skating motion. Move arms side to side from shoulder during each knee bend.

3. Continue for 30 seconds to a minute.

Note: *To make it easier, do this exercise facing the pool wall, holding the edge for stability.*

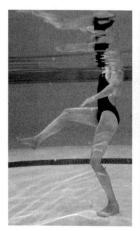 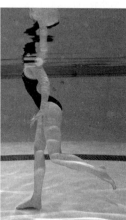

Rocking Horse

1. Stand on your left leg with your right leg extended in front at 45 degrees.

2. Rock forward onto your right leg and bend your left knee to raise left foot to calf height.

3. Lower your left foot and rock back to shift weight to left leg, returning to starting position.

4. Do 8 to 10 reps and repeat with opposite leg in front.

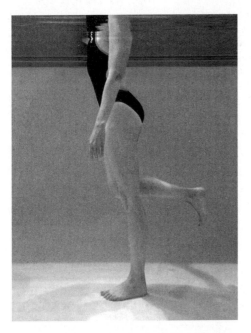

Hamstring Curl

1. Stand next to pool wall and hold on to edge with one hand for stability.

2. Bend one knee and lift your heel toward buttocks.

3. Lower leg to pool floor.

4. Do 8 to 10 reps and repeat with other leg.

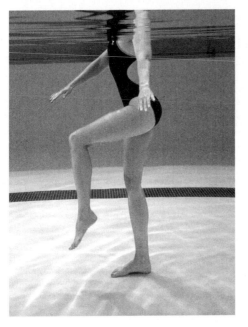

March

1. With feet flexed and fingers and arms loose, lift legs and march forward. (Do not lift knees higher than hip level.)

2. Continue for 30 seconds to a minute.

Pain Centers and Doctors

Multidisciplinary Pain Management Centers

More and more hospitals and medical centers across the nation are establishing multidisciplinary pain management programs that take aim at chronic pain from many directions. The best may include practitioners from many disciplines, including pain specialists, physical therapists, occupational therapists, psychologists, social workers, and practitioners of alternative and complementary therapies.

American Academy of Pain Management

www.aapainmanage.org.
The AAPM accredits five types of pain management centers, from large multidisciplinary programs that give you access to health care practitioners in a wide variety of specialties, to networks of specialists who work together, to centers that specialize in particular types of chronic pain or that offer a single type of therapy (such as biofeedback). You'll find a locator service on its Web site.

If you visit a pain program, these criteria from the American Chronic Pain Association can help you judge whether it's right for you.

- Health care practitioners on the staff share the same beliefs and mission.

- The program is patient- and family-centered.

- Practitioners work together for common, agreed-upon goals.

- The center develops treatment plans based on individual needs.

- Your pain management team displays mutual respect and open communication.

- The pain team communicates frequently with your primary care doctor.

- Your progress is tracked and compared to your pain-relief goals.

- Feedback about your progress and performance is provided to you, caregivers, significant others, and primary care providers.

Alternative and Complementary Therapy

As you've learned throughout this book, the best pain prescriptions are usually a mix of conventional and alternative or complementary therapies, and it's best to work with a doctor who is open to and has experience with both.

American Holistic Medical Association

www. holisticmedicine.org
Founded in 1978, the AHMA is an advocate for the use of holistic and integrative medicine by all licensed health care providers. It supports integrative, complementary, and alternative medicine techniques as well as conventional medical care. You'll find a locator service on this Web site that can help you find a doctor who uses, or is open to, complementary and alternative therapies in addition to standard care.

American Association of Naturopathic Physicians

www.naturopathic.org
This organization advocates for naturopathic medicine and practitioners who are graduates of accredited schools of naturopathic medicine. Naturopathic doctors (NDs) use diet, exercise, lifestyle changes, and cutting-edge natural therapies to enhance the body's ability to heal itself. The AANP Web site includes a locator service for credentialed NDs from recognized naturopathic schools who've also completed 4-year, full-time residency programs.

Second Opinions and Decision Support for Chronic Pain Testing and Treatment

If you're looking for a second opinion or a well-organized, informed way to make a decision about medical treatment for pain, these medical centers can help.

Dartmouth-Hitchcock Medical Center

www.dhmc.org/webpage.cfm?site_id=2&org_id=108&gsec_id=0&sec_id=0&item_id=2486
The Dartmouth-Hitchcock Medical Center (affiliated with Dartmouth Medical School) is home to the nation's first Center for Shared Decision Making in health care. Its Web site includes information that can help you make an informed decision about care for back pain, osteoarthritis, and chronic conditions in general. It also includes links to worksheets you can use to list the information you'll need to make a great decision on the best care for you for any type of chronic pain (or other health condition).

Cleveland Clinic

http://my.clevelandclinic.org/default.aspx
The Cleveland Clinic offers an in-depth, Internet-based second opinion service called MyConsult that gives you access to top health care practitioners. Provide your medical information and for a fee the clinic's staff will review it and make recommendations. This is a good option if you feel you need a second opinion but can't travel to a major medical center, or if you have a rare or complex medical condition not usually treated by doctors near your home. The cost is usually about $565 to $745.

Johns Hopkins International Division

www.hopkinsmedicine.org/international/patients/second_opinions.html
This medical center's international division offers a similar service, called "Remote Medical Second Opinions." After sending in all required information (including, if they pertain to your

condition, pathology reports and slides, and images from x-rays, CT scans, and other radiology checks), you'll receive advice and recommendations in a written report or in a telephone or video conference between Johns Hopkins doctors and your own doctor. The cost is usually $800 to $1,500.

Partners Online Specialty Consultations
https://econsults.partners.org
For a fee ranging from $250 to $495, specialists at Boston-area hospitals affiliated with Harvard Medical School review medical information and provide a second opinion directly to your doctor. Partners Online works with your doctor to explain the process and provide helpful information so you can get the best care close to home.

Food and Supplements

Checking for Drug Supplement Interactions

Before you try any new supplements, check here for any potential interactions with medications you may already be taking.

National Institutes of Health Dietary Supplement Fact Sheets
http://dietary-supplements.info.nih.gov/Health_Information/Information_About_Individual_Dietary_Supplements.aspx
The National Institutes of Health Web site allows you to look up common dietary and herbal supplements and also lists any warnings that have been issued for those types of supplements.

Finding High-Quality Supplements

When shopping for supplements online or at your local drugstore or health food store, look for these seals that indicate they come from reputable manufacturers.

U.S. Pharmacopeia
www.usp.org/USPVerified/
U.S. Pharmacopeia, a nonprofit, sets standards for the purity, potency, and quality of supplements or their ingredients. USP also monitors the manufacturing processes for supplement makers who request it and performs random, off-the-shelf tests of verified products to ensure their continued quality. Look for its seal to ensure that you get high-quality supplements. The program is voluntary and not all supplement makers use it. You can find a list of USP-verified supplements on the Web site.

Natural Products Association
www.npainfo.org
The Natural Products Association will inspect and certify that a supplement maker is adhering to good manufacturing practices. This is a voluntary program. You can learn more about the process and find a list of companies that have the association's GMP (Good Manufacturing Practices) certification at this Web site. The NPA also performs random product testing, using

third-party labs, to see if products from participating supplement makers contain the ingredients and quantities listed on the label. Those that pass earn the "TruLabel" logo from the NPA. More information on this program can also be found at the NPA Web site.

Exercise and Movement Therapies

Physical and Occupational Therapists

Physical and occupational therapists must be licensed by the state in which they practice. Your doctor will usually be able to recommend therapists who have experience with your pain condition, but these resources can also help.

American Physical Therapy Association
www.apta.org
The American Physical Therapy Association is a national network of physical therapists who are especially committed to providing competent and compassionate care. The APTA Web site includes a locator service and information on questions to ask when choosing a physical therapist.

The American Occupational Therapy Association
www.aota.org
The American Occupational Therapy Association is a professional association of occupational therapists. Its Web site gives information on the different ways in which occupational therapy can help.

Certified Personal Trainers

Most gyms and health clubs will either have trainers on staff or can recommend someone. Anyone can advertise personal training services, but your best bet is to work with a trainer who has been certified by a reputable national organization, such as (but not limited to) the ones listed here.

American College of Sports Medicine
www.acsm.org
Working in a wide range of medical specialties, allied health professions, and scientific disciplines, members of the American College of Sports Medicine are committed to the diagnosis, treatment, and prevention of sports-related injuries and the advancement of the science of exercise. From astronauts and athletes to people with chronic diseases or physical challenges, ACSM looks for better methods to allow individuals to live longer and more productive lives. The Web site offers a locator service for certified trainers as well as basic information on preventing injuries while exercising.

American Council on Exercise
www.acefitness.org
Trainers who are certified by the American Council on Exercise must stay up-to-date on the most current research in exercise science and will be able to customize exercise programs for you. The ACE Web site includes a locator service, as well as an exercise library with photos and descriptions of many common exercises, among other resources to help you get fit.

Hydrotherapy

Many multidisciplinary pain centers may also offer hydrotherapy, so check the American Academy of Pain Management site (see page 508) to find one near you. Or check out the Arthritis Foundation's program.

Arthritis Foundation

www.arthritis.org

The Arthritis Foundation has developed water workout classes jointly with the YMCA. You can find your local chapter on the Web site, with information on the closest course to you.

Yoga

There are many different styles of yoga, and even more classes, instructors, and centers. You'll want to try a few to find a routine that suits you. Here are a few resources that are good for beginners.

Yoga Alliance

www.yogaalliance.org

This national organization recognizes yoga teachers who have training and experience that meet a set of strict standards. You can use its locator service to find one. It's wise to talk with a yoga teacher before your first class to explain any limitations created by your chronic pain condition and to find out if the teacher can help you adapt yoga poses to meet your needs safely.

Books

Yoga for Pain Relief: Simple Practices to Calm Your Mind & Heal Your Chronic Pain (Whole Body Healing) by Kelly McGonigal, PhD (New Harbinger Publications)

Healing Yoga for Neck & Shoulder Pain: Easy, Effective Practices for Releasing Tension & Relieving Pain by Carol Krucoff, E-RYT (New Harbinger Publications)

Yoga for Fibromyalgia: Move, Breathe, and Relax to Improve Your Quality of Life by Shoosh Lettick Crotzer (Rodmell Press)

Yoga for Arthritis: The Complete Guide by Loren Fishman, MD, and Ellen Saltonsall (W. W. Norton & Company)

Yoga Heals Your Back: 10-Minute Routines That End Back and Neck Pain by Rita Trieger (Fair Winds Press)

DVDs

Yoga for the Rest of Us: A Step-by-Step Yoga Workout with Peggy Cappy (WGBH Boston)

Yoga Wisdom for Neck Pain and Tight Shoulders by Allison Nolan (Bayview Films)

Healing Yoga for Aches & Pains (Starz/Anchor Bay)

Yoga for Arthritis: Pathways to Better Living with Arthritis & Related Conditions, The Arthritis Foundation (Mobility Limited)

Alexander Technique

The Alexander Technique uses a series of poses and exercises to improve body awareness and help you break habits that stress your muscles, connective tissue, joints, and bones.

Alexander Technique International
www.ati-net.com

The Complete Guide to the Alexander Technique
www.alexandertechnique.com
Learn more on these informative Web sites. Both have locator services that can help you find Alexander Technique teachers and workshops in your area.

Books
How You Stand, How You Move, How You Live: Learning the Alexander Technique to Explore Your Mind-Body Connection and Achieve Self-Mastery by Missy Vineyard (Marlowe & Company)
The Use of the Self by F. M. Alexander (Orion)
The Alexander Technique: A Skill for Life by Pedro de Alcantara (The Crowood Press)

DVDs
Alexander Technique: From Stress to Freedom with Anthony Kingsley (Eclectic DVD Dist.)

Feldenkrais
The Feldenkrais Method is for people who want to reconnect with their natural abilities to move, think, and feel. Whether you want to be more comfortable sitting at your computer, playing with your children and grandchildren, or performing a favorite pastime, these gentle lessons can improve your overall well-being.

Feldenkrais Guild of North America
www.feldenkrais.com
This Web site includes a nationwide locator service for finding Feldenkrais practitioners who trained with method founder Moshe Feldenkrais, PhD, or at an accredited training program. There are also an online bookstore and information on how the method is used for a variety of chronic pain conditions.

Books
Awareness Through Movement: Easy-to-Do Health Exercises to Improve Your Posture, Vision, Imagination, and Personal Awareness by Moshe Feldenkrais (HarperCollins)
Feldenkrais: The Busy Person's Guide to Easier Movement by Frank Wildman (The Intelligent Body Press)

Pilates
The precise, controlled movements of Pilates, whether done on a mat or with specially designed equipment, are intended to boost fitness and build mental alertness.

Pilates Method Alliance
www.pilatesmethodalliance.org
PMA is the certifying organization for Pilates instructors in the United States. Its Web site includes a locator service for finding certified Pilates teachers.

United States Pilates Association
www.unitedstatespilatesassociation.com
The USPA says it certifies teachers in authentic Pilates closest to the type taught by modality
founder Joseph Pilates.

Books
The Pilates Back Book: Heal Neck, Back, and Shoulder Pain with Easy Pilates Stretches by Tia
Stanmore (Fair Winds Press)
*The Pilates Body: The Ultimate At-Home Guide to Strengthening, Lengthening, and Toning Your
Body—Without Machines* by Brooke Siler (Broadway)
Pilates: Body in Motion by Alycea Ungaro (DK Adult)

DVDs
Discovering Pilates with Jon Belanger and Kate Kruuse (JonnyPilates LLC)
Pilates Complete for Inflexible People with Maggie Rhoades (Bodywisdom Media)

Qigong

Qigong is an umbrella term for various ancient Chinese systems of physical and
mental training. Many organizations and schools accredit teachers of Qigong
in the United States, but there are no licensing requirements and there is no
standardized training program.

The National Qigong Association
http://nqa.org
The NQA certifies teachers of qigong at four levels—from Level I instructors, who must have at
least 200 hours of formal training, through Level IV teachers, who must have over 1,000 hours of
training and 10 years of experience training other Qigong teachers. The NQA Web site includes a
locator service.

Books
The Healer Within: Using Traditional Chinese Techniques to Release Your Body's Own Medicine by
Roger Jahnke (HarperOne)
Heal Yourself with Qigong: Gentle Practices to Increase Energy, Restore Health, and Relax the Mind
by Suzanne Friedman (New Harbinger Publications)
Qi Gong for Beginners: Eight Easy Movements for Vibrant Health by Stanley D. Wilson, PhD (Sterling)

DVDs
Getting Started with Qi Gong with Chris Pei (Bodywisdom Media)
Eight Simple Qigong Exercises for Health: The Eight Pieces of Brocade with Dr. Yang, Jwing-Ming
(YMAA Publication Center)
Qigong Beginning Practice with Daisy Lee and Francesco Garripoli (Gaiam)

Tai Chi

Tai chi is a system of slow, gentle, low-impact meditative movements designed
to relieve stress, build fitness. and encourage good health. Many organizations

and schools accredit teachers of tai chi in the United States, but there are no licensing requirements and there is no standardized training program. You can find tai chi classes through a local martial arts center, YMCA or YWCA, senior center, or community education program. To find an instructor with whom you can feel comfortable, ask for recommendations, then ask teachers about their training and experience.

American Tai Chi and Qigong Association
www.americantaichi.org
The American Tai Chi and Qigong Association Web site includes a locator service where you can find tai chi classes in your community.

Books
Tai Chi for Beginners and the 24 Forms by Paul Lam, MD (Tai Chi Productions)
Step-by-Step Tai Chi: The Natural Way to Strength and Health by Master Lam Kam Chuen (Fireside)
T'ai Chi for Seniors: How to Gain Flexibility, Strength, and Inner Peace by Phillipe Bonifonte (Career Press)

DVDs
Tai Chi for Beginners with Samuel Barnes (Starz/Anchor Bay)
Scott Cole: Discover Tai Chi for Beginners (Bayview Entertainment/Widowmaker)
Gentle Tai Chi with Dian Ramirez (Terra Entertainment)

Touch Therapies

Massage Therapy
Most states require that massage therapists be licensed and/or certified. Talk to your doctor before scheduling a massage. Depending on your chronic pain condition, you may need to work with a medical massage therapist or with a therapist with special training in your condition. Here are resources to help you find trained therapists and to learn self-massage techniques that may help.

American Massage Therapy Association
www.amtamassage.org

National Certification Board for Therapeutic Massage and Bodywork
www.ncbtmb.org
The Web sites of these massage organizations allow you to search for certified and licensed massage therapists by technique or specialty and by location. Some massage therapists receive extra training in medical massage. Ask a therapist if he or she has training and experience in treating your type of chronic pain before scheduling a massage.

Books
Massage for Pain Relief: A Step-by-Step Guide by Peijian Shen (Random House)

Products

Thera Cane. This self-massage cane helps ease back, neck, and shoulder pain, and more (www.
theracane.com).
The Knobble II. This knob-shaped device lets you apply more pressure if you're doing pressure
point self-therapy (www.pressurepositive.com).
The Original Backnobber II. This tool helps you reach aching spots on your back (www.
pressurepositive.com).

Acupuncture

Talk with your doctor before you try acupuncture to find out if there are special
limitations you and your acupuncturist should be aware of. It's also important
to find out if the acupuncturist has special training and/or experience working
with people with your type of pain. Plan to go to a trained acupuncturist certified by the National Certification Commission for Acupuncture and Oriental
Medicine. Most, but not all, states require acupuncturists to pass the NCCAOM
exam and/or be certified by the group in order to practice.

National Certification Commission for Acupuncture and Oriental Medicine

www.nccaom.org/find/index.html
The National Certification Commission for Acupuncture and Oriental Medicine is the main
accrediting body for acupuncturists in the United States. Its Web site includes a locator service
for practitioners, including those accredited by AAAOM.

The American Association of Acupuncture and Oriental Medicine

www.aaaomonline.org
Graduates of college programs accredited by the AAAOM have 1,500 to 2,000 hours of acupuncture
training along with additional training in other aspects of Oriental medicine (such as herbs,
nutrition, tai chi, qigong, and meditation). You'll find a locator service on the AAAOM Web site.

Acupressure

Also called trigger point therapy, acupressure involves applying pressure to specific points on the body in order to free up energy—called qi—and improve
health. You can learn acupressure points for your specific pain condition from
a qualified acupuncture practitioner. Some massage therapists also practice
acupressure.

Books

The Trigger Point Therapy Workbook: Your Self-Treatment Guide for Pain Relief by Clair Davies
with Amber Davies (New Harbinger Publications)
The Subtle Body: An Encyclopedia of Your Energetic Anatomy by Cyndi Dale (Sounds True, Inc.)
Acupressure's Potent Points: A Guide to Self-Care for Common Ailments by Michael Reed Gach
(Bantam)

DVD

An Introduction to Acupressure with Lucy Lloyd-Barker and Stephanie Bell (Bodhi)

Chiropractic

Doctors of chiropractic (DCs) take care of people with back pain, neck pain, and headaches as well as those with a wide range of injuries and disorders of the musculoskeletal system involving the muscles, ligaments, and joints. Some states require DCs to be licensed to practice.

American Chiropractic Association
www.acatoday.org
The American Chiropractic Association (ACA) is the largest professional association in the United States representing doctors of chiropractic. You'll find a locator service on the ACA's Web site, along with more information about the practice.

MELT Method

Created by movement instructor Sue Hitzmann, the MELT Method helps prevent pain and eliminate stress. It can easily be done on your own.

MELT
www.meltmethod.com
The MELT Web site will show you where to find instructors and classes. You can also order foam rollers, treatment balls, and an instructional DVD.

Reiki

The Japanese healing art of Reiki involves placing the hands lightly on or over a person receiving treatment to trigger the person's own healing. It is considered energy medicine, and there are no licensing requirements for Reiki in the United States. But it cannot be self-taught. Reiki practitioners study with a master teacher and move through three levels of education. The first two levels may be taught over 2 days.

To find a Reiki practitioner, ask friends and even health care practitioners you know for recommendations. Massage therapists and health care practitioners themselves are sometimes trained in Reiki. Before scheduling an appointment, ask a Reiki practitioner about her level of training, how often she performs Reiki, how long she's been in practice, and whether she practices Reiki on herself daily. Look for someone with solid training and plenty of experience who deepens her knowledge every day through self-Reiki.

TENS

Transcutaneous electrical nerve stimulation (TENS) is the use of electric current produced by a device to stimulate the nerves for therapeutic purposes. It is usually prescribed or recommended by your doctor.

Mind-Body Therapies

Cognitive-Behavioral Therapy

Psychologists, psychiatrists, and clinical social workers may all be trained in cognitive-behavioral techniques. You can find a trained and licensed CBT practitioner through these organizations.

Association for Behavioral and Cognitive Therapies

www.abct.org

The Association for Behavioral and Cognitive Therapies is a multidisciplinary organization that promotes the practice of CBT. Its "Find a Therapist" service allows you to search by location, population, and specific condition.

National Association of Cognitive-Behavioral Therapists

www.nacbt.org

The National Association of Cognitive-Behavioral Therapists trains mental health professionals in CBT. The Web site has a locator service.

Academy of Cognitive Therapy

www.academyofct.org

The Academy of Cognitive Therapy certifies cognitive therapists. The Web site has a locator service.

Books

Feeling Good: The New Mood Therapy Revised and Updated by David D. Burns, MD (Harper)
The Feeling Good Handbook by David D. Burns, MD (Plume)

DVDs

Good Days Ahead by Jesse H. Wright, MD, PhD, Andrew S. Wright, MD, and Aaron T. Beck, MD (Interactive Media Lab)
This self-help cognitive therapy program is aimed at people with depression and/or anxiety, and it could help you if your chronic pain is contributing to stress and low moods.

Guided Imagery

Guided imagery can easily be done on your own, but you may find it helpful to work with a practitioner at first.

Academy for Guided Imagery

www.academyforguidedimagery.com

Log on to find a certified guided imagery practitioner near you. You will also find a listing of CDs and DVDs.

DVDs

Health Journeys

www.healthjourneys.com

This Web site lists various titles for help with pain management, back pain, better sleep, headache, fibromyalgia, chronic fatigue, cancer, stress relief, depression, and more. You can buy guided imagery CDs and DVDs developed by psychotherapist and guided imagery pioneer Belleruth Naparstek (author of *Staying Well with Guided Imagery)* and others at this premiere guided imagery Web site. Naparstek has created a quiet health revolution by convincing big institutions like the U.S. Department of Defense, the American Red Cross, several major insurance companies, and nearly 2,000 hospitals and health centers to distribute guided imagery recordings to their patients and clients, usually free of charge.

Hypnotherapy

Hypnotherapy can be done on your own, but you may find it helpful to work with a practitioner at first.

The American Society of Clinical Hypnosis (ASCH) and The Society for Clinical and Experimental Hypnosis
www.societiesofhypnosis.com
Both groups use the same Web site, at which you can find qualified practitioners. Hypnotherapists in this locator service must hold a doctorate in fields such as medicine, dentistry, podiatry, or psychology, or have advanced degrees and/or training in nursing, social work, or traditional Chinese medicine.

The American Psychotherapy and Medical Hypnosis Association
http://apmha.com
This group awards certificates to licensed medical and mental health professionals who complete a 6- to 8-week hypnotherapy course. Find members, as well as audiotapes, CDs, and self-hypnosis programs, on its Web site.

Books
Hypnotherapy for Dummies by Mike Bryant and Peter Mabbutt (John Wiley)
Working with Hypnotherapy: How to Heal Mind and Body with Self-Hypnosis by Teresa Moorey (Godsfield Press)

DVDs
Hypnotherapy with Shelley Stockwell (Gaiam)

Meditation

There are many different styles of meditation. Here are a few resources that are good for beginners.

Mindfulness Center of the University of Massachusetts Medical School
www.umassmed.edu/cfm/mbsr
You'll find practitioners and mindfulness programs across the United States and around the world by logging on to this Web site.

Books
Full Catastrophe Living: Using the Wisdom of Your Body and Mind to Face Stress, Pain, and Illness. The Program of the Stress Reduction Clinic at the University of Massachusetts Medical Center by Jon Kabat-Zinn, PhD (Delta, 1990)

Wherever You Go, There You Are: Mindfulness Meditation in Everyday Life by Jon Kabat-Zinn, PhD (Hyperion)

Heal Thy Self: Lessons on Mindfulness in Medicine by Saki Santorelli (Three Rivers Press)

CDs

Mindfulness Meditation for Pain Relief: Guided Practices for Reclaiming Your Body and Your Life by Jon Kabat-Zinn, PhD (Sounds True)

Break Through Pain: A Step-by-Step Mindfulness Meditation Program for Transforming Chronic and Acute Pain by Shinzen Young (Sounds True, Inc.)

Defeat Pain: Meditations to Transform Pain to Peace by KRS Edstrom (Soft Stone Publishing)

Biofeedback

Most biofeedback practitioners are licensed health care professionals. It's important also to be sure that the practitioner is trained in the use of biofeedback for your specific pain condition.

Biofeedback Certification International Alliance

www.bcia.org

Practitioners certified by the BCIA are health care practitioners who've also been trained in biofeedback and who meet standards for training and practical experience in this modality. BCIA is recognized as the certification body for the clinical practice of biofeedback by both the Association of Applied Psychophysiology and Biofeedback (AAPB) and the International Society for Neurofeedback and Research (ISNR). You can not only find a practitioner on the site but also learn more about different types of biofeedback.

Books

A Symphony in the Brain by Jim Robbins (Grove Press)

The High-Performance Mind by Anna Wise (Tarcher)

DVDs

The Journey to Wild Divine by Wild Divine Profect (Wild Divine)

Products

Practice biofeedback at home with these devices:

The StressEraser

www.stresseraser.com

This pager-sized device tracks your pulse using a finger sensor. You learn to relax by breathing in sync with your heart rate.

Biodot Skin Thermometers

www.biodots.net

Disposable, stick-on temperature sensors (about the size of a lentil) change color to tell you if the surface of your skin is warm (a sign that you're relaxed) or cool (a sign that you're tense).

Chapter 1

1 Timothy Wiegand, Jingjing Hu and Michele B Delenick, Toxicity, Nonsteroidal Anti-inflammatory Agents. eMedicine, Updated: May 20, 2010 http://emedicine.medscape.com/article/816117-overview

2 Bridget M. Kuehn. "Opioid Prescriptions Soar: Increase in Legitimate Use as Well as Abuse." *JAMA*, 2007, 297: 249–251.

3 www.aapainmanage.org/literature/Articles/PainAnEpidemic.pdf

4 *Ibid.*

5 National Centers for Health Statistics. Chartbook on Trends in the Health of Americans 2006, Special Feature: Pain. http://www.cdc.gov/nchs/data/hus/hus06.pdf.

6 R. J. Gatchel, P. B. Polatin, C. Noe, *et al.* "Treatment and Cost-Effectiveness of Early Intervention for Acute Lowback Pain Patients: A One-Year Prospective Study." *Journal of Occupational Rehabilitation,* 2003 Mar, 13: 1–9.

7 W. Michael Hooten *et al.* "Treatment Outcomes after Multidisciplinary Pain Rehabilitation with Analgesic Medication Withdrawal for Patients with Fibromyalgia." *Pain Medicine*, 2007, 8 (1) 8–16.

8 Timothy S. Clark. "Interdisciplinary Treatment for Chronic Pain: Is It Worth the Money?" *Baylor University Medical Proceedings*, 2000, 13: 240–43.

9 Chantal Berna, Siri Leknes, Emily A. Holmes, *et al.* "Induction of Depressed Mood Disrupts Emotion Regulation Neurocircuitry and Enhances Pain Unpleasantness." *Biological Psychiatry*, 2010, 67 (11):

10 http://www.painmed.org/patient/facts.html#highlights.

11 T. Giesecke *et al.* "The Relationship between Depression, Clinical Pain, and Experimental Pain in a Chronic Pain Cohort." *Arthritis & Rheumatism*, 2005, 52: 1577–1584.

12 John R. Keltner, Ansgar Furst, Catherine Fan, *et al.* "Isolating the Modulatory Effect of Expectation on Pain Transmission: A Functional Magnetic Resonance Imaging Study." *Journal of Neuroscience*, April 19, 2006, Vol. 26, No. 16: 4437–4443.

13 K. J. Sherman *et al.* "Comparing Yoga, Exercise, and a Self-Care Book for Chronic Low Back Pain: A Randomized, Controlled Trial." *Annals of Internal Medicine*, 2005, 143(12): 849–56.

14 C.L. Baird and L. Sands. "A Pilot Study of the Effectiveness of Guided Imagery with Progressive Muscle Relaxation to Reduce Chronic Pain and Mobility Difficulties of Osteoarthritis. *Pain Management Nursing*, 2004 Sep, 5(3): 97–104.

15 S. Bruehl and O. Y. Chung. "Psychological and Behavioral Aspects of Complex Regional Pain Syndrome M." *Clinical Journal of Pain*, 2006, 22(5):430–37.

16 A. R. Drexler, E. J. Mur, and V. C. Günther. "Efficacy of an EMG-Biofeedback Therapy in Fibromyalgia Patients. A Comparative Study of Patients with and without Abnormality in (MMPI) Psychological Scales." *Clinical and Experimental Rheumatology*, 2002 Sep-Oct, 20(5): 677–82.

17 L. L. Hsieh *et al.* "Treatment of Low Back Pain by Acupressure and Physical Therapy: Randomised Controlled Trial." *British Medical Journal*, 2006 Mar 25, 332(7543): 696–700. E-pub 2006 Feb 17.

18 V. R. Aggarwal *et al.* "Reviewing the Evidence: Can Cognitive Behavioral Therapy Improve Outcomes for Patients with Chronic Orofacial Pain?" *Journal of Orofacial Pain*, 2010 Spring, 24(2): 163–71.

19 M.V. Vitiello, B. Rybarczyk, M. Von Korff, *et al.* "Cognitive behavioral therapy for insomnia improves sleep and decreases pain in older adults with co-morbid insomnia and osteoarthritis." *Journal of Clinical Sleep Medicine*, 2009, Aug 15;5(4): 355-62.

20 J. S. Kutner, M. C. Smith, L. Corbin, *et al.* "Massage Therapy Versus Simple Touch to Improve Pain and Mood in Patients with Advanced Cancer: A Randomized Trial." *Annals of Internal Medicine*, 2008 Sep 16, 149(6): 369–79.

21 B. R. Cassileth and A. J. Vickers. "Massage Therapy for Symptom Control: Outcome Study at a Major Cancer Center." *Journal of Pain Symptom Management*, 2004, September, 28, no. 3: 244–49.

22 J. J. Kerssens, P. F. Verhaak, A. I. Bartelds, *et al.* "Unexplained Severe Chronic Pain in General Practice." *European Journal of Pain*, 2002; 6(3): 203–12.

23 http://www.livingwithcrohnsdisease.com/livingwithcrohnsdisease/voices/key_findings.html.

Chapter 2

1   W. Atkinson, T. A. Sheldon, N. Shaath, *et al.* "Irritable Bowel Syndrome: Food Elimination Based on IgG Antibodies in Irritable Bowel Syndrome: A Randomised Controlled Trial." *Gut*, 2004, 53: 1459–1464.

2   G. C. Curhan, W. C. Willett, E. L. Knight, *et al.* "Dietary Factors and the Risk of Incident Kidney Stones in Younger Women: Nurses' Health Study II." *Archives of Internal Medicine*, 2004 Apr 26, 164(8): 885–91.

3   Writing Team for the DCCT/EDIC Research Group. "Effect of Intensive Therapy on the Microvascular Complications of Type 1 Diabetes Mellitus." *JAMA*, 2002, 287: 2563–2569.

4   L. J. Wright *et al.* "Chronic Pain, Overweight, and Obesity: Findings from a Community-Based Twin Registry." *Journal of Pain*, 2010 Mar 23 (E-pub ahead of print).

5   Johns Hopkins Arthritis Center. "Osteoarthritis Weight Management."

6   *Annals of Rheumatic Diseases*, 2003, 62: 208–14.

7   G. Tan *et al.* "Efficacy Of Selected Complementary And Alternative Medicine Interventions For Chronic Pain."

8   G. Tan *et al.* "Efficacy of Selected Complementary and Alternative Medicine Interventions for Chronic Pain." *Journal of Rehabilitation Research & Development*, 2007, Volume 44, Number 2, 195–222.

9   Yi-Hao A. Shen and Richard Nahas. "Complementary and Alternative Medicine for Treatment of Irritable Bowel Syndrome." *Canadian Family Physician,* February 2009, Vol 55.

10   C. J. Bijkerk, N. J. de Wit, J. W. M. Muris, *et al.* "Soluble or Insoluble Fibre in Irritable Bowel Syndrome in Primary Care? Randomised Placebo Controlled Trial." *British Medical Journal*, 2009; 339: b3154.

11   J. M. P. Hyland and I. Taylor. "Does a High Fibre Diet Prevent the Complications of Diverticular Disease?" *British Journal of Surgery*, Volume 67, Issue 2, 77–79.

12   Shen and Nahas. "Complementary and Alternative Medicine for Treatment of Irritable Bowel Syndrome."

13   Lorna Mason, R. Andrew Moore, Sheena Derry, *et al.* "Systematic Review of Topical Capsaicin for the Treatment of Chronic Pain." *British Medical Journal*, 2004, 24 April, 328: 991.

14   D. O. Clegg, D. J. Reda, C. L. Harris, *et al.* "Glucosamine, Chondroitin Sulfate, and the Two in Combination for Painful Knee Osteoarthritis." *New England Journal of Medicine*, 2006 354: 795–808.

15   E. C. Huskisson. "Glucosamine and Chondroitin for Osteoarthritis." *The Journal of International Medical Research*, 2008, 36: 1161–1179 (first published online as 36(6) 6).

16   W. I. Najm *et al.* "S-Adenosyl Methionine (Same) Versus Celecoxib for the Treatment of Osteoarthritis Symptoms: A Double-Blind Cross-Over Trial." *BMC Musculoskeletal Disorders*, 2004, 5: 6.

17   M.K. Turner, M.W. Hooten, J.E. Schmidt *et al.* "Prevalence And Clinical Correlates Of Vitamin D Inadequacy Among Patients With Chronic Pain." *Pain Medicine*, 2008, 9:979–84.

18   Sebastian Straube, R. Andrew Moore, Sheena Derry, *et al.* "Topical Review: Vitamin D and Chronic Pain." *Pain*, 2009, 141: 10–13.

19   M. Ranieri, M. Sciuscio, A. M. Cortese, *et al.* "The Use of Alpha-Lipoic Acid (ALA), Gamma Linolenic Acid (GLA) and Rehabilitation in the Treatment of Back Pain: Effect on Health-Related Quality of Life." *International Journal of Immunopathology and Pharmacology*, 2009 Jul–Sep, 22(3 Suppl): 45–50.

20   G. S. Mijnhout, A. Alkhalaf, N. Kleefstra, *et al.* "Alpha Lipoic Acid: A New Treatment for Neuropathic Pain in Patients with Diabetes?" *Netherlands Journal of Medicine*, 2010 Apr; 68(4): 158–62.

21   G. Di Geronimo, A. F. Caccese, L. Caruso, *et al.* "Treatment of Carpal Tunnel Syndrome with Alpha-Lipoic Acid." *European Review for Medical and Pharmacological Sciences*, 2009 Mar-Apr, 13(2): 133–9.

22   J. M. Zakrzewska, H. Forssell, and A. M. Glenny. "Interventions for the Treatment of Burning Mouth Syndrome." *Cochrane Database of Systematic Reviews*, 2005, Jan 25 (1): CD002779.

23   D. De Grandis and C . Minardi. "Acetyl-L-Carnitine (Levacecarnine) in the Treatment of Diabetic Neuropathy. A Long-Term, Randomised, Double-Blind, Placebo-Controlled Study." *Drugs in R & D*, 2002, 3: 223–231.

24   A. A. Sima, M. Calvani, M. Mehra, *et al.* "Acetyl-L-Carnitine Improves Pain, Nerve Regeneration, and Vibratory Perception in Patients with Chronic Diabetic Neuropathy: An Analysis of Two Randomized Placebo-Controlled Trials." *Diabetes Care*, 2005, 28: 89–94.

25   J. C. Maroon and J.W. Bost. "Omega-3 Fatty Acids (Fish Oil) as an Anti-Inflammatory: An Alternative to Nonsteroidal Anti-Inflammatory Drugs for Discogenic Pain." *Surgical Neurology*, 2006 Apr, 65(4): 326–31.

26   Y. Okuda, M. Mizutani, M. Ogawa, *et al.* "Longterm Effects of Eicosapentaenoic Acid on Diabetic Peripheral Neuropathy and Serum Lipids in Patients With Type II Diabetes Mellitus." *Journal of Diabetes Complications*, 1996, 10: 280–287.

27   B. G. Feagan *et al.* "Omega-3 Free Fatty Acids for the Maintenance of Remission in Crohn Disease." *Journal of the American Medical Association*, April 9, 2008, Vol. 299, No. 14, 1690–1697.

Chapter 3

1   S. Hollinghurst, D. Sharp, K. Ballard, *et al.* "Randomised controlled trial of Alexander technique lessons, exercise, and massage (ATEAM) for chronic and recurrent back pain: economic evaluation." *British Medical Journal*, 2008 Dec 11, 337: a2656. doi: 10.1136/bmj.a2656.

2   G. Gard. "Body Awareness Therapy for Patients with Fibromyalgia and Chronic Pain." *Disability and Rehabilitation*, 2005 Jun 17, 27(12): 725–8.

3   J. K. Freburger, T. S. Carey, G. M. Holmes, *et al.* "Exercise Prescription for Chronic Back or Neck Pain: Who Prescribes It? Who Gets It? What Is Prescribed?" *Arthritis Care Research*, 2009, 61(2): 192–200.

4   K. Williams *et al.* "Evaluation of the Effectiveness and Efficacy of Iyengar Yoga Therapy on Chronic Low Back Pain." *Spine*, 1 September 2009, Volume 34, Issue 19, 2066-2076.

5   L. Altan, N. Korkmaz, U. Bingol, *et al.* "Effect of Pilates Training on People with Fibromyalgia Syndrome: A Pilot Study." *Archives of Physical Medicine and Rehabilitation,* 2009 Dec, 90(12): 1983–88.

6   M. Fransen, L. Nairn, J. Winstanley, *et al.* "Physical Activity for Osteoarthritis Management: A Randomized Controlled Clinical Trial Evaluating Hydrotherapy or Tai Chi Classes." *Arthritis & Rheumatism*, 2007 Apr 15, 57(3): 407–14.

7   R. van Linschoten, M, van Middelkoop, M. Y. Berge, *et al.* "Supervised Exercise Therapy Versus Usual Care for Patellofemoral Pain Syndrome: An Open Label Randomised Controlled Trial." *British Medical Journal* 2009, December 1; 339: b4074.

8   W. H. Ettinger, Jr., R. Burns, S P. Messier, *et al.* "A Randomized Trial Comparing Aerobic Exercise and Resistance Exercise with a Health Education Program in Older Adults with Knee Osteoarthritis." The Fitness Arthritis and Seniors Trial (FAST)." *JAMA*, 1997 Jan 1, 277(1): 25–31.

9   K. Engebretsen, M. Grotle, E. Bautz-Holter, *et al.* "Radial extracorporeal shockwave treatment compared with supervisedexercises in patients with subacromial pain syndrome: single blind randomised study." *British Medical Journal* 2009; 339: b3360.

10   Barbara B. Meyer and Kathy J. Lemley. Clinical Sciences: Clinical Investigations, "Utilizing Exercise to Affect the Symptomology of Fibromyalgia: A Pilot Study." *Medicine & Science in Sports & Exercise,* October 2000, Volume 32, Issue 10, 1691–1697.

11   E. Varkey, A. Cider, J. Carlsson, *et al.* "A Study to Evaluate the Feasibility of an Aerobic Exercise Program in Patients with Migraine." *Headache*, 2009 Apr, 49(4): 563–70. E-pub 2008 Sep 9.

12   E. Varkey, K. Hagen, J. A. Zwart, *et al.* "Physical Activity and Headache: Results from the Nord-Trøndelag Health Study (HUNT)." *Cephalalgia*, 2008 Dec, 28(12): 1292–97.

13   C. P. Loudon, V. Corroll, J. Butcher, *et al.* "The Effects of Physical Exercise on Patients with Crohn's Disease." *American Journal of Gastroenterology*, 1999, 94(3): 697–703. V. Ng, *et al.* "Low-Intensity Exercise Improves Quality of Life in Patients with Crohn's Disease." *Clinical Journal of Sports Medicine*, 2007, 17(5): 384–388.

14   V. Ng, W. Millard, C. Lebrun, *et al.* Low-Intensity Exercise Improves Quality of Life in Patients With Crohn's Disease. *Clinical Journal of Sport Medicine.* 17(5): 384-388, September 2007.

15   M. P. Herring, P. J. O'Connor, and R. K. Dishman. "The Effect of Exercise Training on Anxiety Symptoms Among Patients." *Archives of Internal Medicine*, 2010, 170(4): 321–331.

16   E. M. Bartels, H. Lund, K. B. Hagen, *et al.* "Aquatic Exercise for the Treatment of Knee and Hip Osteoarthritis." *Cochrane Database of Systematic Reviews*, 2007 Oct 17, (4): CD005523.

17   Marcos Renato Assis, Luciana Eduardo Silva, Adriana Martins Barros Alves, *et al.* "A Randomized Controlled Trial of Deep Water Running: Clinical Effectiveness of Aquatic Exercise to Treat Fibromyalgia." *Arthritis & Rheumatism*, published online 6 Feb 2006, Volume 55, Issue 1, 57–65.

18   K. Williams, C. Abildso, L. Steinberg, *et al.* "Evaluation of the Effectiveness and Efficacy of Iyengar Yoga Therapy on Chronic Low Back Pain." *Spine*, 2009, 34(19): 2066-2076.

Chapter 4

1   Jennie C. I. Tsao. "Effectiveness of Massage Therapy for Chronic, Non-Malignant Pain: A Review." *eCAM* 2007, 4(2): 165–179.

2   *Ibid.*

3   Christopher Quinn, Clint Chandler, and Albert Moraska. "Massage Therapy and Frequency of Chronic Tension Headaches." *American Journal of Public Health*, 2002, 92:1657–1661.

4   T. Field, M. Diego, C. Cullen, *et al.* "Fibromyalgia Pain and Substance P Decrease and Sleep Improved after Massage Therapy." *Journal of Clinical Rheumatology*, 2002, 8: 72–6.

5   J. S. Kutner, M. C. Smith, L. Corbin, *et al.* "Massage Therapy Versus Simple Touch to Improve Pain and Mood in Patients with Advanced Cancer: A Randomized Trial." *Annals of Internal Medicine*, 2008 Sep 16, 149 (6): 369–79.

6 B. R. Cassileth and A. J. Vickers. "Massage Therapy for Symptom Control: Outcome Study at a Major Cancer Center." *Journal of Pain Symptom Management*, 2004 September, 28, no. 3: 244–249.

7 *Ibid.*

8 M. Haas, R. Sharma, and M. Stano. "Cost-Effectiveness of Medical and Chiropractic Care for Acute and Chronic Low Back Pain." *Journal of Manipulative Physiological Therapeutics*, 2005 Oct, 28(8): 555–63.

9 J. Shen. "Research on the Neurophysiological Mechanisms of Acupuncture: Review of Selected Studies and Methodological Issues." *Journal of Alternative and Complementary Medicine*, 2001, 7 Suppl 1: S121–7.

10 National Center for Complementary and Alternative Medicine: Magnets for Pain. http://nccam.nih.gov/health/magnet/magnetsforpain.htm#science.

11 A. Hopton and H. MacPherson. "Acupuncture for Chronic Pain: Is Acupuncture More Than an Effective Placebo? A Systematic Review of Pooled Data from Meta-Analyses." *Pain Practice*, 2010 Mar, 10(2): 94–102, E-pub 2010 Jan 8.

12 Richard E. Harris, Jon-Kar Zubieta, David J. Scott, *et al.* "Traditional Chinese Acupuncture and Placebo (Sham) Acupuncture Are Differentiated by Their Effects on Ω-Opioid Receptors (Mors)." *Journal of NeuroImaging*, 2009, 47 (3): 1077–1085.

13 Brain Images Demonstrate that Acupuncture Relieves Pain. Study presented by Huey-Jen Lee, Wen-Ching Liu, Dung-Liang Hung, Barry R. Komisaruk, Andrew Kalnin, and Satyaveni B. Rao at the 85th Scientific Assembly and Annual Meeting of the Radiological Society of North America (RSNA).

13 Carole A. Paley, Michael I. Bennett, Mark I. Johnson. "Acupuncture for Cancer-induced Bone Pain?" *Evidence-Based Complementary and Alternative Medicine*, published online March 24, 2010.

14 David Alimi, Carole Rubino, Evelyne Pichard-Léandri, *et al.* "Analgesic Effect of Auricular Acupuncture for Cancer Pain: A Randomized, Blinded, Controlled Trial." *Journal of Clinical Oncology*, 2003 Nov, Vol 21, Issue 22, 4120–4126.

15 W. E. Mehling, B. Jacobs, M. Acree, *et al.* "Symptom Management with Massage and Acupuncture in Postoperative Cancer Patients: A Randomized Controlled Trial." *Journal of Pain Symptom Management*, 2007 Mar, 33(3): 258–66.

16 D. Cherkin. *Archives of Internal Medicine*, May 11, 2009, vol 169: 858–866.

17 Karen J. Sherman and Remy R. Coeytaux. "Acupuncture for Improving Chronic Back Pain, Osteoarthritis and Headache." *Journal of Clinical Outcomes Management*, 2009 May 1, 16(5): 224–230.

18 D. He, A. T. Høstmark, K. B. Veiersted, *et al.* "Effect of Intensive Acupuncture on Pain-Related Social and Psychological Variables for Women with Chronic Neck and Shoulder Pain—An RCT with Six Month and Three Year Follow Up." *Acupuncture in Medicine*, 2005 Jun, 23(2): 52–61.

19 H. D. Kurland. "Treatment of Headache Pain with Auto-Acupressure." *Diseases of the Nervous System*, 1976, 37(3): 127–129.

20 B. Tu, M. Johnston, and K. K. Hui. "Elderly Patient Refractory to Multiple Pain Medications Successfully Treated with Integrative East-West Medicine." *International Journal of General Medicine*, 2009 Nov 30, 1: 3–6.

21 L. L. Hsieh, C. H. Kuo, L. H. Lee, *et al.* "Treatment of Low Back Pain by Acupressure and Physical Therapy: Randomised Controlled Trial." *British Medical Journal*, 2006 Mar 25, 332(7543): 696–700. E-pub 2006 Feb 17.

22 R. M. Dubinsky and A. Binder. "Assessment: Efficacy of Transcutaneous Electric Nerve Stimulation in the Treatment of Pain in Neurologic Disorders (An Evidence-Based Review). Report of the Therapeutics and Technology Assessment Subcommittee of the American Academy of Neurology" Jan. 12, 2010.

Chapter 5

1 C. Eccleston, A. C. Williams, and S. Morley. "Psychological Therapies for the Management of Chronic Pain (Excluding Headache) in Adults." *Cochrane Database of Systematic Reviews*, 2009, (2): CD007407.

2 V. R. Aggarwal, M. Tickle, H. Javidi, *et al.* "Reviewing the Evidence: Can Cognitive Behavioral Therapy Improve Outcomes for Patients with Chronic Orofacial Pain?" *Journal of Orofacial Pain*, 2010 Spring; 24(2): 163–71.

3 S. van Koulil, W. van Lankveld, F. W. Kraaimaat, *et al.* "Tailored Cognitive-Behavioral Therapy and Exercise Training for High-Risk Fibromyalgia Patients." *Arthritis Care & Research*, 2010 Jun 2 (Hoboken) (E-pub ahead of print).

4 M.V.Vitiello, B.Rybarczyk, M.Von Korff, *et al.* "Cognitive behavioral therapy for insomnia improves sleep and decreases pain in older adults with co-morbid insomnia and osteoarthritis." *Journal of Clinical Sleep Medicine*. 2009 Aug 15;5(4): 355-62.

5 J. M. Lackner, J. Jaccard, S. S. Krasner, *et al.* "Self-Administered Cognitive Behavior Therapy for Moderate to Severe Irritable Bowel Syndrome: Clinical Efficacy, Tolerability, Feasibility." *Clinical Gastroenterology and Hepatology*, 2008 Aug, 6(8): 899–906.

6 Connie A. Luedtke, Jeffrey M. Thompson, John A. Postier, *et al.* "A Description of a Brief Multidisciplinary Treatment Program for Fibromyalgia." *Pain Management Nursing*, June 2005, Vol. 6, Issue 2, 76–80.

7 C. L. Baird and L. P. Sands. "Effect Of Guided Imagery With Relaxation On Health-Related Quality Of Life In Older Women With Osteoarthritis." *Research in Nursing and Health*, 2006 Oct, 29(5): 442–51.

8 ———. "A Pilot Study of the Effectiveness of Guided Imagery with Progressive Muscle Relaxation to Reduce Chronic Pain and Mobility Difficulties of Osteoarthritis." *Pain Management Nursing*, 2004 Sep, 5(3): 97–104.

9 K. L. Kwekkeboom, H. Hau, B. Wanta, *et al.* "Patients' Perceptions of the Effectiveness of Guided Imagery and Progressive Muscle Relaxation Interventions Used for Cancer Pain." *Complementary Therapies in Clinical Practice*, 2008 Aug, 14(3): 185–94.

11 NIH Technology Assessment Panel. "Integration of Behavioral and Relaxation Approaches into the Treatment of Chronic Pain and Insomnia." *JAMA*, 1996, 276: 313–318.

10/12 Brenda L. Stoelb, Ivan R. Molton, Mark P. Jensen, *et al.* "The Efficacy of Hypnotic Analgesia in Adults: A Review of the Literature." *Contemporary Hypnosis*, 2009 March 1, 26(1): 24–39.

13 *Ibid.*

14 *Ibid.*

15 A. Castel, M. Pérez, J. Sala, A. Padrol, *et al.* "Effect of Hypnotic Suggestion on Fibromyalgic Pain: Comparison between Hypnosis and Relaxation." *European Journal of Pain*, 2007, 11: 463–8.

16 G. H. Montgomery, D. H. Bovbjerg, J. B. Schnur, *et al.* "A Randomized Clinical Trial of a Brief Hypnosis Intervention to Control Side Effects in Breast Surgery Patients." *Journal of the National Cancer Institute*, 2007, 99: 1304–12.

17 L. Roberts, S. Wilson, S. Singh, *et al.* "Gut-Directed Hypnotherapy for Irritable Bowel Syndrome: Piloting a Primary Care-Based Randomised Controlled Trial." *British Journal of General Practice*, 2006; 56: 115–21.

18 E. P. Simon and D. M. Lewis. "Medical Hypnosis for Temporomandibular Disorders: Treatment Efficacy and Medical Utilization Outcome." *Oral Surgery, Oral Medicine, Oral Pathology, Oral Radiology, and Endodontics*, 2000, 90: 54–63.

19 I. Kirsch, G. Montgomery, and G. Sapirstein. "Hypnosis as an Adjunct to Cognitive-Behavioral Psychotherapy: A Meta-Analysis." *Journal of Consulting and Clinical Psychology*, 1995 Apr, 63(2): 214–20.

20 L. S. Milling. "Is High Hypnotic Suggestibility Necessary for Successful Hypnotic Pain Intervention?" *Current Pain and Headache Reports*, 2008 Apr, 12(2): 98–102.

21 F. Zeidan, S. K. Johnson, B. J. Diamond, *et al.* "Mindfulness Meditation Improves Cognition: Evidence of Brief Mental Training." *Consciousness and Cognition*, 2010 Jun, 19(2): 597–605. E-pub 2010 Apr 3. http://www.ncbi.nlm.nih.gov/pubmed/20363650.

22 http://www.ncbi.nlm.nih.gov/pubmed/20021599.

23 http://www.ncbi.nlm.nih.gov/pubmed/19900778.

24 http://www.ncbi.nlm.nih.gov/sites/pubmed.

25 http://www.ncbi.nlm.nih.gov/pubmed/18052018.

26 http://www.ncbi.nlm.nih.gov/pubmed/19705417.

27 Sara Fleming, David P. Rabago, Marlon P. Mundt, *et al.* "CAM Therapies among Primary Care Patients Using Opioid Therapy for Chronic Pain." *BMC Complementary and Alternative Medicine*, 2007, 7: 15.

28 http://www.sciencedirect.com/science?_ob=ArticleURL&_udi=B6T0K-504C9JX-2&_user=10&_coverDate=05%2F21%2F2010&_rdoc=1&_fmt=high&_orig=search&_sort=d&_docanchor=&view=c&_acct=C000050221&_version=1&_urlVersion=0&_userid=10&md5=b89e6b8c029258dc65a97b8ffdd06635.

29 "Effects of Relaxation Training on Sleep Quality and Fatigue in Patients with Breast Cancer Undergoing Adjuvant Chemotherapy." www3.interscience.wiley.com/journal/123320487/abstract.

30 Suzanne M. Bertisch, Christina C. Wee, Russell S. Phillips, *et al.* "Alternative Mind-Body Therapies Used by Adults with Medical Conditions." *Journal of Psychosomatic Research*, 2009 June, 66(6): 511–519.

31 S. Rosenzweig, J. M. Greeson, D. K. Reibel, *et al.* "Mindfulness-Based Stress Reduction for Chronic Pain Conditions: Variation in Treatment Outcomes and Role of Home Meditation Practice." *Journal of Psychosomatic Research*, 2010 Jan, 68(1): 29–36.

32 N. S. Porter *et al.* "Alternative Medical Interventions Used in the Treatment and Management of Myalgic Encephalomyyelitis/Chronic Fatigue Syndrome and Fibromyalgia." *Journal of Complementary and Alternative Medicine*, 2010, Vol. 16, No. 3: 235–249.

33 J. Kabat-Zinn, L. Lipworth, and R. Burney. "Four-Year Follow-Up of a Meditation-Based Program for the Self-Regulation of Chronic Pain: Treatment Outcomes and Compliance." *Clinical Journal of Pain*, 1987, 2: 159–73.

34 R. J. Davidson, J. Kabat-Zinn, J. Schumacher, *et al.* "Alterations in Brain and Immune Function Produced by Mindfulness Meditation." *Psychosomatic Medicine*, 2003, 65(4): 564–70.

35 Elizabeth K. Pradhan, Mona Baumgarten, Patricia Langenberg, *et al.* "Effect of Mindfulness-Based Stress Reduction in Rheumatoid Arthritis Patients." *Arthritis & Rheumatism (Arthritis Care & Research),* October 15, 2007, Vol. 57, No. 7, 1134–1142.

36 Based on http://www.rochester.edu/ucc/help/info/meditation.html.

37 Dennis C. Turk, Kimberly S. Swanson, and Eldon R. Tunks. "Psychological Approaches in the Treatment of Chronic Pain Patients—When Pills, Scalpels, and Needles Are Not Enough." *Canadian Journal of Psychiatry*, April 2008, Vol. 53, No. 4.

38 Grant *et al.* "Cortical Thickness and Pain Sensitivity in Zen Meditation." *Emotion*, 2010, 10(1):43.

39 J. Kim *et al.* "Efficacy of Selected Complementary and Alternative Medicine Interventions for Chronic Pain." *Journal of Rehabilitative Research and Development*; *Obesity Surgery*, 17, 920–925.

40 The Smell and Taste Research Foundation. "The Effect of Inhaling Green Apple Fragrance to Reduce Migraine." http://www.smellandtaste.org/index.cfm?action=research.apple

41 A. R. Drexler, E. J. Mur, and V. C. Günther. "Efficacy of an EMG-Biofeedback Therapy in Fibromyalgia Patients. A Comparative Study of Patients with and without Abnormality in (MMPI) Psychological Scales." *Clinical and Experimental Rheumatology*, 2002 Sep-Oct, 20(5): 677–82.

42 N. Kanji, A. R. White, and E. Ernst. "Autogenic Training for Tension Type Headaches: A Systematic Review of Controlled Trials." *Complementary Therapies in Medicine*, 2006, 14(2): 144–50.

43 S. Bruehl and O. Y. Chung. "Psychological And Behavioral Aspects Of Complex Regional Pain Syndrome Management." *Clinical Journal of Pain*, 2006, 22(5): 430–7.

44 National Institutes of Health Technology Assessment Conference Statement. "Integration of Behavioral and Relaxation Approaches Into the Treatment of Chronic Pain and Insomnia." October 16–18, 1995.

45 Charles F. Emery, Christopher R. France, Jennifer Harris, *et al.* "Effects of Progressive Muscle Relaxation Training on Nociceptive Flexion Reflex Threshold in Healthy Young Adults: A Randomized Trial." *Pain*, 31 August 2008, Volume 138, Issue 2, 375–379.

46 C. L. Baird and L. P. Sands. "A Pilot Study of the Effectiveness of Guided Imagery with Progressive Muscle Relaxation to Reduce Chronic Pain and Mobility Difficulties of Osteoarthritis." *Pain Management Nursing*, 2004 Sep, 5(3): 97–104.

47 Y. L. Cheung, A. Molassiotis, and A. M. Chang. "The Effect of Progressive Muscle Relaxation Training on Anxiety and Quality of Life After Stoma Surgery in Colorectal Cancer Patients." *Psychooncology*, 2003 Apr–May, 12(3): 254–66.

48 D. Carroll and K. Seers. "Relaxation for the Relief of Chronic Pain: A Systematic Review." *Journal of Advanced Nursing*, 1998 Mar, 27(3): 476–87.

49 M. W. van Tulder, B. Koes, and A. Malmivaara. "Outcome of Non-Invasive Treatment Modalities on Back Pain: An Evidence-Based Review." *European Spine Journal*, 2006 Jan, 15 Suppl 1:S64-81. E-pub 2005 Dec 1.

50 *Ibid.*

Chapter 6

1 E. L. Fosbol *et al.* "Cause-Specific Cardiovascular Risk Associated with Nonsteroidal Anti-inflammatory Drugs among Healthy Individuals." *Circulation: Cardiovascular Quality and Outcomes*, July 2010, 3:00–00. Published online Jun 8, 2010.

2 G. Singh. "Recent Considerations in NSAID Gastropathy." *American Journal of Medicine*, 1998, 105, 31S–38S.

3 C. David Tollison, John R. Satterthwaite, and Joseph W. Tollison. "Practical Pain Management." 3rd Edition (Lippincott Williams and Wilkins, 2002).

4 N. D. Yeomans, Z. Tulassay, L. Juhasz, *et al.* "A Comparison of Omeprazole with Ranitidine for Ulcers Associated with Nonsteroidal Anti-Inflammatory Drugs." Acid Suppression Trial: Ranitidine vs. Omeprazole for NSAID-Associated Ulcer Treatment (ASTRONAUT) Study Group. *New England Journal of Medicine,* 1998; 338: 719–26.

5 Fosbol, "Cause-Specific Cardiovascular Risk."

6 Wayne A. Ray. "Cardiovascular Risks of Nonsteroidal Anti-inflammatory Drugs in Patients After Hospitalization for Serious Coronary Heart Disease." *Circulation: Cardiovascular Quality and Outcomes*, 2009, 2: 155–163.

7 American College of Gastroenterology. "The Dangers of Aspirin & NSAIDS." http://www.acg.gi.org/patients/women/asprin.asp.

8 M. Reijman, S. M. Bierma-Zeinstra, H. A. Pols, *et al.* "Is There an Association between the Use of Different Types of Nonsteroidal Antiinflammatory Drugs and Radiologic Progression of Osteoarthritis? The Rotterdam Study." *Arthritis & Rheumatism*, 2005 Oct, 52(10): 3137–42.

9 R. D. Altman, R. L. Dreiser, C. L. Fisher, *et al.* "Diclofenac Sodium Gel in Patients with Primary Hand Osteoarthritis: A Randomized, Double-Blind, Placebo-Controlled Trial." *Rheumatology*, 2009 Sep, 36(9): 1991–9. E-pub 2009 Jul 31.

P. A. Baer, L. M. Thomas, and Z. Shainhouse. "Treatment of Osteoarthritis of the Knee with a Topical Diclofenac Solution: A Randomised Controlled, 6-Week Trial." *BMC Musculoskeletal Disorders*, 2005 Aug 8; 6: 44.

10 P. J. Wiffen, H. J. McQuay, and R. A. Moore. "Carbamazepine for Acute and Chronic Pain in Adults." *Cochrane Database of Systematic Reviews*, 2005, Issue 3.

11 S. Friedman and G. R. Lichtenstein. "Ulcerative Colitis." In M. M. Wolfe *et al.*, eds., *Therapy of Digestive Disorders*, 2nd ed., 803–817 (Philadelphia: Saunders, 2006), Elsevier.

12 ———. "Crohn's Disease." In M. M. Wolfe *et al.*, eds., *Therapy of Digestive Disorders*, 2nd ed., 785–801. (Philadelphia: Saunders, 2006), Elsevier.

13 L. Sutherland, J. Singleton, J. Sessions, *et al.* "Double Blind, Placebo Controlled Trial of Metronidazole in Crohn's Disease." *Gut*, 1991, 32: 1071–75.

14 Mark Pimentel, Sandy Park, James Mirocha, *et al.* "The Effect of a Nonabsorbed Oral Antibiotic (Rifaximin) on the Symptoms of the Irritable Bowel Syndrome: A Randomized Trial." *Annals of Internal Medicine*, October 17, 2006, vol. 145, no. 8, 557–563.

15 M. J. Carter, A. J. Lobo, and S. P. L. Travis, on behalf of the IBD Section of the British Society of Gastroenterology, "Guidelines for the Management of Inflammatory Bowel Disease in Adults." *Gut*, 2004, 53 (Suppl V): v1–v16.

16 Roger Cady and David W. Dodick. "Review: Diagnosis and Treatment of Migraine." *Mayo Clinic Procedures*, 2002, 77: 255–261.

17 K. Linde and K. Rossnagel. "Propranolol for Migraine Prophylaxis." *Cochrane Database of Systematic Reviews*, 2004 (2): CD003225.

18 Sumatriptan: MedlinePlus. http://www.nlm.nih.gov/medlineplus/druginfo/meds/a601116.html.

19 Zolmatriptan on MedlinePlus. http://www.nlm.nih.gov/medlineplus/druginfo/meds/a601129.html.

20 Treximet Web site. http://www.treximet.com/.

21 http://www.zomig.com/zomig-zmt-nasal-spray-tablets.aspx#ffinder.

22 http://www.zomig.com/zomig-zmt-nasal-spray-tablets.aspx#ffinder.

23 Group Health Cooperative Center for Health Studies.

24 M. Zenz, M. Strumpf, and M. Tryba. "Long-Term Oral Opioid Therapy in Patients with Chronic Nonmalignant Pain." *Journal of Pain Symptom Management*, 1992, 7: 69–77.

Chapter 7

1 R. B. Lipton, D. Dodick, R. Sadovsky, *et al.* "A Self-Administered Screener For Migraine In Primary Care: The ID Migraine™ Validation Study." *Neurology*, 2003, 61(3): 375–82.

2 Elizabeth K. Seng and Kenneth A. Holroyd. "Dynamics of Changes in Self-Efficacy and Locus of Control Expectancies in the Behavioral and Drug Treatment of Severe Migraine." *Annals of Behavioral Medicine*, 2010, Volume 40, Number 3, 235–247.

3 V. Kirthi, S. Derry, R. A. Moore, *et al.* "Aspirin with or without an Antiemetic for Acute Migraine Headaches in Adults." *Cochrane Database of Systematic Reviews*, 2010, Issue 4, Art. No.: CD008041. DOI: 10.1002/14651858. CD008041.pub2.

4 http://www.nlm.nih.gov/medlineplus/druginfo/meds/a601116.html.

5 http://www.nlm.nih.gov/medlineplus/druginfo/meds/a601129.html.

6 http://www.treximet.com.

7 http://www.zomig.com/zomig-zmt-nasal-spray-tablets.aspx#ffinder.

8 *Ibid.*

9 http://www.elastogel.com/detail.php?product_id=313&category_id=1.

10 R. Noseda, V. Kainz, M. Jakubowski, *et al.* "A Neural Mechanism for Exacerbation of Headache by Light." *Nature Neuroscience*, 2010 Feb, 13(2): 239–45.

11 A. Straube, V. Pfaffenrath, K.-H. Ladwig, *et al.* "Prevalence of Chronic Migraine and Medication Overuse Headache in Germany—The German DMKG Headache Study." *Cephalalgia*, 2010, Vol. 30, No. 2, 207–213. http://cep.sagepub.com/cgi/content/abstract/30/2/207.

12 M. Grossmann and H. Schmidramsl. "An Extract of Petasites Hybridus Is Effective in the Prophylaxis of Migraine." *International Journal of Clinical Pharmacology, Therapy, & Toxicology*, 2000, 38: 430–435. M. Grossmann, H. Schmidramsl. "An Extract of Petasites Hybridus Is Effective in the Prophylaxis of Migraine." *Alternative Medicine Review*, 2001, 6: 303–310.

13 R. B. Lipton, H. Gobel, K. M. Einhaupl, *et al.* "Petasites Hybridus Root (Butterbur) Is an Effective Preventive Treatment for Migraine." *Neurology*, 2004, 63: 2240–2244.

14 http://www.petadolex.com/v2/default.aspx.

15 E. Varkey, K. Hagen, J. A. Zwart, *et al.* "Physical Activity And Headache: Results From The Nord-Trøndelag Health Study (HUNT)." *Cephalalgia*, 2008 Dec, 28(12): 1292–7. E-pub 2008 Sep 11.

16 E. Varkey, A. Cider, J. Carlsson, *et al.* "A Study to Evaluate the Feasibility of an Aerobic Exercise Program in Patients with Migraine." *Headache*, 2009 Apr, 49(4): 563–70. E-pub 2008 Sep 9.

17 S. M. Dittrich. "Aerobic Exercise with Relaxation: Influence on Pain and Psychological Well-Being in Female Migraine Patients." *Clinical Journal of Sport Medicine*, 2008 Jul, 18(4): 363–5.

18 P. J. John. "Effectiveness of Yoga Therapy in the Treatment of Migraine without Aura: A Randomized Controlled Trial." *Headache*, 2007 May, 47(5): 654–61.

19 M. H. Pittler, B. K. Vogler, and E. Ernst. "Feverfew for Preventing Migraine." *Cochrane Database of Systematic Reviews*, Rev. 2004.

20 S. Modi and D. M. Lowder, "Medications for Migraine Prophylaxis", *American Family Physician*, January 1, 2006; 73(1): 72–78.

21 M. F. P. Peres, E. Zukerman, F. da Cunha Tanuri, *et al.* "Melatonin, 3 mg, is effective for migraine prevention" *Neurology*, August 24, 2004 63:757

22 T. E. Whitmarsh, D. M. Coleston-Shields, and T. J. Steiner. "Double-Blind Randomized Placebo-Controlled Study of Homeopathic Prophylaxis of Migraine." *Cephalalgia*, 1997, 17, pp600-604.

23 Randolph W. Evans and Frederick R. Taylor. "'Natural' or Alternative Medications for Migraine Prevention." *Headache*, 2006, 46(6): 1012–1018.

24 *Ibid.*

25 A. J. Vickers, R. W. Rees, C. E. Zollman, *et al.* "Acupuncture of Chronic Headache Disorders in Primary Care: Randomised Controlled Trial and Economic Analysis." *Health Technology Assessment*, 2004 Nov, 8(48): iii, 1–35.

26 R. B. Lipton *et al.* "Migraine Prevalence, Disease Burden, and the Need for Preventive Therapy." *Neurology*, 2007, 68: 343–349.

27 Roger Cady and David W. Dodick. "Review: Diagnosis and Treatment of Migraine." *Mayo Clinic Proceedings*, 2002, 77: 255–261.

28 K. Linde and K. Rossnagel. "Propranolol for Migraine Prophylaxis." *Cochrane Database of Systematic Reviews*, 2004, (2): CD003225.

29 Excedrin migraine ingredients: http://www.excedrin.com/excedrin-migraine-drug-facts.shtml.

30 http://www.mayoclinic.com/health/rebound-headaches/DS00613/DSECTION=causes; and Headache Classification Committee. *Cephalalgia*, 2006, 26: 742–746.

31 P. Rossi, C. Di Lorenzo, J. Faroni, *et al.* "Advice Alone Vs. Structured Detoxification Programmes for Medication Overuse Headache: A Prospective, Randomized, Open-Label Trial in Transformed Migraine Patients with Low Medical Needs." *Cephalalgia*, 2006 Sep, 26(9): 1097-105.

32 Hans-Christoph Diener and Zaza Katsarava. "Medication Overuse Headache." From Current Medical Research and Opinion, www.medscape.com.

33 Michael J. Marmura. "Zolmitriptan and the Triptan Era." *Clinical Medicine: Therapeutics,* 2009 1: 781-785.

34 L. M. Cupini and P. Calabresi. "Medication-Overuse Headache: Pathophysiological Insights." *Journal of Headache Pain*, 2005 Sep, 6(4): 199–202. http://www.ncbi.nlm.nih.gov/pubmed/16362663?ordinalpos=1&itool=EntrezSystem2.PEntrez.Pubmed.Pubmed_ResultsPanel.Pubmed_SingleItemSupl.Pubmed_Discovery_RA&linkpos=5&log$=relatedreviews&logdbfrom=pubmed.

35 "The Triggers or Precipitants of the Acute Migraine Attack." *Cephalalgia*, 27 (5), 394–402.

36 National Headache Foundation survey. "Are Your Headaches Causing You to Miss Out on Life?" September 2007.

37 ———.

38 Goadsby. "Drug for Cluster Headaches May Cause Heart Problems." *Neurology*, August 14, 2007.

39 G. Bussone, M. Leone, C. Peccarisi, *et al.* "Double Blind Comparison of Lithium and Verapamil in Cluster Headache Prophylaxis." *Headache*, 1990, 30: 411–7.

40 H. Gobel, V. Lindner, A. Heinze, *et al.* "Acute therapy for Cluster Headache with Sumatriptan: Findings of a One-Year Long-Term Study." *Neurology*, 1998, 51: 908–11.

41 J. A. Van Vliet, A. Bahra, V. Martin, *et al.* "Intranasal Sumatriptan in Cluster Headache: Randomized Placebo-Controlled Doubleblind Study." *Neurology*, 2003, 60: 630–3.

42 A. U. Cohen, A. S. Burns, and B. Goadsby. "High-Flow Oxygen for Treatment of Cluster Headache: A Randomized Trial." *JAMA*, 2009 Dec 9, 302(22): 2451–7.

43 N. Z. Olson, A. M. Otero, I. Marrero, *et al.* "Onset of Analgesia for Liquigel Ibuprofen 400 mg, Acetaminophen 1000 mg, Ketoprofen 25 mg, and Placebo in the Treatment of Postoperative Dental Pain." *Journal of Clinical Pharmacology*, 2001 Nov, 41(11): 1238–47.

44 B. Packman, E. Packman, G. Doyle, *et al. Headache*, 2000 Jul-Aug, 40(7): 561–7.

45 L. Damen, M. Y. Berger, J. Passchier, *et al.* "Is Any One Analgesic Superior for Episodic Tension-Type Headache?" *Journal of Family Practice*, 2006 Dec, 55(12): 1064–72.

46 Seymour Diamond and Frederick G. Freitag. "The Use of Ibuprofen Plus Caffeine to Treat Tension-Type Headache." *Current Pain and Headache Reports*, 2001 October, vol 5, 472.

47 J. R. Migliardi, J. J. Armellino, M. Friedman, *et al.* "Caffeine as an Analgesic Adjuvant in Tension Headache." *Clinical Pharmacology & Therapeutic*, 1994 Nov, 56(5): 576-86.

48 Lawrence D. Robbins. "Cryotherapy for Headache." *Headache*, 1989, 29 (9), 598–600.

49 H. Gobel, G. Schmidt, and D. Soyka. "Effect of Peppermint and Eucalyptus Oil Preparations on Neurophysiological and Experimental Algesimetric Headache Parameters." *Cephalalgia*, 1994, 14(3): 228–234.

50 B. Kligler and S. Chaudhary. "Peppermint Oil." *American Family Physician*, 2007 Apr 1, 75(7): 1027-30. Review.

51 Seymour Diamond and Frederick G. Freitag. "The Use of Ibuprofen Plus Caffeine to Treat Tension-Type Headache." *Current Pain and Headache Reports*, 2001 October vol 5, 472.

52 Knut Hagen, Kari Thoresen, Lars Jacob Stovner, *et al.* "High Dietary Caffeine Consumption Is Associated with a Modest Increase in Headache Prevalence: Results from the Head-HUNT Study." *Journal of Headache Pain*, 2009, 10: 153-159.

53 E. Varkey, K. Hagen, J. A. Zwart, *et al.* "Physical Activity and Headache: Results from the Nord-Trøndelag Health Study (HUNT)." *Cephalalgia*, 2008 Dec, 28(12): 1292–7.

54 William J. Mullally, Kathryn Hall, and Richard Goldstein. "Efficacy of Biofeedback in the Treatment of Migraine and Tension Type Headaches, Randomized Trial." *Pain Physician*, 2009 December, Vol 12 Issue 6, 1005–1011.

55 P. Zeeberg, J. Olesen, and R. Jensen. "Discontinuation of Medication Overuse in Headache Patients: Recovery of Therapeutic Responsiveness." *Cephalalgia*, 2006 Oct, 26(10): 1192–8.

56 A. U. Diener and H. C. Limmroth. "Medication-Overuse Headache: A Worldwide Problem." *The Lancet Neurology*, 2004 Aug, 3(8): 475-83.

57 R. A. Nicholson. "Differences in Anger Expression between Individuals with and without Headache after Controlling for Depression and Anxiety." *Headache*, 2003 Jun, 43(6): 651-63.

58 E. Torrente Castells, E. Vázquez Delgado, and C. Gay Escoda. "Use of Amitriptyline for the Treatment of Chronic Tension-Type Headache. Review of the Literature." *Medicina Oral, Patología Oral y Cirugía Bucal*, 2008 Sep 1, 13(9): E567–72.

59 *Ibid.*

60 Paul J. Millea and Jonathan J. Brodie. "Tension-Type Headache." Medical College of Wisconsin, Milwaukee, Wisconsin. *American Family Physician*, 2002 Sep 1, 66(5): 797–805.

61 W. F. Yeung, K. F. Chung, and C. Y. Wong. "Relationship between Insomnia and Headache in Community-Based Middle-Aged Hong Kong Chinese Women." *Journal of Headache Pain,* E-pub ahead of print, 2010 Feb 26.

62 Evers S. "Sleep and Headache: The Biological Basis." *Headache*, 2010 Jul, 50(7): 1246–51.

63 J. N. Blau, MD. "Ponytail Headache: A Pure Extracranial Headache." *Headache,* Volume 44 Issue 5, 411–413

64 T. Fukutake, S. Mine, I. Yamakami, *et al.* "Roller Coaster Headache and Subdural Hematoma." *Neurology*, Vol. 54, Issue 1, 264 January 11, 2000.

65 P. B. Prince, A. M. Rapoport, F. D. Sheftell, *et al.* "The Effect of Weather on Headache." *Headache*, 2004, Jun, 44(6): 596–602.

66 L. J. Cooke, M. S. Rose, and W. J. Becker. "Chinook Winds and Migraine Headache." *Neurology*, 2000, 54: 302.

67 K. J. Mukamal, G. A. Wellenius, H. H. Suh, *et al.* "Weather and Air Pollution as Triggers of Severe Headaches." *Neurology*, 2009, Mar 10, 72(10): 922–7.

68 G. Lavigne and S. Palla. "Transient Morning Headache: Recognizing the Role of Sleep Bruxism and Sleep-Disordered Breathing." *Journal of the American Dental Association*, 2010 Mar, 141(3): 297–9.

69 G. Jull, P. Trott, H. Potter, *et al.* "A Randomized Controlled Trial of Exercise and Manipulative Therapy for Cervicogenic Headache." *Spine*, 2002 Sep 1, 27(17): 1835-43, discussion 1843.

70 National Headache Foundation survey. "Headaches and the Workplace." May 2008.

71 Kowacs *et al.* "Critical Flicker Frequency in Migraine. A Controlled Study in Patients without Prophylactic Therapy." *Cephalalgia*, 2005 May, 25(5): 339-43.

72 C. P. Schreiber, S. Hutchinson, C. J. Webster, *et al.* "Prevalence of Migraine in Patients with a History of Self-Reported or Physician-Diagnosed 'Sinus' Headache." *Archives of Internal Medicine*, 2004, Sep 13, 164(16): 1769–72.

73 Dewey C. Scheid. "Acute Bacterial Rhinosinusitis in Adults: Part II. Treatment." *American Family Physician*, November 1, 2004, Vol. 70, Number 9.

74 The National Migraine Association: Treatment and Management. http://www.migraines.org/treatment

75 http://cme.medscape.com/viewarticle/462033_3.

76 http://www.fpnotebook.com/ENT/Pharm/Dcngstnt.htm.

77 L. J. Fagnan. "Acute Sinusitis: A Cost-Effective Approach to Diagnosis and Treatment." *American Family Physician*, 1998 November 15, Vol. 58/No. 8.

78 D. D. Cáceres. "Use of Visual Analogue Scale Measurements (VAS) to Asses the Effectiveness of Standardized Andrographis Paniculata Extract SHA-10 in Reducing The Symptoms of Common Cold. A Randomized Double Blind-Placebo Study." *Phytomedicine*, 1999 Oct, 6(4): 217–23.

79 R. C. Saxena *et al.* "A Randomized Double Blind Placebo Controlled Clinical Evaluation of Extract of Andrographis Paniculata (Kalmcold) in Patients with Uncomplicated Upper Respiratory Tract Infection." *Phytomedicine*, 2010 Mar, 17(3-4): 178–85.

80 J. Liu, Z. T. Wang, L. L. Ji, *et al.* "Inhibitory Effects of Neoandrographolide On Nitric Oxide and Prostaglandin E2 Production in LPS-Stimulated Murine Macrophage." *Molecular and Cellular Biochemistry*, 2007, 298(1-2): 49–57.

81 R. Eccles, M. S. Jawad, S. S. Jawad, *et al.* "Efficacy and Safety of Single and Multiple Doses of Pseudoephedrine in the Treatment of Nasal Congestion Associated with Common Cold." *American Journal of Rhinology*, 2005, 19: 25–31.

82 E. O. Meltzer, C. Bachert, and H. Staudinger. "Treating Acute Rhinosinusitis: Comparing Efficacy and Safety of Mometasone Furoate Nasal Spray, Amoxicillin, and Placebo." *Journal of Allergy and Clinical Immunology*, 2005 Dec, 116(6): 1289–95. E-pub 2005 Oct 24.

83 R. Harvey. "Nasal Saline Irrigations for the Symptoms of Chronic Rhinosinusitis." *Cochrane Database of Systematic Reviews*, 2007 Jul 18, (3): CD006394.

84 *Ibid.*

85 J. M. Gwaltney. "Nose Blowing Propels Nasal Fluid into the Paranasal Sinuses." *Clinical Infectious Diseases*, 2000 Feb, 30(2): 387–91.

Chapter 8

1 A. N. Pearlman and D. B. Conley. "Review of Current Guidelines Related to the Diagnosis and Treatment of Rhinosinusitis." *Current Opinion in Otolaryngology & Head and Neck Surgery*, 2008, 16(3), 226–30.

2 A. Ahovuo-Saloranta, O. V. Borisenko, N. Kovanen, *et al.* "Antibiotics for Acute Maxillary Sinusitis." *Cochrane Database of Systematic Reviews*, 2008, (2), CD000243.

3 W. B. Cherry and J. T. Li. "Chronic Rhinosinusitis in Adults." *American Journal of Medicine*, 2008, 121(3), 185–9.

4 *Ibid.*

5 J. D. Osguthorpe. "Adult Rhinosinusitis: Diagnosis and Management." *American Family Physician*, 2001, 63(1), 69–76.

6 A. C. Chester. "Chronic Sinusitis." *American Family Physician*, 1996, 53(3), 877–87.

7 H. J. Krouse and J. H. Krouse. "Complementary Therapeutic Practices In Patients With Chronic Sinusitis." *Clinical Excellence for Nurse Practitioners*, 1999, 3(6), 346–52.

8 N. A. Cohen. "Sinonasal Mucociliary Clearance in Health and Disease." *Annals of Otology, Rhinology and Laryngology*, 2006, 196, 20–6.

9 R. A. Swain and B. Kaplan. "Upper Respiratory Infections: Treatment Selection for Active Patients." *Physician and Sportsmedicine*, 1998, 26(2), 85–96.

10 E. O. Meltzer, C. Bachert, and H. Staudinger. "Treating Acute Rhinosinusitis: Comparing Efficacy and Safety of Mometasone Furoate Nasal Spray, Amoxicillin, and Placebo." *Journal of Allergy and Clinical Immunology*, 2005, 116(6), 1289–95.

11 J. Young, A. De Sutter, D. Merenstein, *et al.* "Antibiotics for Adults with Clinically Diagnosed Acute Rhinosinusitis: A Meta-Analysis of Individual Patient Data." *The Lancet*, 2008, 371(9616), 908–14.

12 A. Ahovuo-Saloranta, O. V. Borisenko, N. Kovanen, *et al.* "Antibiotics for Acute Maxillary Sinusitis." *Cochrane Database of Systematic Reviews*, 2008 (2), CD000243.

13 G. Mion Ode, R. A. Campos, M. Antila, *et al.* "Futura Study: Evaluation of Efficacy And Safety Of Rupatadine

Fumarate in the Treatment of Persistent Allergic Rhinitis." *Brazilian Journal of Otorhinolaryngology*, 2009, 75(5), 673–9.

14 N. Segall, S. Gawchik, G. Georges, *et al.* "Efficacy and Safety of Levocetirizine in Improving Symptoms and Health-Related Quality of Life in U.S. Adults with Seasonal Allergic Rhinitis: A Randomized, Placebo-Controlled Study." *Annals of Allergy, Asthma and Immunology*, 2010, 104(3), 259–67.

15 N. Bhattacharyya and L. J. Kepnes. "Associations between Fatigue and Medication Use in Chronic Rhinosinusitis." *Ear, Nose and Throat Journal*, 2006, 85(8), 510, 512, 514–5.

16 R. Harvey, S. A. Hannan, L. Badia, *et al.* "Nasal Saline Irrigations for the Symptoms of Chronic Rhinosinusitis." *Cochrane Database of Systematic Reviews*, 2007 (3), CD006394.

17 M. A. Monteil, G. Joseph, C. Chang Kit, *et al.* "Smoking at Home Is Strongly Associated with Symptoms of Asthma and Rhinitis in Children of Primary School Age in Trinidad and Tobago." *Revista Panamericana de Salud Pública*, 2004, 16(3), 193–8.

18 D. D. Reh, S. Y. Lin, S. L. Clipp, *et al.* "Secondhand Tobacco Smoke Exposure and Chronic Rhinosinusitis: A Population-Based Case-Control Study." *American Journal of Rhinology*, 2009, 23(6), 562–7.

19 J. Hellgren. "Occupational Rhinosinusitis." *Current Allergy and Asthma Reports*, 2008, 8(3), 234–9.

20 S. Wadhwa and S. Kapila. "TMJ Disorders: Future Innovations In Diagnostics And Therapeutics." *Journal of Dental Education*, 2008, 72(8), 930–47.

21 S. J. Scrivani, D. A. Keith, and L. B. Kaban. "Temporomandibular Disorders." *New England Journal of Medicine*, 2008, 359(25), 2693–705.

22 S. J. Scrivani, D. A. Keith, and L. B. Kaban. "Temporomandibular Disorders." *New England Journal of Medicine*, 2008, 359(25), 2693–705.

23 R. S. Porter and J. L. Kaplan (eds.). "Arthritis of the Temporomandibular Joint (TMJ)." The Merck Manuals Online, 2008. Retrieved July 24, 2010, from http://merck.com/mmpe/sec08/ch097/ch097c.html.

24 R. H. Poindexter, E. F. Wright, and D. F. Murchison. "Comparison of Moist and Dry Heat Penetration through Orofacial Tissues." *Cranio*, 2002, 20(1), 28–33.

25 J. L. Riley III, C. D. Myers, T. P. Currie, *et al.* "Self-Care Behaviors Associated with Myofascial Temporomandibular Disorder Pain." *Journal of Orofacial Pain*, 2007, 21(3), 194–202.

26 E. F. Wright and E. L. Schiffman. "Treatment Alternatives for Patients with Masticatory Myofascial Pain." *Journal of the American Dental Association*, 1995, 126(7), 1030–9.

27 E. F. Wright, M. A. Domenech, and J. R. Fischer, Jr. "Usefulness of Posture Training For Patients With Temporomandibular Disorders." *Journal of the American Dental Association*, 2000, 131(2), 202–10.

28 J. Fricton, A. Velly, W. Ouyang, *et al.* "Does Exercise Therapy Improve Headache? A Systematic Review with Meta-Analysis." *Current Pain and Headache Reports*, 2009, 13(6), 413–9.

29 E. F. Wright and E. L. Schiffman. "Treatment Alternatives for Patients with Masticatory Myofascial Pain." *Journal of the American Dental Association*, 1995, 126(7), 1030–9.

30 J. L. Riley III, C. D. Myers, T. P. Currie, *et al.* "Self-Care Behaviors Associated with Myofascial Temporomandibular Disorder Pain." *Journal of Orofacial Pain*, 2007, 21(3), 194–202.

31 R. W. Wong and A. B. Rabie. "Local Massage with Topical Analgesic, A Novel Treatment Modality for Temporomandibular Muscular Pain, A Case Study Report of 5 Consecutive Cases." *Open Orthopedics Journal*, 2008, 2, 97–102.

32 A. De Laat, K. Stappaerts, and S. Papy. "Counseling and Physical Therapy as Treatment for Myofascial Pain of the Masticatory System." *Journal of Orofacial Pain*, 2003, 17(1), 42–9.

33 Y. F. Shen and G. Goddard. "The Short-Term Effects of Acupuncture on Myofascial Pain Patients after Clenching." *Pain Practice*, 2007, 7:256–264.

34 P. Smith, D. Mosscrop, S. Davies, *et al.* "The Efficacy of Acupuncture in the Treatment of Temporomandibular Joint Myofascial Pain: A Randomised Controlled Trial." *Journal of Dentistry*, 2007, 35(3), 259–67.

35 M. Schmid-Schwap, I. Simma-Kletschka, A. Stockner, *et al.* "Oral Acupuncture in the Therapy of Craniomandibular Dysfunction Syndrome—A Randomized Controlled Trial." *Wiener Klinische Wochenschrift*, 2006, 118(1–2), 36–42.

36 G. Goddard, H. Karibe, C. McNeill, *et al.* "Acupuncture and Sham Acupuncture Reduce Muscle Pain in Myofascial Pain Patients." *Journal of Orofacial Pain*, 2002, 16(1), 71–6.

37 S. H. Cho and W. W. Whang. "Acupuncture for Temporomandibular Disorders: A Systematic Review." *Journal of Orofacial Pain*, 2010, 24(2), 152–62.

38 R. La Touche, S. Angulo-Diaz-Parreno, J. L. de-la-Hoz, *et al.* "Effectiveness of Acupuncture in the Treatment of Temporomandibular Disorders of Muscular Origin: A Systematic Review of the Last Decade." *Journal of Alternative and Complementary Medicine*, 2010, 16(1), 107–12.

39 J. A. Turner, L. Mancl, and L. A. Aaron. "Short- and Long-Term Efficacy of Brief Cognitive-Behavioral Therapy for Patients with Chronic Temporomandibular Disorder Pain: A Randomized, Controlled Trial." *Pain*, 2006, 121(3), 181–94.

40 Riley III, Myers, Currie, *et al.*

41 D. P. Funch and E. N. Gale. "Biofeedback and Relaxation Therapy for Chronic Temporomandibular Joint Pain: Predicting Successful Outcomes." *Journal of Consulting and Clinical Psychology*, 1984, 52(6), 928–35.

42 A. Crider, A. G. Glaros, and R. N. Gevirtz. "Efficacy of Biofeedback-Based Treatments for Temporomandibular Disorders." *Applied Psychophysiology & Biofeedback*, 2005, 30(4), 333–45.

43 C. M. Ziegler, J. Wiechnik, and J. Muhling. "Analgesic Effects of Intra-Articular Morphine in Patients with Temporomandibular Joint Disorders: A Prospective, Double-Blind, Placebo-Controlled Clinical Trial." *Journal of Oral and Maxillofacial Surgery*, 2010, 68(3), 622–7.

44 P. M. Mountziaris, P. R. Kramer, and A. G. Mikos. "Emerging Intra-Articular Drug Delivery Systems for the Temporomandibular Joint." *Methods*, 2009, 47(2), 134–40.

45 P. C. Song, J. Schwartz, and A. Blitzer. "The Emerging Role of Botulinum Toxin in the Treatment of Temporomandibular Disorders." *Oral Diseases*, 2007, 13(3), 253–60.

46 S. K. Ihde and V. S. Konstantinovic. "The Therapeutic Use of Botulinum Toxin in Cervical and Maxillofacial Conditions: An Evidence-Based Review." *Oral Surgery, Oral Medicine, Oral Pathology, Oral Radiology & Endodontics*, 2007, 104(2), e1–11.

47 C. Mejersjo and B. Wenneberg. "Diclofenac Sodium and Occlusal Splint Therapy in TMJ Osteoarthritis: A Randomized Controlled Trial." *Journal of Oral Rehabilitation*, 2008, 35:729–738.

48 E. Ekberg. "Treatment of Temporomandibular Disorders of Arthrogeneous Origin. Controlled Double-Blind Studies of a Non-Steroidal Anti-Inflammatory Drug and a Stabilisation Appliance." *Swedish Dental Journal Supplement*, 1998, 131:1–57.

49 L. E. Ta and R. A. Dionne. "Treatment of Painful Temporomandibular Joints with a Cyclooxygenase-2 Inhibitor: A Randomized Placebo-Controlled Comparison of Celecoxib to Naproxen." *Pain*, 2004, 111:13–21.

50 B. E. Cairns. "Pathophysiology of TMD Pain-Basic Mechanisms and Their Implications for Pharmacotherapy." *Journal of Oral Rehabilitation*, 2010, 37(6), 391–410.

51 C. R. Herman, E. L. Schiffman, J. O. Look, *et al.* "The Effectiveness of Adding Pharmacologic Treatment with Clonazepam or Cyclobenzaprine to Patient Education and Self-Care for the Treatment of Jaw Pain Upon Awakening: A Randomized Clinical Trial." *Journal of Orofacial Pain*, 2002,16(1), 64–70.

52 S. J. Scrivani, D. A. Keith, and L. B. Kaban. "Temporomandibular Disorders." *New England Journal of Medicine*, 2008, 359(25), 2693–705.

53 C. M. Rizzatti-Barbosa, M. T. Nogueira, E. D. de Andrade, *et al.* "Clinical Evaluation of Amitriptyline for the Control of Chronic Pain Caused by Temporomandibular Joint Disorders." *Cranio*, 2003, 21(3), 221–5.

54 J. Cascos-Romero, E. Vazquez-Delgado, E. Vazquez-Rodriguez, *et al.* "The Use of Tricyclic Antidepressants in the Treatment of Temporomandibular Joint Disorders: Systematic Review of the Literature of the Last 20 Years." *Medicina Oral , Patología Oral y Cirugía Bucal*, 2009, 14(1), E3–7.

55 G. D. Klasser and C. S. Greene. "Oral Appliances in the Management of Temporomandibular Disorders." *Oral Surgery, Oral Medicine, Oral Pathology, Oral Radiology & Endodontics*, 2009, 107(2), 212–23.

56 J. T. Reston and C. M. Turkelson. "Meta-Analysis of Surgical Treatments for Temporomandibular Articular Disorders: A Reply to the Discussants." *Journal of Oral and Maxillofacial Surgery*, 2003, 61(6), 737–8.

57 S.Ingawale and T. Goswami. "Temporomandibular Joint: Disorders, Treatments, and Biomechanics." *Annals of Biomedical Engineering*, 2009, 37(5), 976–96.

58 A. K. Pau, R. Croucher, and W. Marcenes. "Prevalence Estimates and Associated Factors for Dental Pain: A Review." *Oral Health & Preventive Dentistry*, 2003, 1(3), 209–20.

59 A. E. Winston, A. J. Charig, and S. Thong. "Mechanism of Action of a Desensitizing Fluoride Toothpaste Delivering Calcium and Phosphate Ingredients in the Treatment of Dental Hypersensitivity. Part III: Prevention of Dye Penetration Through Dentin Vs, A Calcium- And Phosphate-Free Control." *Compendium of Continuing Education in Dentistry*, 2010, 31(1), 46–8, 50–2.

60 D. E. Myers. "Toothache Referred from Heart Disease and Lung Cancer via the Vagus Nerve." *General Dentistry*, 2010, 58(1), e2–5.

61 T. Nakajima and K. Yamazaki. "Periodontal Disease and Risk of Atherosclerotic Coronary Heart Disease." *Odontology*, 2009, 97(2), 84–91.

62 K. Markowitz and D. H. Pashley. "Discovering New Treatments for Sensitive Teeth: The Long Path from Biology to Therapy." *Journal of Oral Rehabilitation*, 2008, 35(4), 300–15.

63 M. A. Weinberg and J. B. Fine. "Oral Snalgesics for Scute Dental Pain." *Dentistry Today*, 2002, 21(7), 92–7.

64 S. Diernberger, O. Bernhardt, C. Schwahn, *et al.* "Self-Reported Chewing Side Preference and its Associations with Occlusal, Temporomandibular and Prosthodontic Factors: Results from the Population-Based Study of Health in Pomerania (SHIP-0)." *Journal of Oral Rehabilitation*, 2008, 35(8), 613–20.

65 C. Prati, L. Montebugnoli, P. Suppa, *et al.* "Permeability and Morphology of Dentin after Erosion Induced by Acidic Drinks." *Journal of Periodontology*, 2003, 74(4), 428–36.

66 D. L. Zandim, F. O. Correa, C., Rossa Junior, *et al.* "In Vitro Evaluation of the Effect of Natural Orange Juices on Dentin Morphology." *Brazilian Oral Research*, 2008, 22(2), 176–83.

67 ———. "The Influence of Vinegars on Exposure of Dentinal Tubules: A SEM Evaluation." *Brazilian Oral Research*, 2004, 18(1), 63–8.

68 V. Sirimaharaj, L. Brearley Messer, and M. V. Morgan. "Acidic Diet and Dental Erosion among Athletes." *Australian Dental Journal*, 2002, 47(3), 228–36.

69 R. H. Dababneh, A. T. Khouri, and M. Addy. "Dentine Hypersensitivity—An Enigma? A Review of Terminology, Mechanisms, Aetiology and Management." *British Dental Journal*, 1999, 187(11), 606–11, discussion 603.

70 A. V. Ritter, W. de L. Dias, P. Miguez, *et al.* "Treating Cervical Dentin Hypersensitivity with Fluoride Varnish: A Randomized Clinical Study." *Journal of the American Dental Association*, 2006, 137(7), 1013–20, quiz 1029.

71 B. T. Hoang-Dao, H. Hoang-Tu, N. N. Tran-Thi, G. Koubi, J. Camps, I. About. "Clinical Efficiency of a Natural Resin Fluoride Varnish (Shellac F) in Reducing Dentin Hypersensitivity." *Journal of Oral Rehabilitation*, 2009, 36(2), 124–31.

72 M. Goldberg, M. Grootveld, and E. Lynch. "Undesirable and Adverse Effects of Tooth-Whitening Products: A Review." *Clinical Oral Investigations*, 2010, 14(1), 1–10.

73 A. J. van Wijk and J. Hoogstraten. "Experience with Dental Pain and Fear of Dental Pain." *Journal of Dentistry*, 2005, Res, 84(10), 947–50.

74 B. Chanpong, D. A. Haas, and D. Locker. "Need and Demand for Sedation or General Anesthesia in Dentistry: A National Survey of the Canadian Population." *Anesthesia Progress*, 2005,52(1), 3–11.

75 T. Schiff, E. Delgado, Y. P. Zhang, *et al.* "Clinical Evaluation of the Efficacy of an In-Office Desensitizing Paste Containing 8 Percent Arginine and Calcium Carbonate on Providing Instant and Lasting Relief Of Dentin Hypersensitivity." *American Journal of Dentistry*, 2009, 22 Spec No A, 8A–15A.

76 U. Erdemir, E. Yildiz, I. Kilic, *et al.* "The Efficacy of Three Desensitizing Agents Used to Treat Dentin Hypersensitivity." *Journal of the American Dental Association*, 2010, 141(3), 285–96.

77 N. G. Kumar and D. S. Mehta. "Short-Term Assessment of the Nd:YAG Laser with and without Sodium Fluoride Varnish in the Treatment Of Dentin Hypersensitivity—A Clinical and Scanning Electron Microscopy Study." *Journal of Periodontology*, 2005, 76(7), 1140–7.

78 A. C. Aranha, L. A. Pimenta, and G. M. Marchi. "Clinical Evaluation of Desensitizing Treatments for Cervical Dentin Hypersensitivity." *Brazilian Oral Research*, 2009, 23(3), 333–9.

79 T. Schiff, G. N. Wachs, D. M. Petrone, *et al.* "The Efficacy of a Newly Designed Toothbrush to Decrease Tooth Sensitivity." *Compendium of Continuing Education in Dentistry*, 2009, 30(4), 234–6, 238–40.

80 A. Deshpande and A. R. Jadad. "The Impact of Polyol-Containing Chewing Gums on Dental Caries: A Systematic Review of Original Randomized Controlled Trials and Observational Studies." *Journal of the American Dental Association*, 2008, 139(12), 1602–14.

81 B. Tang and B. J. Millar. "Effect of Chewing Gum on Tooth Sensitivity Following Whitening." *British Dental Journal*, 2010, 208(12), 571–7.

82 K. Kamiya, M. Fumoto, H. Kikuchi, *et al.* "Prolonged Gum Chewing Evokes Activation of the Ventral Part p Prefrontal Cortex and Suppression of Nociceptive Responses: Involvement of the Serotonergic System." *Journal of Medical and Dental Sciences*, 2010, 57(1), 35–43.

83 Z. Wang, Y. Sa, S. Sauro, *et al.* "Effect of Desensitising Toothpastes on Dentinal Tubule Occlusion: A Dentine Permeability Measurement and SEM In Vitro Study." *Journal of Dentistry*, 2010, 38(5), 400–10.

84 C. Rivinius. "Burning Mouth Syndrome: Identification, Diagnosis, and Treatment." *Journal of the American Academy of Nurse Practitioners*, 2009, 21(8), 423–9.

85 J. Buchanan and J. Zakrzewska. "Burning Mouth Syndrome." *Clinical Evidence* (Online), 2008.

86 P. Penza, A. Majorana, R. Lombardi, *et al.* "'Burning Tongue' and 'Burning Tip': The Diagnostic Challenge of the Burning Mouth Syndrome." *Clinical Journal of Pain*, 2010, 26(6), 528–32.

87 V. Brailo, V. Vueiaeeviae-Boras, I. Z. Alajbeg, *et al.* "Oral Burning Symptoms and Burning Mouth Syndrome-Significance of Different Variables in 150 Patients." *Medicina Oral, Patología Oral y Cirugía Bucal*, 2006, 11(3), E252–5.

88 H. Terai and M.Shimahara. "Tongue Pain: Burning Mouth Syndrome vs Candida-Associated Lesion." *Oral Diseases*, 2007, 13(4), 440–2.

89 R. Gutta, L. McLain, and S. H. McGuff. "Sjogren Syndrome: A Review for the Maxillofacial Surgeon." 2008, *Oral and Maxillofacial Surgery Clinics of North America*, 20(4), 567–75.

90 F. Femiano, A. Lanza, C. Buonaiuto, *et al.* "Burning Mouth Syndrome and Burning Mouth on Hypothyroidism: Proposal for a Diagnostic and Therapeutic Protocol." *Oral Surgery, Oral Medicine, Oral Pathology, Oral Radiology & Endodontics*, 2008, 105(1), e22–7.

91 N. Matos-Gomes, M. Katsurayama, F. H. Makimoto, *et al.* "Psychological Stress and Its Influence on Salivary Flow Rate, Total Protein Concentration and IgA, IgG and IgM Titers." *Neuroimmunomodulation*, 2010, 17(6), 396–404.

92 P. Maragou and L. Ivanyi. "Serum Zinc Levels in Patients with Burning Mouth Syndrome." *Oral Surgery, Oral Medicine, Oral Pathology*, 1991, 71(4), 447–50.

93 G. S. Cho, M. W. Han, B. Lee, *et al.* "Zinc Deficiency May Be a Cause of Burning Mouth Syndrome as Zinc Replacement Therapy Has Therapeutic Effects." *Journal of Oral Pathology and Medicine*, 2010.

94 J. M. Bourre. "Effects of Nutrients (in Food) on the Structure and Function of the Nervous System: Update on Dietary Requirements for Brain. Part 1: Micronutrients." *The Journal of Nutrition, Health & Aging*, 2006, 10(5), 377–85.

95 Office of Dietary Supplements. National Institutes of Health. Zinc. Health Professional Fact Sheet, 2009. Retrieved from http://ods.od.nih.gov/factsheets/zinc.asp on 9/14/2010.

96 M. Petruzzi, D. Lauritano, M, De Benedittis, *et al.* "Systemic Capsaicin for Burning Mouth Syndrome: Short-Term Results of a Pilot Study." *Journal of Oral Pathology and Medicine*, 2004, 33(2), 111–4.

97 R. Marino, S. Torretta, P. Capaccio, *et al.* "Different Therapeutic Strategies for Burning Mouth Syndrome: Preliminary Data." *Journal Of Oral Pathology and Medicine*, 2010.

98 G. A. Scardina, A. Ruggieri, F. Provenzano, *et al.* "Burning Mouth Syndrome: Is Acupuncture a Therapeutic Possibility?" *British Dental Journal*, 2010, 209(1), E2.

99 H. S. Kho, J. S. Lee, E. J. Lee, *et al.* "The Effects of Parafunctional Habit Control and Topical Lubricant on Discomforts Associated with Burning Mouth Syndrome." BMS, *Archives of Gerontology and Geriatrics*, 2010, 51(1), 95–9.

100 J. M. Zakrzewska, H. Forssell, and A. M. Glenny. "Interventions for the Treatment of Burning Mouth Syndrome." *Cochrane Database of Systematic Reviews*, 2005 (1), CD002779.

101 P. Lopez-Jornet, F. Camacho-Alonso, and S. Leon-Espinosa. "Efficacy of Alpha Lipoic Acid in Burning Mouth Syndrome: A Randomized, Placebo-Treatment Study." *Journal of Oral Rehabilitation*, 2009, 36(1), 52–7.

102 M. Carbone, M. Pentenero, M. Carrozzo, *et al.* "Lack of Efficacy of Alpha-Lipoic Acid in Burning Mouth Syndrome: A Double-Blind, Randomized, Placebo-Controlled Study." *European Journal of Pain*, 2009, 13(5), 492–6.

103 D. R. Cavalcanti and F. R. da Silveira. "Alpha Lipoic Acid in Burning Mouth Syndrome—A Randomized Double-Blind Placebo-Controlled Trial." *Journal of Oral Pathology and Medicine*, 2009, 38(3), 254–61.

104 J. Gao, L. Chen, J. Zhou, *et al.* "A Case-Control Study on Etiological Factors Involved in Patients with Burning Mouth Syndrome." *Journal of Oral Pathology and Medicine*, 2009, 38(1), 24–8.

105 P. Penza, A. Majorana, R. Lombardi, *et al.* "'Burning Tongue' and 'Burning Tip': The Diagnostic Challenge of the Burning Mouth Syndrome." *Clinical Journal of Pain*, 2010, 26(6), 528–32.

106 A. Sardella. "An Up-to-Date View on Burning Mouth Syndrome." *Minerva Stomatologica*, 2007, 56(6), 327–40.

107 I. D. Miziara, B. C. Filho, R. Oliveira, *et al.* "Group Psychotherapy: An Additional Approach to Burning Mouth Syndrome." *Journal of Psychosomatic Research*, 2009, 67(5), 443–8.

108 J. Bergdahl, G. Anneroth, and H. Perris. "Cognitive Therapy in the Treatment of Patients with Resistant Burning Mouth Syndrome: A Controlled Study." *Journal of Oral Pathology and Medicine*, 1995, 24(5), 213–5.

109 D. I. Friedman. "Topirimate-Induced Burning Mouth Syndrome." *Headache*, 2010.

110 M. D. Moura, M. I. Senna, D. F. Madureira, *et al.* "Oral Adverse Effects Due to the Use of Nevirapine." *Journal of Contemporary Dental Practice*, 2008, 9(1), 84–90.

111 C. Salort-Llorca, M. P. Minguez-Serra, and F. J. Silvestre. "Drug-Induced Burning Mouth Syndrome: A New Etiological Diagnosis." *Medicina Oral, Patología Oral y Cirugía Bucal*, 2008, 13(3), E167–70.

112 C. Gremeau-Richard, A. Woda, M. L. Navez, *et al.* "Topical Clonazepam in Stomatodynia: A Randomised Placebo-Controlled Study." *Pain*, 2004,108(1–2), 51–7.

113 J. Buchanan and J. Zakrzewska. "Burning Mouth Syndrome." *Clinical Evidence* (Online), 2008.

114 L. Machet, S. Le Du, A. Bernez, *et al.* "The Value of Allergy Survey in a Retrospective Series of 40 Patients with Burning-Mouth Syndrome (Stomatodynia)." *Annales de Dermatologie et de Venereologie*, 2008, 135(2), 105–9.

115 R. Marino, P. Capaccio, L. Pignataro, and F. Spadari. "Burning Mouth Syndrome: The Role of Contact Hypersensitivity." *Oral Diseases*, 2009, 15(4), 255–8.

116 For the Dental Patient. Burning Mouth Syndrome. *Journal of the American Dental Association*, 2005, 136(8), 1191. Available online at http://jada.ada.org/cgi/content/full/136/8/1191.

Chapter 9

1   Brian Stelter. "8 Hours a Day Spent on Screens, Study Finds." *The New York Times*, March 26, 2009. Available online at http://www.nytimes.com/2009/03/27/business/media/27adco.html.

2   American Pain Foundation. "Pain Facts & Figures." September 9, 2010. Available online at http://www.painfoundation.org/newsroom/reporter-resources/pain-facts-figures.html.

3   Eva Skillgate *et al.* "The Long-Term Effects of Naprapathic Manual Therapy on Back and Neck Pain." *BMC Musculoskeletal Disorders*, 2010, 11. Available online at http://www.biomedcentral.com/1471-2474/11/26/abstract/.

4   Fu Li-Min, Li Ju-Tzu, and Wu Wen-Shuo. "Randomized Controlled Trials of Acupuncture for Neck Pain." The *Journal of Alternative and Complementary Medicine*, 2009 February, Vol. 15, No. 2. Available online at http://www.liebertonline.com/doi/abs/10.1089/acm.2008.0135/.

5   National Pain Foundation. "Overview." Available online at http://www.nationalpainfoundation.org/articles/404/overview.

6   Nicholas Henschke *et al.* "Prevalence of and Screening for Serious Spinal Pathology in Patients Presenting to Primary Care Settings with Acute Low Back Pain." *Arthritis and Rheumatism*, 2009 Oct, vol. 60, 3072–80. Available online at http://onlinelibrary.wiley.com/doi/10.1002/art.24853/abstract.

7   Janet K. Freburger *et al.* "The Rising Prevalence of Chronic Low Back Pain." *Archives of Internal Medicine*, 2009, 169(3): 251–258. Available online at http://archinte.ama-assn.org/cgi/content/abstract/169/3/251.

8   Scott Haldeman. "The Bone and Joint Decade 2000–2010 Task Force on Neck Pain and Its Associated Disorders." *Spine*, 2008 15 February, Volume 33, Issue 4S, S5–S7. Available online at http://journals.lww.com/spinejournal/Fulltext/2008/02151/The_Bone_and_Joint_Decade_2000_2010_Task_Force_on.4.aspx/.

9   "What Is Grade 1 Spondylolisthesis?" Available online at http://www.ehow.com/facts_5630759_grade-spondylolisthesis_.html.

10 K. D. van den Eerenbeemt *et al.* "Total Disc Replacement Surgery for Symptomatic Degenerative Lumbar Disc Disease." *European Spine Journal*, 2010 Aug, 19(8): 1262–80.

11 A. Hopton, H. MacPherson, *et al.* "Acupuncture for Chronic Pain. Is Acupuncture More Than an Effective Placebo?" *Pain Practice*, 2010 Mar, 10(2): 94–102. E-pub 2010 Jan 8. Available online at http://www.painjournalonline.com/article/S0304-3959(99)00304-8/abstract.

12 Karen J. Sherman and Remy R. Coeytaux. "Acupuncture for Improving Chronic Back Pain, Osteoarthritis and Headache." *Journal of Clinical Outcomes Management*, 2009 May 1, 16(5). Available online at http://www.ncbi.nlm.nih.gov/pmc/articles/PMC2863344/.

13 Daisy L. M. Franca *et al.* "Tension Neck Syndrome Treated by Acupuncture Combined with Physiotherapy." *Complementary Therapies in Medicine*, 2008 October, Volume 16, Issue 5, 268–277. Available online at http://www.journals.elsevierhealth.com/periodicals/yctim/article/S0965-2299(08)00011-3/abstract.

14 M. Ranieri, M. Sciuscio, A. M. Cortese, *et al.* "The Use of Alpha-Lipoic Acid (ALA), Gamma Linolenic Acid (GLA) and Rehabilitation in the Treatment of Back Pain." *International Journal of Immunopathology and Pharmacology*, 2009 Jul–Sep 22 (3 Suppl). Available online 45–50. Available online at http://www.ncbi.nlm.nih.gov/pubmed/19887043.

15 G. S. Mijnhout, A. Alkhalaf, N. Kleefstra, *et al.* "Alpha Lipoic Acid. A New Treatment for Neuropathic Pain in Patients with Diabetes?" *Netherlands Journal of Medicine*, 2010 Apr, 68(4): 158–62.

16 *Ibid.*

17 J. J. Gagnier, M. W. van Tulder, B. M. Berman, *et al.* "Herbal Medicine for Low Back Pain." *Cochrane Database of Systematic Reviews*, 2006, Issue 2. Available online 10.1002/14651858.CD004504.pub3.

18 Bruno Massimo Giannetti *et al.* "Efficacy and Safety of a Comfrey Root Extract Ointment in the Treatment of Acute Upper or Low Back Pain." *British Journal of Sports Medicine*. Available online at http://bjsm.bmj.com/content/early/2009/05/21/bjsm.2009.058677.abstract.

19 Michelle Shardell *et al.* "Association of Low Vitamin D Levels with the Frailty Syndrome in Men and Women." *The Journals of Gerontology* Series A. Biological Sciences and Medical Sciences, 2009, 64A (1). Available online at http://biomedgerontology.oxfordjournals.org/content/64A/1/69.abstract.

20 Joseph Charles Maroon *et al.* "Fatty Acids (Fish Oil) as an Anti-Inflammatory: an Alternative to Nonsteroidal Anti-Inflammatory Drugs for Diskogenic Pain." *Surgical Neurology*, 2006, vol. 65, 326–331. Available online at http://cat.inist.fr/?aModele=afficheN&cpsidt=17661611.

21 B. K. L. Choi, J. H. Verbeek, W. W. S. Tam, *et al.* "Exercises for Prevention of Recurrences of Low-Back Pain." *Cochrane Database of Systematic Reviews*, 2010, Issue 1. Available online at http://www.thecochrane library.com/view/0/index.html.

22 J. Hayden, M. W. van Tulder, A. Malmivaara, *et al.* "Exercise Therapy for Treatment of Non-Specific Low Back Pain." *Cochrane Database of Systematic Reviews*, 2005, Issue 3. Available online 10.1002/14651858.CD000335. pub2.

23 J. K. Freburger, T. S. Carey, G. M. Holmes, *et al.* "Exercise Prescription for Chronic Back or Neck Pain. Who Prescribes It? Who Gets It? What Is Prescribed?" *Arthritis Care & Research*, 2009, 61(2): 192–200.

24 D. Chatzitheodorou, C. Kabitsis, P. Malliou, *et al.* "A Pilot Study of the Effects of High-Intensity Aerobic Exercise Versus Passive Interventions on Pain, Disability, Psychological Strain, and Serum Cortisol Concentrations in People with Chronic Low Back Pain." *Physical Therapy*, 2007 Mar, 87(3): 304–12. E-pub 2007 Feb 6. Available online at http://ptjournal.net/cgi/content/abstract/87/3/304.

25 E. L. Hurwitz, H. Morgenstern, G. F. Kominski, *et al.* "A Randomized Trial of Chiropractic and Medical Care for Patients with Low Back Pain. Eighteen-Month Follow-Up Outcomes From The UCLA Low Back Pain Study." *Spine*, 2006 Mar 15, 31(6): 611–21, Available online at http://journals.lww.com/spinejournal/ Abstract/2006/03150/A_Randomized_Trial_of_Chiropractic_and_Medical.2.aspx.

26 J. Hill, M. Lewis, A. C. Papageorgiou, *et al.* "Predicting Persistent Neck Pain. A 1-Year Follow-Up of a Population Cohort." *Spine*, 2004 Aug 1, 29(15): 1648–54. Available online at http://journals.lww.com/spinejournal/ Abstract/2004/08010/Predicting_Persistent_Neck_Pain__A_1_Year.13.aspx.

27 Joel K. Jackson *et al.* "The Influence of Periodized Resistance Training on Recreationally Active Males with Chronic Nonspecific Low Back Pain." *Journal of Strength & Conditioning Research*, 2010 21 January. Available online at http://journals.lww.com/nsca-jscr/Abstract/publishahead/The_Influence_of_Periodized_Resistance_ Training_on.99333.aspx.

28 L. L. Andersen, M. Kjaer, K. Søgaard, *et al.* "Effect of Two Contrasting Types of Physical Exercise on Chronic Neck Muscle Pain." *Arthritis and Rheumatism*, 2008 Jan 15, 59(1): 84–91. Available online at http://onlinelibrary. wiley.com/doi/10.1002/art.23256/abstract.

29 Kimberly Williams. "Evaluation of the Effectiveness and Efficacy of Iyengar Yoga Therapy on Chronic Low Back Pain." *Spine*, 1 September 2009, Volume 34, Issue 19, 2066-2076. Available online at http://journals.lww. com/spinejournal/Abstract/2009/09010/Evaluation_of_the_Effectiveness_and_Efficacy_of.11.aspx.

30 Gail A. Greendale *et al.* "Yoga Decreases Kyphosis in Senior Women and Men with Adult-Onset Hyperkyphosis. Results of a Randomized Controlled Trial." *Journal of the American Geriatrics Society*, 2009 September, Volume 57, Issue 9, 1569–1579. Available online at http://onlinelibrary.wiley.com/doi/10.1111/j.1532-5415.2009.02391.x/abstract.

31 K. J. Sherman, D. C. Cherkin, J. Erro, *et al.* "Comparing Yoga, Exercise, and a Self-Care Book for Chronic Low Back Pain." *Annals of Internal Medicine*, 2005, 143(12): 849–56. Available online at http://www.annals.org/ content/143/12/849.short.

32 S. Hollinghurst, D. Sharp, K. Ballard, *et al.* "Randomised Controlled Trial of Alexander Technique Lessons, Exercise, and Massage (ATEAM) for Chronic and Recurrent Back Pain." *British Medical Journal*, 2008 Dec 11, 337: a2656, doi. Available online at http://www.bmj.com/cgi/content/abstract/337/aug19_2/a884?ijkey=1560c315 3f4cc582721b9640d266d767aad9fde1&keytype2=tf_ipsecsha.

33 Fu Li-Min, Li Ju-Tzu, and Wu Wen-Shuo. "Randomized Controlled Trials of Acupuncture for Neck Pain." *The Journal of Alternative and Complementary Medicine*, 2009 February, Vol. 15, No. 2. Available online at http:// www.liebertonline.com/doi/abs/10.1089/acm.2008.0135.

34 Daniel C. Cherkin *et al.* "A Randomized Trial Comparing Acupuncture, Simulated Acupuncture, and Usual Care for Chronic Low Back Pain." *Archives of Internal Medicine*, 2009 May 11, vol 169. Available online at http:// archinte.ama-assn.org/cgi/content/abstract/169/9/858.

35 D. He, A. T. Høstmark, K. B. Veiersted, *et al.* "Effect of Intensive Acupuncture on Pain-Related Social and Psychological Variables for Women with Chronic Neck and Shoulder Pain—An RCT with Six-Month and Three-Year Follow Up." *Acupuncture Medicine*, 2005 Jun, 23(2): 52–61. Available online at http://aim.bmj.com/ content/23/2/52.abstract.

36 Hsiesh *et al.* "Treatment of Low Back Pain by Acupressure and Physical Therapy." *Pain*, 2008 Feb, 134(3): 310–9.

37 B. F. Walker, S. D. French, W. Grant, *et al.* "Combined Chiropractic Interventions for Low-Back Pain." *Cochrane Database of Systematic Reviews*, 2010, Issue 4. Available online at http://childrenshospital.edu/ emergency/research/CochraneChiropractic.pdf.

38 A. R. Gross, J. L. Hoving, T. A. Haines, *et al.* "A Cochrane Review of Manipulation and Mobilization for Mechanical Neck Disorders." *Spine*, 2004, 29: 1541. Available online at http://journals.lww.com/spinejournal/ Abstract/2004/07150/A_Cochrane_Review_of_Manipulation_and_Mobilization.9.aspx.

39 J. D. Cassidy *et al.* "Risk of Vertebrobasilar Stroke and Chiropractic Care." *Spine*, 2008, 33 (4 Suppl): S176–83. Available online at http://www.ncbi.nlm.nih.gov/pubmed/18204390.

40 Jennie C. I. Tsao. "Effectiveness of Massage Therapy for Chronic, Non-Malignant Pain." *Evidence-Based Complementary and Alternative Medicine*, 2007, February 5, 4(2)165–179. Available online at http://ecam.oxfordjournals.org/cgi/content/abstract/4/2/165.

41 W. P. Hanten, S. L. Olson, N. L. Butts, *et al.* "Effectiveness of a Home Program of Ischemic Pressure Followed by Sustained Stretch for Treatment of Myofascial Trigger Points." *Therapy*, 2000 Oct, 80(10): 997–1003. Available online at http://www.physicaltherapyjournal.net/cgi/content/abstract/80/10/997.

42 Dawn T. Gulick *et al.* "Effect of Ischemic Pressure Using a Backnobber II Device on Discomfort Associated with Myofascial Trigger Points." *Journal of Bodywork and Movement Therapies*, 2010 June.

43 Xuguang (Grant) Tao. "A Randomized Clinical Trial of Continuous Low-Level Heat Therapy for Acute Muscular Low Back Pain in the Workplace." *Journal of Occupational & Environmental Medicine*, 2005 December, Volume 47, Issue 12, 1298–1306. Available online at http://journals.lww.com/joem/Abstract/2005/12000/A_Randomized_Clinical_Trial_of_Continuous.16.aspx.

44 S. D. French, M. Cameron, B. F. Walker, *et al.* "Superficial Heat Or Cold for Low Back Pain." *Cochrane Database of Systematic Reviews*, 2006, Issue 1. Available online at http://researchrepository.murdoch.edu.au/1705/1/Superficial_heat_or_cold_2006.pdf/.

45 G. Garra, A. J. Singer, R. Leno, *et al.* "Heat or Cold Packs for Neck and Back Strain." *Academy of Emergency Medicine*, 2010 May, 17(5): 484–9. Available online at http://onlinelibrary.wiley.com/doi/10.1111/j.1553-2712.2010.00735.x/abstract.

46 N. E. Morone, C. S. Lynch, C. M. Greco, *et al.* "'I Felt Like A New Person.' The Effects of Mindfulness Meditation on Older Adults with Chronic Pain." *Journal of Pain*, 2008 Sep 9(9): 841–8. E-pub 2008 Jun 12. Available online at http://www.jpain.org/article/S1526-5900(08)00544-0/abstract.

47 N. E. Morone, C. M. Greco, and D. K. Weiner. "Mindfulness Meditation for the Treatment of Chronic Low Back Pain In Older Adults." *Pain*, 2008 Feb, 134(3): 310-9. E-pub 2007 Jun 1. Available online at http://www.painjournalonline.com/article/S0304-3959(07)00243-6/abstract.

48 J. Kabat-Zinn, L. Lipworth, and R. Burney. "Four-Year Follow-Up of a Meditation-Based Program for the Self-Regulation of Chronic Pain." *Clinical Journal of Pain*, 1987, 2: 159–73. Available online at http://journals.lww.com/clinicalpain/Abstract/1986/02030/Four_Year_Follow_Up_of_a_Meditation_Based_Program.4.aspx.

49 R. J. Davidson, J. Kabat-Zinn, J. Schumacher, *et al.* "Alterations in Brain and Immune Function Produced by Mindfulness Meditation." *Psychosomatic Medicine*, 2003, 65(4). Available online at http://www.psychosomaticmedicine.org/cgi/content/full/65/4/564?ijkey=ad6454f747329753c6e432b298e4953c38cc6857.

50 M. W. van Tulder, B. Koes, and A. Malmivaara. "Outcome of Non-Invasive Treatment Modalities on Back Pain." *European Spine Journal*, 2006 Jan, 15 Suppl 1: S64–81. E-pub 2005 Dec 1. Available online at http://www.spring erlink.com/content/f454600537287863/.

51 C. R. Jungquist, C. O'Brien, S. Matteson-Rusby, *et al.* "The Efficacy of Cognitive-Behavioral Therapy for Insomnia in Patients with Chronic Pain." *Sleep Medicine*, 2010 Mar, 11(3): 302–9. Epub 2010 Feb 4, Available online at http://www.sleep-journal.com/article/S1389-9457(10)00014-6/abstract.

52 S. E. Lamb, Z. Hansen, R. Lall , *et al.* "Back Skills Training Trial Investigators. Group Cognitive Behavioural Treatment for Low-Back Pain In Primary Care." *The Lancet*. 2010 Mar 13, 375(9718): 916–23. E-pub 2010 Feb 25. Available online at http://www.escardiocontent.org/periodicals/ejcn/article/S0140-6736(09)62164-4/abstract.

53 B. M. Hoffman *et al.* "Meta-Analysis of Psychological Interventions for Chronic Low Back Pain." *Health Psychology*, 2007 Jan 26(1): 1–9. Available online at http://www.ncbi.nlm.nih.gov/pubmed/17209691.

54 K. P. Kapitza *et al.* "First Non-Contingent Respiratory Biofeedback Placebo Versus Contingent Biofeedback in Patients with Chronic Low Back Pain." *Applied Psychophysiology Biofeedback*, March 2010. Available online at http://www.springerlink.com/content/20r53k8728k30qpn/.

55 R. T. Chow, M. I. Johnson, R. A. Lopes-Martins, *et al.* "Efficacy of Low-Level Laser Therapy in the Management of Neck Pain." *The Lancet*, 2009 Dec 5, 374(9705): 1897–908.

56 A. M. Orbai *et al.* "The Effectiveness of Tricyclic Antidepressants on Lumbar Spinal Stenosis." *Joint Diseases*, 2010, 68(1): 22–4. Available online at http://www.ncbi.nlm.nih.gov/pubmed/20345358.

57 S. M. Salerno, R. Browning, and J. L. Jackson. "The Effect of Antidepressant Treatment on Chronic Back Pain." *Archives of Internal Medicine*, 2002, 162(1): 19–24. Available online at http://archinte.ama-assn.org/cgi/content/abstract/162/1/19.

58 Sansone *et al.* "Pain, Pain, Go Away. Antidepressants and Pain Management." *Psychiatry*, 2008 Dec, 5(12): 16–9.

59 H. N. Chan, J. Fam, and B. Y. Ng. "Use of Antidepressants in the Treatment of Chronic Pain." *Annals of the Academy of Medicine*, Singapore, 2009 Nov, 38(11): 974–9. Available online at http://www.ncbi.nlm.nih.gov/pubmed/1723371.

60 J. J. Gagnier, M. W. van Tulder, B. M. Berman, *et al.* "Herbal Medicine for Low Back Pain." *Cochrane Database of Systematic Reviews*, 2006, Issue 2.

61 Eske K. Aasvang *et al.* "The Effect of Wound Instillation of a Novel Purified Capsaicin Formulation on Postherniotomy Pain." *Anesthesia & Analgesia*, 2008 July, vol. 107, 282–291. Available online at http://www.anesthesia-analgesia.org/content/107/1/282.full.

62 Kelvin C. H. Wong. "The Association Between Back Pain and Trunk Posture of Workers In A Special School for the Severe Handicaps." *BMC Musculoskeletal Disorders*, online, April 2009, 10: 43.

63 R. A. Deyo *et al.* "What Can the History and Physical Examination Tell Us about Low Back Pain?" *Journal of the American Medical Association*, 1992, 268. Available online at http://jama.ama-assn.org/cgi/content/summary/268/6/760.

64 S. J. Horton, G. M. Johnson, and M. A. Skinner. "Changes in Head and Neck Posture Using an Office Chair with and without Lumbar Roll Support." *Spine*, 2010 May 20, 35(12): E542–8. Available online at http://journals.lww.com/spinejournal/Abstract/2010/05200/Changes_in_Head_and_Neck_Posture_Using_an_Office.18.aspx.

65 Kim Bergholdt, Rasmus N. Fabricius, and Tom Bendix. "Better Backs by Better Beds?" *Spine*, 2008 April 1, 33 (7): 703–708. Available online at http://www.medscape.com/viewarticle/573670_1.

66 James W. Carson *et al.* "Forgiveness and Chronic Low Back Pain. A Preliminary Study Examining The Relationship of Forgiveness to Pain, Anger, and Psychological Distress." *The Journal of Pain*, 2005 February, Volume 6, Issue 2, 84–91. Available online at http://www.jpain.org/article/S1526-5900(04)01037-5/abstract.

67 Katsouni *et al.* "The Involvement of Substance P in the Induction of Aggressive Behavior." *Peptides*, 2009 Aug, 30(8): 1586–91.

Chapter 10

1 Dennis M. Bramble and Daniel E. Lieberman. "Endurance Running and the Evolution of Homo." *Nature*, 2004, 432: 345–352. Available online at http://www.nature.com/nature/journal/v432/n7015/full/nature03052.html.

2 "Eating Vegetables Slashes Atherosclerosis Risk by 38 Percent, Research Reveals." Available online June 22, 2006 at http://www.naturalnews.com/019449_atherosclerosis_vegetables_eating.html.

3 C. D. Gardner *et al.* "Effect of Ginkgo Niloba (EGb 761) on Treadmill Walking Time among Adults with Peripheral Artery Disease." *Journal of Cardiopulmonary Rehabilitation and Prevention*, 2008, 28, 258–265. Available online at http://www.ncbi.nlm.nih.gov/pubmed/18628657.

4 D. L. Sontheimer. "Peripheral Vascular Disease: Diagnosis and Treatment." *American Family Physician*, 2006 Jun 1, 73(11): 1971–6.

5 Alan T. Hirsch *et al.* "Peripheral Arterial Disease Detection, Awareness, and Treatment in Primary Care." *Journal of the American Medical Association*, 2001 September, vol. 286, 1317–1324. Available online at http://Journal of the American Medical Association.ama-assn.org/cgi/content/abstract/286/11/1317.

6 The Society of Interventional Radiology. "Interventional Radiology Grand Rounds." 2004. Available online at http://www.scvir.org/medical-professionals/GR_PDFs/pad-treatment.pdf.

7 Yao He *et al.* "Passive Smoking and Risk of Peripheral Arterial Disease and Ischemic Stroke in Chinese Women Who Never Smoked." *Circulation*, 2008, 118, 1535–1540. Available online at http://circ.ahajournals.org/cgi/content/abstract/118/15/1535.

8 "Sprains and Strains." *NIAMS*, April 2009. Available online at http://www.niams.nih.gov/Health_Info/Sprains_Strains/default.asp.

9 "Everything about Achilles Tendons." Available online at http://www.achillestendon.com/Injuries.html.

10 Terrence M. Philbin *et al.* "Peroneal Tendon Injuries." *Journal of the American Academy of Orthopaedic Surgeons*, 2009, Vol. 17, 306–317. Available online at http://www.jaaos.org/cgi/content/abstract/17/5/306.

11 Nicola Maffulli *et al.* "Eccentric Calf Muscle Training in Athletic Patients with Achilles Tendinopathy." *Disability and Rehabilitation*, 2008, vol. 30, 1677–1684. Available online at http://informahealthcare.com/doi/abs/10.1080/09638280701786427.

12 M. T. Galloway, P. Dayton, and O. W. Joki. "Achilles Tendon Overuse Injuries." *Journal of Clinical Sports Medicine*, October 1992, Volume 11, 771–782. Available online at http://www.ncbi.nlm.nih.gov/pubmed/1423697.

13 Robert J. De Vos *et al.* "Platelet-Rich Plasma Injection for Chronic Achilles Tendinopathy." *Journal of the American Medical Association*, January 13, 2010, vol. 303, 144–149. Available online at http://www.sonafe.org.br/images_up/prp_achiles_tendon.pdf.

14 Keitaro Kubo *et al.* "Effects of Acupuncture and Heating on Blood Volume and Oxygen Saturation of Human Achilles Tendon in Vivo." *European Journal of Applied Physiology*, June 2010, vol. 109, 545–550. Available online at http://www.springerlink.com/content/1776583888747178/.

15 Shay Tenenbaum *et al.* "The Percutaneous Surgical Approach for Repairing Acute Achilles Tendon Rupture."

Journal of the American Podiatric Medical Association, Volume 100, Number 4, 270-275 2010. Available online at http://www.japmaonline.org/cgi/content/abstract/100/4/270.

16 Nicola Maffulli and Louis C. Almekinders. The Achilles Tendon. 2007, 59–69. Available online at http://books.google.com/books?id=1uZSskDDqCAC&pg=PA93&lpg=PA93&dq=Maffulli,+Nicola+and+Louis+C.+Almekinders&source=bl&ots=nIeHMe250l&sig=uw5cdv6zurXh_ptkzQzMOoFK0EE&hl=en&ei=TJNiTOTQHsOclgf2otSsCg&sa=X&oi=book_result&ct=result&resnum=1&ved=0CBIQ6AEwAA#v=onepage&q=Maffulli%2C%20Nicola%20and%20Louis%20C.%20Almekinders&f=false.

17 "Plantar Fasciitis and Bone Spurs." *American Academy of Orthopaedic Surgeons*, June 2010. Available online at http://orthoinfo.aaos.org/topic.cfm?topic=a00149.

18 "Plantar Fasciitis." Mayo Clinic, March 24, 2009.

19 B. G. Donley, T. Moore, J. Sferra, *et al.* "The Efficacy of Oral Nonsteroidal Anti-Inflammatory Medication (NSAID) in the Treatment of Plantar Fasciitis." *Foot and Ankle International*, 2007, 28: 20–23. Available online at http://cat.inist.fr/?aModele=afficheN&cpsidt=18437701.

20 M. M. Hooper *et al.* "Musculoskeletal Findings in Obese Subjects before and after Weight Loss Following Bariatric Surgery." *International Journal of Obesity*, 2007: 31, 114–120. Available online at http://www.nature.com/ijo/journal/v31/n1/abs/0803349a.html.

21 Wendy J. Pomerantz *et al.* "Injury Patterns in Obese Versus Non-Obese Patients Presenting to a Pediatric Emergency Department." *Pediatrics*, April 2010: Vol. 125, 681–685. Available online at http://pediatrics.aappublications.org/cgi/content/abstract/125/4/681.

22 "Plantar Fasciitis and Bone Spurs." *American Academy of Orthopaedic Surgeons*. June 2010. Available online at http://orthoinfo.aaos.org/topic.cfm?topic=a00149.

23 S. P. Zhang, T. P. Yip, and Q. S. Li. "Acupuncture Treatment for Plantar Fasciitis." *Evidence-Based Complementary and Alternative Medicine*. 2009 Nov 23. Available online at http://ecam.oxfordjournals.org/cgi/content/abstract/nep186.

24 L. Sheridan *et al.* "Plantar Fasciopathy Treated with Dynamic Splinting." *Journal of the American Podiatric Medical Association*, May-June 2010, 100, 161–165. Available online at http://www.ncbi.nlm.nih.gov/pubmed/20479445.

25 Lance D. Barry *et al.* "A Retrospective Study of Standing Gastrocnemius-Soleus Stretching Versus Night Splinting in the Treatment of Plantar Fasciitis." *The Journal of Foot and Ankle Surgery*, Volume 41, Issue 4, July-August 2002, 221–227. Available online at http://www.sciencedirect.com/science?_ob=ArticleURL&_udi=B75DJ-4VPGC25-4&_user=10&_coverDate=08%2F31%2F2002&_rdoc=1&_fmt=high&_orig=search&_origin=search&_sort=d&_docanchor=&view=c&_searchStrId=1480355525&_rerunOrigin=scholar.google&_acct=C000050221&_version=1&_urlVersion=0&_userid=10&md5=cc2ff19554531b0cd72b2e050263139e&searchtype=a.

26 Ludger Gerdesmeyer *et al.* "Radial Extracorporeal Shockwave Therapy Is Safe and Effective." *American Journal of Sports Medicine*, 2008 November, vol. 36, 2100–2109. Available online at http://ajs.sagepub.com/content/36/11/2100.abstract.

27 M. I. Ibrahim *et al.* "Chronic Plantar Fasciitis Treated with Two Sessions of Radial Extracorporeal Shockwave Therapy." *Foot and Ankle International*, 2010 May, 31(5): 391–7.

28 "Down at Their Heels." American Podiatric Medical Association. Available online at http://www.podiatrists.org/cpma_events/2009foothealthawarenessmonth/APMA%20Foot%20Ailments%20Survey.pdf.

29 A. B. Dufour, K. E. Broe, U. S. Nguyen, *et al.* "Foot Pain: Is Current or Past Shoewear a Factor?" *Arthritis & Rheumatism*, 2009 Oct 15, 61(10): 1352–8. Available online at http://onlinelibrary.wiley.com/doi/10.1002/art.24733/abstract.

30 V. Baldassin, C. R. Gomes, and P. S. Beraldo. "Effectiveness of Prefabricated and Customized Foot Orthoses Made from Low-Cost Foam for Noncomplicated Plantar Fasciitis." *Archives of Physical Medicine and Rehabilitation*, 2009 Apr, 90(4): 701–6. Available online at http://www.archives-pmr.org/article/S0003-9993(09)00067-7/abstract.

31 Adel G. Fam, MD. "Gout: Excess Calories, Purines, and Alcohol Intake and Beyond. Response to a Urate-Lowering Diet." *The Journal of Rheumatology*, May 2005. Available online at http://jrheum.com/subscribers/05/05/773.html.

32 T. Neogi *et al.* "Drinking Water Can Reduce the Risk of Recurrent Gout Attacks." *Arthritis & Rheumatism*, 2009, 60: S762–63.

33 Hyon K. Choi *et al.* "Purine-Rich Foods, Dairy and Protein Intake, and the Risk of Gout in Men." *New England Journal of Medicine*, 2004, 350: 1093–1103. Available online at http://www.nejm.org/doi/full/10.1056/NEJMoa035700.

34 Robert Jacobs *et al.* "Consumption of Cherries Lowers Plasma Urate in Healthy Women." *Journal of Nutrition*, 2003. v. 133. 1826-1829. Available online at http://www.ars.usda.gov/research/publications/publications.htm?seq_no_115=151457.

35 Vanisree Mulabagal *et al.* "Anthocyanin Content, Lipid Peroxidation and Cyclooxygenase Enzyme Inhibitory Activities of Sweet and Sour Cherries." *Journal of Agriculture and Food Chemistry*, 2009, 57 (4), pp 1239–1246. Available online at http://pubs.acs.org/doi/abs/10.1021/jf8032039.

36 Hyon K. Choi *et al.* "Vitamin C Intake and the Risk of Gout in Men: A Prospective Study." Archives of Internal Medicine, 2009, 169: 502–507. Available online at http://archinte.ama-assn.org/cgi/content/abstract/169/5/502.

37 Hyon K. Choi. "Coffee Consumption and Risk of Incident Gout in Men: A Prospective Study." *Arthritis & Rheumatism*, Volume 56, Issue 6, 2049–2055. Available online at http://onlinelibrary.wiley.com/doi/10.1002/art.22712/abstract.

38 Pham *et al.* "The Relation of Coffee Consumption to Serum Uric Acid in Japanese Men and Women Aged 49–76 Years." *Nutrition & Metabolism*, 2010, pii: 930757.

39 Paul T. Williams. "Effects of Diet, Physical Activity and Performance, and Body Weight on Incident Gout in Ostensibly Healthy, Vigorously Active Men." *American Journal of Clinical Nutrition*, 2008 May, Vol. 87, No. 5, 1480–1487. Available online at http://www.ajcn.org/cgi/content/abstract/87/5/1480.

40 Yu-feng Xi *et al.* "Clinical Observation on Acupuncture Treatment of Acute Gouty Arthritis in Terms of Clearing Heat, Eliminating Dampness and Stasis." *Acupuncture Research*, 2006-06. Available online at http://en.cnki.com.cn/Article_en/CJFDTOTAL-XCYJ200606013.htm.

41 H. R. Schumacher *et al.* "Effects of Febuxostat Versus Allopurinol and Placebo in Reducing Serum Urate in Subjects With Hyperuricemia and Gout." *Arthritis Care & Research* 2008, 59: 1540–1548. Available online at http://onlinelibrary.wiley.com/doi/10.1002/art.24209/abstract.

42 William Silverman *et al.* "Probenecid, a Gout Remedy, Inhibits Pannexin 1 Channels." *American Journal of Cell Physiology*, 2008, 295: C761–C767. Available online at http://ajpcell.physiology.org/cgi/content/abstract/295/3/C761.

43 Philip Radovic and Ekta Shah. "Nonsurgical Treatment for Hallux Abducto Valgus with Botulinum Toxin A." *Journal of the American Podiatric Medical Association*, 2008, volume 98 Number 1 61–65 2008. Available online at http://www.japmaonline.org/content/abstract/98/1/61.

44 Ali Tehraninasr *et al.* "Effects of Insole with Toe-Separator and Night Splint On Patients with Painful Hallux Valgus." *Prosthetics and Orthotics International*, 2008, vol. 32, 79–83. Available online at http://informahealthcare.com/doi/abs/10.1080/03093640701669074.

45 "Bunion Surgery." *American Academy of Orthopaedic Surgeons*, March 2001. Available online at http://orthoinfo.aaos.org/topic.cfm?topic=a00140.

46 *Ibid.*

47 Y. Yang *et al.* "Diagnosis and Treatment of Post Traumatic Spasmodic Flat Foot." *Zhongguo Gu Shang*, 2008 Dec, 21(12): 917–8. Available online at http://www.ncbi.nlm.nih.gov/pubmed/19146162.

48 W. Brent Edwards. "Foot Joint Pressures during Dynamic Gait Simulation." *Journal of Foot and Ankle Research*, 2008. Available online at http://www.biomedcentral.com/content/pdf/1757-1146-1-S1-O21.pdf.

49 Prasad Gourineni *et al.* "Orthopaedic Deformities Associated With Lumbosacral Spinal Lipomas." *Journal of Pediatric Orthopaedics*, 2009, 29, 932–936. Available online at http://journals.lww.com/pedorthopaedics/Abstract/2009/12000/Orthopaedic_Deformities_Associated_With.19.aspx.

50 Bertil W. Smith *et al.* "Disorders of the Lesser Toes." *Sports Medicine & Arthroscopy Review*, 2009 September, Volume 17, Issue 3, 167–174. Available online at http://journals.lww.com/sportsmedarthro/Abstract/2009/09000/Disorders_of_the_Lesser_Toes.5.aspx.

51 Hylton, B. Menz, and Meg E. Morris. "Footwear Characteristics and Foot Problems in Older People." *Gerontology*, 2005, 51: 346–351. Available online at http://content.karger.com/ProdukteDB/produkte.asp?Aktion=ShowAbstract&ProduktNr=224091&Ausgabe=231181&ArtikelNr=86373.

52 Daniel J. Cuttica *et al.* "New Intramedullary Implant for Proximal Interphalangeal Joint Arthrodesis." *Techniques in Foot & Ankle Surgery*, 2008 September, Volume 7, Issue 3, 203–206. Available online at http://journals.lww.com/techfootankle/Abstract/2008/09000/New_Intramedullary_Implant_for_Proximal.9.aspx.

53 Karen A. Oscar *et al.* "Effectiveness of Splinting on Hammertoe." *The O&P Edge*, 2007 June. Available online at http://www.oandp.com/articles/2007-06_03.asp.

54 M. Kent. "The Oxford Dictionary of Sports Science and Medicine." *Oxford University Press*, 1996, 283.

55 Richard J. Hughes *et al.* "Treatment of Morton's Neuroma with Alcohol Injection Under Sonographic Guidance: Follow-Up of 101 Cases." *American Journal of Roentgenology*, 2007, 188: 1535–1539. Available online at http://www.ajronline.org/cgi/content/abstract/188/6/1535.

56 John D. Mozena and Jared T. Clifford. "Efficacy of Chemical Neurolysis for the Treatment of Interdigital Nerve Compression of the Foot." *Journal of the American Podiatric Medical Association*, 2007, Volume 97, Number 3 203–206 2007. Available online at http://www.japmaonline.org/cgi/content/abstract/97/3/203.

57 C. E. Thomson *et al.* "Interventions for the treatment of Morton's Neuroma." *The Cochrane Collaboration*, 2005, 8. Available online at http://www.shareclevelandla.com/files/Research/Literature_reviews/Mortons_neuroma.pdf.

Chapter 11

1 D. Giugliano, "The Effects of Diet on Inflammation: Emphasis on the Metabolic Syndrome." *Journal of the American College of Cardiology*, 2006, Volume 48, Issue 4, 677–685. Available online at http://linkinghub.elsevier.com/retrieve/pii/S0735109706013350.

2 Riecke *et al.* "Comparing Two Low-Energy Diets for the Treatment of Knee Osteoarthritis Symptoms in Obese Patients." *Osteoarthritis Cartilage*, 2010 Jun, 18(6): 746–54.

3 Ruff *et al.* "Eggshell Membrane in the Treatment of Pain and Stiffness from Osteoarthritis of the Knee." *Clinical Rheumatology*, 2009 Aug, 28(8): 907–14.

4 Alain Jacquet *et al.* "Phytalgic®, a Food Supplement, vs Placebo in Patients with Osteoarthritis of the Knee or Hip." *Arthritis Research & Therapy*, 2009, 11:R192. Available online at http://arthritis-research.com/content/11/6/R192.

5 "Osteoarthritis." *Mayo Clinic*, 2009 October 13. Available online at http://www.mayoclinic.com/health/osteoarthritis/DS00019/DSECTION=alternative-medicine.

6 Daniel O. Clegg *et al.* "Glucosamine, Chondroitin Sulfate, and the Two in Combination for Painful Knee Osteoarthritis." *New England Journal of Medicine*, 2006 February, vol. 354, 795–808. Available online at http://www.contentnejmorg.zuom.info/cgi/content/abstract/354/8/795.

7 Gail D. Deyle. "Effectiveness of Manual Physical Therapy and Exercise in Osteoarthritis of the Knee." *Annals of Internal Medicine*, 2000 February, vol. 132, page 173. Available online at https://www.cebp.nl/media/m549.pdf.

8 Terry K. Selfe. "Mind-Body Therapies and Osteoarthritis of the Knee." *Current Rheumatology Reviews*, 2009 November, Volume 5, Number 4, 204–211(8). Available online at http://www.ingentaconnect.com/content/ben/crr/2009/00000005/00000004/art00006.

9 Luciana E. Silva *et al.* "Hydrotherapy Versus Conventional Land-Based Exercise for the Management of Patients With Osteoarthritis of the Knee." *Physical Therapy*, Vol. 88, No. 1, 2008 January, 21. Available online at http://www.physther.net/cgi/content/abstract/88/1/12.

10 Susan L. Murphy. "Effects of Activity Strategy Training on Pain and Physical Activity in Older Adults with Knee or Hip Osteoarthritis." *Arthritis Care & Research*, 2009 September, vol. 59, 1480–7. Available online at http://www3.interscience.wiley.com/journal/121425835/abstract?CRETRY=1&SRETRY=0.

11 Adam I. Perlman. "Massage Therapy for Osteoarthritis of the Knee." *Archives of Internal Medicine*, 2006 September, vol. 166, 2533–2539. Available online at http://www.stanford.edu/~jhilton/Perlman.2006.pdf.

12 E. Manheimer *et al.* "Acupuncture for Peripheral Joint Osteoarthritis." The Cochrane Collaboration, 2010, Available online at http://mrw.interscience.wiley.com/cochrane/clsysrev/articles/CD001977/image_n/CD001977_abstract.pdf.

13 T. Towheed *et al.* "Acetaminophen for Osteoarthritis." *Cochrane Database of Systematic Reviews*, 2010, Issue 9. Available online at http://www2.cochrane.org/reviews/en/ab004257.html.

14 Jon G. Divine *et al.* "Viscosupplementation for Knee Osteoarthritis." *Clinical Orthopaedics & Related Research*, 2007, February, Volume 455, 113–122. Available online at http://journals.lww.com/corr/Abstract/2007/02000/Viscosupplementation_for_Knee_Osteoarthritis__A.19.aspx.

15 Alexandra Kirkley *et al.* "A Randomized Trial of Arthroscopic Surgery for Osteoarthritis of the Knee." *New England Journal of Medicine*, 2008 September 11, Volume 359: 1097–1107. Available online at http://www.contentnejmorg.zuom.info/cgi/content/abstract/359/11/1097.

16 Mary Beth Hamel *et al.* "Joint Replacement Surgery in Elderly Patients with Severe Osteoarthritis of the Hip or Knee." *Archives of Internal Medicine*, 2008, 168(13): 1430–1440. Available online at http://archinte.ama-assn.org/cgi/content/abstract/168/13/1430.

17 Hegedus *et al.* "The effect of low-level laser in knee osteoarthritis." *Photomedicine and Laser Surgery*, 2009 Aug, 27(4): 577–84.

18 Roy D. Altman *et al.* "Improving Long-Term Management of Osteoarthritis: Strategies for Primary Care Physicians." *Journal of Family Practice*, 2009 February, Vol. 58, No. 2 Suppl: S17–S24. Available online at http://www.jfponline.com/Pages.asp?AID=7347.

19 "Ganglion Cysts." *Mayo Clinic*, 2010 July 1. Available online at http://www.mayoclinic.com/health/ganglion-cysts/DS00767/DSECTION=treatments-and-drugs.

20 Mavilde Arantes *et al.* "Spontaneous Hemorrhage in a Lumbar Ganglion Cyst." *Spine*, 2008 1 July, Volume 33, Issue 15, E521–E524. Available online at http://journals.lww.com/spinejournal/Abstract/2008/07010/Spontaneous_Hemorrhage_in_a_Lumbar_Ganglion_Cyst.23.aspx.

21 Statistics on Lupus. Lupus Foundation of America. Available online at http://www.lupus.org/webmodules/webarticlesnet/templates/new_newsroomreporters.aspx?articleid=247&zoneid=60.

22 Minami *et al.* "Diet and Systemic Lupus Erythematosus: A 4-Year Prospective Study of Japanese Patients." *Journal of Rheumatology*, 2003 Apr, 30(4): 747–54.

23 Amital, *et al.* "Serum Concentrations of 25-OH Vitamin D in Patients with Systemic Lupus Erythematosus (SLE) Are Inversely Related to Disease Activity: Is It Time to Routinely Supplement Patients with SLE with Vitamin D?" *Annals of Rheumatic Diseases*, 2010 Jun, 69(6): 1155–7.

24 S. A. Wright *et al.* "A Randomised Interventional Trial of Ω-3-Polyunsaturated Fatty Acids on Endothelial Function and Disease Activity in Systemic Lupus Erythematosus." *Annals of the Rheumatic Diseases*, 2008, 67: 841–848. Available online at http://ard.bmj.com/content/67/6/841.abstract.

25 Walton *et al.* "Dietary Fish Oil and the Severity of Symptoms in Patients with Systemic Lupus Erythematosus." *Annals of Rheumatic Diseases*, 1991 Jul, 50(7): 463–6.

26 Duffy *et al.* "The Clinical Effect of Dietary Supplementation with Omega-3 Fish Oils and/or Copper in Systemic Lupus Erythematosus." *Journal of Rheumatology*, 2004 Aug, 31(8): 1551–6.

27 Jill Nicole Barnes. "Habitual Exercise Is Associated with Reduced Arterial Stiffness in Systemic Lupus Erythematosus." *FASEB Journal*, 2010, 804.7. Available online at http://www.fasebj.org/cgi/content/meeting_abstract/24/1_MeetingAbstracts/804.7.

28 Chung-E Tseng. "The Effect of Moderate-Dose Corticosteroids in Preventing Severe Flares in Patients with Serologically Active, But Clinically Stable, Systemic Lupus Erythematosus." *Arthritis & Rheumatism*, 2006 October, Volume 54, Issue 11, 3623–3632. Available online at http://www3.interscience.wiley.com/journal/113446023/abstract?CRETRY=1&SRETRY=0.

29 Richard K. Burt *et al.* "Nonmyeloablative Hematopoietic Stem Cell Transplantation for Systemic Lupus Erythematosus." *Journal of the American Medical Association*, 2006, 295: 527–535. Available online at http://jama.ama-assn.org/cgi/content/abstract/295/5/527.

30 D. Crosbie, C. Black, L. McIntyre, *et al.* "Dehydroepiandrosterone for Systemic Lupus Erythematosus." *Cochrane Database of Systematic Reviews*, 2007, Issue 4. Available online at http://www2.cochrane.org/reviews/en/ab005114.html.

31 Iva Gunnarsson. "Histopathologic and Clinical Outcome of Rituximab Treatment in Patients with Cyclophosphamide-Resistant Proliferative Lupus Nephritis." *Arthritis & Rheumatism*, 2007, October, Volume 56, Issue 4, 1263–1272. Available online at http://www3.interscience.wiley.com/journal/114203625/abstract.

32 M. Hvatum *et al.* "The Gut–Joint Axis: Cross Reactive Food Antibodies in Rheumatoid Arthritis." *Gut Immunology*, 2006, 55: 1240–1247. Available online at http://gut.bmj.com/content/55/9/1240.abstract.

33 F. R. Pérez-López *et al.* "Effects of the Mediterranean Diet on Longevity and Age-Related Morbid Conditions." *Maturitas*, 2009 Oct 20, 64(2): 67–79.

34 Gillian E. Caughey *et al.* "Fish Oil Supplementation Increases the Cyclooxygenase Inhibitory Activity of Paracetamol in Rheumatoid Arthritis Patients." *Complementary Therapies in Medicine*, 2010. Available online at http://www.sciencedirect.com/science?_ob=ArticleURL&_udi=B6WCS-50G0F01-1&_user=10&_coverDate=07%2F05%2F2010&_rdoc=1&_fmt=high&_orig=search&_sort=d&_docanchor=&view=c&_searchStrId=1420057353&_rerunOrigin=scholar.google&_acct=C000050221&_version=1&_urlVersion=0&_userid=10&md5=97da5808e2b011b16d26f6949650f848.

35 Cheol Park *et al.* "Curcumin Induces Apoptosis and Inhibits Prostaglandin E2 Production in Synovial Fibroblasts of Patients with Rheumatoid Arthritis." *International Journal of Molecular Medicine*, 2007, vol. 20, no 3, 365–372. Available online at http://cat.inist.fr/?aModele=afficheN&cpsidt=19007328.

36 Lis Eversden *et al.* "A Pragmatic Randomised Controlled Trial of Hydrotherapy and Land Exercises on Overall Well Being and Quality of Life in Rheumatoid Arthritis." *BMC Musculoskeletal Disorders*. 2007, 8. Available online at http://www.biomedcentral.com/1471-2474/8/23/.

37 Mary J. Bell *et al.* "A Randomized Controlled Trial to Evaluate the Efficacy of Community Based Physical Therapy in the Treatment of People with Rheumatoid Arthritis." *Journal of Rheumatology*, 1998, 25: 231–7. Available online at https://www.cebp.nl/media/m951.pdf.

38 "The Chinese Herbal Remedy Tripterygium wilfordii Hook F in the Treatment of Rheumatoid Arthritis." *Annals of Internal Medicine*, 2009 August 18, vol. 151, no. 4, I-36. Available online at http://www.annals.org/content/151/4/I-36.full.

39 Till Uhlig. "Exploring Tai Chi in Rheumatoid Arthritis." *BMC Musculoskeletal Disorders*, 2010. Available online at http://www.biomedcentral.com/1471-2474/11/43/abstract/.

40 Alyssa M. Macedo *et al.* "Functional and Work Outcomes Improve in Patients with Rheumatoid Arthritis Who Receive Targeted, Comprehensive Occupational Therapy." *Arthritis Care & Research*, October 2009, Volume 61, Issue 11, 1522–1530. Available online at http://www3.interscience.wiley.com/journal/122666515/abstract.

41 Tiffany Field *et al.* "Hand Arthritis Pain Is Reduced by Massage Therapy." *Journal of Bodywork and Movement Therapies*, 2007 January, Volume 11, Issue 1, 21–24. Available online at http://www.bodyworkmovementthera-pies.com/article/S1360-8592(06)00108-2/abstract.

42 Masoumeh Bagheri-Nesami. "The Effect of Benson Relaxation Technique on Rheumatoid Arthritis Patients." *International Journal of Nursing Practice*, June 2006, Volume 12, Issue 4, 214–219. Available online at http://www3.interscience.wiley.com/journal/118584629/abstract.

43 D. L. Scott *et al.* "Tumor Necrosis Factor Inhibitors for Rheumatoid Arthritis." *New England Journal of Medicine*, 2006, vol. 355, 704–712. Available online at http://www.nejm.org/doi/full/10.1056/NEJMct055183.

44 "Adult Still's Disease." *Medline Plus*, 2009 February. Available online at http://www.nlm.nih.gov/medlineplus/ency/article/000450.htm.

45 M. B. Jacobsen, P. Aukrust, E. Kittang, *et al.* "Relation between Food Provocation and Systemic Immune Activation in Patients with Food Intolerance." *The Lancet*, 2000, 356:400–401.

46 Timo A. Lakka *et al.* "Exercise and Inflammation: Reply." *European Heart Journal*, 2006. 27 (11): 1385–1386. Available online at http://eurheartj.oxfordjournals.org/content/27/11/1385.2.full.

47 Sampalis *et al.* "Risk Factors for Adult Still's Disease." *Journal of Rheumatology*, 1996 Dec, 23(12): 2049–54. Available online at http://www.ncbi.nlm.nih.gov/pubmed/8970040.

48 Jacques Wouters *et al.* "Adult-Onset Still's Disease, Clinical and Laboratory Features, Treatment and Progress of 45 Cases." *Quarterly Journal of Mathematics*, (1986) 61 (2): 1055–1065.

49 Takao Fujii *et al.* "Methotrexate Treatment in Patients with Adult Onset Still's Disease—Retrospective Study of 13 Japanese Cases." *Annals of the Rheumatic Diseases*, 1997, 56:144–148. Available online at http://ard.bmj.com/content/56/2/144.abstract.

50 T. Babacan, *et al.* "Successful Treatment of Refractory Adult Still's Disease and Membranous Glomerulone-phritis with Infliximab." *Clinical Rheumatology*, 2010 Apr, 29(4): 423–6. E-pub 2010 Jan 26. Available online at http://www.ncbi.nlm.nih.gov/pubmed/20101429.

51 Lawrence H. Brent. "Ankylosing Spondylitis and Undifferentiated Spondyloarthropathy." May 6, 2010. Available online at http://emedicine.medscape.com/article/332945-overview.

52 Mazen Elyan and Muhammad Asim Khan. "Does Physical Therapy Still Have a Place in the Treatment of Ankylosing Spondylitis?" *Current Opinion in Rheumatology*, May 2008, Volume 20, Issue 3, 282–286. Available online at http://journals.lww.com/co-rheumatology/Abstract/2008/05000/Does_physical_therapy_still_have_a_place_in_the.10.aspx.

53 Sundstrom *et al.* "Supplementation of Omega-3 Fatty Acids in Patients with Ankylosing Spondylitis." *Scandinavian Journal of Rheumatology*, 2006 Sep-Oct, 35(5):359–62.

54 J. Braun *et al.* "Efficacy of Sulfasalazine in Patients with Inflammatory Back Pain Due to Undifferentiated Spondyloarthritis and Early Ankylosing Spondylitis." *Annals of the Rheumatic Diseases*, 2006, 65:1147–1153. Available online at http://ard.bmj.com/content/65/9/1147.abstract.

55 Désirée van der Heijde *et al.* "Efficacy and Safety of Adalimumab in Patients with Ankylosing Spondylitis." *Arthritis & Rheumatism*, Volume 54, Issue 7, 2136–2146, July 2006. Available online at http://onlinelibrary.wiley.com/doi/10.1002/art.21913/abstract.

56 Alexander A. Khalessi *et al.* "Medical Management of Ankylosing Spondylitis." *Neurosurgery Focus*, 2008 January, Volume 24. Available online at http://thejns.org/doi/pdf/10.3171/FOC/2008/24/1/E4.

Chapter 12

1 MarathonGuide.com. "USA Marathoning: 2007 Overview." Available online at http://www.marathonguide.com/features/Articles/2007RecapOverview.cfm.

2 Jean-Louis Croisier *et al.* "An Isokinetic Eccentric Programme for the Management of Chronic Lateral Epicondylar Tendinopathy." *British Journal of Sports Medicine*, 2007, 41: 269–275. Available online at http://bjsm.bmj.com/content/41/4/269.abstract.

3 N. Maffulli. "How Do Eccentric Exercises Work in Tendinopathy?" *Rheumatology*, 2008 Oct, 47(10): 1444–5.

4 Yang Gao. "Observations on the Efficacy of Acupuncture Plus Tuina Therapy in Treating Supraspinatus Tendonitis." *Journal of Acupuncture and Tuina Science*, 2009 April, Volume 7, Number 2, 94–97. Available online at http://www.springerlink.com/content/38771t8646708834/.

5 L. Brosseau *et al.* "Deep Transverse Friction Massage for Treating Tendinitis." *The Cochrane Library*, 2009, issue 1. Available online at http://onlinelibrary.wiley.com/store/mrw_content/cochrane/clsysrev/articles/CD003528/image_n/CD003528_abstract.pdf?v=1&t=ged2j8qq&s=8ae656e5e255ab2386578aaaca65421a2cc38e70.

6 C. Gaujoux-Viala. "Efficacy and Safety of Steroid Injections for Shoulder and Elbow Tendonitis." *Annals of the Rheumatic Diseases*, 2009, 68: 1843–1849. Available online at http://ard.bmj.com/content/68/12/1843.short.

7 *Ibid.*

8 O. Oken, "The Short-Term Efficacy of Laser, Brace, and Ultrasound Treatment in Lateral Epicondylitis." *Journal of Hand Therapy*, 2008 Jan–Mar, 21(1): 63–8. Available online at http://www.healinglightseminars.com/listing/Arthritis%20-%20Elbow.pdf.

9 *Ibid.*

10 National & International Statistics for Carpal Tunnel Syndrome and Repetitive Strain Injuries of the Upper Extremity. Available online at http://www.repetitive-strain.com/national.html.

11 Milly Ryan-Harshman. "Carpal Tunnel Syndrome and Vitamin B6." *Canadian Family Physician*, 2007 July, Vol. 53, No. 7, 1161–1162. Available online at http://www.cfp.ca/cgi/content/abstract/53/7/1161.

12 G. Di Geronimo. "Treatment of Carpal Tunnel Syndrome With Alpha-Lipoic Acid." *European Review for Medical and Pharmacological Sciences*, 2009 Mar–Apr, 13(2): 133–9. Available online at http://www.ncbi.nlm.nih.gov/pubmed/19499849.

13 O. Baysal *et al.* "Comparison of Three Conservative Treatment Protocols In Carpal Tunnel Syndrome." *International Journal of Clinical Practice*, May 2006, Volume 60, Issue 7, 820–828. Available online at http://www3.interscience.wiley.com/journal/118555981/abstract?CRETRY=1&SRETRY=0.

14 Bo Povlsen. "Managing Type II Work-Related Upper Limb Disorders in Keyboard and Mouse Users Who Remain at Work." *Journal of Hand Therapy*, 2008, 21: 69–79. Available online at http://www.handconsult.com/pubs/Managing%20Type%20II%20Work%20Related%20Upper%20Limb%20Disorders.pdf.

15 Moraska *et al.* "Comparison of a Targeted and General Massage Protocol on Albert Strength, Function, and Symptoms Associated with Carpal Tunnel Syndrome." *Journal of Alternative and Complementary Medicine*, 2008 April, 14(3): 259–267 Available online at http://www.liebertonline.com/doi/abs/10.1089/acm.2007.0647.

16 Yang *et al.* "Acupuncture in Patients with Carpal Tunnel Syndrome." *Clinical Journal of Pain*, 2009 May, 25(4): 327–33.

17 V. Napadow *et al.* "Hypothalamus and Amygdala Response To Acupuncture Stimuli In Carpal Tunnel Syndrome." *Pain*, 2007 August, Volume 130, Issue 3, 254–266. Available online at http://www.painjournalonline.com/article/S0304-3959(06)00668-3/abstract.

18 S. Marshall *et al.* "Local Corticosteroid Injection for Carpal Tunnel Syndrome." *The Cochrane Library*, 2008, Issue 4. Available online at http://www.unilim.fr/campus-neurochirurgie/IMG/cochrane__corticoides_locaux__syndrome_du_canal_carpien.pdf.

19 R. J. Verdugo *et al.* "Surgical Versus Non-Surgical Treatment for Carpal Tunnel Syndrome." *The Cochrane Collaboration*, 2008, issue 4. Available online at http://mrw.interscience.wiley.com/cochrane/clsysrev/articles/CD001552/image_n/CD001552_abstract.pdf

20 Stacey H. Berner *et al.* "Pain from Carpal Tunnel Syndrome Reduce with Dynamic Splinting." *Journal of Clinical Medicine and Research*, 2009, vol. 1, 22–25. Available online at http://www.dynasplint.com/uploads/references/12.%20Berner%20et%20al%20Carpal%20Tunnel_1.pdf/

21 Joan Lappe *et al.* "Calcium and Vitamin D Supplementation Decreases Incidence of Stress Fractures in Female Navy Recruits." *Journal of Bone and Mineral Research*, 2008 February, vol. 23, 741–749. Available online at http:// onlinelibrary.wiley.com/doi/10.1359/jbmr.080102/abstract/.

22 W. Brent Edwards. "Effects of Reducing Stride Length and Shoe Stiffness on the Probability of Tibial Stress Fracture." *Medicine & Science in Sports & Exercise*, 2009 May, Volume 41, Issue 5, 4–5. Available online at http://journals.lww.com/acsm-msse/Citation/2009/05001/Effects_Of_Reducing_Stride_Length_And_Shoe.735.aspx.

23 David A. Porter *et al.* "Intramedullary Screw Fixation for Chronic Proximal Fourth Metatarsal Stress Fractures: A New Technique for the Fourth Metatarsal 'Jones.'" *Techniques in Foot & Ankle Surgery*, 2010 September,Volume 9, Issue 3, 147–153. Available online at http://journals.lww.com/techfootankle/Abstract/2010/09000/Intramedullary_Screw_Fixation_for_Chronic_Proximal.12.aspx.

24 Joseph S. Torg *et al.* "Management of Tarsal Navicular Stress Fractures." *American Journal of Sports Medicine*, 2010 May, vol. 38, no. 5, 1048–1053. Available online at http://ajs.sagepub.com/content/38/5/1048.abstract.

25 Rebecca A. Snyder. "Does Shoe Insole Modification Prevent Stress Fractures?" Hospital for Special Surgery Journal, 2009 September, vol. 5, 92–98. Available online at http://www.springerlink.com/content/2225pl1lx24563p1/.

26 Gamze Senbursa *et al.* "Comparison of Conservative Treatment with and without Manual Physical Therapy for Patients with Shoulder Impingement Syndrome." *Knee Surgery, Sports Traumatology, Arthroscopy*, 2007 28 February, Vol. 15, 915–21. Available online at http://www.springerlink.com/content/u5153h56t8763115/.

27 J. I. Jian-you. "Treatment of Shoulder Impingement Syndrome by Tuina and Acupuncture Plus Functional Training." *Journal of Acupuncture and Tuina Science*, 2008 February, Volume 6, Number 1, 56–57. Available online at http://www.springerlink.com/content/6170txv0525j7353/.

28 Paul A van den Dolder and David L Roberts. "A Trial into the Effectiveness of Soft Tissue Massage in the Treatment of Shoulder Pain." *Australian Journal of Physiotherapy*, 2003, Vol. 49, 183–8. Available online at http://svc019.wic048p.server-web.com/AJP/vol_49/3/AustJPhysiotherv49i3Van%20Den%20Dolder.pdf.

29 S. Karthikeyan *et al.* "Randomised Controlled Study Comparing Subacromial Nsaid (Tenoxicam) and Steroid (Methylprednisolone) Injection in Patients with Shoulder Impingement Syndrome." *Journal of Bone and Joint Surgery* (British volume), Vol 91-B, Issue SUPP_I, 121–122. Copyright © 2009. Available online at http://proceedings.jbjs.org.uk/cgi/content/abstract/91-B/SUPP_I/121-d.

30 Simon W. Young *et al.* "The SMR Reverse Shoulder Prosthesis in the Treatment of Cuff-Deficient Shoulder Conditions." *Journal of Shoulder and Elbow Surgery*, 2009 July, Volume 18, Issue 4, 622–62. Available online at http://www.jshoulderelbow.org/article/S1058-2746(09)00082-2/abstract.

31 Peter Miller, *et al.* "Does Scapula Taping Facilitate Recovery for Shoulder Impingement Symptoms?" *Journal of Manual & Manipulative Therapy*, 2009, 17(1): E6–E13. Available online at http://www.ncbi.nlm.nih.gov/pmc/articles/PMC2704341/.

32 B. Orlando *et al.* "Efficacy of Physical Therapy in the Treatment of Masticatory Myofascial Pain." *Minerva Stomatologica*, 2006 Jun, 55(6): 355–66. Available online at http://www.ncbi.nlm.nih.gov/pubmed/16971881.

33 Johannes Fleckenstein *et al.* "Discrepancy between Prevalence and Perceived Effectiveness of Treatment Methods in Myofascial Pain Syndrome." *BMC Musculoskeletal Disorders*, 2010, 11: 32. Available online at http://www.biomedcentral.com/1471-2474/11/32/abstract/.

34 John Paolini. "Review of Myofascial Release as an Effective Massage Therapy Technique." *Athletic Therapy Today*, 2009 September, 30–34. Available online at http:// hk.humankinetics.com/eJournalMedia/pdfs/17347.pdf.

35 Meltem Esenyel *et al.* "Myofascial Pain Syndrome: Efficacy of Different Therapies." *Journal of Back and Musculoskeletal Rehabilitation*, 2007, Volume 20, Number 1, 43–47. Available online at http://iospress.metapress.com/content/k87h0g723x20070l/.

36 Phil Smith *et al.* "The Efficacy of Acupuncture in the Treatment of Temporomandibular Joint Myofascial Pain." *Journal of Dentistry*, 35 (3), 259–267. Available online at http://research-archive.liv.ac.uk/455/.

37 Giannapia Affaitati *et al.* "A Randomized, Controlled Study Comparing a Lidocaine Patch, a Placebo Patch, and Anesthetic Injection for Treatment of Trigger Points in Patients with Myofascial Pain Syndrome." *Clinical Therapeutics*, 2009 April, Volume 31, Issue 4, 705–720. Available online at http://www.sciencedirect.com/science?_ob=ArticleURL&_udi=B6VRS-4W90NCX-3&_user=10&_coverDate=04%2F30%2F2009&_rdoc=1&_fmt=high&_orig=search&_origin=search&_sort=d&_docanchor=&view=c&_searchStrId=1478573363&_rerunOrigin=scholar.google&_acct=C000050221&_version=1&_urlVersion=0&_userid=10&md5=3bb4e5d5a9a4ece76b601ac0901697ec&searchtype=a.

38 Mayo Clinic. "Acupuncture And Myofascial Trigger Therapy Treat Same Pain Areas." *Science Daily*, 2008 May 14. Available online at http://www.sciencedaily.com /releases/2008/05/080513101614.htm.

39 G. Syme *et al.* "Disability in Patients with Chronic Patellofemoral Pain Syndrome: A Randomised Controlled Trial of VMO Selective Training Versus General Quadriceps Strengthening." *Manual Therapy*, 2009 June, Volume 14, Issue 3, 252–263. Available online at http://www.manualtherapyjournal.com/article/S1356-689X(08)00053-2/abstract.

40 Guy Hains. "Patellofemoral Pain Syndrome Managed by Ischemic Compression to the Trigger Points Located in the Peri-Patellar and Retro-Patellar Areas." *Clinical Chiropractic*, 2010, doi: 10.1016/j.clch.2010.05.001. Available online at http://www.sciencedirect.com/science?_ob=ArticleURL&_udi=B758B-50H1HHB-1&_user=10&_coverDate=07%2F10%2F2010&_rdoc=1&_fmt=high&_orig=search&_sort=d&_docanchor=&view=c&_searchStrId=1423229295&_rerunOrigin=scholar.google&_acct=C000050221&_version=1&_urlVersion=0&_userid=10&md5=b31f8a0168056180d648d84a1ee35b51.

41 G. J. Tang *et al.* "Clinical Observation of Arthroscopic Medial Patellofemoral Ligament Overlap and Lateral Patellar Retinaculum Release in Treatment of Patellofemoral Pain Syndrome." *Zhongguo Gu Shang*, 2008 Jul, 21(7): 507–9. Available online at http://www.ncbi.nlm.nih.gov/pubmed/19102149.

42 Jyrki A. Kettunen *et al.* "Knee Arthroscopy and Exercise Versus Exercise Only for Chronic Patellofemoral Pain Syndrome." *BMC Medicine*, 2007, 5: 38doi: 10.1186/1741-7015-5-38. Available online at http://www.biomedcentral.com/1741-7015/5/38/.

43 Aditya Derasari. "McConnell Taping Shifts the Patella Inferiorly in Patients with Patellofemoral Pain: A Dynamic Magnetic Resonance Imaging Study." *Physical Therapy*, Vol. 90, No. 3, March 2010, 411–419. Available online at http://physicaltherapyjournal.com/cgi/content/abstract/90/3/411.

Chapter 13

1 M. M. Collins, J. B. Meigs, M. J. Barry, *et al.* "Prevalence and Correlates of Prostatitis in the Health Professionals Follow-Up Study Cohort." *Journal of Urology*, 2002, 167(3), 1363–6.

2 J. Q. Clemens, R. T. Meenan, M. C. O'Keeffe Rosetti, *et al.* 2005, "Prevalence of Interstitial Cystitis Symptoms in a Managed Care Population." *Journal of Urology*, 174(2), 576–80.

3 P. Latthe, M. Latthe, L. Say, M. Gulmezoglu, K. S. Khan. "WHO Systematic Review of Prevalence of Chronic Pelvic Pain: A Neglected Reproductive Health Morbidity." *BMC Public Health*, 2006, 6, 177.

4 J. Abbott. "Gynecological Indications for the Use of Botulinum Toxin in Women with Chronic Pelvic Pain." *Toxicon*, 2009, 54(5), 647–53.

5 X. Zhu, M. Proctor, A. Bensoussan, *et al.* "Chinese Herbal Medicine for Primary Dysmenorrhoea." *Cochrane Database of Systematic Reviews*, 2008, (2), CD005288.

6 A. H. Clayton. "Symptoms Related to the Menstrual Cycle: Diagnosis, Prevalence, and Treatment." *Journal of Psychiatric Practice*, 2008, 14(1), 13–21.

7 N. F. Woods, A. Most, and G. K. Dery. "Prevalene of Perimenstrual Symptoms." *American Journal of Public Health*, 1982, 72(11), 1257–64.

8 V. Lundstrom, K. Green, and K. Svanborg. "Endogenous Prostagland ins in Dysmenorrhea and the Effect of Prostagland in Synthetase Inhibitors (PGSI) on Uterine Contractility." *Acta Obstetricia et Gynecologica Scandinavica* Supplement, 1979, 87, 51–6.

9 J. Marjoribanks, M. Proctor, C. Farquhar, *et al.* "Nonsteroidal Anti-Inflammatory Drugs for Dysmenorrhoea." *Cochrane Database of Systematic Reviews*, 2010, (1), CD001751.

10 M. D. Akin, K. W. Weingand , D. A. Hengehold, *et al.* "Continuous Low-Level Topical Heat in the Treatment of Dysmenorrhea." *Obstetrics & Gynecology*, 2001, 97(3), 343–9.

11 L. Wang, X. Wang, W. Wang, *et al.* 2004. Stress and dysmenorrhoea: a population based propective study. *Occup Environ Med.* 61(12), 1021-6.

12 L. B. Gordley, G. Lemasters, S. R. Simpson, *et al.* "Menstrual Disorders and Occupational, Stress, and Racial Factors among Military Personnel." *Journal of Occupational & Environmental Medicine*, 2000, 42(9), 871–81.

13 M. L. Proctor, C. A. Smith, C. M. Farquhar, *et al.* "Transcutaneous Electrical Nerve Stimulation and Acupuncture for Primary Dysmenorrhoea." *Cochrane Database of Systematic Reviews*, 2002, (1), CD002123.

14 J. Brown and S. Brown. "Exercise for Dysmenorrhoea." *Cochrane Database of Systematic Reviews*, 2010, 2, CD004142.

15 S. Ziaei, M. Zakeri, and A. Kazemnejad. "A Randomised Controlled Trial of Vitamin E in the Treatment of Primary Dysmenorrhoea." *British Journal of Obstetrics and Gynecology*, 2005, 112(4), 466–9.

16 M. L. Proctor and P. A. Murphy. "Herbal and Dietary Therapies for Primary and Secondary Dysmenorrhoea." *Cochrane Database of Systematic Reviews*, 2001, (3), CD002124.

17 W. Jia, X. Wang, D. Xu, *et al.* "Common Traditional Chinese Medicinal Herbs for Dysmenorrhea." *Phytotherapy Research*, 2006, 20(10), 819–24.

18 C. L. Wong, C. Farquhar, H. Roberts, *et al.* "Oral Contraceptive Pill for Primary Dysmenorrhoea." *Cochrane Database of Systematic Reviews*, 2009, (4), CD002120.

19 A. L. Nelson. "Communicating with Patients about Extended-Cycle and Continuous Use of Oral Contraceptives." *Journal of Women's Health (Larchmt)*, 2007, 16(4), 463–70.

20 X. Zhu, M. Proctor, A. Bensoussan, *et al.* "Chinese Herbal Medicine for Primary Dysmenorrhoea." *Cochrane Database of Systematic Reviews*, 2008, (2), CD005288.

21 W. Jia, X. Wang, D. Xu, *et al.*

22 M. L. Proctor and P. A. Murphy. "Herbal and Dietary Therapies for Primary and Secondary Dysmenorrhoea." *Cochrane Database of Systematic Reviews*, 2001, (3), CD002124.

23 K. B. Lloyd and L. B. Hornsby. "Complementary and Alternative Medications for Women's Health Issues." *Nutrition in Clinical Practice*, 2009, 24(5), 589–608.

24 Office of Dietary Supplements, National Institutes of Health 2009. "Magnesium." Retrieved from http://ods.od.nih.gov/factsheets/magnesium.aspon 8/6/2020.

25 N. Suzuki, K. Uebaba, T. Kohama, *et al.* "French Maritime Pine Bark Extract Significantly Lowers the Requirement for Analgesic Medication on Dysmenorrhea." *Journal of Reproductive Medicine*, 2008, 53(5), 338–46.

26 R. Canali, R. Comitato, F. Schonlau, *et al.* "The Anti-Inflammatory Pharmacology of Pycnogenol in Humans Involves COX-2 and 5-LOX mRNA Expression in Leukocytes." *International Immunopharmacology*, 2009, 9(10), 1145–9.

27 E. S. Ford, U. A. Ajani, A. H. Mokdad. "Brief Communication: The Prevalence of High Intake of Vitamin E from the Use of Supplements among U.S. Adults." *Annals of Internal Medicine*, 2005, 143,116–20.

28 S. Ziaei, M. Zakeri, A. Kazemnejad. "A Randomised Controlled Trial of Vitamin E in the Treatment of Primary Dysmenorrhoea." *British Journal of Obstetrics and Gynecology*, 2005, 112(4), 466–9.

29 Office of Dietary Supplements, National Institutes of Health. "Vitamin E." 2009 Health Professional Fact Sheet. Retrieved from http://ods.od.nih.gov/factsheets/vitamine.asp on 8/6/2020.

30 M. K. Jahromi, A. Gaeini, Z. Rahimi. "Influence of a Physical Fitness Course on Menstrual Cycle Characteristics." Gynecological Endocrinology, 2008, 24(11), 659–62.

31 J. Brown and S. Brown. "Exercise for Dysmenorrhoea." *Cochrane Database of Systematic Reviews*, 2, 2010, CD004142.

31 A. Daley. "The Role of Exercise in the Treatment of Menstrual Disorders: The Evidence." *British Journal of General Practice*, 2009, 59(561), 241–2.

33 M. D. Akin, K. W. Weingand , D. A. Hengehold, *et al.* "Continuous Low-Level Topical Heat in the Treatment of Dysmenorrhea." *Obstetrics & Gynecology*, 2001, 97(3), 343–9.

34 M. Akin, W. Price, G. Rodriguez, Jr., *et al.* "Continuous, Low-Level, Topical Heat Wrap Therapy as Compared to Acetaminophen for Primary Dysmenorrhea." *Journal of Reproductive Medicine*, 2004, 49(9), 739–45.

35 S. H. Han, M. H. Hur, J. Buckle, *et al.* "Effect of Aromatherapy on Symptoms of Dysmenorrhea in College Students." *Journal of Alternative and Complementary Medicine*, 2006, 12(6), 535–41.

36 M. L. Proctor, W. Hing, T. C. Johnson, and P. A. Murphy. "Spinal Manipulation for Primary and Secondary Dysmenorrhoea." *Cochrane Database of Systematic Reviews*, 2006, 3, CD002119.

37 L. B. Gokhale. "Curative Treatment of Primary (Spasmodic) Dysmenorrhoea." *Indian Journal of Medical Research*, 1996, 103, 227–31.

38 G. A. Eby. "Zinc Treatment Prevents Dysmenorrhea." *Med Hypotheses*, 2007, 69(2), 297–301.

39 H. A. Schiotz, M. Jettestad, and D. Al-Heeti. "Treatment of Dysmenorrhoea with w New TENS Device (OVA)." *American Journal of Obstetrics & Gynecology*, 2007, 27(7), 726–8.

40 M. L. Proctor, C. A. Smith, C. M. Farquhar, R. W. Stones. "Transcutaneous Electrical Nerve Stimulation and Acupuncture for Primary Dysmenorrhoea." *Cochrane Database of Systematic Reviews*, 2002, (1), CD002123.

41 D. Taylor, C. Miaskowski, and J. Kohn. "A Randomized Clinical Trial of the Effectiveness of an Acupressure Device (Relief Brief) for Managing Symptoms of Dysmenorrhea." *Journal of Alternative and Complementary Medicine*, 2002, 8(3), 357–70.

42 S. H. Cho and E. W. Hwang. "Acupuncture for Primary Dysmenorrhoea: A Systematic Review." *British Journal of Obstetrics and Gynecology*, 2010, 117(5), 509–21.

43 S. H. Cho and E. W. Hwang. "Acupuncture Primary Dysmenorrhoea: A Systematic Review." *Complementary Therapies in Medicine*, 2010, 18(1), 49–56.

44 L. Wang, X. Wang, W. Wang, *et al.* "Stress and dysmenorrhoea: a population based prospective study." *Occup Environ Med*, 61(12), 1021-6.

45 L. B. Gordley, G. Lemasters, S. R. Simpson, *et al.* "Menstrual Disorders and Occupational, Stress, and Racial Factors among Military Personnel." *Journal of Occupational & Environmental Medicine*, 2000, 42(9), 871–81.

46 M. L. Proctor, P. A. Murphy, H. M. Pattison, *et al.*"Behavioural Interventions for Primary and Secondary Dysmenorrhoea." *Cochrane Database of Systematic Reviews*, 2007, (3), CD002248.

47 J. Marjoribanks, M. Proctor, C. Farquhar, *et al.* "Nonsteroidal Anti-Inflammatory Drugs for Dysmenorrhea." *Cochrane Database of Systematic Reviews*, 2010, (1), CD001751.

48 H. P. Zahradnik, A. Hanjalic-Beck, and K. Groth. "Nonsteroidal Anti-Inflammatory Drugs and Hormonal Contraceptives for Pain Relief from Dysmenorrhea." *Contraception*, 2010, 81(3), 185–96.

49 C. L. Wong, C. Farquhar, H. Roberts, *et al.* "Oral Contraceptive Pill for Primary Dysmenorrhoea." *Cochrane Database of Systematic Reviews*, 2009, (4), CD002120.

50 D. F. Archer. "Menstrual-Cycle-Related Symptoms: A Review of the Rationale for Continuous Use of Oral Contraceptives." *Contraception*, 2006, 74(5), 359–66.

51 K. Stein and C. Ascher-Walsh. "A Comprehensive Approach to the Treatment of Uterine Leiomyomata." *Mount Sinai Journal of Medicine*, 2009, 76(6), 546–56.

52 H. Divakar. "Asymptomatic Uterine Fibroids." *Best Practice & Research Clinical Obstetrics & Gynaecology*, 22(4), 2008, 643–54.

53 P. Evans and S. Brunsell. "Uterine Fibroid Tumors: Diagnosis and Treatment." *American Family Physician*, 75(10), 2007, 1503–8.

54 J. Askew. "A Qualitative Comparison of Women's Attitudes toward Hysterectomy and Myomectomy." *Health Care for Women International*, 2009, 30(8), 728–42.

55 K. L. Terry, I. De Vivo, S. E. Hankinson, *et al.* "Reproductive Characteristics and Risk of Uterine Leiomyomata." *Fertility and Sterility*, 2010.

56 V. L. Jacoby, V. Y. Fujimoto, L. C. Giudice, *et al.* "Racial and Ethnic Disparities in Benign Gynecologic Conditions and Associated Surgeries." *American Journal of Obstetrics & Gynecology*, 2010, 202(6), 514–21.

57 L. A. Wise, R. G. Radin, J. R. Palmer, *et al.* "A Prospective Study of Dairy Intake and Risk of Uterine Leiomyomata." *American Journal of Epidemiology*, 2010, 171(2), 221–32.

58 R. G. Radin, J. R. Palmer, L. Rosenberg, *et al.* "Dietary Glycemic Index and Load in Relation to Risk of Uterine Leiomyomata in the Black Women's Health Study." *American Journal of Clinical Nutrition*, 2010, 91(5), 1281–8.

59 F.Chiaffarino, F. Parazzini, C.La Vecchia, *et al.* Diet and Uterine Myomas." *Obstetrics & Gynecology*, 1999, 94(3), 395–8.

60 C. Nagata, K. Nakamura, S. Oba, *et al.* "Association of Intakes of Fat, Dietary Fibre, Soya Isoflavones and Alcohol with Uterine Fibroids in Japanese Women." *British Journal of Nutrition*, 2009, 101(10), 1427–31.

61 D. D. Baird, D. B. Dunson, M. C. Hill, *et al.* "Association of Physical Activity with Development of Uterine Leiomyoma." *American Journal of Epidemiology*, 2007, 165(2), 157–63.

62 A. M. Kaunitz. "Progestin-Releasing Intrauterine Systems and Leiomyoma." *Contraception*, 2007, 75(6 Suppl), S130-3.

63 S.Soysal and M. E. Soysal. "The Efficacy of Levonorgestrel-Releasing Intrauterine Device in Selected Cases of Myoma-Related Menorrhagia." *Gynecologic and Obstetric Investigation*, 2005, 59(1), 29–35.

64 R. Varma, D. Sinha, and J. K. Gupta. "Non-Contraceptive Uses of Levonorgestrel-Releasing Hormone System (LNG-IUS)—A Systematic Enquiry and Overview." *European Journal of Obstetrics & Gynecology and Reproductive Biology*, 2006, 125(1), 9–28.

65 S. Venkatachalam, J. S. Bagratee, and J. Moodley. "Medical Management of Uterine Fibroids with Medroxyprogesterone Acetate (Depo-Provera)." *American Journal of Obstetrics & Gynecology*, 2004, 24(7), 798–800.

66 F. Chiaffarino, F. Parazzini, C. La Vecchia, *et al.* "Use of Oral Contraceptives and Uterine Fibroids: Results from a Case-Control Study." *British American Journal of Obstetrics & Gynecology*, 1999, 106(8), 857–60.

67 M. Bagaria, A. Suneja, N. B. Vaid, *et al.* "Low-Dose Mifepristone in Treatment of Uterine Leiomyoma." *Australian and New Zealand Journal of Obstetrics & Gynecology*, 2009, 49(1), 77–83.

68 G. K. Hesley, J. P. Felmlee, J. B. Gebhart, *et al.* "Noninvasive Treatment of Uterine Fibroids: Early Mayo Clinic Experience with Magnetic Resonance Imaging-Guided Focused Ultrasound." *Mayo Clinic Proceedings*, 2006, 81(7), 936–42.

69 J. P. Pelage, O. Le Dref, J. P. Beregi, *et al.* "Limited Uterine Artery Embolization with Tris-Acryl Gelatin Microspheres for Uterine Fibroids." *Journal of Vascular and Interventional Radiology*, 2003, 14(1), 15–20.

70 N. Berkane and C. Moutafoff-Borie. "Impact of Previous Uterine Artery Embolization on Fertility." *Current Opinion in Obstetrics & Gynecology*, 2010, 22(3), 242–7.

71 B. S. Levy. "Modern Management of Uterine Fibroids." *Acta Obstetricia et Gynecologica Scandinavica*, 2008, 87(8), 812–23.

72 A. Khaund and M. A. Lumsden. "Impact of Fibroids on Reproductive Function." *Best Practice & Research Clinical Obstetrics & Gynaecology*, 2008, 22(4), 749–60.

73 E. A. Pritts, W. H. Parker, and D. L. Olive. "Fibroids and Infertility: An Updated Systematic Review of the Evidence." *Fertility and Sterility*, 2009, 91(4), 1215–23.

74 A. Singh and S. Bansal. "Comparative Study of Morbidity and Mortality Associated with Nondescent Vaginal Hysterectomy and Abdominal Hysterectomy Based on Ultrasonographic Determination of Uterine Volume." *International Surgery*, 2008, 93(2), 88–94.

75 C. Schindlbeck, K. Klauser, D. Dian, *et al.* "Comparison of Total Laparoscopic, Vaginal and Abdominal Hysterectomy." *Archives of Gynecology and Obstetrics*, 2008, 277(4), 331–7.

76 I. M. Spitz. "Clinical Utility of Progesterone Receptor Modulators and Their Effect on the Endometrium." *Current Opinion in Obstetrics & Gynecology*, 2009, 21(4), 318–24.

77 C. Feng, S. Meldrum, and K. Fiscella. "Improved Quality of Life Is Partly Explained by Fewer Symptoms after Treatment of Fibroids with Mifepristone." *International Journal of Gynecology & Obstetrics*, 2010, 109(2), 121–4.

78 S. G. Hilario, N. Bozzini, R. Borsari, *et al.* "Action of Aromatase Inhibitor for Treatment of Uterine Leiomyoma in Perimenopausal Patients." *Fertility and Sterility*, 2009, 91(1), 240–3.

79 P. Vercellini, L. Trespidi, B. Zaina, *et al.* "Gonadotropin-Releasing Hormone Agonist Treatment before Abdominal Myomectomy." *Fertility and Sterility*, 2003, 79(6), 1390–5.

80 H. Divakar. "Asymptomatic Uterine Fibroids." *Best Practice & Research Clinical Obstetrics & Gynaecology*, 2008, 22(4), 643–54.

81 K. Arisawa, H. Takeda, and H. Mikasa. "Background Exposure to PCDDs/PCDFs/PCBs and Its Potential Health Effects: A Review of Epidemiologic Studies." *Journal of Investigative Medicine*, 2005, 52(1-2), 10–21.

82 W. G. Foster and S. K. Agarwal. "Environmental Contaminants and Dietary Factors in Endometriosis." *Annals of the New York Academy of Sciences*, 2002, 955, 213–29; discussion 230–2, 396–406.

83 P. C. Klatsky, N. D. Tran, A. B. Caughey, *et al.* "Fibroids and Reproductive Outcomes: A Systematic Literature Review from Conception to Delivery." *American Journal of Obstetrics & Gynecology*, 2008, 198(4), 357–66.

84 L. C. Giudice. "Clinical practice. Endometriosis." *New England Journal of Medicine*, 2010, 362(25), 2389–98.

85 S. Simoens, L. Hummelshoj, and T. D'Hooghe. "Endometriosis: Cost Estimates and Methodological Perspective." *Human Reproduction Update*, 2007,13(4), 395–404.

86 B. S. McLeod and M. G. Retzloff. "Epidemiology of Endometriosis: An Assessment of Risk Factors." *Clinical Obstetrics & Gynecology*, 2010, 53(2), 389–96.

87 K. Hansen, A. Chalpe, and K. Eyster. "Management of Endometriosis-Associated Pain." *Clinical Obstetrics & Gynecology*, 2010, 53(2), 439–448.

88 X. Gao, J. Outley, M. Botteman, *et al.* "Economic Burden of Endometriosis." *Fertility and Sterility*, 2006, 86(6), 1561–72.

89 I. C. Green, S. L. Cohen, D. Finkenzeller, *et al.* "Interventional Therapies for Controlling Pelvic Pain: What Is the Evidence?" *Current Pain and Headache Reports*, 2010, 14(1), 22–32.

90 C. Allen, S. Hopewell, A. Prentice, *et al.* "Nonsteroidal Anti-Inflammatory Drugs for Pain in Women with Endometriosis." *Cochrane Database of Systematic Reviews*, 2009, (2), CD004753.

91 P. Sepulcri Rde and V. F. do Amaral. "Depressive Symptoms, Anxiety, and Quality of Life in Women with Pelvic Endometriosis." *European Journal of Obstetrics & Gynecology and Reproductive Biology*, 2009, 142(1), 53–6.

92 C. Lorencatto, C. A. Petta, M. J. Navarro, *et al.* "Depression in Women with Endometriosis with and without Chronic Pelvic Pain." *Acta Obstetricia et Gynecologica Scandinavica*, 2006, 85(1), 88–92.

93 C. D. Greco. "Management of Adolescent Chronic Pelvic Pain from Endometriosis: A Pain Center Perspective." Journal of Pediatric and Adolescent Gynecology, 2003, 16(3 Suppl), S17–9.

94 C. J. Sutton, A. S. Pooley, S. P. Ewen, *et al.* "Follow-Up Report on a Randomized Controlled Trial of Laser Laparoscopy in the Treatment pf Pelvic Pain Associated with Minimal to Moderate Endometriosis." *Fertility and Sterility*, 1997, 68(6), 1070–4.

95 S. Ferrero, V. Remorgida, P. L. Venturini. "Current Pharmacotherapy for Endometriosis." *Expert Opinion on Pharmacotherapy*, 2010, 11(7), 1123–34.

96 P. P. Yeung, Jr., J. Shwayder, and R. P. Pasic. "Laparoscopic Management of Endometriosis." *Journal of Minimally Invasive Gynecology*, 2009, 16(3), 269–81.

97 S. W. Guo. "Emerging Drugs for Endometriosis." *Expert Opinion on Emerging Drugs*, 2008, 13(4), 547–71.

98 F. Wieser, M. Cohen, A. Gaeddert, *et al.* "Evolution of Medical Treatment for Endometriosis: Back to the Roots?" *Human Reproduction Update*, 2007, 13(5), 487–99.

99 S. A. Missmer, J. E. Chavarro, S. Malspeis, *et al.* "A Prospective Study of Dietary Fat Consumption and Endometriosis Risk." *Human Reproduction*, 2010, 25(6), 1528–35.

100 T. Kohama, K. Herai, and M.Inoue. "Effect of French Maritime Pine Bark Extract on Endometriosis as Compared with Leuprorelin Acetate." *Journal of Reproductive Medicine*, 2007, 52(8), 703–8.

101 F. Parazzini, F. Chiaffarino, M. Surace, *et al.* "Selected Food Intake and Risk of Endometriosis." *Human Reproduction*, 2004, 19(8), 1755–9.

102 A. Flower, J. P. Liu, S. Chen, *et al.* "Chinese Herbal Medicine for Endometriosis." *Cochrane Database of Systematic Reviews*, 2009, (3), CD006568.

103 F. Sesti, A. Pietropolli, T. Capozzolo, *et al.* "Hormonal Suppression Treatment or Dietary Therapy Versus Placebo in the Control of Painful Symptoms after Conservative Surgery for Endometriosis Stage III-IV." *Fertility and Sterility*, 2007, 88(6), 1541–7.

104 F. B. Lockhat, J. O. Emembolu, and J. C. Konje. "The Efficacy, Side-Effects and Continuation Rates in Women with Symptomatic Endometriosis Undergoing Treatment with an Intra-Uterine Administered Progestogen (Levonorgestrel): A 3- Year Follow-Up." *Human Reproduction*, 2005, 20(3), 789–93.

105 A. M. Abou-Setta, H. G. Al-Inany, and C. M. Farquhar. "Levonorgestrel-Releasing Intrauterine Device (LNG-IUD) for Symptomatic Endometriosis Following Surgery." *Cochrane Database of Systematic Reviews*, 2006, (4), CD005072.

106 W. D. Schlaff, S. A. Carson, A. Luciano, *et al.* "Subcutaneous Injection of Depot Medroxyprogesterone Acetate Compared with Leuprolide Acetate in the Treatment of Endometriosis-Associated Pain." *Fertility and Sterility*, 2006, 85(2), 314–25.

107 K. W. Schweppe. "Long-Term Use of Progestogens—Effects on Endometriosis, Adenomyosis and Myomas." *Gynecological Endocrinology*, 2007, 23 Suppl 1, 17–21.

108 R. Seracchioli, M. Mabrouk, C. Frasca, *et al.* "Long-Term Oral Contraceptive Pills and Postoperative Pain Management after Laparoscopic Excision of Ovarian Endometrioma." *Fertility and Sterility*, 2010, 94(2), 464–71.

109 P. Vercellini, G. Frontino, O. De Giorgi, *et al.* "Continuous Use of an Oral Contraceptive for Endometriosis-Associated Recurrent Dysmenorrhea That Does Not Respond to a Cyclic Pill Regimen." *Fertility and Sterility,* 2003, 80(3), 560–3.

110 –––. "Treatment of Symptomatic Rectovaginal Endometriosis with an Estrogen-Progestogen Combination Versus Low-Dose Norethindrone Acetate." *Fertility and Sterility,* 2005, 84(5), 1375–87.

111 J. S. Sanfilippo and H. C. Hur. "Oral Contraceptives for Endometriosis-Associated Pain." *Journal of Minimally Invasive Gynecology,* 2006, 13(6), 525–7.

112 A. M. Dlugi, J. D. Miller, and J. Knittle. "Lupron Depot (Leuprolide Acetate for Depot Suspension) in the Treatment of Endometriosis: A Randomized, Placebo-Controlled, Double-Blind Study. Lupron Study Group." *Fertility and Sterility,* 1990, 54(3), 419–27.

113 D. L. Olive. "Gonadotropin-Releasing Hormone Agonists for Endometriosis." *New England Journal of Medicine,* 2008, 359(11), 1136–42.

114 V. Selak, C. Farquhar, A. Prentice, *et al.* "Danazol for Pelvic Pain Associated with Endometriosis." *Cochrane Database of Systematic Reviews,* 2007, (4), Cd000068.

115 D. C. Martin. "Hysterectomy for Treatment of Pain Associated with Endometriosis." *Journal of Minimally Invasive Gynecology,* 2006, 13(6), 566–72.

116 A. Nawathe, S. Patwardhan, D. Yates, *et al.* "Systematic Review of the Effects of Aromatase Inhibitors on Pain Associated with Endometriosis." *British Journal of Obstetrics and Gynecology,* 2008, 115(7), 818–22.

117 S. Ferrero, P. L. Venturini, N. Ragni, *et al.* "Pharmacological Treatment of Endometriosis: Experience with Aromatase Inhibitors." Drugs, 2009, 69(8), 943–52.

118 J. A. Abbott, J. Hawe, R. D. Clayton, *et al.* "The Effects and Effectiveness of Laparoscopic Excision of Endometriosis: A Prospective Study with 2–5 Year Follow-Up." *Human Reproduction,* 2003, 18(9), 1922–7.

119 M. Catenacci, S. Sastry, and T. Falcone. "Laparoscopic Surgery for Endometriosis." *Clinical Obstetrics & Gynecology,* 2009, 52(3), 351–61.

120 E. Taylor and C. Williams. "Surgical Treatment of Endometriosis: Location and Patterns of Disease at Reoperation." *Fertility and Sterility,* 93(1), 2010, 57–61.

121 K. Shakiba, J. F. Bena, K. M. Mcgill, *et al.* "Surgical Treatment pf Endometriosis: A 7-Year Follow-Up on the Requirement for Further Surgery." *Obstetrics & Gynecology,* 2008, 111(6), 1285–92.

122 B. D. Reed. "Vulvodynia: Diagnosis and Management." *American Family Physician,* 2006, 73(7), 1231–8.

123 L. D. Arnold, G. A. Bachmann, R. Rosen, *et al.* "Assessment of Vulvodynia Symptoms in a Sample of U.S. Women: A Prevalence Survey with a Nested Case Control Study." *American Journal of Obstetrics & Gynecology,* 2007, 196(2), 128.E1–6.

124 J. T. Sutton. G. A. Bachmann, L. D. Arnold, *et al.* "Assessment of Vulvodynia Symptoms in a Sample of U.S. Women: A Follow-Up National Incidence Survey." *Journal of Women's Health (Larchmt),* 2008, 17(8), 1285–92.

125 M. Ponte, E. Klemperer, A. Sahay, *et al.* "Effects of Vulvodynia on Quality of Life." *Journal of the American Academy of Dermatology,* 2009, 60(1), 70–6.

126 D. C. Foster, M. B. Kotok, L. S. Huang, *et al.* "The Tampon Test for Vulvodynia Treatment Outcomes Research: Reliability, Construct Validity, and Responsiveness." *Obstetrics & Gynecology,* 2009, 113(4), 825–32.

127 B. L. Harlow and E. G. Stewart. "A Population-Based Assessment of Chronic Unexplained Vulvar Pain: Have We Underestimated the Prevalence of Vulvodynia?" *Journal of the American Medical Women's Association,* 2003, 58(2), 82–8.

128 P. Nyirjesy. "Vulvar Vestibulitis Syndrome: A Post-Infectious Entity?" *Current Infectious Disease Reports,* 2000, 2(6), 531–535.

129 H. K. Haefner, M. E. Collins, G. D. Davis, *et al.* "The Vulvodynia Guideline." *Journal of Lower Genital Tract Disease,* 2005, 9(1), 40–51.

130 G. Desrochers, S. Bergeron, S. Khalife, *et al.* "Fear Avoidance and Self-Efficacy in Relation to Pain and Sexual Impairment in Women with Provoked Vestibulodynia." *Clinical Journal of Pain,* 2009, 25(6), 520–7.

131 I. Danielsson, T. Torstensson, G. Brodda-Jansen, *et al.* "EMG Biofeedback Versus Topical Lidocaine Gel: A Randomized Study for the Treatment of Women with Vulvar Vestibulitis." *Acta Obstetricia et Gynecologica Scandinavica,* 2006, 85(11), 1360–7.

132 S. Bergeron, Y. M. Binik, S. Khalife, *et al.* "A Randomized Comparison of Group Cognitive–Behavioral Therapy, Surface Electromyographic Biofeedback, and Vestibulectomy in the Treatment of Dyspareunia Resulting from Vulvar Vestibulitis." *Pain,* 2001, 91(3), 297–306.

133 J. Powell and F. Wojnarowska. "Acupuncture for Vulvodynia." *Journal of the Royal Society of Medicine,* 1999, 92(11), 579–81.

134 S. Ventegodt, B. Clausen, H. A. Omar, *et al.* "Clinical Holistic Medicine: Holistic Sexology and Acupressure through the Vagina (Hippocratic Pelvic Massage)." *Scientific World Journal*, 2006, 6, 2066–79.

135 H. Yoon, W. S. Chung, and B. S. Shim. "Botulinum Toxin A for the Management of Vulvodynia." *International Journal of Impotence Research*, 2007, 19(1), 84–7.

136 A. C. Steinberg, I. A. Oyama, A. E. Rejba, *et al.* "Capsaicin for the Treatment of Vulvar Vestibulitis." *American Journal of Obstetrics & Gynecology*, 2005, 192(5), 1549–53.

137 B. Ben-David and M. Friedman. "Gabapentin Therapy for Vulvodynia." *Anesthesia & Analgesia*, 1999, 89(6), 1459–60.

138 L. A. Boardman, A. S. Cooper, L. R. Blais, *et al.* "Topical Gabapentin in the Treatment of Localized and Generalized Vulvodynia." *Obstetrics & Gynecology*, 2008, 112(3), 579–85.

139 F. Murina, R. Bernorio, and R. Palmiotto. "The Use of Amielle Vaginal Trainers as Adjuvant in the Treatment of Vestibulodynia: An Observational Multicentric Study." *Medscape Journal of Medicine*, 2008, 10(1), 23.

140 E. Ripoll and D. Mahowald. "Hatha Yoga Therapy Management of Urologic Disorders." *World Journal of Urology*, 2002, 20(5), 306–9.

141 ACOG Committee Opinion. "Vulvodynia." October 2006, Number 345, 2006, *Obstetrics & Gynecology*, 108(4), 1049–52.

142 H. I. Glazer. "Dysesthetic Vulvodynia. Long-Term Follow-Up after Treatment with Surface Electromyography-Assisted Pelvic Floor Muscle Rehabilitation." *Journal of Reproductive Medicine*, 2000, 45(10), 798–802.

143 H. L. Forth, M. C. Cramp, and W. I. Drechsler. "Does Physiotherapy Treatment Improve the Self-Reported Pain Levels and Quality of Life of Women with Vulvodynia? A Pilot Study." *American Journal of Obstetrics & Gynecology*, 2009, 29(5), 423–9.

144 S. Bergeron, C. Brown, M. J. Lord, *et al.* "Physical Therapy for Vulvar Vestibulitis Syndrome: A Retrospective Study." *Journal of Sex & Marital Therapy*, 2002, 28(3), 183–92.

145 D. Hartmann, M. J. Strauhal, and C. A. Nelson. "Treatment of Women in the United States with Localized, Provoked Vulvodynia: Practice Survey of Women's Health Physical Therapists." *Journal of Reproductive Medicine*, 2007, 52(1), 48–52.

146 G. Desrochers, S. Bergeron, S. Khalife, *et al.* "Fear Avoidance and Self-Efficacy in Relation to Pain and Sexual Impairment in Women with Provoked Vestibulodynia." *Clinical Journal of Pain*, 2009, 25(6), 520–7.

147 S. Bergeron, Y. M. Binik, S. Khalife, *et al.*

148 R. M. Masheb, R. D. Kerns, C. Lozano, *et al.* "A Randomized Clinical Trial for Women with Vulvodynia: Cognitive-Behavioral Therapy vs. Supportive Psychotherapy." *Pain*, 2009, 141(1-2), 31–40.

149 M. S. Baggish, E. H. Sze, and R. Johnson. "Urinary Oxalate Excretion and Its Role in Vulvar Pain Syndrome." *American Journal of Obstetrics & Gynecology*, 1997, 177(3), 507–11.

150 B. L. Harlow, H. A. Abenhaim, A. F. Vitonis, *et al.* "Influence of Dietary Oxalates on the Risk of Adult-Onset Vulvodynia." *Journal of Reproductive Medicine*, 2008, 53(3), 171–8.

151 H. K. Haefner, M. E. Collins, G. D. Davis, *et al.* "The Vulvodynia Guideline." *Journal of Lower Genital Tract Disease*, 2005, 9(1), 40–51.

152 B. D. Reed, A. M. Caron, D. W. Gorenflo, *et al.* "Treatment of Vulvodynia with Tricyclic Antidepressants: Efficacy and Associated Factors." *J Journal of Lower Genital Tract Disease*, 2006, 10(4), 245–51.

153 J. L. Jackson, P. G. O'malley, and K. Kroenke. "Antidepressants and Cognitive-Behavioral Therapy for Symptom Syndromes." *CNS Spectrums*, 2006, 11(3), 212–22.

154 P. J. Lynch. "Vulvodynia as a Somatoform Disorder." *Journal of Reproductive Medicine*, 2008, 53(6), 390–6.

155 M. F. Goetsch, T. K. Morgan, V. B. Korcheva, *et al.* "Histologic and Receptor Analysis of Primary and Secondary Vestibulodynia and Controls: A Prospective Study." *American Journal of Obstetrics & Gynecology*, 2010, 202(6), 614.E1–8.

156 C. W. Butrick. "Pelvic Floor Hypertonic Disorders: Identification and Management." *Obstetrics & Gynecology Clinics of North America*, 2009, 36(3), 707–22.

157 D. A. Zolnoun, K. E. Hartmann, and J. F. Steege. "Overnight 5% Lidocaine Ointment for Treatment of Vulvar Vestibulitis." *Obstetrics & Gynecology*, 2003, 102(1), 84–7.

158 I. Danielsson, T. Torstensson, G. Brodda-Jansen, *et al.* "EMG Biofeedback Versus Topical Lidocaine Gel: A Randomized Study for the Treatment of Women with Vulvar Vestibulitis." *Acta Obstetricia et Gynecologica Scandinavica*, 2006, 85(11), 1360–7.

159 D. C. Foster, M. B. Kotok, L. S. Huang, *et al.* "Oral Desipramine and Topical Lidocaine for Vulvodynia." 2010, *Obstetrics & Gynecology*, 116(3), 583–93.

160 D. E. Soper. "Pelvic Inflammatory Disease." *Obstetrics & Gynecology*, 2010, 116(2 Pt 1), 419–28.

161 S. Barrett and C. Taylor. "A Review On Pelvic Inflammatory Disease." *International Journal of STD & AIDS*, 2005, 16(11), 715–20;

162 A. J. Pavletic, P. Wolner-Hanssen, J. Paavonen, *et al.* "Infertility Following Pelvic Inflammatory Disease." *Infect Dis Obstetrics & Gynecology*, 1999, 7(3), 145–52.

163 C. L. Chan and C. Wood. "Pelvic Adhesiolysis —The Assessment of Symptom Relief by 100 Patients." *Australian and New Zealand Journal of Obstetrics & Gynecology*, 1985, 25(4), 295–8.

164 S. El Sahwi. "Laparoscopic Pelvic Adhesiolysis Using CO2 Laser." *Journal of the American Association of Gynecologic Laparoscopists*, 1994, 1(4, Part 2), S10–1.

165 L. Abatangelo, L. Okereke, C. Parham-Foster, *et al.* "If Pelvic Inflammatory Disease Is Suspected Empiric Treatment Should Be Initiated." *Journal of the American Academy of Nurse Practitioners*, 2010, 22(2), 117–22.

166 D. E. Soper. "Pelvic Inflammatory Disease."

167 M. J. Hopkins, L. J. Ashton, F. Alloba, *et al.* "Validation of a Laboratory-Developed Real-Time PCR Protocol for Detection of Chlamydia Trachomatis and Neisseria Gonorrhoeae in Urine." *Sexually Transmitted Infections*, 2010, 86(3), 207–11.

168 A. Mindel and S. Sawleshwarkar. "Condoms for Sexually Transmissible Infection Prevention: Politics Versus Science." *Journal of Sexual Health*, 2008, 5(1), 1–8.

169 H. Verstraelen, R. Verhelst, M. Vaneechoutte, *et al.* "The Epidemiology of Bacterial Vaginosis in Relation to Sexual Behaviour." *BMC Infectious Diseases*, 2010, 10, 81.

170 B. H. Cottrell. "An Updated Review of Evidence to Discourage Douching." *MCN American Journal of Maternal Child Nursing*, 2010, 35(2), 102–7.

171 S. D. Hillis, R. Joesoef, P. A. Marchbanks, *et al.* "Delayed Care of Pelvic Inflammatory Disease as a Risk Factor for Impaired Fertility." *American Journal of Obstetrics & Gynecology*, 1993, 168(5), 1503–9.

172 D. T. Evans, H. Jaleel, M. T. Kinsella, *et al.* "A Retrospective Audit of The Management and Complications of Pelvic Inflammatory Disease." *International Journal of STD & AIDS*, 2008, 19(2), 123–4.

173 W. Stones, Y.C. Cheong, and F.M. Howard. "Interventions for Treating Chronic Pelvic Pain in Women." *Cochrane Database of Systematic Reviews*, 2005, Cd000387.

174 R. B. Ness, D. E. Soper, R. L. Holley, *et al.* "Effectiveness of inpatient and outpatient treatment strategies for women with pelvic inflammatory disease: results from the Pelvic Inflammatory Disease Evaluation and Clinical Health (PEACH) Randomized Trial." *Am J Obstet Gynecol*, 186(5), 929-37.

175 S. M. Lareau and R. H. Beigi. "Pelvic Inflammatory Disease and Tubo-Ovarian Abscess." *Infectious Disease Clinics of North America*, 2008, 22(4), 693–708,

176 J. Q. Clemens, R. T. Meenan, M. C. O'Keeffe Rosetti, *et al.* "Prevalence of Interstitial Cystitis Symptoms in a Managed Care Population." *Journal of Urology*, 2005, 174(2), 576–80.

177 I. A. Ibrahim, A. C. Diokno, K. A. Killinger, *et al.* "Prevalence of Self-Reported Interstitial Cystitis (IC) and Interstitial-Cystitis-Like Symptoms among Adult Women in the Community." *International Urology and Nephrology*, 2007, 39(2), 489–95.

178 M. T. Rosenberg and M. Hazzard. "Prevalence of Interstitial Cystitis Symptoms in Women: A Population-Based Study in the Primary Care Office." *Journal of Urology*, 2005, 174(6), 2231–4.

179 S. H. Berry, L. M. Bogart, C. Pham, *et al.* "Development, Validation and Testing of an Epidemiological Case Definition of Interstitial Cystitis/Painful Bladder Syndrome." *Journal of Urology*, 2010, 183(5), 1848–52.

180 J. M. Teichman. "The Role of Pentosan Polysulfate in Treatment Approaches for Interstitial Cystitis." *Reviews in Urology*, 2002, 4 Suppl 1, S21–7.

181 K. M. Peters, D. J. Carrico, S. E. Kalinowski, *et al.* "Prevalence of Pelvic Floor Dysfunction in Patients with Interstitial Cystitis." *Urology*, 2007, 70(1), 16–8.

182 T. C. Theoharides and G. R. Sant. "Immunomodulators for Treatment of Interstitial Cystitis." *Urology*, 2005, 65(4), 633–8.

183 S. H. Berry, L. M. Bogart, C. Pham, *et al.* "Development, Validation and Testing of an Epidemiological Case Definition of Interstitial Cystitis/Painful Bladder Syndrome." *Journal of Urology*, 2010, 183(5), 1848–52.

184 National Kidney and Urologic Diseases Information Clearinghouse. "Interstitial Cystitis/Painful Bladder Syndrome." NIH Publication No. 10-3220. 2009. Accessed at http://kidney.niddk.nih.gov/kudiseases/pubs/interstitialcystitis/on 8/8/10.

185 C. W. Butrick, F. M. Howard, and P. K. Sand. "Diagnosis and Treatment of Interstitial Cystitis/Painful Bladder Syndrome." *Journal of Women's Health (Larchmt)*, 2010, 19(6), 1185–93.

186 J. R. Dell, M. L. Mokrzycki, and C. J. Jayne. "Differentiating Interstitial Cystitis from Similar Conditions Commonly Seen in Gynecologic Practice." *European Journal of Obstetrics & Gynecology and Reproductive Biology*, 2009, 144(2), 105–9.

187 The Interstitial Cystitis Association. Available online at http://www.ichelp.org.

188 M. D. Akin, K. W. Weingand , D. A. Hengehold, *et al.* "Continuous Low-Level Topical Heat in the Treatment of Dysmenorrhea." *Obstetrics & Gynecology*, 2001, 97(3), 343–9.

189 E. B. Cornel, E. P. Van Haarst, R. W. Schaarsberg, *et al.* "The Effect of Biofeedback Physical Therapy in Men with Chronic Pelvic Pain Syndrome Type III." *European Urology*, 2005, 47(5), 607–11.

190 J. Q. Clemens, R. T. Meenan, M. C. O'Keeffe Rosetti, *et al.* "Prevalence of Interstitial Cystitis Symptoms in a Managed Care Population." *Journal of Urology*, 2005, 174(2), 576–80.

191 J. B. Forrest and S. Schmidt. "Interstitial Cystitis, Chronic Nonbacterial Prostatitis and Chronic Pelvic Pain Syndrome in Men: A Common and Frequently Identical Clinical Entity." *Journal of Urology*, 2004, 172(6 Pt 2), 2561–2.

192 C. L. Parsons, M. T. Rosenberg, P. Sassani, *et al.* "Quantifying Symptoms in Men with Interstitial Cystitis/Prostatitis, and Its Correlation with Potassium-Sensitivity Testing." *British Journal of Urology International*, 2005, 95(1), 86–90.

193 R. J. Evans. "Treatment Approaches for Interstitial Cystitis: Multimodality Therapy." *Reviews in Urology*, 2002, 4 Suppl 1, S16–20.

194 N. E. Rothrock, S. K. Lutgendorf, K. J. Kreder, *et al.* "Stress and Symptoms in Patients with Interstitial Cystitis: A Life Stress Model." *Urology*, 2001, 57(3), 422–7.

195 J. Sairanen, M. Leppilahti, T. L. Tammela, *et al.* "Evaluation of Health-Related Quality of Life in Patients with Painful Bladder Syndrome/Interstitial Cystitis and the Impact of Four Treatments on It." *Scand Journal of Urology and Nephrology*, 2009, 43(3), 212–9.

196 Kennedy, C. M. Bradley, C. S. Galask, *et al.* "Risk Factors for Painful Bladder Syndrome in Women Seeking Gynecologic Care." *International Urogynecology Journal and Pelvic Floor Dysfunction*, 2006, 17(1), 73–8.

197 T. C. Theoharides, D. Kempuraj, S. Vakali, *et al.* "Treatment of Refractory Interstitial Cystitis/Painful Bladder Syndrome with Cystoprotek—An Oral Multi-Agent Natural Supplement." *Canadian Journal of Urology*, 2008, 15(6), 4410–4.

198 T. C. Theoharides and G. R. Sant. "A Pilot Open Label Study of Cystoprotek in Interstitial Cystitis." *International Journal of Immunopathology and Pharmacology*, 2005, 18(1), 183–8.

199 C. Iavazzo, S. Athanasiou, E. Pitsouni, *et al.* "Hyaluronic Acid: An Effective Alternative Treatment of Interstitial Cystitis, Recurrent Urinary Tract Infections, and Hemorrhagic Cystitis?" *European Urology*, 2007, 51(6), 1534–40; Discussion 1540–1.

200 J. C. Nickel, R. B. Egerdie, G. Steinhoff, *et al.* "A Multicenter, Randomized, Double-Blind, Parallel Group Pilot Evaluation of the Efficacy and Safety of Intravesical Sodium Chondroitin Sulfate Versus Vehicle Control in Patients with Interstitial Cystitis/Painful Bladder Syndrome." *Urology*, 2010.

201 M. P. Fitzgerald, R. U. Anderson, J. Potts, *et al.* "Randomized Multicenter Feasibility Trial of Myofascial Physical Therapy for the Treatment of Urological Chronic Pelvic Pain Syndromes." *Journal of Urology*, 182(2), 570–80.

202 J. M. Weiss. "Pelvic Floor Myofascial Trigger Points: Manual Therapy for Interstitial Cystitis and the Urgency-Frequency Syndrome." *Journal of Urology*, 2001, 2009, 166(6), 2226–31.

203 D. J. Carrico, K. M. Peters, and A. C. Diokno. "Guided Imagery for Women with Interstitial Cystitis." *Journal of Alternative and Complementary Medicine*, 2008,14(1), 53–60.

204 J. M. Teichman. "The Role of Pentosan Polysulfate in Treatment Approaches for Interstitial Cystitis." *Reviews in Urology*, 2002, 4 Suppl 1, S21–7.

205 V. R. Anderson and C. M. Perry. "Pentosan Polysulfate: A Review of Its Use in the Relief of Bladder Pain or Discomfort in Interstitial Cystitis." *Drugs*, 2006, 66(6), 821–35.

206 A. Giannantoni, M. Porena, E. Costantini, *et al.* "Botulinum A Toxin Intravesical Injection in Patients with Painful Bladder Syndrome: 1-Year Followup." *Journal of Urology*, 2008, 179(3), 1031–4.

207 S. Tirumuru, D. Al-Kurdi, and P. Latthe. "Intravesical Botulinum Toxin A Injections in the Treatment of Painful Bladder Syndrome/Interstitial Cystitis." *International Urogynecology Journal and Pelvic Floor Dysfunction*, 2010.

208 A. Van Ophoven, S. Pokupic, A. Heinecke, *et al.* "A Prospective, Randomized, Placebo Controlled, Double-Blind Study of Amitriptyline for the Treatment of Interstitial Cystitis." *Journal of Urology*, 2004, 172(2), 533–6.

209 H. E. Foster, Jr., P. M. Hanno, J. C. Nickel, *et al.* "Effect of Amitriptyline on Symptoms in Treatment Naive Patients with Interstitial Cystitis/Painful Bladder Syndrome." *Journal of Urology*, 2010, 183(5), 1853–8.

210 A. Van Ophoven and L. Hertle. "Long-Term Results of Amitriptyline Treatment for Interstitial Cystitis." *Journal of Urology*, 2005, 174(5), 1837–40.

211 S. Nishijima, K. Sugaya, T. Yamada, *et al.* "Efficacy of Tricyclic Antidepressant Is Associated with Beta2-Adrenoceptor Genotype in Patients with Interstitial Cystitis." *Biomedical Research*, 2006,27(4), 163–7.

212 T. E. Dawson and J. Jamison. "Intravesical Treatments for Painful Bladder Syndrome/Interstitial Cystitis." *Cochrane Database of Systematic Reviews*, 2007, (4), Cd006113.

213 K. M. Peters. "Neuromodulation for the Treatment of Refractory Interstitial Cystitis." *Reviews in Urology*, 2002, 4 Suppl 1, S36–43.

214 C. R. Powell and K. J. Kreder. "Long-Term Outcomes of Urgency-Frequency Syndrome Due to Painful Bladder Syndrome Treated with Sacral Neuromodulation and Analysis of Failures." *Journal of Urology*, 2010, 183(1), 173–6.

215 S. E. Bristow, S. T. Hasan, and D. E. Neal. "TENS: A Treatment Option for Bladder Dysfunction." *International Urogynecology Journal and Pelvic Floor Dysfunction*, 1996, 7(4), 185–90.

216 C. H. Hsieh, S. T. Chang, C. J. Hsieh, *et al.* "Treatment of Interstitial Cystitis with Hydrodistention and Bladder Training." *International Urogynecology Journal and Pelvic Floor Dysfunction*, 2008, 19(10), 1379–84.

217 R. S. Hanley, J. T. Stoffel, R. M. Zagha, *et al.* "Multimodal Therapy for Painful Bladder Syndrome/Interstitial Cystitis: Pilot Study Combining Behavioral, Pharmacologic, and Endoscopic Therapies." *International Brazilian Journal of Urology*, 2009, 35(4), 467–74.

218 M. M. Collins, J. B. Meigs, M. J. Barry, *et al.* "Prevalence and Correlates of Prostatitis in the Health Professionals Follow-Up Study Cohort." *Journal of Urology*, 2002, 167(3), 1363–6.

219 M. Marszalek, C. Wehrberger, W. Hochreiter, *et al.* "Symptoms Suggestive of Chronic Pelvic Pain Syndrome in an Urban Population: Prevalence and Associations with Lower Urinary Tract Symptoms and Erectile Function." *Journal of Urology*, 2007, 177(5), 1815–9.

220 M. A. Pontari. "Chronic Prostatitis/Chronic Pelvic Pain Syndrome." *Urologic Clinics of North America*, 2008, 35(1), 81–9; Vi.

221 J. Q. Clemens, R. B. Nadler, A. J. Schaeffer, *et al.* "Biofeedback, Pelvic Floor Re-Education, and Bladder Training for Male Chronic Pelvic Pain Syndrome." *Urology*, 2000, 56(6), 951–5.

222 G. M. Habermacher, J. T. Chason, and A. J. Schaeffer. "Prostatitis/Chronic Pelvic Pain Syndrome." *Annual Review of Medicine*, 2006, 57, 195–206.

223 A. J. Schaeffer. "Etiology and Management of Chronic Pelvic Pain Syndrome in Men." *Urology*, 2004, 63(3 Suppl 1), 75–84.

224 B. V. Le and A. J. Schaeffer." Genitourinary Pain Syndromes, Prostatitis, and Lower Urinary Tract Symptoms." *Urologic Clinics of North America*, 2009, 36(4), 527–36, Vii.He

225 J. C. Nickel. "Treatment of Chronic Prostatitis/Chronic Pelvic Pain Syndrome." *International Journal of Antimicrobial Agents*, 2008, 31 Suppl 1, S112–6.

226 W. P. Zhao, Z. G. Zhang, X. D. Li, *et al.* "Celecoxib Reduces Symptoms in Men with Difficult Chronic Pelvic Pain Syndrome (Category IIIA)." *Brazilian Journal of Medical and Biological Research*, 2009, 42(10), 963–7.

227 S. W. Lee, M. L. Liong, K. H. Yuen, *et al.* "Acupuncture Versus Sham Acupuncture for Chronic Prostatitis/Chronic Pelvic Pain." *American Journal of Medicine*, 2008, 121(1), 79.E1–7.

228 L. Sikiru, H. Shmaila, and S. A. Muhammed. "Transcutaneous Electrical Nerve Stimulation (TENS) in the Symptomatic Management of Chronic Prostatitis/Chronic Pelvic Pain Syndrome." *International Brazilian Journal of Urology*, 2008, 34(6), 708–13;

229 M. P. Fitzgerald, R. U. Anderson, J. Potts, *et al.* "Randomized Multicenter Feasibility Trial of Myofascial Physical Therapy for the Treatment of Urological Chronic Pelvic Pain Syndromes." *Journal of Urology*, 2009, 182(2), 570–80.

230 M. A. Pontari. "Chronic Prostatitis/Chronic Pelvic Pain Syndrome and Interstitial Cystitis: Are They Related?" *Current Urology Reports*, 2006, 7(4), 329–34.

231 M. Marszalek, C. Wehrberger, C. Temml, *et al.* "Chronic Pelvic Pain and Lower Urinary Tract Symptoms in Both Sexes: Analysis of 2749 Participants of an Urban Health Screening Project." *European Urology*, 2009, 55(2), 499–507.

232 J. Q. Clemens, R. B. Nadler, A. J. Schaeffer, *et al.* "Biofeedback, Pelvic Floor Re-Education, and Bladder Training for Male Chronic Pelvic Pain Syndrome." *Urology*, 2000, 56(6), 951–5.

233 J. M. Potts. "Chronic Pelvic Pain Syndrome: A Non-Prostatocentric Perspective." *World Journal of Urology*, 2003, 21(2), 54–6.

234 M. A. Pontari. "Chronic Prostatitis/Chronic Pelvic Pain Syndrome."

235 F. M. Wagenlehner, H.Schneider, M. Ludwig, *et al.* "A Pollen Extract (Cernilton) in Patients with Inflammatory Chronic Prostatitis-Chronic Pelvic Pain Syndrome." *European Urology*, 2009, 56(3), 544–51.

236 J. Elist. "Effects of Pollen Extract Preparation Prostat/Poltit on Lower Urinary Tract Symptoms in Patients with Chronic Nonbacterial Prostatitis/Chronic Pelvic Pain Syndrome." *Urology*, 2006, 67(1), 60–3.

237 A. E. Gordon and A. F. Shaughnessy. "Saw Palmetto for Prostate Disorders." *American Family Physician*, 2003, 67(6), 1281–3.

238 G. Morgia, G. Mucciardi, A.Gali, *et al.* "Treatment of Chronic Prostatitis/Chronic Pelvic Pain Syndrome Category IIIA with Serenoa Repens Plus Selenium and Lycopene (Profluss) Versus S. Repens Alone." *Urologia Internationalis*, 2010, 84(4), 400–6.

239 J. Yang and A. E. Te. "Saw Palmetto and Finasteride in the Treatment of Category-III Prostatitis/Chronic Pelvic Pain Syndrome." *Current Urology Reports*, 2005, 6(4), 290–5.

240 S. A. Kaplan, M. A. Volpe, and A. E. Te. "A Prospective, 1-Year Trial Using Saw Palmetto Versus Finasteride in the Treatment of Category III Prostatitis/Chronic Pelvic Pain Syndrome." *Journal of Urology*, 2004, 171(1), 284–8.

241 S. W. Lee, M. L. Liong, K. H.Yuen, *et al.* "Acupuncture Versus Sham Acupuncture for Chronic Prostatitis/Chronic Pelvic Pain." *American Journal of Medicine*, 2008, 121(1), 79.E1–7.

242 H. Honjo, K. Kamoi, Y. Naya, *et al.* "Effects of Acupuncture for Chronic Pelvic Pain Syndrome with Intrapelvic Venous Congestion." *International Journal of Urology*, 2004, 11(8), 607–12.

243 Fitzgerald, Anderson, and Potts. "Randomized Multicenter Feasibility Trial of Myofascial Physical Therapy for the Treatment of Urological Chronic Pelvic Pain Syndromes."

244 R. U. Anderson, D. Wise, T. Sawyer, C. A. Chan. "Sexual Dysfunction in Men with Chronic Prostatitis/Chronic Pelvic Pain Syndrome: Improvement after Trigger Point Release and Paradoxical Relaxation Training." *Journal of Urology*, 2006, 176(4 Pt 1), 1534–8;

245 J. Q. Clemens, R. B. Nadler, A. J. Schaeffer, *et al.* "Biofeedback, Pelvic Floor Re-Education, and Bladder Training for Male Chronic Pelvic Pain Syndrome." *Urology*, 2000, 56(6), 951–5.

246 E. B. Cornel, E. P. Van Haarst, R. W. Schaarsberg, *et al.* "The Effect of Biofeedback Physical Therapy in Men with Chronic Pelvic Pain Syndrome Type III." *European Urology*, 2005, 47(5), 607–11.

247 Y. Evliyaoglu and R. Burgut. "Lower Urinary Tract Symptoms, Pain and Quality of Life Assessment in Chronic Non-Bacterial Prostatitis Patients Treated with Alpha-Blocking Agent Doxazosin Versus Placebo." *International Urology and Nephrology*, 2002, 34(3), 351–6.

248 A. B. Murphy and R. B. Nadler. "Pharmacotherapy Strategies in Chronic Prostatitis/Chronic Pelvic Pain Syndrome Management." *Expert Opinion on Pharmacotherapy*, 2010, 11(8), 1255–61.

249 S. Kabay, S. C. Kabay, M. Yucel, *et al.* "Efficiency of Posterior Tibial Nerve Stimulation in Category IIIB Chronic Prostatitis/Chronic Pelvic Pain: A Sham-Controlled Comparative Study." *Urologia Internationalis*, 2009, 83(1), 33–8.

250 A. B. Murphy and R. B. Nadler. "Pharmacotherapy Strategies in Chronic Prostatitis/Chronic Pelvic Pain Syndrome Management." *Expert Opinion on Pharmacotherapy*, 2010, 11(8), 1255–61.

251 S. A. Kaplan, M. A. Volpe, and A. E. Te. "A Prospective, 1-Year Trial Using Saw Palmetto Versus Finasteride in the Treatment of Category III Prostatitis/Chronic Pelvic Pain Syndrome." *Journal of Urology*, 2004, 171(1), 284–8.

252 L. Sikiru, H. Shmaila, and S. A. Muhammed. "Transcutaneous Electrical Nerve Stimulation (TENS) in the Symptomatic Management of Chronic Prostatitis/Chronic Pelvic Pain Syndrome." *International Brazilian Journal of Urology*, 2008, 34(6), 708–13;

253 S. H. Lee and B. C. Lee. "Electroacupuncture Relieves Pain in Men with Chronic Prostatitis/Chronic Pelvic Pain Syndrome." *Urology*, 2009, 73(5), 1036–41.

254 C. R. Powell and K. J. Kreder. "Long-Term Outcomes of Urgency-Frequency Syndrome Due to Painful Bladder Syndrome Treated with Sacral Neuromodulation and Analysis of Failures." *Journal of Urology*, 2010, 183(1), 173–6.

256 J. C. Nickel, J. B. Forrest, K. Tomera, *et al.* "Pentosan Polysulfate Sodium Therapy for Men with Chronic Pelvic Pain Syndrome." *Journal of Urology*, 2005, 173(4), 1252–5.

255 S. I. Zeitlin. "Heat Therapy in the Treatment of Prostatitis." *Urology*, 2002, 60 (6 Suppl), 38–40, Discussion 41.

Chapter 14

1 S. Lydeard and R. Jones. "Factors Affecting the Decision to Consult with Dyspepsia: Comparison of Consulters and Non-Consulters." *Journal of the Royal College of General Practice*, 1989, 39: 495–8.

2 R. Fass. "Proton Pump Inhibitor Therapy in Patients with Gastro-Oesophageal Reflux Disease: Putative Mechanisms of Failure." *Drugs*, 2007, 67: 1521–30

3 M. Nilsson, R Johnsen, W. Ye *et al.* "Lifestyle related risk factors in the aetiology of gastro-oesophageal reflux." *Gut* 2004; 53: 1730-1735

4 Tonya Kaltenbach, Seth Crockett, and Lauren B. Gerson. "Are Lifestyle Measures Effective in Patients with Gastroesophageal Reflux Disease?" *Archives of Internal Medicine*, 2006, May 8, 166:965–971.

5 M. Nilsson, R. Johnsen, W. Ye, *et al.* "Lifestyle-Related Risk Factors in the Aetiology of Gastro-Oesophageal Reflux." *Gut*, 2004, 53:1730–1735.

6 R. Dickman, E.Schiff, A. Holland, *et al.* "Clinical Trial: Acupuncture Vs. Doubling the Proton Pump Inhibitor Dose in Refractory Heartburn." *Alimentary Pharmacology & Therapeutics*, 2007 Nov 15, 26(10): 1333–44. E-pub 2007 Sep 17.

7   Duowu Zou, Wei Hao Chen, Katsuhiko Iwakiri, *et al.* "Inhibition of Transient Lower Esophageal Sphincter Relaxations by Electrical Acupoint Stimulation." *American Journal of Physiology-Gastrointestinal and Liver Physiology*, 2005 August.

8   G. Holtmann, R. Kriebel, and M. Singer. "Mental Stress and Gastric Acid Secretion. Do Personality Traits Influence the Response?" *Digestive Diseases and Sciences*, 1990, 35: 998–1007.

9   L. A. Bradley, J. E.Richter, T. J. Pulliam, *et al.* "The Relationship between Stress and Symptoms of Gastroesophageal Reflux: The Influence of Psychological Factors." *American Journal of Gastroenterology*, 1993, 88: 11–9.

10   J. McDonald-Haile, L. A. Bradley, M. A. Bailey, *et al.* "Relaxation Training Reduces Symptom Reports and Acid Exposure in Patients with Gastroesophageal Reflux Disease." *Gastroenterology*, 1994 Jul, 107(1): 61–9.

11   R. W. Shaw. "Randomized Controlled Trial of Syn-Ergel and an Active Placebo in the Treatment of Heartburn of Pregnancy." *Journal of International Medical Research*, 1978, 6:147–51.

12   B. Van Pinxteren *et al.* "Short-Term Treatment with Proton Pump Inhibitors, H2-Receptor Antagonists and Prokinetics for Gastrooesophageal Reflux Disease-Like Symptoms and Endoscopy Negative Reflux Disease." *Cochrane Database of Systematic Reviews*, 2006.

13   M. Robinson, S. Rodriguez-Stanley, A. A. Ciociola, *et al.* "Synergy between Low-Dose Ranitidine and Antacid in Decreasing Gastric and Oesophageal Acidity and Relieving Meal-Induced Heartburn." *Alimentary Pharmacology & Therapeutics*, Volume 15, Issue 9, 1365–1374. Published online 2001 20 Dec.

14   W. Rayburn, E. Liles, H. Christensen, *et al.* "Antacids Vs. Antacids Plus Non-Prescription Ranitidine for Heartburn during Pregnancy." *International Journal of Gynecology & Obstetrics*, 1999, 66: 35–37.

15   "Overprescribing Proton Pump Inhibitors." *British Medical Journal*, 2008, 336:2–3 (5 January).

16   Johan Brun and Heléne Sörngårda. "High Dose Proton Pump Inhibitor Response as an Initial Strategy for a Clinical Diagnosis of Gastro-Oesophageal Reflux Disease (GERD)." *Family Practice*, Vol. 17, No. 5, 401–404.

17   B. Kaplan-Machlis, G. E. Spiegler, M. W. Zodet, *et al.* "Effectiveness and Costs of Omeprazole Vs. Ranitidine for Treatment of Symptomatic Gastroesophageal Reflux Disease in Primary Care Clinics in West Virginia." *Archives of Family Medicine*, 2000 Jul, 9(7): 624–30.

18   R. Fiocca, L. Mastracci, C. Engström, *et al.* "Long-Term Outcome of Microscopic Esophagitis in Chronic GERD Patients Treated with Esomeprazole or Laparoscopic Antireflux Surgery in the LOTUS Trial." *American Journal of Gastroenterology*, 2010 May, 105(5): 1015–23. E-pub 2009 Nov 10.

19   M. Nocon, J. Labenz, and S. N. Willich. "Lifestyle Factors and Symptoms of Gastro-Oesophageal Reflux—A Population-Based Study." *Alimentary Pharmacology & Therapeutics*, 2006 Jan 1, 23(1): 169–74.

20   Jacobson *et al.* "Body-Mass Index and Symptoms of Gastroesophageal Reflux in Women." *New England Journal of Medicine*, 2006 Jun 1, 354(22): 2340–8.

21   M. Nilsson, R. Johnsen, W. Ye, *et al.* "Lifestyle Related Risk Factors in the Aetiology of Gastro-Oesophageal Reflux." *Gut*, 2004 Dec, 53(12): 1730–5.

22   J. P. Waring, T. F. Eastwood, J. M. Austin, *et al.* "The Immediate Effects of Cessation of Cigarette Smoking on Gastroesophageal Reflux." *American Journal of Gastroenterology*, 1989, 84: 1076–1078.

23   Christiaan W. Sies and Jim Brooker. "Could These Be Gallstones?" *The Lancet*, Volume 365, Issue 9468, 1388, 16 April 2005.

24   O. Alimoglu, O. V. Ozkan, M. Sahin, *et al.* "Timing of Cholecystectomy for Acute Biliary Pancreatitis: Outcomes of Cholecystectomy on First Admission and after Recurrent Biliary Pancreatitis." *World Journal of Surgery*, 2003, 27: 256–9.

25   S. Syngal, E. H. Coakley, W. C. Willett, *et al.* "Long-Term Weight Patterns and Risk for Cholecystectomy in Women." *Annals of Internal Medicine*, 1999, 130:471–7.

26   V. K. Li, N. Pulido, P. Fajnwaks, *et al.* "Predictors of Gallstone Formation after Bariatric Surgery: A Multivariate Analysis of Risk Factors Comparing Gastric Bypass, Gastric Banding, and Sleeve Gastrectomy." *Surgical Endoscopy*, 2009 Jul, 23(7): 1640–4. E-pub 2008 Dec 5.

27   M. F. Leitzmann, E. L. Giovannucci, E. B. Rimm, *et al.* "The Relation of Physical Activity to Risk for Symptomatic Gallstone Disease in Men." *Annals of Internal Medicine*, 1998, 128: 417–25.

28   Chung-Jyi Tsai, Michael F. Leitzmann, Walter C. Willett, *et al.* "The Effect of Long-Term Intake of CIS Unsaturated Fats on the Risk for Gallstone Disease in Men." *Annals of Internal Medicine*, October 5, 2004, vol. 141 no. 7 514–522.

29   Chung-Jyi Tsai, Michael F. Leitzmann, Frank B. Hu1, *et al.* "A Prospective Cohort Study of Nut Consumption and the Risk of Gallstone Disease in Men." *American Journal of Epidemiology*, 2004 160(10): 961–968.

30   Chung-Jyi Tsai, Michael F. Leitzmann, Frank B. Hu1, *et al.* "Frequent Nut Consumption and Decreased Risk of Cholecystectomy in Women." *American Journal of Clinical Nutrition*, 2004 July, Vol. 80, No. 1, 76–81.

31   Nahum Méndez-Sánchez, Verónica González, Patricia Aguayo, *et al.* "Fish Oil (n-3) Polyunsaturated Fatty

Acids Beneficially Affect Biliary Cholesterol Nucleation Time in Obese Women Losing Weight." *Journal of Nutrition*, 2001, 131: 2300–2303.

32 M. D. Yago, V.González, P. Serrano, *et al.* "Effect of the Type of Dietary Fat on Biliary Lipid Composition and Bile Lithogenicity in Humans with Cholesterol Gallstone Disease." *Nutrition*, 2005 Mar, 21(3): 339–47.

33 C. J. Tsai, M. F. Leitzmann, W. C. Willett, *et al.* "Long-Term Intake of Dietary Fiber and Decreased Risk of Cholecystectomy in Women." *Gastroenterology*, 2004 Jul, 99(7):1364–70.

34 M. F. Leitzmann, E. L. Giovannucci, E. B. Rimm, *et al.* "The Relation of Physical Activity to Risk for Symptomatic Gallstone Disease in Men." *Annals of Internal Medicine*, 1998, 128:417–25. Available online at http://www.annals.org/cgi/content/full/128/6/417.

35 http://content.nejm.org/cgi/content/abstract/341/11/777.

36 "Endurance Exercise Training Reduces Gallstone 2 Development in Mice." Available online at http://jap.physiology.org/cgi/reprint/01292.2007v1.

37 Hart *et al.* "Hormone Replacement Therapy and Symptomatic Gallstones—A Prospective Population Study in the EPIC-Norfolk Cohort." *Digestion*, 2008, 77(1): 4–9.

38 http://www.British Medical Journal.com/cgi/content/abstract/337/jul10_2/a386.

39 M. L. Petroni, R. P. Jazrawi, P. Pazzi, *et al.* "Ursodeoxycholic Acid Alone or with Chenodeoxycholic Acid for Dissolution of Cholesterol Gallstones. The British-Italian Gallstone Study Group." *Alimentary Pharmacology & Therapeutics*, 2001, 15:123–8.

40 K. A. Hood, D. Gleeson, D. C. Ruppin, *et al.* "Gallstone Recurrence and Its Prevention: The British/Belgian Gall Stone Study Group's Postdissolution Trial." *Gut*, 1993, 34:1277–88.

41 E. Lionetti. "Lactobacillus Reuteri Therapy to Reduce Side-Effects During Anti-Helicobacter Pylori Treatment in Children." *Alimentary Pharmacology & Therapeutics*. 2006 Nov 15, 24(10): 1461–8.

42 University of Michigan Health System. "Guidelines for Clinical Care: Peptic Ulcer Disease."

43 T. Stupnicky, M. Taufer, H. Denk, *et al.* "Triple Therapy with Sucralfate, Amoxicillinc and Metronidazole for Healing Duodenal Ulcer and Eradicating Helicobacter Pylori Infection." *Alimentary Pharmacology & Therapeutics*, Volume 10, Issue 2, 193–197. Published online 2003 28 Nov.

44 Yasuki Habua, Shigeto Mizunob, Seiichi Hiranoc, *et al.* "Triple Therapy with Omeprazole, Amoxicillin and Clarithromycin Is Effective against Helicobacter Pylori Infection in Gastric Ulcer Patients as well as in Duodenal Ulcer Patients." *Digestion*, 1998, Vol. 59, No. 4.

45 G. Treiber, J. Wittig, S. Ammon, *et al.* "Clinical Outcome and Influencing Factors of a New Short-Term Quadruple Therapy for Helicobacter Pylori Eradication: A Randomized Controlled Trial (MACLOR Study)." *Archives of Internal Medicine*, 2002, 162:153–60.

46 Andrea Morgner, Stephan Miehlke, and Joachim Labenz. "Esomeprazole: Prevention and Treatment of NSAID-Induced Symptoms and Ulcers." *Expert Opinion on Pharmacotherapy*, 2007 May, Vol. 8, No. 7, 975–988.

47 Frank L. Lanza, Francis K. L. Chan, and Eamonn M. M. Quigley. "Guidelines for Prevention of NSAID-Related Ulcer Complications." *American Journal of Gastroenterology*, 2009, 104: 728–738.

48 M. J. Langman. "Risk of Peptic Ulcer Hospitalizations in Users of NSAIDs with Gastroprotective Cotherapy Versus Coxibs." *Gastroenterology*, 2007 September. "Risks of Bleeding Peptic Ulcer Associated with Individual Non-Steroidal Anti-Inflammatory *Drugs*." *The Lancet*, 1994 Apr 30, 343(8905): 1075–8.

49 http://www.gi.org/patients/women/aspirin.asp.

50 A. Rostom, C. Dube, G. Wells, *et al.* "Prevention of NSAID-Induced Gastroduodenal Ulcers." *Cochrane Database of Systematic Reviews,* 2002, 4: CD002296.

51 *American Family Physician*, 2007, 76: 1005–1012.

52 T. Poynard, M. Lemaire, and H. Agostini. "Meta-Analysis of Randomized Clinical Trials Comparing Lansoprazole with Ranitidine or Famotidine in the Treatment of Acute Duodenal Ulcer." *European Journal of Gastroenterology & Hepatology*, 1995, 7: 661–5.

53 *American Family Physician*, 2007, 76:1005–1012.

54 Robert F. Anda, David F. Williamson, Luis G. Escobedo, *et al.* "Smoking and the Risk of Peptic Ulcer Disease Among Women in the United States." *Archives of Internal Medicine*. 1990, 150(7): 1437–1441.

55 P. Maity, K. Biswas, S. Roy, *et al.* "Smoking and the Pathogenesis of Gastroduodenal Ulcer—Recent Mechanistic Update." *Molecular and Cellular Biochemistry*, 2003 Nov, 253(1–2): 329–38.

56 Vivian Y. Shin, Edgar S. L. Liu, Marcel W. L. Koo, *et al.* "Cigarette Smoke Extracts Delay Wound Healing in the Stomach: Involvement of Polyamine Synthesis." *Experimental Biology and Medicine*, 2002, 227: 114–124.

57 I. Heymann-Monnikes, R. Arnold, I. Florin, *et al.* "The Combination of Medical Treatment Plus Multicomponent Behavioral Therapy Is Superior to Medical Treatment Alone in the Therapy of Irritable Bowel Syndrome." *American Journal of Gastroenterology*, 2000, 95: 981–94.

58 Philip S. Schoenfeld. "New Developments in the Treatment of Irritable Bowel Syndrome." Available online at http://cme.medscape.com/viewarticle/540226.

59 S. Zar. "Elimination Diets." *American Journal of Gastroenterology*, July 2005, vol 100: 1550–1557. *Gut*, October 2004.

60 W. Atkinson, T. A. Sheldon, N. Shaath, *et al.* "Food Elimination Based on IgG Antibodies in Irritable Bowel Syndrome." *Gut*, 2004, 53: 1459–1464.

61 Zar. "Elimination Diets."

62 C. J. Bijkerk. "Systematic Review: The Role of Different Types of Fibre in the Treatment of Irritable Bowel Syndrome." *Alimentary Pharmacology & Therapeutics*, 2004 Feb 1, 19(3): 245–51.

63 C. J. Bijkerk, N. J. de Wit, J. W. M. Muris, *et al.* "Soluble or Insoluble Fibre in Irritable Bowel Syndrome in Primary Care?" 2009, *British Medical Journal*, 2009 27 August, 339: b3154.

64 S. Merat, S. Khalili, P. Mostajabi, *et al.* "The Effect of Enteric-Coated, Delayed-Release Peppermint Oil on Irritable Bowel Syndrome." *Digestive Diseases and Sciences*, 2010 May, 55(5): 1385–90. E-pub 2009 Jun 9.

65 G. Cappello, M. Spezzaferro, L. Grossi, *et al.* "Peppermint Oil (Mintoil) in the Treatment of Irritable Bowel Syndrome." *Digestive Liver Diseases*, 2007 Jun, 39(6): 530–6. E-pub 2007 Apr 8.

66 K. S. Hong, H. W. Kang, J. P. Im, *et al.* "Effect of Probiotics on Symptoms in Korean Adults with Irritable Bowel Syndrome." *Gut and Liver*, 2009 Jun, 3(2): 101–7. E-pub 2009 Jun 30.

67 *Ibid.*

68 Vid Sutto *et al.* "Anorectal Biofeedback Therapy Is Effective for Non-Diarrhea Predominant Irritable Bowel Syndrome as for Functional Constipation." Presented at Digestive Disease Week 2007, Washington, DC, May 19–23, 2007.

69 I. Taneja, K K. Deepak, G. Poojary, *et al.* "Yogic Versus Conventional Treatment in Diarrhea-Predominant Irritable Bowel Syndrome: A Randomized Control Study." *Applied Psychophysiology & Biofeedback*, 2004 Mar, 29(1): 19–33.

70 V. P. Suttor, G. M. Prott, R. D. Hansen, *et al.* "Evidence for Pelvic Floor Dyssynergia in Patients with Irritable Bowel Syndrome." *Diseases of the Colon & Rectum*, 2010 Feb, 53(2): 156–60.

71 J. M. Lackner, J. Jaccard, S. S. Krasner, *et al.* "Self-Administered Cognitive Behavior Therapy for Moderate to Severe Irritable Bowel Syndrome: Clinical Efficacy, Tolerability, Feasibility." *Clinical Gastroenterology and Hepatology*, 2008 Aug, 6(8): 899–906.

72 Mark Pimentel, Sandy Park, James Mirocha, *et al.* "The Effect of a Nonabsorbed Oral Antibiotic (Rifaximin) on the Symptoms of the Irritable Bowel Syndrome." *Annals of Internal Medicine*, October 17, 2006, vol. 145 no. 8 557–563.

73 E. B. Blanchard, B. Greene, L. Scharff, *et al.* "Relaxation Training as a Treatment for Irritable Bowel Syndrome." *Biofeedback and Self-Regulation*, 1993 Sep, 18(3): 125–32.

74 R. E. Clouse. "Antidepressants for Functional Gastrointestinal Syndromes." *Digestive Diseases and Sciences*, 1994, 39: 2352–2363.

75 http://www.gi.org/patients/gihealth/diverticular.asp.

76 http://www.ncbi.nlm.nih.gov/pubmed/964566.

77 W. H. Aldoori, E. L. Giovannucci, H. R. Rockett, *et al.* "A Prospective Study of Dietary Fiber Types and Symptomatic Diverticular Disease in Men." *Journal of Nutrition*, 1998, 128(4): 714–719.

78 J. M. P. Hyland and I. Taylor. "Does a High Fibre Diet Prevent the Complications of Diverticular Disease?" *British Journal of Surgery*, Volume 67, Issue 2, 77–79.

79 B. J. Smits, A. M. Whitehead, and P. Prescott. "Lactulose in the Treatment of Symptomatic Diverticular Disease: A Comparative Study with High-Fibre Diet." *British Journal of Clinical Practice*, 1990, 4: 314–318.

80 D. Makola. "Diverticular Disease: Evidence for Dietary Intervention?" *Practical Gastroenterology*, Feb 2007: 41–46.

81 I. Taylor and H. L. Duthie. "Bran Tablets and Diverticular Disease." *British Medical Journal*, 1976, 1(6016): 988–990.

82 M. H. Ornstein, E. R. Littlewood, I. M. Baird, *et al.* "Are Fibre Supplements Really Necessary in Diverticular Disease of the Colon?" *British Medical Journal*, (Clin Res Ed) 1981, 282: 1353–1356. A. J. Brodribb and D. M. Humphreys. "Diverticular Disease: Three Studies. Part II—Treatment with Bran." *British Medical Journal*, 1976, 1(6007): 425–428.

83 W. H. Aldoori, E. L. Giovannucci, E. B. Rimm, *et al.* "A Prospective Study of Diet and the Risk of Symptomatic Diverticular Disease in Men." *American Journal of Clinical Nutrition*, 1994 Nov, 60(5): 757–64.

84 W. H. Aldoori, E. L. Giovannucci, H. R. Rockett, *et al.* "A Prospective Study of Dietary Fiber Types and Symptomatic Diverticular Disease in Men." *Journal of Nutrition*, 1998, 128(4): 714–719.

85 O. Manousos, N. E. Day, A. Tzonou, *et al.* "Diet and Other Factors in the Aetiology of Diverticulosis: An Epidemiological Study in Greece." *Gut*, 1985, 26: 544–549.

86 Lin *et al.* "Dietary Habits and Right-Sided Colonic Diverticulosis." *Diseases of the Colon and Rectum*, 2000 Oct, 43(10): 1412–8.

87 W. H. Aldoori, E. L. Giovannucci, E B. Rimm, *et al.* "A Prospective Study of Diet and the Risk of Symptomatic Diverticular Disease in Men."

88 A. Tursi, G. Brandimarte, G. M. Giorgetti, *et al.* "Mesalamine and/or Lactobacillus Casei in Maintaining Long-Term Remission of Symptomatic Uncomplicated Diverticular Disease of the Colon." *Hepato-Gastroenterology*, 2008 May–Jun, 55(84): 916–20.

89 Antonio Tursi, Giovanni Brandimarte, Gian Marco Giorgetti, *et al.* "Balsalazide and/or High-Potency Probiotic Mixture (VSL#3) in Maintaining Remission after Attack of Acute, Uncomplicated Diverticulitis of the Colon." *International Journal of Colorectal Disease*, 22(9) September 2007.

90 Strate *et al.* "Physical Activity Decreases Diverticular Complications." *American Journal of Gastroenterology*, 2009 May, 104(5): 1221–30.

91 Aldoori *et al.* "Prospective Study of Physical Activity and the Risk of Symptomatic Diverticular Disease in Men." *Gut*, 1995 Feb, 36(2): 276–82.

92 A. Colecchia, A. Vestito, F. Pasqui, *et al.* "Efficacy of Long Term Cyclic Administration of the Poorly Absorbed Antibiotic Rifaximin in Symptomatic, Uncomplicated Colonic Diverticular Disease." *World Journal of Gastroenterology*, 2007 Jan 14, 13(2): 264–9. G. Latella, C. Scarpignato. "Rifaximin in the Management of Colonic Diverticular Disease." *Expert Review of Gastroenterology & Hepatology*, 2009 Dec, 3(6): 585–98.

93 A. Tursi, G. Brandimarte, G. M. Giorgetti, *et al.* "Assessment of Small Intestinal Bacterial Overgrowth in Uncomplicated Acute Diverticulitis of the Colon." *World Journal of Gastroenterology*, 2005 May 14, 11(18): 2773–6.

94 G. Latella and C. Scarpignato. "Rifaximin in the Management of Colonic Diverticular Disease." *Expert Review of Gastroenterology & Hepatology*, 2009 Dec, 3(6): 585–98.

95 Luigi Gatta, Nimish Vakil, Dino Vaira, *et al.* "Efficacy of 5-ASA in the Treatment of Colonic Diverticular Disease." *Journal of Clinical Gastroenterology*, 2010 February, 44(2): 113–119.

96 G. Comparato, L. Fanigliulo, L. G. Cavallaro, *et al.* "Prevention of Complications and Symptomatic Recurrences in Diverticular Disease with Mesalamine: A 12-Month Follow-Up." *Digestive Diseases and Sciences*, 2007 Nov, 52(11): 2934–41.

97 A. Tursi, G. Brandimarte, and R. Daffinà. "Long-Term Treatment with Mesalamine and Rifaximin Versus Rifaximin Alone for Patients with Recurrent Attacks of Acute Diverticulitis of Colon." *Digestive and Liver Disease*, 2002 Jul, 34(7): 510–5.

98 D. Collins and D. C. Winter. "Elective Resection for Diverticular Disease: An Evidence-Based Review." *World Journal of Surgery*, 2008 Nov, 32(11): 2429–33.

99 W. H. Aldoori, E. L. Giovannucci, E. B. Rimm, *et al.* "Use of Acetaminophen and Nonsteroidal Anti-Inflammatory Drugs: A Prospective Study and the Risk of Symptomatic Diverticular Disease in Men." *Archives of Family Medicine*, 1998 May–Jun, 7(3): 255–60.

100 C. Andeweg, J. Peters, R. Bleichrodt, *et al.* "Incidence and Risk Factors of Recurrence after Surgery for Pathology-Proven Diverticular Disease." *World Journal of Surgery*, 2008 Jul, 32(7): 1501–6.

101 B. R. Klarenbeek, M. Samuels, M. A. van der Wal, *et al.* "Indications for Elective Sigmoid Resection in Diverticular Disease." *Annals of Surgery*, 2010 Apr, 251(4): 670–4.

102 A. Tursic, G. Brandimartec, and R. Daffinà. "Long-Term Treatment with Mesalamine and Rifaximin Versus Rifaximin Alone for Patients with Recurrent Attacks of Acute Diverticulitis of Colon."

103 Eram Zaidi and Barry Daly. "CT and Clinical Features of Acute Diverticulitis in an Urban U.S. Population: Rising Frequency in Young, Obese Adults." *American Journal of Roentgenology*, 2006 October 12, 187(3): 689–694.

104 Lisa L. Strate, Yan L. Liu, Sapna Syngal, *et al.* "Obesity Increases the Risks of Diverticulitis and Diverticular Bleeding." *Gastroenterology*, 2009 January, 136(1): 115–122.e1.

105 http://www.urocit-k.com.

106 Gary C. Curhan, Walter C. Willett, Eric B. Rimm, *et al.* "A Prospective Study of Dietary Calcium and Other Nutrients and the Risk of Symptomatic Kidney Stones." *New England Journal of Medicine*, 1993 March 25, 328(12): 833–838.

107 Gary C. Curhan, Walter C. Willett, E. L. Knight, *et al.* "Dietary Factors and the Risk of Incident Kidney Stones in Younger Women: Nurses' Health Study II." *Archives of Internal Medicine*, 2004 Apr 26, 164(8): 885–91.

108 G. C. Curhan, W. C. Willett, E. B. Rimm, *et al.* (1996). "Prospective Study of Beverage Use and the Risk of Kidney Stones." *American Journal of Epidemiology*, 143(3), 240–247.

109 E. N. Taylor, M. J. Stampfer, and G. C. Curhan. "Dietary Factors and the Risk of Incident Kidney Stones in Men: New Insights after 14 Years of Follow-Up." *Journal of the American Society of Nephrology*, 2004 Dec, 15(12): 3225–32.

110 D. E. Kang, R. L. Sur, G. E. Haleblian, *et al.* "Long-Term Lemonade Based Dietary Manipulation in Patients with Hypocitraturic Nephrolithiasis." *Journal of Urology*, 2007, 177: 1358–1362.

111 S. G. Koff, E. L. Paquette, J. Cullen, *et al.* "Comparison Between Lemonade and Potassium Citrate and Impact on Urine Ph and 24-Hour Urine Parameters in Patients with Kidney Stone Formation." *Urology*, 2007 Jun, 69(6): 1013–6.

112 *Journal of Urology*, 2010, 183(6): 2419–2423.

113 K. L. Penniston, T. H. Steele, and S. Y. Nakada. "Lemonade Therapy Increases Urinary Citrate and Urine Volumes in Patients with Recurrent Calcium Oxalate Stone Formation." *Urology*, 2007 Nov, 70(5): 856–60. E-pub 2007 Oct 24.

114 E. N. Taylor *et al.* "DASH-Style Diet Associates with Reduced Risk for Kidney Stones." *Journal of the American Society of Nephrology*, 2009 Aug 13.

115 Gary C. Curhan, Walter C. Willett, Eric B. Rimm, *et al.* "A Prospective Study of Dietary Calcium and Other Nutrients and the Risk of Symptomatic Kidney Stones."

116 A. Nouvenne, T. Meschi, B. Prati, *et al.* "Effects of a Low-Salt Diet on Idiopathic Hypercalciuria in Calcium-Oxalate Stone Formers: A 3-Mo Randomized Controlled Trial." *American Journal of Clinical Nutrition*, 2010 Mar, 91(3): 565–70. E-pub 2009 Dec 30.

117 L. Borghi, T. Schianchi, T. Meschi, *et al.* "Comparison of Two Diets for the Prevention of Recurrent Stones in Idiopathic Hypercalciuria." *New England Journal of Medicine*, 2002 Jan 10, 346(2): 77–84.

118 D. A. Spector. 2007. "Urinary Stones." In N. H. Fiebach *et al.*, eds., *Principles of Ambulatory Medicine*, 7th ed., 754–766 (Philadelphia: Lippincott Williams and Wilkins).

119 http://www.livingwithcrohnsdisease.com/livingwithcrohnsdisease/voices/key_findings.html.

120 Voices of Ulcerative Colitis survey. Available online at http://www.livingwithuc.com/livingwithuc/voices/index.html.

121 Voices of Crohn's survey. Available online at http://www.livingwithcrohnsdisease.com/livingwithcrohnsdisease/voices/key_findings.html.

122 "ASGE Guideline: Endoscopy in the Diagnosis and Treatment of Inflammatory Bowel Disease." *Gastrointestinal Endoscopy,* Volume 63, No. 4 : 2006.

123 P. Jantchou, S. Morois, F. Clavel-Chapelon, *et al.* "Animal Protein Intake and Risk of Inflammatory Bowel Disease: The E3N Prospective Study." *American Journal of Gastroenterology*, 2010 May 11. E-pub ahead of print.

124 W. Kruis, P. Fric, J. Pokrotnieks, *et al.* "Maintaining Remission of Ulcerative Colitis with the Probiotic Escherichia Coli Nissle 1917 Is as Effective as with Standard Mesalazine." *Gut*, 2004, 53: 1617–1623.

125 A. Ulitsky. Presented at the 73rd Annual Meeting of the American College of Gastroenterology, 2008.

126 B. G. Feagan *et al.* "Omega-3 Free Fatty Acids for the Maintenance of Remission in Crohn's Disease." *Journal of the American Medical Association*, 2008 April 9, Vol. 299, No. 14, 1690–1697.

127 S. L. Jowett, C J. Seal, M. S. Pearce, *et al.* "Influence of Dietary Factors on the Clinical Course of Ulcerative Colitis: A Prospective Cohort Study." *Gut*, 2004 Oct, 53(10): 1479–84.

128 M. G. Russel, L. G. Engels, J. W. Muris, *et al.* "'Modern Life' in the Epidemiology of Inflammatory Bowel Disease: A Case-Control Study with Special Emphasis on Nutritional Factors." *European Journal of Gastroenterology & Hepatology*, 1998, vol. 10, no3, 243–249.

129 C. P. Loudon, V. Corroll, J. Butcher, *et al.* "The Effects of Physical Exercise on Patients with Crohn's Disease." *American Journal of Gastroenterology*, 94(3), 697–703 (1999). V. Ng, W. Millard, C. Lebrun, *et al.* "Low-Intensity Exercise Improves Quality of Life in Patients with Crohn's Disease." *Clinical Journal of Sports Medicine*, 17(5), 384–388 (2007).

130 W. Millard. *Clinical Journal of Sports Medicine*, 2007.

131 C. B. Bernstein, S. Singh, L. A. Graff, *et al.* "A Prospective Population-Based Study of Triggers of Symptomatic Flares in IBD," *American Journal of Gastroenterology*, 2010; 105:1994–2002.

132 E. García-Vega and C. Fernandez-Rodriguez. "A Stress Management Programme for Crohn's Disease." *Behaviour Research and Therapy*, 2004 Apr, 42(4): 367–83.

133 J. L. Kiebles, B. Doerfler, and L. Keefer. "Preliminary Evidence Supporting a Framework of Psychological Adjustment to Inflammatory Bowel Disease." *Inflammatory Bowel Disease*, 2010 Feb 12. E-pub ahead of print.

134 A. Shetty, C. Kalantzis, D. Polymeros, *et al.* "Hypnotherapy for Inflammatory Bowel Disease." *Gut*, 53 (2004). L. Keefer and A. Keshavarzian. "Feasibility and Acceptability of Gut-Directed Hypnosis on Inflammatory Bowel Disease." *International Journal of Clinical and Experimental Hypnosis*, 55(4), 457–466 (2007).

135 V. Miller and P. J. Whorwell. "Treatment of Inflammatory Bowel Disease: A Role for Hypnotherapy?" *International Journal of Clinical and Experimental Hypnosis*, 2008 Jul, 56(3): 306–17.

136 Paul Rutgeerts, Robert Lofberg, Helmut Malchow, *et al.* "A Comparison of Budesonide with Prednisolone for Active Crohn's Disease." *New England Journal of Medicine,* Volume 331: 842–845, September 29, 1994, Number 13.

137 R. J. Farrell and D. Kelleher. "Mechanisms of Steroid Action and Resistance in Inflammation. Glucocorticoid Resistance in Inflammatory Bowel Disease." *Journal of Endocrinology,* (2003) 178, 339–346.

138 S. Friedman and G. R. Lichtenstein. "Ulcerative Colitis." 2006. In M. M. Wolfe *et al.*, eds. *Therapy of Digestive Disorders*, 2nd ed., 803–817 (Philadelphia: Saunders Elsevier).

139 ———. "Crohn's Disease." 2006. In M. M. Wolfe, *et al.*, eds. *Therapy of Digestive Disorders*, 2nd ed., 785–801 (Philadelphia: Saunders Elsevier).

140 L. Sutherland, J. Singleton, J. Sessions, *et al.* "Double Blind, Placebo Controlled Trial of Metronidazole in Crohn's Disease." *Gut*, 1991, 32: 1071–5.

141 C. Prantera, F. Zannoni, M. L. Scribano, *et al.* "An Antibiotic Regimen for the Treatment of Active Crohn's Disease: A Randomized, Controlled Clinical Trial of Metronidazole Plus Ciprofloxacin." *American Journal of Gastroenterology*, 1996, 91: 328–32.

142 K. Takeuchi, S.Smale, P. Premchand, *et al.* "Prevalence and Mechanism of Nonsteroidal Anti-Inflammatory Drug-Induced Clinical Relapse in Patients with Inflammatory Bowel Disease." *Clinical Gastroenterology and Hepatology*, 2006 Feb, 4(2): 157–9.

143 Din *et al.* "Use of Methotrexate in Refractory Crohn's Disease: The Edinburgh Experience." *Inflammatory Bowel Disease*, 2008 Jun, 14(6): 756–62.

144 B. G. Feagan *et al.* "Omega-3 Free Fatty Acids for the Maintenance of Remission in Crohn Disease: The EPIC Randomized Controlled Trials."

145 William J. Sandborn. "Transdermal Nicotine for Mildly to Moderately Active Ulcerative Colitis." *Annals of Internal Medicine*, March 1, 1997, 126(5): 364–371.

146 M. J. Carter, A. J. Lobo, and S. P. L. Travis. "Guidelines for the Management of Inflammatory Bowel Disease in Adults." On behalf of the IBD Section of the British Society of Gastroenterology, *Gut*, 2004, 53(Suppl V): v1–v16.

147 *Ibid.*

148 T. Tanaka, K. Takahama, T. Kimura, *et al.* "Effect of Concurrent Elemental Diet on Infliximab Treatment for Crohn's Disease." *Journal of Gastroenterology and Hepatology*, 2006 Jul, 21(7): 1143–9.

149 F. Casellas, J. López-Vivancos, X. Badia, *et al.* "Impact of Surgery for Crohn's Disease on Health-Related Quality of Life." *American Journal of Gastroenterology*, 2000 Jan, 95(1): 177–82.

150 S. R. Nordgren, S. B. Fasth, T. O. Oresland, *et al.* "Long-Term Follow-Up in Crohn's Disease. Mortality, Morbidity, and Functional Status." *Scandinavian Journal of Gastroenterology*, 1994 Dec, 29(12): 1122–8.

Chapter 15

1 The Neuropathy Association Inc. Available online at http://www.neuropathy.org/site/PageServer?pagename=About_Facts.

2 D. M. Nathan. "Some Answers, More Controversy, from UKPDS: U.K. Prospective Diabetes Study." The Lancet, 1998, 12: 832–833.

3 W. H. Herman and L. Kennedy. "Underdiagnosis of Peripheral Neuropathy in Type 2 Diabetes." Diabetes Care, 2005, 28: 1480–1481.

4 T. S. Jensen, M. M. Backonja, S. Hernández Jiménez, *et al.* "New Perspectives on the Management of Diabetic Peripheral Neuropathic Pain." *Diabetes and Vascular Disease Research*, 2006, Vol. 3, No. 2, 108–119.

5 Nicola Torrancea, Blair H. Smitha, Margaret C. Watsona, *et al.* "Medication and Treatment Use in Primary Care Patients with Chronic Pain of Predominantly Neuropathic Origin." *Family Practice,* published online on 2007 August 1.

6 *GfK HealthCare*. "Attitudes towards Neuropathic Pain: Consumer Survey." 2008 July.

7 B. Thompson *et al.* "Behavioral and Pharmacologic Interventions: The Raynaud's Treatment Study." *Controlled Clinical Trials,* 1999 Feb;20(1): 52–63.

8 Raynaud's Treatment Study Investigators, "Comparison of sustained-release nifedipine and temperature biofeedback for treatment of primary Raynaud phenomenon. Results from a randomized clinical trial with 1-year follow-up." *Archives of Internal Medicine*, 2000 Apr 24;160(8):1101-8.

9 L. Li, "The Effect of Neuragen PN® on Neuropathic Pain." *BMC Complementary and Alternative Medicine*, 2010, 10: 22.

10 F. T. Scott, M. E. Leedham-Green, W. Y. Barrett-Muir, *et al.* "A Study of Shingles and the Development of Postherpetic Neuralgia in East London." *Journal of Medical Virology*, 2003, 70 Suppl 1: S24–30.

11 *Ibid.*

12 B. S. Galer and R. K. Portenoy. "Acute Herpetic and Postherpetic Neuralgia: Clinical Features and Management." *Mt. Sinai Journal of Medicine*, 1991 May, 58(3): 257–66.

13 *Ibid.*

14 S. K. Tyring, K. R. Beutner, B. A. Tucker, *et al.* "Antiviral Therapy for Herpes Zoster: Randomized, Controlled Clinical Trial of Valacyclovir and Famciclovir Therapy in Immunocompetent Patients 50 Years and Older." *Archives of Family Medicine*, 2000 Sep–Oct, 9(9): 863–9.

15 K. R. Beutner. "Antivirals in the Treatment of Pain." *Journal of Geriatric Dermatology*, 1994, 6(2 suppl): 23A–28A.

16 Ian Gilron, C. Peter N. Watson, Catherine M. Cahill, *et al.* "Neuropathic Pain: A Practical Guide for the Clinician." *Canadian Medical Association Journal,* August 1, 2006, 175 (3).

17 Ralf Baron. "Therapy of Zoster Pain, Postherpetic Neuralgia and Other Neurological Complications." *Monographs in Virology*, 2006, vol 26, 143–153.

18 Ian Gilron, C. Peter N. Watson, Catherine M. Cahill, *et al.* "Neuropathic Pain: A Practical Guide for the Clinician." *Canadian Medical Association Journal,* August 1, 2006, 175 (3).

19 R. Baron. "Therapy of Zoster Pain, Postherpetic Neuralgia and Other Neurological Complications."

20 U. S. Department of Justice. "Tramadol." http://www.deadiversion.usdoj.gov/drugs_concern/tramadol.htm.

21 R. M. Duehmke, J. Hollingshead, and D. R. Cornblath. "Tramadol for Neuropathic Pain." *Cochrane Database of Systematic Reviews*, 2006, Issue 3, Art. No. CD003726.

22 H. W. Baik and R. M. Russell. "Vitamin B12 Deficiency in the Elderly." *Annual Review of Nutrition*, 1999, 19: 357–377.

23 K. El-Salem, F. Ammari, Y. Khader, *et al.* "Elevated Glycosylated Hemoglobin Is Associated with Subclinical Neuropathy in Neurologically Asymptomatic Diabetic Patients: A Prospective Study." *Journal of Clinical Neurophysiology*, 2009 Feb, 26(1): 50–3.

24 Writing Team for the DCCT/EDIC Research Group. "Effect of Intensive Therapy on the Microvascular Complications of Type 1 Diabetes Mellitus." *Journal of the American Medical Association*, 2002, 287: 2563–2569.

25 G. Negrisanu, M. Rosu, B. Bolte, *et al.* "Effects of 3-Month Treatment with the Antioxidant Alpha-Lipoicacid in Diabetic Peripheral Neuropathy." *Romanian Journal of Internal Medicine*, 1999, 37: 297–306. K. J. Ruhnau, H. P. Meissner, J. R. Finn, *et al.* "Effects of 3-Week Oral Treatment with the Antioxidant Thioctic Acid (Alpha-Lipoic Acid) in Symptomatic Diabetic Polyneuropathy." *Diabetic Medicine*, 1999, 16: 1040–1043.

26 A. Poorabbas, F. Fallah, J. Bagdadchi, *et al.* "Determination of Free L-Carnitine Levels in Type II Diabetic Women with and without Complications." European Journal of Clinical Nutrition, 2007 Jul, 61(7): 892–5.

27 M. Youle. "Acetyl-L-Carnitine in HIV-Associated Antiretroviral Toxic Neuropathy." CNS Drugs, 2007, 21 Suppl 1: 25–30, discussion 45–6.

28 A. A. Sima, M. Calvani, M. Mehra, *et al.* "Acetyl-L-Carnitine Improves Pain, Nerve Regeneration, and Vibratory Perception in Patients with Chronic Diabetic Neuropathy: An Analysis of Two Randomized Placebo-Controlled Trials." Acetyl-L-Carnitine Study Group. *Diabetes Care*, 2005 Jan, 28(1): 89–94.

29 *Ibid.*

30 Angelo Cacchio. "Mirror Therapy for Chronic Complex Regional Pain Syndrome, Type 1 and Stroke." *New England Journal of Medicine*, 2009 August 6, 361, 634–635.

31 Ruud W. Selles, Ton A. R. Schreuders, and Henk J. Stam. "Mirror Therapy in Patients with Causalgia (Complex Regional Pain Syndrome Type II) Following Peripheral Nerve Injury: Two Cases." *Journal of Rehabilitation Medicine*, 2008, 40: 312–314.

32 Benjamin H. Lee. "Physical Therapy and Cognitive-Behavioral Treatment for Complex Regional Pain Syndromes." *Journal of Pediatrics*, 2002, 141: 135–40.

33 G. Singh, S. N. Willen, M. V. Boswell, *et al.* "The Value of Interdisciplinary Pain Management in Complex Regional Pain Syndrome Type I: A Prospective Outcome Study." *Pain Physician*, 2004 Apr, 7(2): 203–9.

34 B. B. Abuaisha, J. B. Costanzi, and A. J. Boulton. "Acupuncture for the Treatment of Chronic Painful Peripheral Diabetic Neuropathy: A Long-Term Study." *Diabetes Research and Clinical Practice*, 1998, 39: 115–121.

35 Paul J. Goodnick, Karen Breakstone, Xue/Lan Wen, *et al.* "Acupuncture and Neuropathy." *American Journal of Psychiatry*, 2000 August, 157: 1342–1343.

36 J. Fleckenstein. "Acupuncture In Acute Herpes Zoster Pain Therapy (Acuzoster)." *BMC Complementary and Alternative Medicine*, 2009 Aug 12, 9: 31.

37 M. I. Korpan, *et al.* "Acupuncture in the Treatment of Post Traumatic Pain Syndrome." *Acta Orthopedica Belgica*, 1999, Vol 65-2, 197–201.

38 The Capsaicin Study Group. "Treatment of Painful Diabetic Neuropathy with Topical Capsaicin." *Archives of Internal Medicine*, 1991 Nov, 151(11): 2225–9.

39 N. Ellison *et al.* "Phase III Placebo-Controlled Trial of Capsaicin Cream in the Management of Surgical Neuropathic Pain in Cancer Patients." *Journal of Clinical Oncology*, 1997, 15: 2974–80.

40 M.Nolano, D. A. Simone, G. Wendelschafer-Crabb, *et al.* "Topical Capsaicin in Humans: Parallel Loss of Epidermal Nerve Fibers and Pain Sensation." *Pain*, 1999, 81: 135–45.

41 J. A. Paice *et al.* "Topical Capsaicin in the Management of HIV-Associated Peripheral Neuropathy." *Journal of Pain Symptom Management*, 2000, 19: 45–52

42 VA Pharmacy Benefits Management Services. "National Drug Monograph Capsaicin 8% Patch (Qutenza)."

43 Baron. "Therapy of Zoster Pain, Postherpetic Neuralgia and Other Neurological Complications."

44 N. Garroway, S. Chhabra, S. Landis, *et al.* "Clinical Inquiries: What Measures Relieve Postherpetic Neuralgia?" *Journal of Family Practice*, 2009 Jul, 58(7): 384d–f.

45 M. C. Rowbotham, P. S. Davies, C. Verkempinck, *et al.* "Lidocaine Patch: Double-Blind Controlled Study of a New Treatment Method for Post-Herpetic Neuralgia." *Pain*, 1996, 65(1): 39–44. B. S. Galer, M. P. Jensen, T. Ma, *et al.* "The Lidocaine Patch 5% Effectively Treats All Neuropathic Pain Qualities: Results of a Randomized, Double-Blind, Vehicle-Controlled, 3-Week Efficacy Study with Use of the Neuropathic Pain Scale." *Clinical Journal of Pain*, 2002, 18(5): 297–301.

46 E. Eisenberg, E. D. McNicol, and D. B. Carr. "Opioids for Neuropathic Pain." Chapter 16.

47 R. Baron *et al.* "5% Lidocaine Medicated Plaster Vs. Pregabalin in Patients with Painful Diabetic Polyneuropathy (DPN)." *Diabetologia*, 52: S452.

48 T. Saarto and P. J. Wiffen. "Antidepressants for Neuropathic Pain." *Cochrane Database of Systematic Reviews*, 2007, Issue 4. Art. No. CD005454.

49 H. J. McQuaya, M. Traméra, B. A. Nyea, *et al.* "A Systematic Review of Antidepressants in Neuropathic Pain." *Pain*, 1996 December, Volume 68, Issues 2–3, 217–227.

50 M. Max. *New England Journal of Medicine*, 1982.

51 A. Sultan, H. Gaskell, S. Derry, and R. A. Moore. "Duloxetine for Painful Diabetic Neuropathy and Fibromyalgia Pain." *BMC Neurology*, 2008 Aug 1, 8: 29.

52 P. J. Wiffen, H. J. McQuay, and R. A. Moore. "Carbamazepine for Acute and Chronic Pain in Adults." *Cochrane Database of Systematic Reviews*, 2005, Issue 3, Art. No. CD005451.

53 FDA. "Information for Healthcare Professionals: Dangerous or Even Fatal Skin Reactions— Carbamazepine."

54 E. Eisenberg, E. D. McNicol, and D. B. Carr. "Opioids for Neuropathic Pain." *Cochrane Database of Systematic Reviews*, 2006, Issue 3. Art. No. CD006146.

55 Michael C. Rowbotham, Lisa Twilling, Pamela S. Davies, *et al.* "Oral Opioid Therapy for Chronic Peripheral and Central Neuropathic Pain." *New England Journal of Medicine*, 2003 March 27, Volume 348, Number 13, 1223–1232.

56 I. Gilron, J. M. Bailey, D. Tu, *et al.* "Morphine, Gabapentin, or Their Combination for Neuropathic Pain." *New England Journal of Medicine*, 2005, 352, 1324–1334.

Chapter 16

1 http://www.ncbi.nlm.nih.gov/pubmed/17196904.

2 Nora Janjan. "Do We Need to Improve Pain Management in the Radiation Oncology Department?" *Nature Clinical Practice Oncology*, 2005, 2, 130–131.

3 Ana Blasco, Miguel Berzosa, Vega Iranzo, *et al.* "Update in Cancer Pain." *Cancer & Chemotherapy Reviews*, 2009.

4 J. B. Streisand, J. R. Varvel, D. R. Stanski, *et al.* "Absorption and Bioavailability of Oral Transmucosal Fentanyl Citrate." *Anesthesiology*, 1991, 75: 223–9.

5 T. D. Egan, A. Sharma, M. A. Ashburn, *et al.* "Multiple Dose Pharmacokinetics of Oral Transmucosal Fentanyl Citrate in Healthy Volunteers." *Anesthesiology*, 2000, 92: 665–73.

6 N. Y. Gabrail. "The Efficacy, Tolerability, and Speed of Onset of Fentanyl Pectin Nasal Spray (FPNS) in the Treatment of Breakthrough Cancer Pain (BTCP)." *Journal of Clinical Oncology*, 2009, 27: 15s.

7 M. D. David and A. Fishbain. "Pharmacotherapeutic Management of Breakthrough Pain in Patients with Chronic Persistent Pain." *FAPA, American Journal of Managed Care*, 2008, 14: S123–S128.

8 S. Mercadante. "Breakthrough Pain in Oncology: A Longitudinal Study." *Journal of Pain Symptom Management*, 2010 May 4. E-pub ahead of print.

9 K. L. Kwekkeboom, H. Hau, B. Wanta, *et al.* "Patients' Perceptions of the Effectiveness of Guided Imagery and Progressive Muscle Relaxation Interventions Used for Cancer Pain." *Complementary Therapies in Clinical Practice*, 2008 Aug, 14(3): 185–94.

10 *Ibid.*

11 Elizabeth M. Thomas and Sharlene M. Weiss. "Nonpharmacological Interventions with Chronic Cancer Pain in Adults." *Cancer Control,* 2000 March/April, Vol. 7, No. 2, 157–164.

12 J. W. Carson, K. M. Carson, L. S. Porter, *et al.* "Yoga for Women with Metastatic Breast Cancer: Results from a Pilot Study." *Journal of Pain Symptom Management,* 2007 Mar, 33(3): 331–41.

13 S. C. Danhauer, J. A. Tooze, D. F. Farmer, *et al.* "Restorative Yoga for Women with Ovarian or Breast Cancer: Findings from a Pilot Study." *Journal of the Society for Integrative Oncology,* 2008 Spring, 6(2): 47–58.

14 Julienne E. Bower, Alison Woolery, Beth Sternlieb, *et al.* "Yoga for Cancer Patients and Survivors." *Cancer Control,* July 2005, Vol. 12, No. 3.

15 Carole A. Paley, Michael I. Bennett, and Mark I. Johnson. "Acupuncture for Cancer-Induced Bone Pain?" *Evidence-Based Complementary and Alternative Medicine,* 2010. Published online 2010 March 24.

16 David Alimi, Carole Rubino, Evelyne Pichard-Léandri, *et al.* "Analgesic Effect of Auricular Acupuncture for Cancer Pain." *Journal of Clinical Oncology,* Vol 21, Issue 22 (November), 2003: 4120–4126.

17 W. E. Mehling, B. Jacobs, M. Acree, *et al.* "Symptom Management with Massage and Acupuncture in Postoperative Cancer Patients." *Journal of Pain Symptom Management,* 2007 Mar, 33(3): 258–66.

18 Carole A. Paley, Michael I. Bennett, and Mark I. Johnson. "Acupuncture for Cancer-Induced Bone Pain?" *Evidence-Based Complementary and Alternative Medicine,* 2010. Published online 2010 March 24.

19 Carole A. Paley, Michael I. Bennett, and Mark I. Johnson. "Investigating Acupuncture Using Brain Imaging Techniques: The Current State of Play." *Evidence-Based Complementary and Alternative Medicine,* 2005 2(3): 315–319.

20 Carole A. Paley, Michael I. Bennett, and Mark I. Johnson. "Acupuncture for Cancer-Induced Bone Pain?" *Evidence-Based Complementary and Alternative Medicine,* 2010. Published online March 24, 2010.

21 B. R. Cassileth, A. J. Vickers. "Massage Therapy for Symptom Control: Outcome Study at a Major Cancer Center." *Journal of Pain Symptom Management,* 2004 September, 28, no. 3: 244–249.

22 J. S. Kutner, M. C. Smith, L. Corbin, *et al.* "Massage Therapy Versus Simple Touch to Improve Pain and Mood in Patients with Advanced Cancer." *Annals of Internal Medicine,* 2008 Sep 16, 149(6): 369–79.

23 Janice Post-White, Mary Ellen Kinney, Kay Savik, *et al.* "Therapeutic Massage and Healing Touch Improve Symptoms in Cancer." *Integrative Cancer Therapies,* 2003, Vol. 2, No. 4, 332–344.

24 Gary Deng and Barrie R. Cassileth. "Integrative Oncology: Complementary Therapies for Pain, Anxiety, and Mood Disturbance." *CA: A Cancer Journal for Clinicians,* 2005 March/April, 55: 109–116, Volume 55Y, Number 2Y.

25 J. S. Kutner, M. C. Smith, L. Corbin, *et al.* "Massage Therapy Versus Simple Touch to Improve Pain and Mood in Patients with Advanced Cancer." *Annals of Internal Medicine,* 2008 Sep 16, 149(6): 369–79.

26 D. Spiegel, J. R. Bloom, and I. Yalom. "Group Support for Patients with Metastatic Cancer." *Archives of General Psychiatry,* 1981, 38: 527–533.

27 D. Spiegel and J. R. Bloom. "Group Therapy and Hypnosis Reduce Metastatic Breast Carcinoma Pain." *Psychosomatic Medicine,* 1983, 45: 333–339.

28 K. L. Syrjala, G. W. Donaldson, M. W. Davis, *et al.* "Relaxation and Imagery and Cognitive-Behavioral Training Reduce Pain during Cancer Treatment." *Pain,* 1995 Nov, 63(2): 189–98.

29 L. D. Butler, C. Koopman , E. Neri, *et al.* "Effects of Supportive-Expressive Group Therapy on Pain in Women with Metastatic Breast Cancer." *Health Psychology,* 2009 Sep, 28(5): 579–87.

30 G. Montgomery, D. Bovbjerg, J. B. Schnur, *et al.* "A Randomized Clinical Trial of a Brief Hypnosis Intervention to Control Side Effects in Breast Surgery Patients." *Journal of the National Cancer Institute* (2007) 99 (17): 1304-1312.

31 L. E. Carlson, M. Speca, K. D. Patel, *et al.* "Mindfulness-Based Stress Reduction in Relation to Quality of Life, Mood, Symptoms of Stress, and Immune Parameters in Breast and Prostate Cancer Outpatients." *Psychosomatic Medicine,* 2003 Jul–Aug, 65(4): 571–81.

32 S. M. Bauer-Wu and E. Rosenbaum. "Facing the Challenges of Stem Cell/Bone Marrow Transplantation with Mindfulness Meditation." *Psycho-Oncology,* 13, S10–S11.

33 *Ibid.*

34 L. Witek-Janusek, K. Albuquerque, K. Rambo Chroniak, *et al.* "Effect of Mindfulness Based Stress Reduction on Immune Function, Quality of Life and Coping in Women Newly Diagnosed with Early Stage Breast Cancer." *Brain, Behavior, and Immunity,* 2008, 22: 969–981.

35 L. E. Carlson and S. N. Garland. "Impact of Mindfulness-Based Stress Reduction (MBSR) on Sleep, Mood, Stress and Fatigue Symptoms in Cancer Outpatients." *International Journal of Behavioral Medicine,* 2005, 12: 278–285.

36 Kristine L. Kwekkeboom, Britt Wanta, and Molly Bumpus. "Individual Difference Variables and the Effects of Progressive Muscle Relaxation and Analgesic Imagery Interventions on Cancer Pain." *Journal of Pain Symptom Management,* 2008 Dec, 36(6): 604-15. Volume 36, Issue 6, Pages 604-615.

37 *Ibid.*

38 Kwekkeboom, Wanta, and Bumpus.

39 Hee J. Yoo, Se H. Ahn, Sung B. Kim, *et al.* "Efficacy of Progressive Muscle Relaxation Training and Guided Imagery in Reducing Chemotherapy Side Effects in Patients with Breast Cancer and in Improving Their Quality of Life." *Supportive Care in Cancer*, 2005 October, Volume 13, Number 10, 826–833.

40 Meral Demiralp, Fahriye Oflaz, and Seref Komurcu. "Effects of Relaxation Training on Sleep Quality and Fatigue in Patients with Breast Cancer Undergoing Adjuvant Chemotherapy." *Journal of Clinical Nursing*, published online, 2010 12 Mar, Volume 19, Issue 7–8, 1073–1083.

41 E. D. McNicol, S. Strassels, L. Goudas, *et al.* "NSAIDS or Paracetamol, Alone or Combined with Opioids, for Cancer Pain." *Cochrane Database of Systematic Reviews*, 2005, Issue 1. Art. No. CD005180.

42 Ana Blasco, Miguel Berzosa, Vega Iranzo, *et al.* "Update in Cancer Pain." *Cancer & Chemotherapy Reviews*, 2009, 4(2): 95–109.

43 V. Ventafridda, M. Tamburini, A. Caraceni, *et al.* "A Validation Study of the WHO Method for Cancer Pain Relief." *Cancer*, 1987, 59: 850–6.

44 Ana Blasco, Miguel Berzosa, Vega Iranzo, *et al.* "Update in Cancer Pain."

45 T. Saarto and P. J. Wiffen. "Antidepressants for Neuropathic Pain." *Cochrane Database of Systematic Reviews*, 2007, Issue 4. Art. No. CD005454.

46 A. Jacox, D. B. Carr, R. Payne, *et al.* "Clinical Practice Guideline Number 9: Management of Cancer Pain." Rockville, MD: U.S. Department of Health and Human Services, Agency for Health Care Policy and Research, 1994. AHCPR publication no. 94-0592.

47 M. H. Levy. "Pharmacologic Treatment of Cancer Pain." *New England Journal of Medicine*, 1996, 335: 1124–32.

48 K. Keskinbora, A. F. Pekel, and I. Aydinli. "Gabapentin and an Opioid Combination Versus Opioid Alone for the Management of Neuropathic Cancer Pain." *Journal of Pain Symptom Management*, 2007, 34: 183–189.

49 T. Donovan-Rodríguez, A. H. Dickenson, and C. E. Urch. "Gabapentin Normalizes Spinal Neuronal Responses That Correlate with Behavior in A Rat Model of Cancer-Induced Bone Pain." *Anesthesiology*, 2005, 102: 132–140.

50 D. P. Petrylak, C. M. Tangen, M. H. Hussain, *et al.* "Docetaxel and Estramustine Compared with Mitoxantrone and Prednisone for Advanced Refractory Prostate Cancer." *New England Journal of Medicine*, 2004, 351: 1513–1520.

51 O. O. Zaidat and R. L. Ruff. "Treatment of Spinal Epidural Metastasis Improves Patient Survival and Functional State." *Neurology*, 2002, 58: 1360–1366.

52 K. K. Yuen, M. Shelley, W. M. Sze, T. J. Wilt. Mason M. "Bisphosphonates for Advanced Prostate Cancer." *Cochrane Database of Systematic Reviews*, 2006, Issue 4. Art. No. CD006250.

53 "Double-Blinded Controlled Study Comparing Clodronate Versus Placebo in Patients with Breast Cancer Bone Metastases." *Bulletin of Cancer*, 2001 Jul, 88(7): 701–7.

54 D. Taylor, V. Galan, S. M.Weinstein, *et al.* "Fentanyl Pectin Nasal Spray in Breakthrough Cancer Pain." *Journal of Supportive Oncology*, 2010 Jul–Aug, 8(4): 184–90.

Chapter 17

1 J. Rohrbeck, K. Jordan, and P. Croft. "The Frequency and Characteristics of Chronic Widespread Pain in General Practice: A Case-Control Study." *British Journal of General Practice*, 2007, 57(535), 109-15.

2 V. R. Aggarwal, J. McBeth, J. M. Zakrzewska, *et al.* "The Epidemiology of Chronic Syndromes That Are Frequently Unexplained: Do They Have Common Associated Factors?" *International Journal of Epidemiology*, 2006, 35(2), 468-76.

3 P. Henningsen, S. Zipfel, and W. Herzog. "Management of Functional Somatic Syndromes." *The Lancet*, 2007, 369(9565), 946-55.

4 D. L. Goldenberg. "Pain/Depression Dyad: A Key to a Better Understanding and Treatment of Functional Somatic Syndromes." *American Journal of Medicine*, 2010, 123(8), 675–682.

5 D. Maquet, C. Demoulin, and J. M. Crielaard. "Chronic Fatigue Syndrome: A Systematic Review." *Annales de Réadaptation et de Médecine Physique*, 2006,49(6), 337–47, 418–27.

6 A. Avellaneda Fernandez, A. Perez Martin, M. Izquierdo Martinez, *et al.* "Chronic Fatigue Syndrome: Aetiology, Diagnosis and Treatment." *BMC Psychiatry*, 2009, 9 Suppl 1, S1.

7 I. Hickie, T. Davenport, S. D. Vernon, *et al.* "Are Chronic Fatigue and Chronic Fatigue Syndrome Valid Clinical Entities Across Countries and Health-Care Settings?" *Australian and New Zealand Journal of Psychiatry*, 2009, 43(1), 25–35.

8 K. Fukuda, S. E. Straus, I. Hickie, *et al.* "The Chronic Fatigue Syndrome: A Comprehensive Approach to Its

Definition and Study." International Chronic Fatigue Syndrome Study Group. *Annals of Internal Medicine*, 1994, 121(12), 953–9.

9 D. Maquet, C. Demoulin, and J. M. Crielaard. "Chronic Fatigue Syndrome: A Systematic Review."

10 B. Van Houdenhove, C. U. Pae, and P. Luyten. "Chronic Fatigue Syndrome: Is There A Role for Non-Antidepressant Pharmacotherapy?" *Expert Opinion on Pharmacotherapy*, 2010, 11(2), 215–23.

11 L. Jason, K. Muldowney, and S. Torres-Harding. "The Energy Envelope Theory and Myalgic Encephalomyelitis/Chronic Fatigue Syndrome." *American Association of Occupational Health Nurses*, 2008, 56(5), 189–95.

12 J. Nijs, I. van Eupen, J. Vandecauter, *et al.* "Can Pacing Self-Management Alter Physical Behavior and Symptom Severity in Chronic Fatigue Syndrome?" *Journal of Rehabilitation Research and Development*, 2009, 46(7), 985–96.

13 N. S. Porter, L. A. Jason, A. Boulton, *et al.* "Alternative Medical Interventions Used in the Treatment and Management of Myalgic Encephalomyelitis/Chronic Fatigue Syndrome and Fibromyalgia." *Journal of Alternative and Complementary Medicine*, 2010, 16(3), 235–49.

14 I. M. Cox, M. J. Campbell, and D. Dowson. "Red Blood Cell Magnesium and Chronic Fatigue Syndrome." *The Lancet*, 1991, 337(8744), 757–60.

15 Y. Manuel, B. Keenoy, G. Moorkens, *et al.* "Magnesium Status and Parameters of the Oxidant-Antioxidant Balance in Patients with Chronic Fatigue: Effects of Supplementation with Magnesium." *Journal of the American College of Nutrition*, 2000, 19(3), 374–82.

16 Office of Dietary Supplements, National Institutes of Health 2009, "Magnesium." Health Professional Fact Sheet. Available online at http: //ods.od.nih.gov/factsheets/magnesium.asp.

17 P. O. Behan, W. M. Behan, and D. Horrobin. "Effect of High Doses of Essential Fatty Acids on the Postviral Fatigue Syndrome." *Acta Neurologica Scandinavica*, 1990, 82: 209–16.

18 G. Warren, M. McKendrick, and M. Peet. "The Role of Essential Fatty Acids in Chronic Fatigue Syndrome. A Case-Controlled Study of Red-Cell Membrane Essential Fatty Acids (EFA) and a Placebo-Controlled Treatment Study with High Dose of EFA." *Acta Neurologica Scandinavica*, 1999, 99: 112–6.

19 N. J. Temple. "The Marketing of Dietary Supplements in North America: The Emperor Is (Almost) Naked." *Journal of Alternative and Complementary Medicine*, 2010, 16(7), 803–6.

20 F. Lesperance, N. Frasure-Smith, E. St-Andre, *et al.* "The Efficacy of Omega-3 Supplementation for Major Depression: A Randomized Controlled Trial." *Journal of Clinical Psychiatry*, 2010.

21 R. C. Vermeulen and H. R. Scholte. "Exploratory Open Label, Randomized Study of Acetyl- and Propionyl-carnitine in Chronic Fatigue Syndrome." *Psychosomatic Medicine*, 2004, 66(2), 276–82.

22 M. Edmonds, H. McGuire, and J. Price, "Exercise Therapy for Chronic Fatigue Syndrome." *Cochrane Database of Systematic Reviews*, 2004, (3), CD003200.

23 T. M. Field, W. Sunshine, M. Hernandez-Reif, *et al.* "Massage Therapy Effects On Depression and Somatic Symptoms in Chronic Fatigue Syndrome." *Journal of Chronic Fatigue Syndrome*, 1997, 3: 43–52.

24 J. H. Wang, T. Q. Chai, G. H. Lin, *et al.* "Effects of the Intelligent-Turtle Massage on the Physical Symptoms and Immune Functions in Patients with Chronic Fatigue Syndrome." *Journal of Traditional Chinese Medicine*, 2009, 29(1), 24–8.

25 T. Field, M. Hernandez-Reif, M. Diego, *et al.* "Cortisol Decreases and Serotonin and Dopamine Increase Following Massage Therapy." *International Journal of Neuroscience*, 2005, 115(10): 1397–1413.

26 N. S. Porter, L. A. Jason, A. Boulton, *et al.* "Alternative Medical Interventions Used in the Treatment and Management of Myalgic Encephalomyelitis/Chronic Fatigue Syndrome and Fibromyalgia." *Journal of Alternative and Complementary Medicine*, 2010, 16(3), 235–49.

27 T. Wang, Q. Zhang, X. Xue, *et al.* "A Systematic Review of Acupuncture and Moxibustion Treatment for Chronic Fatigue Syndrome in China." *American Journal of Chinese Medicine*, 2008, 36(1), 1–24.

28 L. Yuemei, L. Hongping, F. Shulan, *et al.* "The Therapeutic Effects of Electrical Acupuncture and Auricular-Plaster in 32 Cases of Chronic Fatigue Syndrome." *Journal of Traditional Chinese Medicine*, 2006, 26(3), 163–4.

29 J. R. Price, E. Mitchell, E. Tidy, *et al.* "Cognitive Behaviour Therapy for Chronic Fatigue Syndrome in Adults." *Cochrane Database of Systematic Reviews*, 2008, (3), CD001027.

30 C. U. Pae, D. M. Marks, A. A. Patkar, *et al.* "Pharmacological Treatment of Chronic Fatigue Syndrome: Focusing on the Role of Antidepressants." *Expert Opinion on Pharmacotherapy*, 2009, 10(10), 1561–70.

31 A.-M. Bagnall, S. Hempel, D. Chambers, *et al.* 2007, "The Treatment and Management of Chronic Fatigue Syndrome (CFS)/Myalgic Encephalomyelitis (ME) in Adults and Children." CRD Report 35. York: University of York. Available online at http: //www.york.ac.uk/inst/crd/CRD_Reports/crdreport35.pdf.

32 B. Van Houdenhove, C. U. Pae, and P. Luyten. "Chronic Fatigue Syndrome: Is There a Role for Non-Antidepressant Pharmacotherapy?" *Expert Opinion on Pharmacotherapy*, 2010, 11(2), 215–23.

33 N. G. Klimas and A. O. Koneru. "Chronic Fatigue Syndrome: Inflammation, Immune Function, and Neuroendocrine Interactions." *Current Rheumatology Reports*, 2007, 9(6), 482–7.

34 J. K. Chia. "The Role of Enterovirus in Chronic Fatigue Syndrome." *J Clin Pathol*, 2005, 58(11), 1126–32.

35 A. L. Komaroff. "Is Human Herpesvirus-6 a Trigger for Chronic Fatigue Syndrome?" *Journal of Clinical Virology*, 2006, 37 Suppl 1, S39–46.

36 L. D. Devanur and J. R. Kerr. "Chronic fatigue syndrome." *Journal of Clinical Virology*, 2006, 37(3), 139–50.

37 S. C. Lo, N. Pripuzova, B. Li, *et al.* "Detection of MLV-Related Virus Gene Sequences in Blood of Patients with Chronic Fatigue Syndrome and Healthy Blood Donors." *Proceedings of the National Academy of Sciences of the United States of America*, 2010, 107(36), 15874–9.

38 K. P. White and M. Harth. "Classification, Epidemiology, and Natural History of Fibromyalgia." *Current Pain Headache Reports*, 2001, 5(4), 320–9.

39 E. Choy, S. Perrot, T. Leon, *et al.* "A Patient Survey of the Impact of Fibromyalgia and the Journey to Diagnosis." *BMC Health Services Research*, 2010, 10, 102.

40 F. Wolfe, H. A. Smythe, M. B. Yunus, *et al.* "The American College of Rheumatology 1990 Criteria for the Classification of Fibromyalgia. Report of the Multicenter Criteria Committee." *Arthritis & Rheumatism*, 1990, 33(2), 160–72.

41 F. Wolfe, D. J. Clauw, M. A. Fitzcharles, *et al.* "The American College of Rheumatology Preliminary Diagnostic Criteria for Fibromyalgia and Measurement of Symptom Severity." *Arthritis Care & Research* (Hoboken), 2010, 62(5), 600–10.

42 R. M. Bennett. "Clinical Manifestations and Diagnosis of Fibromyalgia." *Rheumatic Disease Clinics of North America*, 2009, 35(2), 215–32.

43 J. Langhorst, F. Musial, P. Klose, *et al.* "Efficacy of Hydrotherapy in Fibromyalgia Syndrome." *Rheumatology (Oxford)*, 2009, 48(9), 1155–9.

44 F. Wolfe, H. A. Smythe, M. B Yunus, *et al.* "The American College of Rheumatology 1990 Criteria for the Classification of Fibromyalgia. Report of the Multicenter Criteria Committee." *Arthritis & Rheumatism*, 1990, 33(2), 160–72.

45 J. E. Sumpton and D. E. Moulin. "Fibromyalgia: Presentation and Management with a Focus On Pharmacological Treatment." *Pain Research & Management*, 2008, 13(6), 477–83.

46 W. Hauser, P. Klose, J. Langhorst, *et al.* "Efficacy of Different Types of Aerobic Exercise in Fibromyalgia Syndrome." *Arthritis Research & Therapy*, 2010, 12(3), R79.

47 K. B. Jensen, F. Petzke, S. Carville, *et al.* "Anxiety and Depressive Symptoms in Fibromyalgia Are Related to Low Health Esteem But Not to Pain Sensitivity Or Cerebral Processing of Pain." *Arthritis & Rheumatism*, 2010.

48 L. Kalichman. "Massage Therapy for Fibromyalgia Symptoms." *Rheumatology International*, 2010, 30(9), 1151–7.

49 R. A. Targino, M. Imamura, H. H. Kaziyama, *et al.* "A Randomized Controlled Trial of Acupuncture Added to Usual Treatment for Fibromyalgia." *Journal of Rehabilitation Medicine*, 2008, 40(7), 582–8.

50 A. Castel, M. Perez, J. Sala, *et al.* "Effect of Hypnotic Suggestion On Fibromyalgic Pain: Comparison between Hypnosis and Relaxation." *European Journal of Pain*, 2007, 11(4), 463–8.

51 J. Langhorst, F. Musial, P. Klose, *et al.* "Efficacy of Hydrotherapy in Fibromyalgia Syndrome."

52 W. Hauser, F. Petzke, and C. Sommer. "Comparative Efficacy and Harms of Duloxetine, Milnacipran, and Pregabalin in Fibromyalgia Syndrome." *Journal of Pain*, 2010, 11(6), 505–21.

53 S. Jacobsen, B. Danneskiold-Samsoe, and R. B. Andersen. "Oral S-Adenosylmethionine in Primary Fibromyalgia." *Scandinavian Journal of Rheumatology*, 1991, 20(4), 294–302.

54 R. J. Reiter, D. Acuna-Castroviejo, and D. X. Tan. "Melaton in therapy in Fibromyalgia." *Current Pain Headache Reports*, 2007, 11(5), 339–42.

55 L. Brosseau, G. A. Wells, P. Tugwell, *et al.* "Ottawa Panel Evidence-Based Clinical Practice Guidelines for Strengthening Exercises in the Management of Fibromyalgia: Part 2." *Physical Therapy*, 2008, 88(7), 873–86.

56 *Ibid.* 857–71.

57 W. Hauser, P. Klose, J. Langhorst, *et al.* "Efficacy of Different Types of Aerobic Exercise in Fibromyalgia Syndrome."

58 A. J. Busch, C. L. Schachter, T. J. Overend, *et al.* "Exercise for Fibromyalgia." *Journal of Rheumatology*, 2008, 35(6), 1130–44.

59 D. Munguia-Izquierdo and A. Legaz-Arrese. "Assessment of the Effects of Aquatic Therapy on Global Symptomatology in Patients with Fibromyalgia Syndrome." *Archives of Physical Medicine and Rehabilitation*, 2008, 89(12), 2250–7.

60 G. D. da Silva, G. Lorenzi-Filho, and L. V. Lage, "Effects of Yoga and the Addition of Tui Na in Patients with Fibromyalgia." *Journal of Alternative and Complementary Medicine*, 2007, 13(10), 1107–13.

61 L. Altan, N. Korkmaz, U. Bingol, *et al.* "Effect of Pilates Training On People with Fibromyalgia Syndrome." *Archives of Physical Medicine and Rehabilitation*, 2009, 90(12), 1983–8.

62 H. M. Taggart, C. L. Arslanian, S. Bae, *et al.* "Effects of T'ai Chi Exercise On Fibromyalgia Symptoms and Health-Related Quality of Life." *Orthopaedic Nursing*, 2003, 22(5), 353–60.

63 D. P. Martin, C. D. Sletten, B. A. Williams, *et al.* "Improvement in Fibromyalgia Symptoms with Acupuncture." *Mayo Clin Proceedings*, 2006, 81(6), 749–57.

64 J. Langhorst, P. Klose, F. Musial, *et al.* "Efficacy of Acupuncture in Fibromyalgia Syndrome." *Rheumatology (Oxford)*, 2010, 49(4), 778–88.

65 E. Martin-Sanchez, E. Torralba, E. Diaz-Dominguez, *et al.* "Efficacy of Acupuncture for the Treatment of Fibromyalgia." *Open Rheumatology Journal*, 2009, 3, 25–9.

66 E. Mayhew and E. Ernst. "Acupuncture for Fibromyalgia." *Rheumatology* (Oxford), 2007, 46(5), 801–4.

67 I. Citak-Karakaya, T. Akbayrak, F. Demirturk, *et al.* "Short and Long-Term Results of Connective Tissue Manipulation and Combined Ultrasound Therapy in Patients with Fibromyalgia." *Journal of Manipulative and Physiological Therapeutics*, 2006, 29(7), 524–8.

68 L. Kalichman, "Massage Therapy for Fibromyalgia Symptoms." Rheumatology International, 2010, 30(9), 1151–7.

69 J. Langhorst, F. Musial, P. Klose, *et al.* "Efficacy of Hydrotherapy in Fibromyalgia Syndrome." *Rheumatology* (Oxford), 2009, 48(9), 1155–9.

70 A. Fioravanti, G. Perpignano, G. Tirri, *et al.* "Effects of Mud-Bath Treatment On Fibromyalgia Patients." *Rheumatology International*, 2007, 27(12), 1157–61.

71 D. F. Vitorino, L. B. Carvalho, and G. F Prado. "Hydrotherapy and Conventional Physiotherapy Improve Total Sleep Time and Quality of Life of Fibromyalgia Patients." *Sleep Medicine*, 2006, 7(3), 293–6.

72 S. van Koulil, W. van Lankveld, F. W. Kraaimaat, *et al.* "Tailored Cognitive-Behavioral Therapy and Exercise Training for High-Risk Fibromyalgia Patients." *Arthritis Care & Research* (Hoboken) 2010.

73 P. J. Keel, C. Bodoky, U. Gerhard, *et al.* "Comparison of Integrated Group Therapy and Group Relaxation Training for Fibromyalgia." *Clinical Journal of Pain*, 1998, 14(3), 232–8.

74 L. Lipworth, R. E. Tarone, and J. K. McLaughlin. "Breast Implants and Fibromyalgia: A Review of the Epidemiologic Evidence." *Annals of Plastic Surgery*, 2004, 52(3), 284–7.

75 J. P. Fryzek, L. Holmich, and J. K. McLaughlin, L. Lipworth, R. E. Tarone, T. Henriksen, K. Kjoller, S. Friis. "A Nationwide Study of Connective Tissue Disease and Other Rheumatic Conditions Among Danish Women with Long-Term Cosmetic Breast Implantation." *Annals of Epidemiology*, 2007, 17(5), 374–9.

76 S. L. Brown, G. Pennello, W. A. Berg, *et al.* "Silicone Gel Breast Implant Rupture, Extracapsular Silicone, and Health Status in a Population of Women." *Journal of Rheumatology*, 2001, 28(5), 996–1003.

77 L. R. Holmich, K. Kjoller, J. P. Fryzek, *et al.* "Self-Reported Diseases and Symptoms by Rupture Status Among Unselected Danish Women with Cosmetic Silicone Breast Implants." *Plastic and Reconstructive Surgery*, 2003, 111(2), 723–32, discussion 733–4.

78 S. van Koulil, M. Effting, F. W. Kraaimaat, *et al.* "Cognitive-Behavioural Therapies and Exercise Programmes for Patients with Fibromyalgia." *Annals of the Rheumatic Diseases*, 2007, 66(5), 571–81.

79 G. Elkins, M. P. Jensen, and D. R. Patterson. "Hypnotherapy for the Management of Chronic Pain." *International Journal of Clinical and Experimental Hypnosis*, 2007, 55(3), 275–87.

80 A. Castel, M. Perez, J. Sala, *et al.* "Effect of Hypnotic Suggestion On Fibromyalgic Pain: Comparison between Hypnosis and Relaxation." *European Journal of Pain*, 2007, 11(4), 463–8.

81 G. Wik, H. Fischer, B. Bragee, *et al.* "Functional Anatomy of Hypnotic Analgesia: A PET Study of Patients with Fibromyalgia." *European Journal of Pain*, 1999, 3(1), 7–12.

82 S. W. Derbyshire, M. G. Whalley, and D. A. Oakley. "Fibromyalgia Pain and Its Modulation by Hypnotic and Non-Hypnotic Suggestion: an fMRI Analysis." *European Journal of Pain*, 2009, 13(5), 542–50.

83 S. W. Derbyshire, M. G. Whalley, V. A. Stenger, *et al.* "Cerebral Activation During Hypnotically Induced and Imagined Pain." *Neuroimage*, 2004, 23(1), 392–401.

84 S. E. Sephton, P. Salmon, I. Weissbecker, *et al.* "Mindfulness Meditation Alleviates Depressive Symptoms in Women with Fibromyalgia." *Arthritis & Rheumatism*, 2007, 57(1), 77–85.

85 A. S. Babu, E. Mathew, D. Danda, *et al.* "Management of Patients with Fibromyalgia Using Biofeedback." *Indian Journal of Medical Sciences*, 2007, 61(8), 455–61

86 S. P. Buckelew, R. Conway, J. Parker, *et al.* "Biofeedback/Relaxation Training and Exercise Interventions for Fibromyalgia." *Arthritis Care & Research*, 1998, 11(3), 196–209.

87 A. L. Hassett, D. C. Radvanski, E. G. Vaschillo, *et al.* "A Pilot Study of the Efficacy of Heart Rate Variability (HRV) Biofeedback in Patients with Fibromyalgia." *Applied Psychophysiology and Biofeedback*, 2007, 32(1), 1–10.

88 L. M. Arnold, D. J. Clauw, M. M. Wohlreich, *et al.* "Efficacy of Duloxetine in Patients with Fibromyalgia." *Primary Care Companion, Journal of Clinical Psychiatry*, 2009, 11(5), 237–44.

89 J. C. Branco, O. Zachrisson, S. Perrot, *et al.* "A European Multicenter Randomized Double-Blind Placebo-Controlled Monotherapy Clinical Trial of Milnacipran in Treatment of Fibromyalgia." *Journal of Rheumatology*, 2010, 37(4), 851–9.

90 I. J. Russell, P. J. Mease, T. R. Smith, *et al.* "Efficacy and Safety of Duloxetine for Treatment of Fibromyalgia in Patients with or without Major Depressive Disorder." *Pain*, 2008, 136(3), 432–44.

91 M. E. Geisser, R. H. Palmer, R. M. Gendreau, *et al.* "A Pooled Analysis of Two Randomized, Double-Blind, Placebo-Controlled Trials of Milnacipran Monotherapy in the Treatment of Fibromyalgia." *Pain Practice*, 2010.

92 L. J. Crofford, M. C. Rowbotham, P. J. Mease, *et al.* "Pregabalin for the Treatment of Fibromyalgia Syndrome: Results of a Randomized, Double-Blind, Placebo-Controlled Trial." *Arthritis & Rheumatism*, 2005, 52(4), 1264–73.

93 L. M. Arnold, I. J. Russell, E. W. Diri, *et al.* "A 14-week, Randomized, Double-Blinded, Placebo-Controlled Monotherapy Trial of Pregabalin in Patients with Fibromyalgia." *Journal of Pain*, 2008, 9(9), 792–805.

94 L. J. Crofford, P. J. Mease, S. L. Simpson, *et al.* "Fibromyalgia Relapse Evaluation and Efficacy for Durability of Meaningful Relief (FREEDOM): A 6-Month, Double-Blind, Placebo-Controlled Trial with Pregabalin." *Pain*, 2008, 136(3), 419–31.

95 W. Hauser, F. Petzke, and C. Sommer. "Comparative Efficacy and Harms of Duloxetine, Milnacipran, and Pregabalin in Fibromyalgia Syndrome." *Journal of Pain*, 2010, 11(6), 505–21.

96 A. J. Holman and R. R. Myers. "A Randomized, Double-Blind, Placebo-Controlled Trial of Pramipexole, a Dopamine Agonist, in Patients with Fibromyalgia Receiving Concomitant Medications." *Arthritis & Rheumatism*, 2005, 52(8), 2495–505.

97 N. Uceyler, W. Hauser, and C. Sommer. "A Systematic Review on the Effectiveness of Treatment with Antidepressants in Fibromyalgia Syndrome." *Arthritis & Rheumatism*, 2008, 59(9), 1279–98.

98 R. M. Bennett, M. Kamin, R. Karim, *et al.* "Tramadol and Acetaminophen Combination Tablets in the Treatment of Fibromyalgia Pain." *American Journal of Medicine*, 2003, 114(7), 537–45.

99 FDA MedWatch. "Ultram (tramadol hydrochloride), Ultracet (tramadol hydrochloride/acetaminophen): Label Change." Available online at http: //www.fda.gov/Safety/MedWatch/SafetyInformation/SafetyAlerts forHumanMedicalProducts/ucm213264.htm. Accessed online 7/31/2010.

100 M. Lofgren and C. Norrbrink. "Pain Relief in Women with Fibromyalgia: A Cross-Over Study of Superficial Warmth Stimulation and Transcutaneous Electrical Nerve Stimulation." *Journal of Rehabilitation Medicine*, 2009, 41(7), 557–62.

101 A. S. Lichtbroun, M. M. Raicer, and R. B. Smith, "The Treatment of Fibromyalgia with Cranial Electrotherapy Stimulation." *Journal of Clinical Rheumatology*, 2001, 7(2), 72–8, discussion 78.

102 S. T. Sutbeyaz, N. Sezer, F. Koseoglu, *et al.* "Low-Frequency Pulsed Electromagnetic Field Therapy in Fibromyalgia." *Clinical Journal of Pain*, 2009, 25(8), 722–8.

103 C. Usui, N. Doi, M. Nishioka, *et al.* "Electroconvulsive Therapy Improves Severe Pain Associated with Fibromyalgia." *Pain*, 2006, 121(3), 276–80.

104 J. Rohrbeck, K. Jordan, and P. Croft. "The Frequency and Characteristics of Chronic Widespread Pain in General Practice." *British Journal of General Practice*, 2007, 57(535), 109–15.

105 V. R. Aggarwal, J. McBeth, J. M. Zakrzewska, *et al.* "The Epidemiology of Chronic Syndromes That Are Frequently Unexplained: Do They Have Common Associated Factors?" *International Journal of Epidemiology*, 2006, 35(2), 468–76.

106 N. Egloff, M. E. Sabbioni, C. Salathé, *et al.* "Nondermatomal Somatosensory Deficits in Patients with Chronic Pain Disorder: Clinical Findings and Hypometabolic Pattern in FDG-PET." *Pain*, 2009, 145(1–2),252–8.

107 M. Valet, H. Gündel, T. Sprenger, *et al.* "Patients with Pain Disorder Show Gray-Matter Loss in Pain-Processing Structures: A Voxel-Based Morphometric Study." *Psychosomatic Medicine*, 2009, 71(1),49–56.

108 R. J. Brown. "Introduction to the Special Issue on Medically Unexplained Symptoms: Background and Future Directions." *Clinical Psychology Review*, 2007, 27(7), 769–80.

109 G. E. Simon, M. VonKorff, M. Piccinelli, *et al.* "An International Study of the Relation between Somatic Symptoms and Depression." *New England Journal of Medicine*, 1999, 341(18), 1329–35.

110 K. Kroenke. "Patients Presenting with Somatic Complaints: Epidemiology, Psychiatric Comorbidity and Management." *International Journal of Methods in Psychiatric Research*, 2003,12(1), 34–43.

111 P. Henningsen, S. Zipfel, and W. Herzog. "Management of Functional Somatic Syndromes." *The Lancet*, 2007, 369(9565), 946–55.

112 B. Saletu, W. Prause, P. Anderer, *et al.* "Insomnia in Somatoform Pain Disorder: Sleep Laboratory Studies On Differences to Controls and Acute Effects of Trazodone, Evaluated by the Somnolyzer 24 X 7 and the Siesta Database." *Neuropsychobiology*, 2005, 51(3), 148–63.

113 T. Muller, M. Mannel, H. Murck, *et al.* "Treatment of Somatoform Disorders with Saint-John's-Wort." *Psychosomatic Medicine*, 2004, 66(4), 538–47.

114 National Institutes of Health National Center on Complementary and Alternative Medicine. "Get the Facts: Saint-John's-Wort and Depression. Available online at http: //nccam.nih.gov/health/stjohnswort/sjw-and-depression.htm.

115 Q. Ma. "Beneficial Effects of Moderate Voluntary Physical Exercise and Its Biological Mechanisms on Brain Health." *Neuroscience Bulletin*, 2008, 24(4), 265–70.

116 S. Peters, I. Stanley, M. Rose, *et al.* "A Randomized Controlled Trial of Group Aerobic Exercise in Primary Care Patients with Persistent, Unexplained Physical Symptoms." *Family Practice*, 2002, 19(6), 665–74.

117 J. M. Glass, A. K. Lyden, F. Petzke, *et al.* "The Effect of Brief Exercise Cessation on Pain, Fatigue, and Mood Symptom Development in Healthy, Fit Individuals." *Journal of Psychosomatic Research*, 2004, 57(4), 391–8.

118 J. I. Escobar, M. A. Gara, A. M. Diaz-Martinez, *et al.* "Effectiveness of a Time-Limited Cognitive Behavior Therapy Type Intervention Among Primary Care Patients with Medically Unexplained Symptoms." *Annals of Family Medicine*, 2007, 5(4), 328–35.

119 C. Masia Warner, L. C. Reigada, P. H. Fisher, *et al.* "CBT for Anxiety and Associated Somatic Complaints in Pediatric Medical Settings." *Journal of Clinical Psychology in Medical Settings*, 2009, 16(2), 169–77.

120 M. Baetz and R. Bowen. "Chronic Pain and Fatigue: Associations with Religion and Spirituality." *Pain Research & Management*, 2001, 3(5), 383–8.

121 A. K. Nickel, T. Hillecke, H. Argstatter, *et al.* "Outcome Research in Music Therapy: A Step on the Long Road to an Evidence-Based Treatment." *Annals of the New York Academy of Sciences*, 2005, 1060, 283–93.

122 A. Hennings, P. Zill, and W. Rief. "Serotonin Transporter Gene Promoter Polymorphism and Somatoform Symptoms." *Journal of Clinical Psychiatry*, 2009, 70(11), 1536–9.

123 S. K. Brannan, C. H. Mallinckrodt, E. B. Brown, *et al.* "Duloxetine 60 mg Once-Daily in the Treatment of Painful Physical Symptoms in Patients with Major Depressive Disorder." *Journal of Psychiatric Research*, 2005, 39(1), 43–53.

124 M. W. Jann and J. H. Slade. "Antidepressant Agents for the Treatment of Chronic Pain and Depression." *Pharmacotherapy*, 2007, 27(11), 1571–87.

125 K. A. Davies, G. J. Macfarlane, B. I. Nicholl, *et al.* "Restorative Sleep Predicts the Resolution of Chronic Widespread Pain: Results from the EPIFUND Study." *Rheumatology (Oxford)*, 2008, 47(12), 1809–13.

126 J. I. Gold, N. E. Mahrer, J. Yee, *et al.* "Pain, Fatigue, and Health-Related Quality of Life in Children and Adolescents with Chronic Pain." *Clinical Journal of Pain*, 2009, 25(5), 407–12.

Boldface page references indicate photographs. Underscored references indicate boxed text.

Biofeedback *(cont.)*
  resources, 520
  for specific conditions
    back, neck, and shoulder pain, 166–67
    chronic prostatitis/chronic pelvic pain in
      men, 340
    fibromyalgia, 475
    temporomandibular disorders, 126–27
    vulvodynia, 316, 318
Biofreeze, 69
Biologics
  for adult Still's disease, 249–50
  for inflammatory bowel disease, Crohn's
    disease, and ulcerative colitis, 414–15
  overview, 68
Bisphosphonates, for cancer pain, 453
Bladder instillation/intravesical therapy, 332
Bladder pain. *See* Interstial cystitis/painful
    bladder syndrome
Bladder training, 333
Blood sugar control, for nerve pain, 424–25
Body awareness techniques, for cancer pain, 443
Bonefos (clodronate), 453
Bone pain, in cancer, 435
Boniva (ibandronate), 453
Boots, for stress fractures, 274
Botox
  for bunions, 202
  for interstial cystitis/painful bladder
    syndrome, 331
  for migraines, 84
  for myofascial pain, 282
  for temporomandibular disorders, 128
  for vulvodynia, 317
Bovine cartilage, 24
Bowels, clearing with clear liquid diet, 384
Braces
  for bursitis and tendinitis, 262
  for patellofemoral pain syndrome, 288
  for stress fractures, 274
Brain, effect of pain on, 6–7
Brain waves, 54–55
Breakthrough pain, cancer, 436
Breast implants, as potential cause of
    fibromyalgia, 473
Breaststroke, 505, **505**
Breathing techniques
  for gout, 194
  for rheumatoid arthritis, 237
Breath test, for *Helicobacter pylori*, 370
Bromelain, 24
Budesonide (Entocort), 411
Bunion pads, 200
Bunions
  diagnosis, 199
  fast relief, 199–200
  overview of, 198–99
  pain prevention strategies, 201–3
    Botox, 202
    shoe choice, 203

splint, 202
surgery, 202–3
toe-stretching exercises, 201–2
when to call the doctor, 200
Bupropion (Wellbutrin), 67, 430, 465
Burning mouth syndrome
  diagnosis, 139
  fast pain relief, 139–40
  medications as cause of, 144
  overview of, 138–39
  pain prevention strategies, 141–45
    acupuncture, 142
    capsaicin, 142
    clonazepam, 143–44
    medications, 143–44
    mind-body therapies, 142–43
    psychotherapy, 142–43
    supplements, 141–42
    zinc, 141–42
  symptoms, 139
  when to call the doctor, 140
  your pain prescription, 140–41
Bursitis and tendinitis. *See also* Achilles
    tendinitis; Rotator cuff injuries and
    impingement syndrome
  causes of, 256
  diagnosis, 257–58
  fast relief, 258
  overview, 256–57
  pain prevention strategies
    acupuncture, 260
    braces, pads, and splints, 262
    corticosteroid injections, 261
    eccentric stretching, 259, 259–60
    exercise and movement therapies, 259–60
    laser therapy, 262
    massage, 260
    medications, 261
    NSAIDs, 261
    touch therapies, 260
    ultrasound therapy, 261–62
  symptoms, 256, 257
  when to call the doctor, 257
  your new pain prescription, 258–59
Butterbur, for migraines, 85
Bypass surgery, 179–80

Caffeine
  in inflammatory bowel disease, 407
  as irritable bowel syndrome trigger, 21
  reducing for headache prevention, 98
  for tension headaches, 95, 97
Calan (verapamil), 69
Calcium
  calcium rich foods for kidney stones, 395,
    397
  in kidney stones, 393, 395, 396, 398,
    398–400
  for stress fractures, 271–72
Calf stretch, 189

Transcendental meditation, <u>54</u>
Transcutaneous electrical nerve stimulation
    (TENS), <u>41</u>
  for cancer pain, 439
  for chronic prostatitis/chronic pelvic pain in
    men, <u>341</u>
  described, <u>41</u>
  for interstial cystitis/painful bladder
    syndrome, 333
  for menstrual cramps, 292, 295–96
  resources, 517
Transrectal microwave hyperthermia, <u>342</u>
Transurethral microwave hyperthermia, <u>342</u>
Transurethral needle abalation (TUNA), <u>342</u>
Tree Pose, 504, **504**
Trexall. *See* Methotrexate
Treximet (sumatriptan plus naproxen), 70
Triamcinolone (Nasacort), 109
Trigeminal neuralgia, 416, 418. *See also* Nerve
    pain
Trigger foods, 20–21, 491–92
Trigger point injections, for myofascial pain, 283
Trigger points, 39
Trigger point therapy
  for chronic prostatitis/chronic pelvic pain in
    men, 339–40
  for interstial cystitis/painful bladder
    syndrome, 330
  for myofascial pain, 281, 282
  for patellofemoral pain syndrome, 286–87
Trileptal (oxcarbazepine), 67, 431
Triptans, 70, 83, <u>89</u>
TruLabel seal, 25
Tuina therapy, 277
TUNA, <u>342</u>
Turmeric, 27, 239
Tylenol. *See* Acetaminophen
Types of pain, 5–6
Tysabri (natalizumab), 68, 414

Ulcerative colitis, 34, 67, 68, 400–415. *See
    also* Inflammatory bowel disease (IBD)
Ulcers
  causes of, 61, 64, 364–66
  diagnosis, 366–67
  fast pain relief, 367–68
  milk effects on, <u>369</u>
  odds of recurrence, <u>370</u>
  pain prevention strategies
    antibiotics, 369–70
    food and supplements, 368–69
    H2 blockers, 371–72
    medications, 369–72
    NSAIDs cessation, 371
    probiotics, 368–69
    proton pump inhibitor, 371–72
    smoking cessation, 372
    triple therapy, 369–70
  symptoms, 366

  when to call the doctor, <u>367</u>
  your new pain prescription, 368
Ultram. *See* Tramadol
Ultrasound therapy, for bursitis and tendinitis,
    261–62
Unifiber, 386
Upright row, <u>159</u>
Uric acid
  in gout, 192
  kidney stones, 393, 399
Urinary tract infection, interstial cystitis
    distinguished from, <u>327</u>
Uroxatrol (alfuzosin), 340
Ursodeoxycholic acid (Actigall), <u>357</u>, 364
U.S. Pharmacopeia, <u>25</u>
Uterine artery embolism, for fibroids, <u>304</u>

Vaginal dilators, for vulvodynia, <u>317</u>
Vaginal odor, 323
Valacyclovir (Valtrex), for shingles, 422
Valium (diazepam), 69
Venlafaxine (Effexor), 67, 430
Verapamil (Calan, Verelan), 69
Vertebrae
  fractured, 150–51
  slipped, 151
Vicodin (hydrocodone), 70, 449
Vioxx, 64, 133
Viscosupplementation, for osteoarthritis,
    222–23
Visualization, for rheumatoid arthritis, 237
Vitamin B_1, for menstrual cramps, <u>296</u>
Vitamin B_6, for carpal tunnel syndrome, 265
Vitamin B_{12}, for nerve pain, 424
Vitamin C, for gout, 196
Vitamin D
  for back, neck, and shoulder pain, <u>156</u>
  benefits of, <u>27</u>
  for inflammatory bowel disease, Crohn's
    disease, and ulcerative colitis, 408
  for stress fractures, 271–72
Vitamin E, for menstrual cramps, 294
Voltaren (diclofenac), 11, 64, <u>65</u>, 70
Vulvodynia
  diagnosis, 314–15
  fast pain relief
    anticipating problems, 315–16
    local anesthetic cream, 315
    lubrication, 315
  incidence of, 314
  pain prevention strategies
    acupuncture and acupressure, <u>317</u>
    antidepressants, 320
    biofeedback, 316, 318
    Botox, <u>317</u>
    capsaicin, <u>317</u>
    cognitive-behavioral therapy, 319
    exercise and movement therapies, 316,
      318–19